FIFTH EDITION

ETHICAL & LEGAL ISSUES
IN CANADIAN NURSING

T0073704

MARGARET KEATINGS, RN(Ret)., MHSc

PAMELA ADAMS, RN, BN, MScN, PhD, JD
Member of the Law Society of Ontario

ELSEVIER

ETHICAL & LEGAL ISSUES IN CANADIAN NURSING, FIFTH EDITION

ISBN: 978-0-32382-746-1

Copyright © 2024 Elsevier Inc. All Rights Reserved

Notice

Senior Content Strategist (Acquisitions, Canada): Roberta A. Spinosa-Millman
Content Development Manager: Lenore Gray-Spence
Content Development Specialist: Toni Chahley
Publishing Services Manager: Deepthi Unni
Senior Project Manager: Umarani Natarajan/Manchu Mohan
Design Direction: Patrick Ferguson

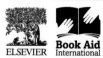

I would like to dedicate this edition to the compassionate and caring nurses who continue to make a difference every day, as they demonstrated so well despite the many challenges during and beyond the COVID-19 pandemic.

In memory of my family members who inspired my commitment to compassionate nursing care.

MARGARET KEATINGS

I want to recognize the nursing students who have provided me with the opportunity to see the world through their eyes. Your passion, interest, and excellence aligns with the nursing profession's accomplishments, professionalism, and competence. We need you!

For you, my loved ones, thanks.

PAMELA ADAMS

PREFACE

Since the first edition of this book was published in 1994, the influence of ethics in the everyday practice of nurses has grown significantly. Nurses are more aware of what constitutes ethical issues in their practice, and as they acquire greater ethical knowledge, they become more competent in addressing more complex ethical issues. Nurses are confident participants in the important dialogue surrounding these issues and in reaching a consensus on the best course of action or approach to challenging situations. At the same time, the ethical issues facing nurses, and the interprofessional team, have increased in complexity and frequency. These challenges became prominent during the COVID-19 pandemic, including the ethical issues associated with individual versus collective rights, and the experience of nurses that led to an increased awareness of the consequences of moral distress. Ethics and the law are becoming increasingly intertwined as new legislation is introduced that ensures ethical standards are met. In other words, previously common or best practices are now being regulated (e.g., the regulations for consent to treatment and privacy which were formerly embedded in common law and standards of practice). A significant illustration of the integration between ethics and the law, and how values evolve over time, is demonstrated in the legislation related to Medical Assistance in Dying (MAiD) and its ongoing evolution.

As with the previous editions, *Ethical & Legal Issues in Canadian Nursing* is by no means a comprehensive or exhaustive text. Chapters are arranged to facilitate both class discussion and individual study. Case scenarios, integrated within many of the chapters, help focus discussion of the issues raised and encourage class participation and deliberation. Additional case scenarios at the end of most chapters encourage critical thinking and debate among students or between nurses and other members of the interprofessional team. Also included are questions for discussion, which are intended to consolidate the key concepts introduced in the chapter. Narratives that further exemplify central themes are woven throughout selected chapters. Relevant current Canadian case law and legislation has been updated, and additional references are provided as sources for further investigation. Previous content with respect to the experience of the Indigenous Peoples in Canada has been enhanced throughout this edition with specific attention to issues associated with health equity, racism, and the ongoing consequences of colonialism.

This edition includes Evolve® online resources to accompany the text, for both students and instructors, and these can be found at http://evolve.elsevier.com/Canada/Keatings/ethical. These include additional case scenarios, a table—*Overview of Provincial Legislation and Regulatory Bodies and the Category of Nurses Represented*—review questions, critical thinking scenarios that further explore chapter themes, a test bank, TEACH manual, and PowerPoint® presentation slides.

The authors of this text recognize and acknowledge the diverse histories of the First Peoples of the lands now referred to as Canada. It is recognized that individual communities identify themselves in various ways; within this text, the term *Indigenous* is used to refer to all First Nations, Inuit, and Métis people within Canada unless there are research findings that are presented uniquely to a population.

In this text, gender-neutral language is used as much as possible to be respectful of an consistent with the values of equality recognized in the *Canadian Charter of Rights and Freedoms*. Using gender-neutral language is professionally responsible and mandated by the Canadian Federal Plan for Gender Equality. Knowledge and language concerning sex, gender, and identity are fluid and continually evolving. The language and terminology presented in this text endeavour to be inclusive of all people and reflect what is to the best of our knowledge current at the time of manuscript development. However, legislation, case law and original documents may not reflect current usage and the text may reflect the original language.

Chapter 1 introduces ethics and the law and offers nursing perspectives that assist in grounding the remaining chapters. Chapter 2 delves into ethical theory and thought. There is expanded content related to moral distress, social justice, virtue ethics, and additional insights and reflections on the ways of knowing and moral perspectives of the Indigenous Peoples in Canada. Chapter 3 examines the resources available to support nurses when dealing with ethical challenges, such as those revealed during the COVID-19 pandemic, including the International Council of Nurses (ICN) *Code of Ethics for Nurses* (2012), and concludes with a discussion of the values expressed in the Canadian Nurses Association (CNA) *Code of Ethics for Registered Nurses* (2017). Specific scenarios associated with each value are examined to highlight their relevance to nursing practice. To encourage further deliberation, additional case scenarios have been provided and can be found at http://evolve.elsevier.com/Canada/Keatings/ethical. Chapter 4 introduces the evolution and fundamentals of the Canadian legal system, including a review of Indigenous legal traditions, the differences between common law and civil law traditions, and how legislation evolves over time. Chapter 5 reviews the provincial regulatory systems that govern the nursing profession and clarifies entry to the profession, standards of practice, the various categories and definitions of nurses and how nurses are held accountable for their actions, across the country. Chapter 6 focuses on respectful and ethical strategies for obtaining informed consent to treatment, and introduces new material that considers the experience of Indigenous persons in Indian hospitals, reinforcing the role of nurses in ensuring the rights of patients, especially those most vulnerable, are protected. Chapter 7 examines the legal accountabilities of nurses (i.e., professional competence, misconduct, and malpractice) and provides recent examples of cases that illustrate these legal issues. Chapter 8 addresses the multifaceted issues associated with death and dying, and the ethical issues associated with the delivery of compassionate care. An update on the legislation related to MAiD is provided, and the

discussion related to nurses' rights to conscientious objection and their experience with MAiD is enhanced. Chapter 9 explores the rapidly advancing world of science and technology and provides updates in such areas as genetics and genomics and their influence on disease prevention, diagnostics, and treatment. Chapter 10 expands on the rights of patients, particularly those most vulnerable, such as older persons, children, the Indigenous Peoples in Canada, members of the 2SLGBTQI+ (Two-Spirit, Lesbian, Gay, Bisexual, Transgender, Queer, Intersex, Plus) community, and the mentally ill. It explores the ethical issues associated with quality improvement and safety, and the rights of persons during the COVID-19 pandemic, such as those in long-term care. Chapter 11 concentrates on some specific rights of nurses, emphasizing how individual nurses and leaders alike must pay attention to the critical issues associated with ensuring a healthy, safe, and violence-free work environment, and how moral distress can arise when ethical issues are not addressed. And, finally, Chapter 12 discusses leadership and organizational ethics and explores the ethical and legal complexities related to issues such as systemic racism and the need for a comprehensive and a sustained human resource strategy. Furthermore, it reinforces the importance of patient- and family-centred care and ethical approaches to structures and processes such as recruitment. Also explored are the challenges associated with cultural safety so that nurses are in a better position to understand, respect, and support those with beliefs and values that may differ from their own.

The goal throughout this book is to explain current ethical and legal concepts in Canadian nursing in as clear and reasoned a style as possible. To this end, tables and figures are included to illustrate pertinent concepts. Boxes highlight information of interest, such as the key points of historical codes of ethics or the health beliefs and practices of various cultural groups. Key terms are indicated in bold type and are further defined and explained in the Glossary.

Throughout the book, the term "patient" rather than "client" has been primarily used. This has principally been done to reduce duplication and improve clarity. In many cases "client" could have been used instead of "patient." In addition, the term *resident* is used when referring to persons living in long-term care facilities.

Ethical & Legal Issues in Canadian Nursing continues to be a work in progress. Many of the issues discussed continue to be debated in Parliament, provincial legislatures, the courts, and health care institutions. We welcome feedback, specifically suggestions, criticism, and comments from readers, which will inform the continuing effort to improve this work.

The fifth edition of *Ethical & Legal Issues in Canadian Nursing* states the law as it stood at the time of publication in December 2023. Although every attempt has been made to ensure the accuracy of the information given, the authors and publisher emphasize that they are not engaged in providing medical, legal, or other professional advice. Those desiring such advice are encouraged to seek the assistance of appropriate professionals.

ELSEVIER eBOOKS

This exciting program is available to faculty who adopt a number of Elsevier texts, including *Ethical & Legal Issues in Canadian Nursing*, fifth edition. Elsevier eBooks is an integrated electronic study centre consisting of a collection of textbooks made available online. It is carefully designed to "extend" the textbook for an easier and more efficient teaching and learning experience. It includes study aids such as highlighting, e-note taking, and cut-and-paste capabilities. Even more importantly, it allows students and instructors to do a comprehensive search within the specific text or across a number of titles. Please check with your Elsevier Educational Solutions Consultant for more information.

ACKNOWLEDGEMENTS

Preparing the fifth edition of this book was no less of a challenge than writing the previous editions. During preparation of the manuscript, we relied on the help, support, and encouragement of people too numerous to mention.

We wish to thank Roberta Spinosa-Millman, Lenore Spence and Toni Chahley at Elsevier Inc. for their support, patience, and understanding during the development of the fifth edition. We also acknowledge and thank those who reviewed the manuscript and provided helpful comments, constructive criticism, and suggestions for improvements:

Monique Bacher, RN, BScN, MSN/Ed
Professor
Practical Nursing Program
Sally Horsfall Eaton School of Nursing
George Brown College

Michael Yeo, BA, MA, PhD
Professor Emeritus, Philosophy
Laurentian University

Siobhan Bell, RN – Forensic Nurse Examiner, BScN, MN
Professor of Nursing
School of Nursing
Seneca Polytechnic

Laura Bulmer, RN, BScN, MEd
Professor
School of Nursing
George Brown College

Kim Tekakwitha Martin, RN, BScN
Dean of Indigenous Education
CEGEP John Abbott College

Tia Nymark, RN, BScN
Instructor
John Abbott College

Kristin Zelyck, RN, BScN, Masters Bioethics
Assistant Lecturer
Faculty of Nursing
University of Alberta

We wish to thank those nurses who shared their stories with us, so that the case scenarios would more accurately reflect real practice situations. In particular, Margaret would like to acknowledge not only her own family members and friends but also the patients and families she has met over the years, whose experiences in the health care system inspired many of the case scenarios and added a new dimension to her appreciation of what constitutes ethical nursing practice.

Margaret would also like to acknowledge the support, guidance, and input she received for this edition from colleagues and researchers who constantly strive to improve the care of older persons and those living in long-term care, nurse practitioners and nurses working in primary care, the community and hospice settings, and the nurses from 6ES at Toronto General Hospital, who continued to provide compassionate care as they faced many challenges during the COVID-19 pandemic, and welcomed her as a volunteer in their setting. She continues to thank her colleagues at the Hospital for Sick Children and Hamilton Health Sciences, and Kathleen Keatings, Robert Boucher, and Morgan Hempinstall who provided input into the literature review. Also much appreciated were the insights provided by Dr. Michael Szego, Director Centre for Clinical Ethics (St. Michael's Hospital, St. Joseph's Health Centre & Providence

Healthcare, Toronto), and Cheryl Shuman, the previous Director, Genetic Counselling, Hospital for Sick Children, Toronto, for clarifying the science and complex ethical issues associated with genetics and genomics. Thanks to Dr. Katherine McGilton, RN, Senior Scientist, Toronto Rehabilitation Institution, University Health Network; Joanne Dykeman, Executive Vice President, Operations; and Lois Cormack, President and Chief Executive Officer, Sienna Living, for giving insight into the real everyday challenges faced by older adults and vulnerable persons living in long-term care. Also many thanks to Dr. Hilary Whyte, Neonatologist at the Hospital for Sick Children, for her sensitive perspectives on the extremely complex ethical issues related to fragile neonates. A special thanks to Carol Taylor, Community Member, Curve Lake First Nation, for reviewing earlier sections of the book related to

Indigenous Peoples in Canada. Carol's insights and perspectives were very much appreciated, as was the opportunity to learn more from her about the culture, traditions, and history of Indigenous communities. Finally, the insights of Jacob van Haaften related to the experiences of Indigenous peoples within the health care system were very much appreciated. The resources he shared, especially those related to "Indian Hospitals" in Canada reveal why there is much to do to gain the trust of Indigenous Peoples in the Canadian Health Care system. To everyone, your insights, stories, and ideas have enabled a deeper comprehension of the complex ethical and legal challenges faced in nursing and health care today.

Margaret Keatings RN(Ret), MHSc
Pamela Adams RN, BN, MScN, PhD, JD
Member of the Law Society of Ontario

CONTENTS

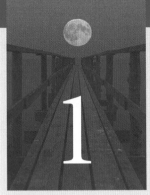

1

AN INTRODUCTION TO ETHICS AND THE LAW: A PERSPECTIVE FOR NURSES

LEARNING OBJECTIVES

This chapter provides an overview of this book and creates a foundation for the chapters to come by clarifying:

■ Why nurses must be familiar with ethics and the law

■ What knowledge nurses require to practise in accordance with the ethical and legal standards of the profession

■ Nursing's professional role in serving the public interest

■ How and why the field of ethics has transformed in response to evolving situations in health care

■ The challenges nurses face when managing complex ethical and legal issues

■ Fundamental ethical and legal issues that arise in the practice of nursing

■ How societal values influence and shape the law over time

INTRODUCTION

A century or more ago, before the regulation of the profession of nursing, and prior to the many advances in science and technology that resulted in a highly complex health care environment, nurses had little autonomy or authority to address the ethical and legal issues in their practice. Conceivably, there would have been incidents that today would constitute a violation of the law. Nurses were less likely to face complex ethical dilemmas, but principles of respect, integrity, and good character influenced the practice of compassionate and caring nursing practice. Although these values continue to guide nursing today, much has changed over the past century.

Until the 1950s there was no universal medicare system, and because patients had to pay for care, this created inequities that posed moral conflicts for nurses concerned about social justice. At the time, nursing curricula did not focus on the resolution of ethical challenges and dilemmas but, rather, on the virtues, character, and behaviour of the professional nurse (LaSala, 2009).

Florence Nightingale (1820–1910), recognized as a significant visionary for modern nursing, placed importance on nurses' accountability for personal moral conduct and emphasized responsibility for knowing what is right and wrong in their practice. She called attention to nursing's role in advocacy, highlighting the obligation of nurses to bring forward concerns regarding safe practices (LaSala, 2009). Safe practice is now the cornerstone of high-quality nursing care where accountability for patient safety continues to focus on minimizing risks, and avoiding errors and harm. Nightingale viewed the ethical principle of care as being an interpersonal process where caring and healing advanced the concept of nurses as role models in the practice setting.

Nightingale was an early proponent of social justice, advocating for care for all, regardless of class or the ability to pay. She promoted respect for diversity, cultural differences, and the health beliefs and values of others. As an ethical leader, she addressed important issues related to the treatment of nurses at the time, including workload, work hours, and abuse by employers (LaSala, 2009; Nurse.com, 2010). Furthermore,

1

she recognized that to be compassionate and kind, nurses also needed to care for themselves. Nightingale transitioned nursing into being an ethical profession, and her legacy is apparent today in the values, principles, and theories that guide nursing as a profession (Chapter 2).

Today, nurses are required to think critically, to offer evidence-informed solutions, and to engage in interprofessional collaboration with members of the health care team, patients, and families to deliver the best possible patient outcomes.

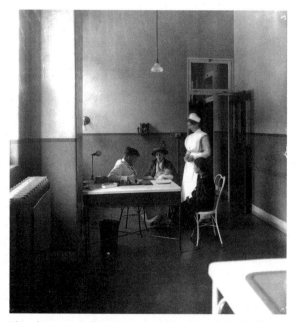

This photograph from the early 1900s shows the lack of interprofessional collaboration in that the physician is engaged with the patient while the nurse stands in the background. *Source: Reproduced by permission of Hospital Archives, The Hospital for Sick Children, Toronto.*

Relationships with physicians were very different in the nineteenth and early twentieth centuries. The following exerpt from a textbook on nursing ethics first published in 1916 by Charlotte Aikens, an early nursing educator, highlights the nature of such relationships (Aikens, 1926):

Loyalty to the physician is one of the duties demanded of every nurse, not only because the physician is her superior officer, but chiefly because the confidence of the patient in his physician is one of the important elements in the management of

his illness, and nothing should be said or done that would weaken this faith or create doubts as to the character or ability or methods of the physician on whom he is depending. (p. 25)

Today the professional nurse is seen as a crucial colleague within the interprofessional health care team, having a deeper understanding of patients and being able to participate fully in a complex health care environment where ethical values are challenged within a system striving for equity and inclusivity.

Nurses as professionals operate within a set of standards as well as a framework of legal rules and ethical guidelines. Such structures are aimed at ensuring consistent, quality, competent, and safe health services while preserving respect for individual rights and human dignity. Within their professional role, nurses make and act on decisions that relate to both independent practice and collaborative partnerships with other professionals; patients, and their families; government agencies; and others. For all of these decisions and actions, the nursing professional answers to individual patients, their families, fellow health care team members, regulatory bodies, employers, their communities, the profession, and society in general. These multiple accountabilities may, at times, be in conflict, posing difficulties and perhaps distress for nurses if left unresolved. Nurses benefit from a sound knowledge base, which includes familiarity with ethical values and principles, ethical theory, and the workings of Canada's legal system (Akhtar-Danesh et al., 2011; Battié & Steelman, 2014; Baumann et al., 2014; Blythe et al., 2008; Chesterton et al., 2021; Milton, 2008; Registered Nurses' Association of Ontario [RNAO], 2007; Wynd, 2003).

NURSING, ETHICS, AND THE LAW

Background

Members of professional groups have an obligation through a regulatory structure to serve the public interest and the common good because their roles, missions, and ethical foundations focus not only on the individuals they serve but also on society as a whole. Professionals have this authority, and they accept this responsibility because of their unique body of knowledge, skills, and expertise. Society has traditionally depended on professionals as custodians of such fields of knowledge as health, law, and education. They are placed in a position of respect and are accordingly given the power to engage in decisions that influence and shape public policy, law, and societal norms. As technology advances and the issues society faces become more complex, existing professions are becoming more specialized, and new professions are emerging (Brennan & Monson, 2014; Jennings et al., 1987).

In recent decades, greater attention has been paid to the interplay of ethics and the law in health care due to the growing complexity of the legal and ethical challenges that arise from advances in science and technology, the important emphasis on human rights, expanding diversity of the population, and shifts in the culture, norms, and values of Canadian society. Many of these issues have been accentuated through the COVID-19 pandemic and the revelations of the Truth and Reconciliation Commission of Canada (TRC) (Government of Canada, 2021).

The COVID-19 pandemic highlighted issues related to the protection of vulnerable persons in health care, the rights of the individual versus the collective, health equity and other related factors. These issues are explored throughout this book.

The TRC acknowledges the injustices and harms suffered by Indigenous people and the need for ongoing healing arising out of the Indian Residential Schools Settlement Agreement. The TRC was established in 2007 and concluded its final report in 2015 (Government of Canada, 2021). The full report is available on the National Centre for Truth and Reconciliation website (https://nctr.ca/records/reports/). The implications of the TRC report for Canada, and the relationship between Canada and Indigenous peoples, will be highlighted throughout this book.

The relationship between Indigenous peoples in Canada and non-Indigenous people has been evolving since Europeans began colonizing North America. Often hostile and fractious, the relationship is a combination of nation-to-nation rights, compromise, authoritarian state action, xenophobia, cultural and ethnic misunderstanding, and discrimination.

The path to reconciliation with Indigenous peoples changed in 1982 with the recognition of the rights of "Aboriginal Peoples" in the *Constitution Act* and the *Canadian Charter of Rights and Freedoms*, then continued with the Statement of Reconciliation in 1998 in which the federal government acknowledged the

damage to Indigenous peoples, the apology from then-Prime Minister Stephen Harper in 2008, the introduction of the Truth and Reconciliation Commission of Canada in 2007, and the publication of the Commission's final report in 2015, which included 94 Calls to Action (Joseph & Joseph, 2019). The nursing profession is committed to addressing these issues and to making the achievement of those Calls to Action that are specific to nursing and health care a priority of the profession across the country.

In the TRC report, there was a discussion about the graves of Indigenous children at many residential school sites. Evidence provided to the TRC indicated that there were likely at least 3,213 students who had died (Hamilton, 2021). The graves of children who died at the residential schools were often poorly documented, the grounds abandoned, and the records damaged or lost. At least one cemetery was deliberately disturbed to prevent graves from being identifiable. The discovery of more than 200 unmarked graves in 2021 at a former Kamloops residential school site sparked outrage in many Canadians and spurred on our collective accountability for reconciliation.

Since ethical and legal issues with respect to Indigenous peoples in Canada are discussed throughout this book. Indigenous peoples in Canada include, First Nations, Inuit, and Métis. "First Nations" is an umbrella term that replaced the term "Indian Bands" in the 1970s and refers to the 634 First Nation communities across Canada. Métis and Inuit are distinct and separate groups. The Métis are descended from Europeans (Scottish, French) and First Nation (Ojibway, Cree) ancestors from the early years of colonization. They are recognized as a group under the *Constitution Act*. The Inuit live above the tree line in Nunavut (Nunavik), Northwest Territories (Inuvialuit), northern Quebec, and Labrador (Nunatsiavut). Inuit means "people" in the language of Inuktitut. Previously referred to as *Eskimo* (meaning "meat eater"), this term is viewed as offensive today. First Nations, Inuit, and Metis have diversity in values, lifestyles, and perspectives across and within their communities (The Canadian Encyclopedia, 2017).

In this text, the term *Indigenous* will be used to refer to the first inhabitants of this country. Both terms *Indigenous and Aboriginal* are derived from Latin and mean the original inhabitants of the land. Most Indigenous people prefer the term *Indigenous. Aboriginal* is viewed in a less positive light, as its prefix "ab" can mean "not" or "away from." The term *Indian* is considered pejorative (Joseph & Joseph, 2019). When *Aboriginal* and *Indian* are used in this text, these words reflect usage in a publication or historical legal document (e.g., the *Indian Act* and the *Constitution Act, 1982*) being referenced.

There has been a strong focus on assimilation policies related to Indian residential schools, but the health system also engaged in systemic racism through the adoption of policies associated such racist policies with the establishment of "Indian hospitals." The tragic legacy of Indian hospitals, which segregated and isolated Indigenous people, is discussed in this book (Lux, 2016). Today, systemic racism and discrimination continues in health care. Recent examples, such as the treatment of Joyce Echaquan, who died in a Quebec hospital while being racially profiled and verbally abused (Friesen, 2020), demonstrate systemic racism observed in the behaviour of certain members of the nursing profession and others within the interprofessional team. These issues, the legacy of the *Indian Act*, and opportunities for a better future will be explored throughout this book.

There is ongoing debate about how ethics, morality, and the law are related. Nurses consider these questions while reflecting on the values and beliefs that govern them as persons and as professionals. The ethical nurse may ask, "What should I do?" or "How do I provide the best care?" For example, how does a nurse respond to a patient who is refusing what would likely be life-saving treatment? The law can be described as having a narrower scope, guiding the nurse to act within a certain set of decided and established rules. For example, the law sets out rules on informed consent and the right of competent persons to control their own health care decisions. These rules do not always fall within the values and beliefs of all nurses as individuals, such as with abortion or the law related to Medical Assistance in Dying (MAiD), and as members of a professional group. The law is supportive when nurses' actions fall within the rules established by law. However, this is not always the case, particularly when the answers to the questions "What should I do?" and "How do I provide the best care?" present an ethical challenge. That is, what is ethical may not always be legal. In a similar manner, what is legal may not always

be considered ethical by some. As ethical and moral issues in health care become more apparent and nurses' answers to the questions "What should I do?" and "How do I provide the best care?" become more informed, they may seek to challenge the established rules or standards in law. For example, some health care professionals supported legislation on medical assistance in dying.

Many situations that nurses face are complex and complicated, requiring them to decide the morally correct thing to do from many possible alternative courses of action. Nurses may face situations in which what they believe to be the most ethically correct course of action may not be supported by the law, and thus, they are unable to act upon what they believe to be right. An illustration of the tension between ethics and the law was the issue of medical assistance in dying. Until 2016, when MAiD legislation was introduced, the *Criminal Code* of Canada made it an offence for a person to assist another person in taking their own life (*Criminal Code*, 1985). Leading up to the legislation, many argued that there were times when providing assistance in dying was the most compassionate and ethical approach if death was imminent or is continued suffering was unbearable. Others disagreed and held to their belief in the sanctity of life and upholding the laws against contributing to the death of another. The courts interpreted patients' rights as including the right to medical assistance in dying and considered frameworks within which the right could be safely exercised. The challenging and emotional debate around MAiD legislation and subsequent changes to the *Criminal Code* guided the development of the legislation in 2016 and its subsequent revisions. This is a good example of an action that might have been considered ethical but was not legal and how the shifting values and beliefs in society over time came to influence and shape the law. The MAiD legislation attempts to balance legal issues with the social issues and concerns raised by various human rights groups and stakeholders.

The introduction of MAiD has not eliminated all of the debate around medically assistance in dying, and there continues to be areas of controversy. For example, would nurses and doctors with personal moral opposition to MAiD be required to participate in this process, and could they refuse to refer patients to health care practitioners prepared to provide MAiD?

The complex issues related to MAiD and conscientious objection are discussed in Chapter 8.

The law means different things to different people. Legal philosophers have conceived of the types of law that can be used to capture different legal concepts: natural law (inherent rights), positive law (enacted government), Roman law, civil law, or God's law. The consistent theme is that what are described as laws are rules and principles established to create and support justice within a particular society. Laws are created by governing authorities, judicial decisions, and customs. Laws only function to the extent that they are accepted, respected, and observed by members of society. Where laws are not respected and accepted, the government has three choices—to use compulsion (force, threats, humiliation), to seek a compromise, or to change the law, which will then be respected.

In Canada, one of the most well-known examples of the public's refusal to accept a law relates to abortion. Abortion rights were very restricted in the 1960s and 1970s. Even as the public's moral perspectives on abortion were shifting, performing an abortion remained an offence under the *Criminal Code*. Dr. H. Morgentaler, a general practitioner who originally specialized in family planning and later provided abortions in his private clinic, brought an unsuccessful court challenge to the constitutionality of this law in 1975. A similar proceeding in 1988 the legal prohibition of abortion was successful in obtaining an order that the law was unconstitutional. He also challenged by setting up abortion clinics across the country and inviting criminal charges. The Crown charged him with providing illegal abortion services. However, in a series of criminal trials, juries refused to convict him. Juries were unwilling to convict persons for providing what they considered socially necessary abortion services. In due course, the federal government stopped filing criminal charges against Dr. Morgentaler and tried to develop a legal framework under which abortions could be provided legally. Attempts to revise the law failed, and eventually, the federal government stopped trying to regulate abortions through criminal law.

The federal government, through the *Canada Health Act* (1985), expects that there will be reasonable access to publicly funded health care. Consider how this relates to what is ethical or legal. A nurse may believe that all Canadians have an ethical right to health care; for example, that a specific treatment should be available to all persons in need of such care. However, the legal right to health care is not specified in the *Canada Health Act* or any other Canadian law. The federal government has no jurisdiction over health care, but only over the conditions under which it will fund health care as specified in the Act. Nurses who believe appropriate care is being denied to some patients may decide to operate an illegal safe injection site (Kerr et al., 2017) or volunteer to provide primary care to undocumented immigrants, funded through donations, when the *legal* health care system cannot or will not act.

Nurses face an increasing number of ethical and legal concerns in their everyday practice, which became even more apparent during the COVID-19 pandemic (Haslam-Larmer et al., 2022; Savage et al., 2022). Consider the requirement of having to enforce public health rules related to family visits. In relation to this requirement, nurses faced ethical dilemmas associated with the conflicts between the ethical principles of beneficence, nonmaleficence, fidelity, and justice. Nurses must address these conflicts while providing quality, ethical care to patients within the context of a health care system challenged by limited funds and resources. Nurses fulfill the important task of supporting patients and their families, as well as intervening or advocating on behalf of those patients, when necessary. The nursing role involves building professional and trusting relationships with people throughout the life continuum. All of this must be achieved within the requirements of legal and ethical principles.

To aid them in the difficult decisions they have to make, nurses must have knowledge of ethics and the law. Chapter 2 explores theories, principles, and decision frameworks that guide nurses' ethical choices. This material is not exhaustive, but it is intended to provide an introductory foundation in ethics. In Chapter 3, these theories will be applied to nursing codes of ethics, including the Canadian Nurses Association (CNA) *Code of Ethics for Registered Nurses* (CNA, 2017). In Chapter 4, the Canadian legal system is described. This introduction to ethics and the law will begin the process of lifelong professional learning and provide a framework for the specific ethical and legal themes discussed in later chapters.

Why Should Nurses Study Ethics?

Nurses function within a health care team and collaborate with many other health care professionals. Today, nurses practise in many different contexts beyond traditional health care settings—in the community or the home; in continuing care or rehabilitation; in business or industry; in the academic environment, in adult and pediatric long-term care facilities; in government or public policy; and many other areas. In some situations, nurses may interact with other professionals who do not share the same perspective about or understanding of nursing or health care in general. Each member of the team may have a different perspective on an ethical issue, and some may share similar positions. However, with a strong ethical framework, similarities—as well as differences—can be clarified. Without transparent team discussions that clarify various positions, ethical decisions and actions may be misinterpreted and considered wrong by others. If the reasons, values, and perspectives behind decisions and actions are explained, they would more readily be understood and respected, if not accepted. Nurses practise within the context of interprofessional teams, so strong collaboration and communication are essential. Interprofessional practice is discussed in detail in Chapter 12.

Most importantly, nurses must study ethics because morality (i.e., doing good) is at the heart of nursing theory and practice. Many nursing theorists consider "care" to be a moral imperative, not only a key dimension of nursing practice but at the very core of it (Benner, 1990, 1994, 1996, 2000; Leininger, 1988a, 1988b; Roach, 1992; Watson, 1988). They view nurses as "moral agents," charged with nurturing the humanity of those for whom they care (Cloyes, 2002). These theories are discussed in Chapter 2.

Within health care, choices are often not easy—it may be difficult to determine, from among many alternatives, which one is right or the "least wrong." Consider, for example, the major public health policies that were introduced during the COVID-19 pandemic, specifically the restriction of visitors in hospitals and long-term care settings. Some viewed this restriction as wrong because it conflicted with the values and positive outcomes associated with person and family-centred care and resulted in emotional, psychological, and physical harm to residents in long-term care, patients, and family members (Johnston et al., 2022).

Others supported this restriction as a necessary infection control strategy and less harmful than the spread of the COVID-19 infection itself. Still others saw a middle ground that limited general visiting but offered some access to essential family members. Opportunities for leaders and team members to clarify their positions to each other might not have altered individual perspectives, but through sharing their positions, nurses and other team members better understood the values and reasons underlying each perspective. Such clarification reduced the moral conflict and distress experienced by nurses who ultimately were the ones to enforce these rules. There might also have been the opportunity to look at alternatives that would have addressed the concerns held by all involved, from policymakers to the team at the point of care (Johnston et al., 2022).

When challenging ethical issues arise in the care setting, it is imperative that patients, families, physicians, nurses, and other team members discuss such issues together and attempt to reach a consensus on a course of action. Because many ethical qestions do not have clear-cut answers, collaboration and effective communication, as well as a respect for each other's values and beliefs, can facilitate the resolution process. The communication that is necessary to clarify and justify moral actions and choices to other professional colleagues is improved through a shared language grounded in a solid foundation of ethical theory. This shared language also involves the interplay of the law relative to such difficult dilemmas, such as withdrawal of treatment and the use of advance directives.

The study of ethics provides nurses with the knowledge and tools to better facilitate or contribute to such discussions. Knowledge of abstract philosophical theories and terminologies does not always provide solutions to ethical problems; however, such knowledge can serve to achieve a better understanding of the moral context and the values and beliefs for ourselves and others.

Nurses face ethical choices every day in practice. These choices may be about challenges related to pain management, patient comfort, restraints, consent, and family involvement in care. The everyday issues nurses face do not always make headlines. For example, ethics is involved when nurses decide how to allocate time and nursing care to patients; whose needs are met first; and how to show respect to patients, families, each other, and members of the interprofessional team.

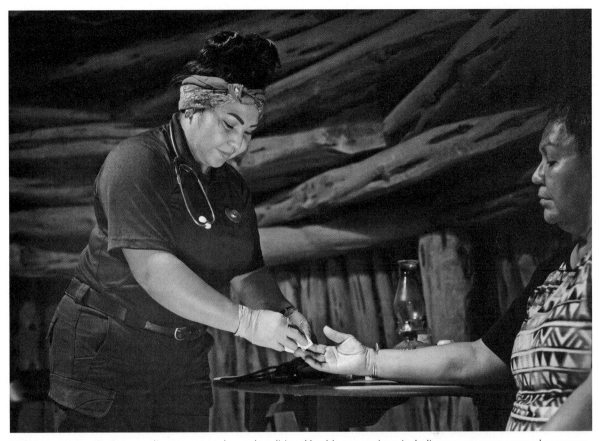

Today, nurses practise in many diverse contexts beyond traditional health care settings, including remote areas across the country. *Source: iStock.com/THEPALMER.*

Nurses not only deal with ethical issues and challenges in the clinical context of the individual, they are also impacted by—and are in a position to influence—ethical decisions regarding policy, the wider context of health care, and the health care system.

As the role of nurses expands, they are being given more autonomy and, with that, more authority and responsibility. However, nurses and health care teams do not function in isolation. They work within organizations and are supported by leaders who have a significant influence on the practice and outcomes of care. Many factors influence a moral organization, such as leadership behaviours and values, as well as the strategy, processes, and operations of the organization. Supportive and ethical leaders enable a healthy and open culture that supports the ethical practice of nurses and ensures that the needs of patients are met. They influence

approaches to care by ensuring that the appropriate resources are in place; determining how teams are organized; introducing ethical models, such as person-centred and family-centred care; and enabling many other strategies that are explored in Chapter 12.

Nurses cannot manage the complexities of ethical and legal issues independent of their leaders and organizations. A moral organizational climate is essential and necessary to give nurses the support they need to address the complex and challenging ethical issues related to care.

Moral Justification

Those involved in the field of ethics draw upon ethical theories and principles, not only to identify the most ethical approach to an issue but also to justify and defend their positions to others. Points of view, especially in controversial areas, should be open to criticism and debate and require justification, an argued defence of one's perspective. Theories and principles of ethics can clarify relationships between reasons and conclusions. Positions on an issue can be justified through reasoned arguments and evidence that is subject to criticism and counterexamples. It is important for nurses to have this knowledge because there is the risk that arguments can be cloaked in rhetoric, irrelevancies, redundancies, and connections with other arguments that can mislead those not comfortable with ethical language and theory (Beauchamp & Walters, 2003). In recent years, moral problems in the health care environment have become more frequent and more intense, and, therefore, it is critical that nurses have knowledge of ethical theory and some skill in justifying and defending their positions to others.

Ethical theory is the study of the nature and justification of general ethical principles, duties and obligations, and character, that can be applied to moral problems (Armstrong, 2006; Beauchamp & Walters, 2003; Keller, 2009). Ethical theory aims to provide a more rigorous and systematic approach to how to make decisions about what is right or wrong. Many theories have been developed over the centuries in an attempt to provide more rigorous and systematic approaches to how decisions are made about what is

right and wrong. These theories provide frameworks for the exploration of the ethical questions and moral issues faced in health care and guide how morality is understood within the sphere of nursing practice and the nurse–patient relationship. Furthermore, they assist in clarifying expectations regarding the character and behaviour of nurses and the role of the nurse as a moral agent.

Everyday Ethical Issues Faced by Nurses

Nurses have the opportunity to defend and protect patient rights, to promote compassionate care, and to enhance the dignity and autonomy of their patients. They are often required to choose from among a number of good or "least wrong" alternatives and to assess and defend the choices made or actions taken; however, they may not even be aware of the ethical nature of their choices. Because options are not always clear, how does one decide what the right thing to do is? To address ethical challenges, nurses first need to be aware that these challenges exist and be able to identify them as being ethical in nature.

Within the context of a health care system strained by limited funds and resources, nurses face challenges every day in providing high-quality and ethical care to patients. The following scenarios are not uncommon (Box 1.1).

BOX 1.1
EVERYDAY ETHICAL CHALLENGES

An infant in a pediatric centre has been diagnosed with a malignant cerebral tumour. The infant is comatose, nonresponsive, and on life support. There is nothing the team can do to halt the progress of this terminal disease. They believe it would be in the baby's best interests to discontinue what they consider futile treatment and to let a peaceful natural death occur. The parents disagree and want all measures taken to save their baby.

■ *Who decides what the best interests of the infant and the family are? Do patients or families have the right to expensive but futile health care? How should nurses support the parents through this crisis and the imminent death of their baby? How do nurses ensure supportive quality care throughout the dying process?*

A 20-year-old diagnosed with schizophrenia at age 16 years is admitted to the mental health unit of a community hospital. They are agitated and express a wish to "end all this pain." They refuse all medications to deal

with their symptoms. They want to be left alone and to go home.

■ *What rights does a patient have in this situation? What might it mean when a person expresses a wish to "end all this pain?" What options are available to patients and the team in this type of situation? What is your role as a nurse?*

A patient with end-stage cancer of the liver is receiving palliative care at home. The patient's spouse and children are the primary caregivers, with some support from home care and community nurses. As the patient's condition deteriorates, their symptoms become more difficult to manage. Physically and emotionally drained, the family questions whether the patient might be better off in a hospital. The patient, however, has always stated the preference to die at home.

■ *How does the community nurse manage the conflicting interests of this patient and their family? What is society's role in ensuring adequate resources to address the needs of a dying patient at home?*

BOX 1.1—cont'd
EVERYDAY ETHICAL CHALLENGES

A 40-year-old single person is recovering from surgery to their lower back. Although they are still in pain and continue to have difficulty with mobility, the hospital needs the bed, and the patient completed the expected length of stay. The hospital nurse discusses the patient's transition to the community with the home care case manager. The case manager determines that the patient not qualify for homemaker support, even though they do not have family or friends to help at home.

■ *How do these nurses ensure the safe transition from hospital to home? How do they respond to the rules that place limitations on the needed resources in the community?*

An occupational health nurse in an industrial setting is managing the case of a worker who was injured at work. The worker has recovered and is functionally able to return to work. The employer is eager to have the worker return as soon as possible. However, the worker confides to the nurse that the manager constantly harasses the employees; and the worker believes that it was the stressful work environment that led to the accident in the first place. The worker asks the nurse to keep this information confidential, fearing repercussions from the manager.

■ *How does the nurse balance the responsibility to ensure this worker's safe return to work—and concern about the safety of other workers in this hostile environment—with the obligation to honour the worker's request for confidentiality?*

An older person living in a long-term care setting has mobility issues, a result of complications after the repair of a fractured hip. The prosthesis they used has migrated into the resident's pelvis. The resident has dementia and (due to the injury) is not able to walk, but keeps forgetting this and constantly tries to get out of the wheelchair. This has resulted in a number of falls, with the resident sustaining numerous lacerations and bruising. The family would like the staff to use a seat belt to prevent falls and more serious injury. The staff refuse to do this, citing the employer's least restraint policy.

■ *How do nurses caring for this resident balance the risks and benefits of the options available to them? What are those options? Which option do you think is the most ethical?*

It is the middle of an evening shift on a busy medical unit. A patient is dying; and the patient's family and friends are not around.

■ *What options should be available to ensure that the patient does not die alone? Does it matter? Priorities and resources*

are reorganized if an emergency arises; should dying be considered in the same light?

A child is dying. The clearly distressed parents, who have been with the child for weeks, are seriously sleep deprived. One parent, who has grown increasingly agitated, goes to the nursing station to request additional pain medication for the child. When 10 minutes pass and there has been no response to this request, the parent becomes enraged and yell at the team, using profanity, aggressive language, and other threatening behaviours.

■ *How does the nursing team balance the needs of the parents and the child with the rights of the nurses and staff to a safe work environment? How could the situation have been avoided?*

A male nurse has recently begun working as a nurse in a small hospital located in a rural community. He moved there with his male partner, who was recently appointed as a manager in a nearby mine. Because he started only a few months earlier, he has found it difficult to engage with other staff members. They routinely fail to help him if he is busy and have never invited him to join them on a break. Already feeling marginalized, he overhears three of the nurses discussing his personal relationship and speculating on why a man would ever become a nurse.

■ *What is happening here? What options does this nurse have to address this uncomfortable prejudicial situation?*

During the COVID-19 pandemic, a province had imposed strict rules on visiting. Only one designated person, usually a family member, was permitted to visit for a maximum of 2 hours on a daily basis. One evening, the charge nurse on a medical unit received a call from the family of an older patient receiving palliative care who was not expected to live beyond a few days, requesting that they receive an additional visit from their child who had just arrived from another city. The family reassured the nurse that the child was fully vaccinated and was demonstrating no signs of infection. This patient had already received a visit that day from their designated essential family member and, according to the rules, the charge nurse was required to refuse this request.

■ *What are the ethical conflicts facing the nurse in this scenario? Do the rules make sense to you? What are the potential consequences for the nurse, the patient, and the family if the policy is followed? What if the nurse disregarded the policy and permitted the visit?*

These are only a few examples of the types of complex and challenging situations faced by nurses on a daily basis. It is not uncommon for nurses to be confronted with a number of these ethical issues and questions simultaneously. Knowledge of ethical theory, a greater ability to identify the ethical issues and respond

to them, and appropriate system supports may assist nurses in managing these challenges.

Now, take some time to reflect on the above scenarios. What choices would you make? What are your reasons for making them? Is your rationale consistent from one scenario to the next, or does your approach vary depending on the situation or your past experience? Are you able to defend your approach to your colleagues?

After you review the theoretical perspectives discussed in Chapter 2, return to these scenarios. Was your approach to these problems consistent with any of Chapter 2's theories? Did your views change as you read through the chapter? Did these perspectives provide you with arguments to assist in defending your position? Are you better able to identify the ethical issues in these scenarios? Do the theories help you decide on a course of action?

Why Must Nurses Know the Law?

Society holds nurses to high standards of professional, moral, and ethical competence, but it also affords them certain rights and privileges. The law strives to keep these competing interests in balance. It regulates the education and credentials of nurses; the conditions of their employment; their collective bargaining rights; their rights, duties, and responsibilities toward patients, their professional colleagues, the public, and each other; and a host of other matters. Furthermore, the legal system provides a forum for resolving disputes and conflicts, which inevitably arise when divergent interests clash.

Thus, for example, under occupational health and safety legislation, a nurse who is being made to work in conditions that are unsafe or even dangerous has recourse against the employer (Manitoba Nurses Union, 2018; *The Workplace Safety and Health Act,* n.d.). Over recent years, this protection has advanced through human rights and prevention of violence in the workplace legislation described in Chapters 10 and 11. There is now acknowledgement that nurses' work environments must be healthy and that employers must ensure a work culture that is ethical, safe, supportive, and free of discrimination. The ultimate aim is to provide a workplace with a low tolerance for disrespect, especially among nurses and within the health care team. Signifying the critical importance of this issue and consistent views across disciplines, the Canadian Nurses Association (CNA) and the Canadian Federation of Nurses Unions (CFNU) issued a joint statement endorsing a Canadian Medical Association (CMA) policy related to the identification, implementation, and evaluation

of quality practice environments guided by the principles of providing the right care to the right person, at the right time, by the right providers.

It was easier to remove the quote and summarize the principles. The references apply to this whole section. (CMA, 2013; CNA and CFNU, 2014)

Legal processes are in place for a patient who suffers injury or harm as a result of the negligence of a nurse. Patients can, alleging negligence, commence a civil suit in the courts for damages against that nurse and the responsible health care facility.

Not all errors or mistakes made by nurses lead to a finding of negligence. For negligence to occur, a person must owe a duty of care to another, that duty of care must be breached or the standard of care not be met, and harm must result. Negligence and the implications for nurses are described in Chapter 7.

Today, much more attention is given to patient safety and the prevention of harm. In the past, nurses frequently met with discipline or reprimands when they made mistakes. The climate within the health care environment is shifting to a "just culture" and a system-oriented approach to transparency. This approach recognizes that errors are often system related; therefore, it is important to understand their root cause so that changes to design and processes can be made. There is also policy, guidelines, and (in some provinces) legislation in place related to disclosure to patients and families (Canadian Medical Protective Association [CMPA], 2013). When there is transparency, full disclosure, and sincere apologies offered, patients and families are less likely to take on adversarial roles and engage in legal processes. However, as discussed in Chapter 7, justice obliges appropriate compensation in some circumstances. Approaches to patient safety and disclosure are described in Chapter 10.

Canada is a culturally diverse society. Correspondingly, patients and interprofessional teams reflect this diversity. Nurses need to welcome, understand, and respect the differences, divergent values and beliefs. Nurses have to be sensitive to cultural differences, the interplay of human rights, privacy and confidentiality legislation, and the implications of the *Canadian Charter of Rights and Freedoms,* discussed in Chapter 4.

A growing awareness of patients' ethical and legal rights and a greater emphasis on individual autonomy have led to the establishment of advocacy groups to represent the interests of various constituencies. Consider the goals of the Alliance for Healthier Communities: to foster change within the primary health care sector to promote a more accepting environment for members of Two-Spirit, Lesbian, Gay, Bisexual, Transgender, Queer, Intersex, Plus (2SLGBTQI+) communities; and to ensure that health care professionals are aware and knowledgeable about their issues (AOHC, 2018). The nonprofit organization Dying With Dignity Canada played a key role in lobbying for a person's right to die (Dying With Dignity Canada, 2018). The subsequent MAiD legislation attempts to balance legal issues with the social issues and ethical concerns raised by various human rights groups and stakeholders.

There are many other reasons why nurses should have a basic understanding of Canada's legal system. Provinces and territories have legislation that governs the profession, including the establishment of regulatory bodies that impose requirements with respect to nurses' level of professional knowledge and skill. Failure to meet these requirements or undertaking the practice of nursing without adequate education leaves the nurse open to disciplinary action from the governing body and, if the conduct is serious enough, from the courts, by way of either criminal prosecution (in cases in which the conduct involves a breach of criminal law), or a lawsuit (in which the nurse is sued for negligence or some other misconduct resulting from breach of an accepted standard of nursing care). Chapter 4 outlines the principles of Canada's legal system to provide nurses with a basic understanding of what often seems an obscure and confusing institution. The roles of legislatures and the executive branch of government are briefly discussed, as are some of the legal concepts and principles applicable to nursing. These provide a framework for the chapters that follow. Chapter 5 describes the structure, role, and workings of various provincial/territorial professional regulatory bodies and institutions. Against this background, nurses can begin to appreciate how the profession is regulated and, in particular, how the concept of self-governance is integrated into this regulatory structure and into professional codes of ethics.

In Canada, legal authority is divided between the federal government and the provinces. Consequently, legal authority often requires laws to be put in place both federally and provincially. For example, to grant Nurse Practitioners (NPs) authority to prescribe certain controlled drugs required federal regulations (New Classes of Practitioners Regulations, 2012) under the *Controlled Drugs and Substances Act*, and in the province, companion legislation setting out the legal requirements of the province to authorize NPs (such as the Nova Scotia *Prescription Monitoring Act* and *Regulations* [2004]).

Not only civil consequences but also criminal consequences can flow from a breach of such laws. Chapter 7 deals with issues of negligence and standards of care in the nursing profession. It describes how nurses' conduct and professionalism in carrying out their duties are measured in relation to the law and current ethical standards.

Chapter 7 also explores the legal, ethical, and practical aspects of proper documentation. Ensuring a high standard of documentation is important in maintaining effective communication, which is key to safe care. The nurse's assessment and progress notes monitor, on a continuing basis, the course of a patient's treatment and the effect of interventions. Documentation provides evidence in any complaint or lawsuit against the nursing staff and the institution; therefore, they should always be created with the understanding that they may be subject to review and examination. Inadequate documentation or the failure to review patient information and history has a negative influence on the quality of care. Given that multiple caregivers are involved in care, it is impossible to achieve effective communication and continuity of care without clear and accurate documentation.

The legal rights of patients influence the everyday actions and decisions made by nurses. These actions and decisions may involve going beyond the usual barriers to consent. For instance, a patient who needs an injection may readily consent by holding out an arm to the nurse who administers it. However, if a patient is unable to consent to a procedure because of physical or mental incapacity, including impairment by illness or the effects of medication, the nurse bears the onus of ensuring that any action taken or treatment administered is in the patient's best interests and is consistent with that patient's wishes. At times, it is a challenge to determine whether the patient is truly capable of giving consent; however, failure to do so leaves the nurse open to the risk of a civil suit by a nonconsenting patient or the next of kin. There are also complexities with respect to consent from those who are most vulnerable, including children, persons who are cognitively impaired, and those with mental illness. Further challenges arise when the team questions the validity or the sincerity of substitute decision makers. Most provinces and territories have enacted legislation that clearly defines the parameters of consent, the patient's capacity, the manner of giving consent, express versus implied consent, and so forth. This legislation is discussed in detail in Chapter 6. Furthermore, health care professionals are legally obligated to ensure that the patient understands the nature of the illness, the need for treatment, and all the attendant risks and benefits of such treatment if that patient is to give fully informed consent. Issues of consent to treatment and the many sub-issues arising from this area are also addressed in Chapter 6.

Recent, extraordinary advances in medical technology have made it possible both to manipulate the reproductive process at one end of the life continuum and to extend life at the other end in cases where death would once have been certain. These advances force questions about how these resources are used, and, indeed, whether this technology should be used at all.

Chapter 8 discusses the challenging legal and ethical issues associated with the end of life. Topics such as assistance in dying and organ donation and transplantation, are explored. These issues have gained public prominence in recent years and hold profound implications for nurses. Science and technology have focused on finding ways to extend life. Yet, a heavy price is paid when extending someone's life diminishes the quality and dignity that give life its meaning. As a means of dealing with death and the dying process change, nurses are challenged to find new ways to preserve patients' human values, autonomy, and dignity.

Chapter 9 explores complex technologies, such as those related to reproductive and genetic science. Currently, there are technologies that not only overcome infertility but also have the capacity to identify and correct genetic anomalies, predict future disease, and control the characteristics of offspring during the embryonic stage of development. This power to manipulate the creation of life has the potential to reshape society and to redefine future generations.

The Human Genome Project (HGP), launched in 1990 and completed in 2003, identified approximately 20,500 genes in human DNA. The results of the initiative provided scientists with the ability to identify genetic diseases, create strategies for their cure and prevention, and even identify guilty persons in previously unsolved criminal cold cases. In some situations, it is now possible to predict the response of a patient with cancer to particular treatment interventions. Many ethical questions arise out of this advancing science: Just because we can do this, should we? What impact will these interventions have on future generations? What are we to do with the knowledge and information gained from this evolving science?

Often, these possibilities arise before laws can be made to deal with them. The law, therefore, is not an exhaustive source of guidance and direction in such matters and is sometimes slow to adapt legal solutions for them, as in the case of MAiD. Through knowledge of our legal system, the nurse will see that the law is also, not infrequently, out of step with current societal values. Law is usually perceived as unequivocal, whereas ethical situations—such as assistance in dying, as mentioned earlier—are vastly more complicated and nuanced. Today, the single biggest challenge facing lawmakers and the legal system is the attempt to come to terms with the grey areas and to provide more realistic and practical guidelines for dealing with ethical problems. Law often evolves from the ethical principles that guide practice and common sense. For example, ethical practices associated with consent existed in health care, before these rules were established in law. This stems from the principle of autonomy, that persons have the ethical right to control what is done to their body and person. The law now recognizes that a person's consent is essential before a health care professional initiates any physical contact.

Also, autonomy guided practices associated with privacy and confidentialy, and this is now established in legislation. Nurses have both legal and ethical obligations to keep all patient information confidential and not to divulge it without the patient's consent. When that consent cannot be obtained, they may reveal only as much as is absolutely necessary in the interests of the patient, and only to persons whose participation in the patient's treatment is necessary (i.e., the "circle of care"). There may be cases in which nurses are required to disclose such information in court in the form of testimony or when it is essential to prevent harm to the patient or others. (See, for example, the Alberta *Personal Information Protection Act* [2003, ss. 5 and 19]) Federal and provincial governments have enacted strict privacy legislation governing health records that clearly delineates the responsibilities of the custodians of such records, the use that may be made of confidential patient information, who may consent to its release, and to whom such information can be disclosed. This legislation is discussed in Chapter 10. Sharing information and consulting with family members, friends, and others has become much more complex with the implementation of this legislation. Health care institutions are required to maintain privacy pursuant to the legislation, and the consequences can be very serious for staff, both nurses and others, if a breach occurs. See, for example, the federal *Personal Information Protection and Electronic Documents Act*, (2000).

Knowledge of the workings of the law, the rules of evidence, ethics, and the judicial system provides a framework when determining whether to disclose sensitive and confidential information about a particular patient. Ill or injured patients are in a vulnerable state and are not always able to protect their rights as citizens. To ensure that the interests of their patients are represented, nurses must understand the rights of their patients and their own professional obligations to protect or respect these rights. These issues are explored in Chapter 10.

If nurses have obligations to their patients, they also have rights regarding what they can expect as professionals. Like all other Canadians, under the Charter, nurses have the right to privacy and respect, and to freedom of expression—the right to think, say, write, or otherwise act in accordance with their beliefs. However, these rights must be considered in the context of nurses' responsibilities as professionals and of their obligations to patients. Chapter 11 focuses on the balance between these rights and obligations.

The introduction to the law begins in Chapter 4, with a historical perspective of the evolution of the legal system in Canada. The Indigenous peoples inhabited this land centuries before the arrival of the first Europeans and subsequent colonization, and they had their own legal systems that, though varied, had common elements across their communities. Canada began as a confederation of the British and French colonizers, who without consideration of the existing Indigenous systems, used the legal structures, rules, and principles of their home countries as the foundation of the Canadian legal system.

SUMMARY

Clearly, the impact of the law and ethics on the nursing profession is widespread and significant. An understanding of the law's structures, terminology, and mechanisms is essential to the nurse's ability to operate within society's expectations and standards; similarly, familiarity with, and willingness to be guided by, the values and ethical standards of the nursing profession is essential to practising within a system that delivers high standards of patient care. This chapter provided a foundation for understanding the material presented in the chapters that follow.

This chapter conveyed the reasons nurses must be familiar with the law and ethics and have the knowledge to practise according to these standards. Professionals have a significant role in serving the interests of the public and must be sure they have their trust. As we have seen from the scenarios and examples provided, the complexity of ethical issues has grown alongside the increasing reliance on ethics in guiding and supporting decisions. It is clear that ethics and the law intersect on many levels, and a strong understanding of both is essential to exemplary nursing practice.

CRITICAL THINKING

Discussion Points

The goal of this chapter is to provide an overview of the interplay of ethics and the law and to introduce the issues and concepts that are discussed in future chapters. The following questions are intended to encourage reflection prior to acquiring knowledge of the ethical and legal concepts outlined in this book. You may also discuss these questions as a group and share your reflections with one another.

1. What informed your decision to become a professional nurse?

2. Identify what personal values you share with the nursing profession.

3. Describe an ethical dilemma you have experienced in your life or as a student or nurse. What position did you take, and why? Did your personal values help you address this issue?

4. Prior to becoming a nursing student, were you expecting to face the significant ethical and legal challenges associated with nursing?

5. Describe an encounter that you or your family have had with the health care system. Examine you or your family's experience with this encounter. Was this a positive or a negative experience? What factors influenced this perspective? How might this experience inform your practice as a nurse?

6. In your opinion, what is the most significant legal issue that nurses may encounter? What do you think are the two most significant ethical issues that a nurse may face?

7. If you were a patient, what would you expect from the nurses caring for you? If a member of your family was a patient, what would be your expectations? As a nurse or a nursing student, do you believe you meet these standards?

REFERENCES

Statutes

Canada Health Act, R.S.C. 1985, c. C-6, as amended.

Criminal Code, R.S.C. 1985, c. C-46 (Canada), s. 241; R.S., 1985, c. 27 (1st Supp.), s. 7.

Personal Information Protection Act, SA 2003, c. P-6.5, ss. 5 and 19.

Personal Information Protection and Electronic Documents Act, S.C 2000, c. 5, as amended.

Prescription Monitoring Act and Regulations, NSS 2004, c. 32.

The Workplace Safety and Health Act, Manitoba Statutes c. W210. 10/02 (2002) as amended.

Regulations

New Classes of Practitioners Regulations (Controlled Drugs and Substances Act) (2012), SOR/2012-230.

Texts and Articles

Aikens, C. A. (1926). Studies in ethics for nurses (2nd ed.). W.B. Saunders Company.

Akhtar-Danesh, N., Baumann, A., Kolotylo, C., et al. (2011). Perceptions of professionalism among nursing faculty and nursing students. Western Journal of Nursing Research, 35(2), 248–271. https://doi.org/10.1177/0193945911408623

Alliance for Healthcare Communities. (2018). https://www.allianceon.org

Armstrong, A. E. (2006). Towards a strong virtue ethics for nursing practice. Nursing Philosophy, 7(3), 110–124. https://doi.org/10.1111/j.1466-769X.2006.00268.x. PMID: 16774598

Battié, M., & Steelman, V. M. (2014). Accountability in nursing practice: Why it is important for patient safety. Association of perioperative Registered Nurses, 100(5), 537–541. https://doi.org/10.1016/j.aorn.2014.08.008

Baumann, A., Norman, P., Blythe, J., et al. (2014). Accountability: the challenge for medical and nursing regulators [Special issue]. Healthcare Policy, 10, 121–131.

Beauchamp, T. L., & Walters, L. (2003). Contemporary issues in bioethics (6th ed.). Wadsworth Publishing Company.

Benner, P. (1990). The moral dimensions of caring. In J. S. Stevenson & T. Tripp-Reimer (Eds.), Knowledge about care and caring: State of the art and future developments (pp. 5–17). American Academy of Nursing.

Benner, P. (1994). Discovering challenges to ethical theory in experience-based narratives of nurses' everyday ethical comportment. In J. F. Monagle & D. C. Thomasma (Eds.), Health care ethics: Critical issues (pp. 401–411). Aspen Publishers.

Benner, P. (1996). The primacy of caring and the role of experience, narrative, and community in clinical and ethical expertise. In P. Benner, C. A. Tanner, & C. A. Chesla (Eds.), Expertise in nursing practice: Caring, clinical judgment, and ethics (pp. 232–237). Springer Publishing Company.

Benner, P. (2000). The roles of embodiment, emotion and lifeworld for rationality and agency in nursing practice. Nursing Philosophy, 1(1), 5–19.

Blythe, J., Baumann, A., Zeytinoglu, I. U., et al. (2008). Nursing generations in the contemporary workplace. Public Personnel Management, 37(2), 137–159. https://doi.org/10.1177/009102600803700201

Brennan, M., & Monson, V. (2014). Professionalism: Good for patients and for health care organizations. Mayo Clinic Proceedings, 89(5), 644–652. https://doi.org/10.1016/j.mayocp.2014.01.011

The Canadian Encyclopedia. (2017). Treaties with Indigenous Peoples in Canada. https://www.thecanadianencyclopedia.ca/en/article/aboriginal-treaties

Canadian Medical Association. (2013). Physicians taking lead on appropriateness of care. Ottawa: Author.

Canadian Medical Protective Association. (2013). Apology legislation in Canada. https://www.cmpa-acpm.ca/en/advice-publications/browse-articles/2008/apology-legislation-in-canada-what-it-means-for-physicians

Canadian Nurses Association. (2017). Code of Ethics for Registered Nurses.

Canadian Nurses Association and Canadian Federation of Nurses Unions (2014). Practice environments: Maximizing outcomes for clients, nurses and organizations.

Chesterton, L., Tetley, J., Cox, N., et al. (2021). A hermeneutical study of professional accountability in nursing. Journal of Clinical Nursing, 30(1–2), 188–199.

Cloyes, K. G. (2002). Agonizing care: Care ethics, agonistic feminism and a political theory of care. Nursing Inquiry, 9(3), 203–214.

Dying With Dignity Canada. (2018). Dying with dignity. https://www.dyingwithdignity.ca

Friesen, P. (2020). Trust in health care after the death of Joyce Echaquan. *Impact Ethics: Making a Difference in Bioethics.* https://impactethics.ca/2020/11/09/trust-in-health-care-after-the-death-of-joyce-echaquan/

Government of Canada (2021). *Truth and Reconciliation Commission of Canada.* https://www.rcaanc-cirnac.gc.ca/eng/1450124405592/1529106060525

Hamilton, S. (2021). *Where are the children buried?* https://ehprnh2mwo3.exactdn.com/wp-content/uploads/2021/05/AAA-Hamilton-cemetery-FInal.pdf

Haslam-Larmer, L., Grigorovich, A., Quirt, H., et al. (2022). Prevalence, causes, and consequences of moral distress in healthcare providers caring for people living with dementia in long-term care during a pandemic. *Dementia, 22*(1), 5–27. https://doi.org/10.1177/14713012221124995

Jennings, B., Callahan, D., & Wolf, S. M. (1987, February). The professions: Public interest and common good [Special supplement]. *Hastings Center Report*, 3–4.

Johnston, P., Keatings, M., & Monk, A. (2022, December). Experiences of essential care partners during the COVID-19 pandemic [Special issue]. *Healthcare Quarterly, 25*, 41–47. https://doi.org/10.12927/hcq.2022.26979

Joseph, B., & Joseph, C. F. (2019). Indigenous relations: Insights, tips and suggestions to make reconciliation a reality. Indigenous Relations Press.

Keller, D. (2009). *A brief overview of basic ethical theory.* Wiley-Blackwell.

Kerr, T., Mitra, S., Kennedy, M. C., et al. (2017). Supervised injection facilities in Canada: Past, present, and future. *Harm Reduction Journal, 14*, 28. https://doi.org/10.1186/s12954-017-0154-1

LaSala, C. A. (2009). Moral accountability and integrity in nursing practice. *Nursing Clinics of North America, 44*(4), 423–434.

Leininger, M. M. (1988a). Care: The essence of nursing and health. In M. M. Leininger (Ed.), *Care: The essence of nursing* (pp. 3–15). Wayne State University Press.

Leininger, M. M. (1988b). *Caring: An essential human need.* Wayne State University Press.

Lux, M. K. (2016). *Separate beds: A history of Indian hospitals in Canada, 1920s–1980s.* University of Toronto Press.

Manitoba Nurses Union. (2018). *Workplace health and safety: Health and safety rights are legislated.* https://manitobanurses.ca/workplace-health-safety

Milton, C. L. (2008). Accountability in nursing: Reflecting on ethical codes and professional standards of nursing practice from a global perspective. *Nursing Science Quarterly, 21*(4), 300–303. https://doi.org/10.1177/0894318408324314

Nurse.com. (2010, June 29). What would Nightingale say about ethical dilemmas facing nurses? *Nurse.com.* https://www.nurse.com/blog/what-would-nightingale-say-about-ethical-dilemmas-facing-nurses/

Registered Nurses' Association of Ontario. (2007). *Best practice guidelines: Professionalism in nursing.* https://rnao.ca/bpg/guidelines/professionalism-nursing

Roach, M. S. (1992). *The human act of caring: A blueprint for the health professions.* Canadian Hospital Association.

Savage, A., Young, S., Titley, H., et al. (2022). This was my Crimean War: COVID-19 experiences of nursing home leaders. *Journal of the American Medical Directors Association, 23*(11), 1827–1832. https://www.ncbi.nlm.nih.gov/pmc/articles/PMC9371982/

Watson, M. J. (1988). New dimensions of human caring theory. *Nursing Science Quarterly, 1*(4), 175–181.

Wynd, C. A. (2003). Current factors contributing to professionalism in nursing. *Journal of Professional Nursing, 19*(5), 251–261.

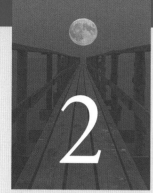

2 ETHICAL THEORIES: THEIR MEANING FOR NURSES

LEARNING OBJECTIVES

The purpose of this chapter is to enable you to understand:

- The moral complexity of the practice environment and the role of nurses as moral agents
- The challenging ethical choices nurses face
- The influence of values on ethical decision making
- The need for nurses to have a solid understanding of ethical theory and principles
- The application of traditional and contemporary ethical theory to challenging moral situations
- The evolution of present-day ethical thinking in nursing
- The value of the narrative in moral discourse
- The moral and oral traditions of Indigenous peoples in Canada

INTRODUCTION

Nurses enjoy a position of extraordinary responsibility. Their actions, both independent and collaborative, contribute to the well-being of persons living in Canada and across the world. Whether nurses are influencing the quality of a person's death, protecting the vulnerable (such as children, older persons, and the disadvantaged), promoting the health of the community, or advocating for policy and legislation, they do so with the trust of individuals, communities, and society at large, who view nurses as moral agents. Nurses are considered to be professionals who are able to differentiate between right and wrong, and be held accountable for their actions and decisions.

Nurses are present during many life transitions, during which time society expects them to meet high standards of ethical care. Because of these expectations and the trust bestowed upon them, nurses must be able to understand, clarify, and justify their choices and actions to others: patients, colleagues, the profession, employers, the justice system, and society. To do this effectively, nurses must have a strong foundation in ethics and acquire the skills and tools to make and defend complex moral decisions.

Every day, nurses make complex choices within the context of a challenging health care environment. They may not always be aware, however, that the many issues and challenges they face, and their subsequent decisions, are ethical in nature (Oddi et al., 2016). How do nurses identify the option that is best for everyone concerned, and one that ensures an optimal level of care? How do they choose a course of action from several alternatives when the relative merit of these options may be unclear? How are nurses confident that the decisions they make and the actions they take are the right ones? How are ethical dilemmas and violations identified? When are moral violations the result of poor communication, inadequate system support and resources, or substandard patient care processes? Within this complex health care environment, how are nurses supported in their moral relationships with patients, family members, and the community? How do they maintain and sustain, throughout all challenges and adversity, their own integrity (the quality of possessing and acting on high moral principles) as a person and as a professional, and that they have, to the best they are able, done what is best and what is right?

16

Nurses who demonstrate professional integrity in all circumstances contribute to the relationship of trust between themselves and those they serve.

This chapter is designed to guide nurses in their ethical practice and to introduce them to the tools, methods, and ethical theory and principles that can facilitate and guide the process of making and defending ethical choices. To begin this chapter, reflect on the ethical challenge faced in the following scenario.

CASE SCENARIO 2.1

MY STORY

Years ago, when I was a novice nurse working an evening shift on a busy medical unit, I returned from break to find the unit in utter chaos. One of my patients, a gentleman with heart failure, had and the team was attempting resuscitation. Meanwhile, I heard loud screams and observed my colleagues making attempts to prevent his wife from entering the room. I tried to reassure her and to explain the situation, describing the chaos in the room and how disturbing it would be for her to observe the resuscitation efforts. The wife insisted that she wanted to be with her husband and promised to stay focused on him and not on the team, and she understood they were trying to help him.

I was very conflicted and distressed and didn't know what to do. The usual practice, thinking we were protecting them, was to have family members leave during emergency situations. However, I explained the wife's wishes and assurances to the team, and I asked whether we could allow her to be present with her husband.

The senior nurse participating in the resuscitation attempts expressed concern that the wife would find it too disturbing and might interfere with the team's efforts. The team members also refused, saying they would be uncomfortable with the wife watching them. I explained this to the wife, who, while making intense eye contact, replied, "He is my husband, not yours. If he is dying, I want to be with him."

This story raises several issues and challenges, which include:

- The nurse's professional and moral obligations to the patient and his family
- The well-being and best interests of the patient
- The rights of the team caring for the patient
- The rights and well-being of the wife
- The effect of policies, rules, and routine practices inhibiting nurses from doing what they consider to be the right action
- The potential for moral distress when nurses are unable to act on what they believe is right

As you begin this chapter, reflect on your reaction to my dilemma. What are the most important ethical issues and challenges in this story? If you were me, what would you do? As various ethical theories and principles are discussed in this chapter, we will revisit my story and consider how these may guide my actions. At the conclusion of this chapter, the ultimate choice I made will be revealed, and you can debate whether it was the right one.

To understand the moral issues that arise in nursing and health care, it is essential to have knowledge of the most significant ethical theories, principles, and methods applicable to such moral issues; that is, those that help guide moral decision making. The extent to which moral issues are understood and addressed enhances the quality of health care, both practised and received.

Canada is a pluralistic society. Therefore, the notion of respecting differences in values and beliefs, and understanding the influence of culture in ethics, is vital. Given the significant history and position of Indigenous peoples in Canada (First Nations, Inuit, and Métis), it is important that their moral traditions be shared, understood, and honoured. Not all Indigenous communities hold the same philosophical view, religious belief, or moral code. There are differences in moral and ethical value systems across and within First Nations, Inuit, and Métis communities.

AN INTRODUCTION TO ETHICAL THEORY

Many factors influence our thinking about what is right or wrong, good or bad. These factors may include the norms, beliefs, and expectations of the society and culture within which we live; gender, age, and our personal characteristics; the context of the situation; previous experiences with similar situations; the potential outcomes or consequences of actions; the relationship of the individuals involved; and professional and individual values and beliefs. Over the centuries, many philosophers have tried to uncover the foundations of morality to understand the key moral considerations that guide our behaviour and our decisions about what is right and what is wrong. Believing that decisions about morality transcend our emotions, philosophers of the past developed theories and identified principles grounded in a "reasoned" or "rational" approach to ethical decision making. These thinkers related **rationality** to the notion of logical thinking and reasoning. Being rational was associated with intelligence, comprehension, or inference, particularly when an inference or a conclusion resulted from such a (rational or reasoned) thought process. Rationality was considered being able to explain and justify, that is provide good grounds or motives behind a decision or an action. "Irrationality," on the other hand, arose when the thinking behind a decision or action could not be explained or justified according to reason or logic (Internet Encyclopedia of Philosophy [IEP], n.d.; Landauer & Rowlands, 2001; Wilson, 1970).

In recent decades, thinking about morality has advanced beyond these "rationalistic" views to acknowledge the influence of emotion, caring, relationships, and experience. Early ethical theories were developed by men, who did not at the time consider women's input relevant. However, recent theories established by both men and women consider gender and the value of emotion and moral relationships (Gilligan, 1982; Norlock, 2019).

A body of work has emerged in nursing where ethical theories integrate nursing concepts and values, such as caring and compassion, and view nurses as moral agents within the context of professional relationships. Although rationalistic approaches devalue the role of emotion and instinct, some contemporary thinkers consider our emotional responses to be important guides for moral decisions and actions.

To better appreciate contemporary perspectives, one must understand the evolution of ethical theory, so some of the well-known historical and contemporary views, and their application to nursing, will be discussed.

Key Terms

Prior to describing the evolution of ethical theory, it is important to understand some of the key terms and concepts used in the field of ethics.

Morality is the tradition of beliefs and norms within a culture, religion, or society about right or wrong human conduct, often guided by explicit codes of conduct and rules governing behaviour. A well-known example is the "golden rule": Do unto others as you would have them do unto you. This rule implies that by following it, the right or moral action will follow. As children develop, they observe and learn the moral principles and values significant to their culture and society (Beauchamp & Walters, 2003; IEP, n.d.).

Ethics is the philosophical study of morality, or the systematic exploration of what is morally right or morally wrong. The study of ethics focuses on the recognition and evaluation of the variables that influence moral decisions and obligations, one's character, and the nature of the good life (Armstrong, 2006; BBC, 2014; Grassian, 1992; Landauer & Rowlands, 2001). The field of **biomedical ethics** explores ethical and moral questions associated with health-related issues, including research. **Nursing ethics** focuses on the moral questions and issues within the sphere of nursing practice, the nurse–patient relationship, the moral character of nurses, and nurses as moral agents (Fry, 1989). **Feminist ethics** attempts to reframe traditional ethics that devalue the experience and contribution of women. It is committed to eliminating the subordination of women and raising the moral question about what this means for women (Keller, 2009; Noddings, 1984).

Ethical theory is the study of the nature and justification of general ethical principles, duties and obligations, and character, and how they apply to moral problems (Armstrong, 2006; Beauchamp & Walters, 2003; Keller, 2009). Ethical theories are intended to guide what we ought to do when faced with an ethical dilemma. The intent is to provide a more rigorous and systematic approach to how we make decisions about what is right or wrong, or why one decision seems right and the other wrong (Frederiksen et al., 2013).

Applied ethics is the field of ethics in where theories and principles are applied to actual moral problems, for example, in health care, business and science (Almond, 1995; Beauchamp & Walters, 2003). The focus is on moral situations that arise in practice, and whether ethical theories can offer guidance to their resolution (Beauchamp, 2007; Singer, 2011). The scenarios included in this chapter illustrate actual moral problems and are intended to encourage the application of theories and principles.

Ethical dilemmas arise when the best course of action is unclear, when strong moral reasons support each position (i.e., when good reasons for mutually exclusive alternatives can be cited) (Beauchamp & Walters, 2003; IEP, n.d.; Keller, 2009), and when the only choice is the most right or the least wrong (Box 2.1).

Ethical processes, resources, and laws are in place to guide the nurse through such challenges and can assist in achieving the best outcome for both the patient and the family.

Categories of Ethical Study

There are two main categories of ethical study: nonnormative and normative. **Non-normative ethics** involves analyzing morality without taking a moral position, whereas **normative ethics** attempts to answer questions of what is right or what is wrong (Amer, 2019; Beauchamp & Walters, 2003; Frederiksen et al., 2013).

Non-normative studies include the fields of descriptive ethics and metaethics. **Descriptive ethics** is a field of ethics that encompasses factual descriptions and explanations of moral behaviours and beliefs. By looking at a wide range of moral beliefs and behaviours, this field of study attempts to explain how moral attitudes, rules, and beliefs differ from person to person and across societies and cultures. **Metaethics** is the field of ethics that analyzes the meanings of such key terms as *right, obligation, good,* and *virtue* and attempts to distinguish between what is moral and what is not—for example, the difference between a moral rule and a social rule. These include questions such as, *What is the meaning of the language used in specific instances of moral discourse, whether practical or theoretical? What is meant by a specific moral concept?* and many others. Further, metaethics analyzes the structure or logic of moral reasoning and justification and explores the nature of morality and the meanings and interrelationships of the fundamental concepts of moral language (Amer, 2019; Copp, 2007; Grassian, 1992). For example, in metaethics, answers to the following questions are pursued:

- How is a moral principle different from a nonmoral one?
- What do we mean when we say an act is right?
- What does it mean to have "free will" or to be "morally responsible" (Grassian, 1992)?

In normative ethics, attempts are made to identify the basic principles and **virtues** that guide morality and provide coherent, systematic, and justifiable answers to moral questions (Grassian, 1992). Through the development of ethical theory, normative ethics provides a system of moral principles or virtues and focuses on the reasons or arguments that guide decisions about what is right and what is wrong (Grassian, 1992, Keller, 2009).

MORAL DISTRESS

It is important for members of the interprofessional health care team, including the patient and family, to collaborate and communicate effectively to address difficult ethical issues. When ethical challenges, such as the one described, are not addressed, and when nurses

---

BOX 2.1
COMPETING INTERESTS: A DILEMMA FOR NURSES

An example of an ethical dilemma was shared by a nurse working in an acute care setting whose patient with a terminal illness expressed a wish to die and to have all treatment stopped. Before an advance directive could be established, the patient lost consciousness, and distressed, family members pleaded for all possible interventions. Presented with this situation, the nurse was torn between the expressed wishes of the patient and the emotional distress of family members not yet prepared for the death of their family member.

do not receive appropriate support with these ethical challenges, there is the risk of moral distress and moral residue. **Moral distress** can result when we are not able to recognize ethical issues or to deal with them effectively, or when we believe that a particular course of action is right but are not permitted or able to pursue it (Burston & Tuckett, 2013; Jameton, 1984; Lamiani & Borghi, 2017; Peter, 2013; Rushton, 2008; Wallis, 2015). Nurses are at a high risk for moral distress when they are unable to act on what they judge to be the best course of action, such as when an excessive workload prevents them from providing compassionate care to dying patients and to support families in distress (Rodney, 2017). The emotional and psychological pain that occurs is "the feeling of being unable to be yourself in a situation in which you feel that you should (but are not) able to do the right thing" (Batho & Pitton, 2018, p. 21). These frustrating experiences can result in feelings of anger and powerlessness (Holtz et al., 2018; Rodney, 2017).

The lingering feelings and personal discord from moral distress can continue long after the event is over. When nurses are repeatedly not able to act on what they think is morally right, this can result in moral residue and long-term consequences, such as lack of engagement, resignation from their place of employment, or leaving the nursing profession entirely. These risks are greater in circumstances where nurses are not supported or empowered to do what they think is right (Epstein & Delgado, 2010). Moral resilience—the ability to recover or adapt to moral adversity or trauma—is enhanced when the systems and processes are in place to support nurses in their response to morally complex situations. Nurses can learn to respond positively to ethically challenging situations by building their capacity for moral resilience, for example by gaining more knowledge about ethics; and when organizations and leaders can support nurses by creating a culture of ethical practice (Holtz et al., 2018; Rushton et al., 2017). The potential for moral distress in nurses who were at the "front lines" of the COVID-19 pandemic was significant (Haslam-Larmer et al., 2022; White et al., 2021). Consider their role in enforcing public health rules that restricted the presence of family members in acute, convalescent, and long-term care settings. Many nurses experienced moral conflict in situations where they were obligated to deny family access,

while knowing the negative consequences this would have for the patient and family (Institute for Patient and Family-Centered Care, 2021).

Reflect on the potential for moral distress in My Story (Case Scenario 2.1). How might it be mitigated or prevented in this situation and in similar ones in the future? Examples of the supports and resources available to nurses in these circumstances are described in Chapters 3 and 12.

Ethical theories provide a framework of **principles** and guidelines to help identify ethical issues and reconcile problems or conflicts. Although the solutions to these moral problems may not always be clear, these theories offer some guidance and facilitate ethical discussions. Although the many theories and principles available to guide ethical reflection may not be able to help resolve ethical conflict in every circumstance, nevertheless, they serve as a template or guide to assist nurses in justifying their moral position to others.

VALUES

A **value** is an ideal that has significant meaning or importance to individuals, cultural groups, and societies. Values influence morality and the norms, rules, and laws of a society. For example, Canadian society values individual freedom, health, fairness, honesty, and integrity. Evidence of these values is found in Canada's laws, in the *Canadian Charter of Rights and Freedoms,* and in individual and collective actions and behaviours. The structure of the Canadian health care system is grounded in core values of equality, individual rights, health and well-being, quality of life, and human dignity. Equality is evident in the principle of universality contained in the *Canada Health Act*—that is, the attempt to provide equal access to health care for all Canadians, regardless of where they live and their socioeconomic status.

Values influence our own individual beliefs, our views of others, and our opinions related to not only our moral judgements but also other areas, such as literature and art. Values emerge through our associations with others—family, friends, classmates, teachers, colleagues—and life experiences, religious beliefs, and the environment in which we live. Gender, age, and cultural beliefs are all relevant in shaping our values—but how significant are they in guiding moral judgements and decision making? Gender is said by some to affect the development of values in individuals and groups (Brown & Gilligan, 1992; Gilligan, 1982); women are considered more empathetic, and men are considered more likely to value certain outcomes when looking at a specific moral situation, though this may shift with age and experience (Arutyunova et al., 2016).

In recent times, the media have had a strong influence on value development. In particular, social media have become a vehicle through which values, beliefs, and attitudes are shaped, but social media pose risks associated with privacy and truthfulness (Cha et al., 2010; Inglehart, 1977; Salwin & Dupagne, 1999). We adapt our behaviours according to social expectations. Our behaviours, rituals, symbols, structures, rules, and laws represent the collective values and beliefs of our society.

Values within a culture can shift over time. For example, in recent years, Canadian society has shifted to a focus on the meaning and quality of life rather than on prolonging life at all costs. This shift led, in part, to the legislation on Medical Assistance in Dying (MAiD) discussed in Chapter 8. Greater respect for individual rights and freedoms has emerged just in the past couple of centuries. Evolving values around individual rights have led to legislation regarding consent to treatment, confidentiality, and so forth. The experience of the COVID-19 pandemic, however, has highlighted the rights of the collective community and society as a whole, versus those of the individual.

Though some values are universal, there is variation in conventional rules and how they are demonstrated across cultures. For example, as most cultures and societies value human life and therefore outlaw killing or murder, the punishment for such crimes may differ. Capital punishment has been abolished in Canada, but it is permitted in other countries, including China, India, and in certain jurisdictions across the United States.

There are further differences in how various cultures hold individuals accountable and impose sanctions for breaking the laws within a society. For example, in some countries, flogging is used as a form of punishment (Tiwari & Agarwal, 2020). In Canada, Indigenous healing lodges prepare offenders for reintegration into society. These settings offer culturally appropriate interventions that are guided by the values, beliefs, and traditions of Indigenous communities

in Canada. The focus is on Indigenous teaching, ritual and ceremony, dialogue with Elders, and connection with nature (Correctional Services Canada, 2021).

The tension between individualism and collectivism, and independence and interdependence can be observed across cultures and societies. In North America, there is a strong focus on independence and individual rights, whereas in other cultures greater value is placed on collective rights, duties, and the notion of social harmony (Arutyunova et al., 2016) For example, though we put value on helping others, in Canadian law (except in Quebec), there is no general legal obligation to assist others. This differs from "good Samaritan" laws in force in other countries, where individuals can face legal consequences for failing to provide assistance in emergencies (Linden, 2016). Though in Canada there is great respect for the rights of individuals, it is recognized that with these rights come responsibilities. Tension between individual rights versus social responsibility came into focus during the COVID-19 pandemic with the establishment of public health restrictions and vaccine mandates.

Not all values are moral, or good. Consider the experience of colonialism. Nations that considered exploitation and subjugation of other territories as a morally acceptable attribute valued the expansion of their wealth and power over any sense of obligation to the Indigenous peoples of the lands they claimed. This sense of entitlement was manifest in the total disregard for the cultural integrity of Indigenous peoples and a lack of respect for their spiritual and cultural traditions (Bufacchi, 2017). Consider the negative consequences of ethnocentric values (placing a higher value on one's own culture), which led to attempts to extinguish the culture of Indigenous peoples in Canada. Although Britain had entered into treaties with some Indigenous nations on a nation-to-nation basis, neither the Crown nor its successor, the Canadian state, seemed to respect these obligations. Settler culture in nineteenth-century Canada promoted the assimilation of Indigenous peoples into the European culture. Residential schools in Canada were conceived to provide Indigenous children with the skills to survive and earn their way in the world of "white" people. These institutions were established without any consultation with Indigenous communities and without any consideration of their culture and traditions. These institutions and the policies around them were used to erode and destroy Indigenous culture. For example, in some circumstances, if a family renounced their "Indian" status, then their children could attend a local school and not be required to go to a residential school.

Indifference and neglect exacerbated the negative legacy of these schools. The involuntary attendance of children from young ages, kilometres away from their families, forbidden to speak their own languages or associate with their siblings, and often exposed to physical, mental and sexual abuse, created a lasting legacy that Canada is still coming to terms with (Canada, 1996; Hanson et al., 2020).

Consider views regarding white supremacy, where there is greater value placed on white people over others. This explicit form of racism fosters a culture where white people are considered superior, and as such should be the dominant force in society (Beliso-De Jesús & Pierre, 2020).

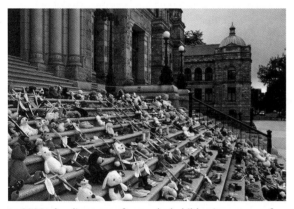

In 2021, the discovery of unmarked children's graves at former residential schools led to public protests, with children's shoes being left on display in public spaces. *Source: iStock.com/Wirestock.*

Influence of Values on Nursing Practice and Ethical Decision Making

Professional values build on and expand personal values and emerge as nurses are socialized into the profession. Nurses sometimes experience a struggle between their personal beliefs and professional responsibilities. Facing life-altering experiences, such as those associated with end of life, being present through the joy, pain, and sorrow of others, and witnessing inequity and hardship may alter their perspectives and reframe and reprioritize their values.

Codes of ethics for nurses in Canada, including the Canadian Nurses Association (CNA) *Code of Ethics for Registered Nurses* (described in Chapter 3) and the Canadian Council for Practical Nurse Regulators (CCPNR) *Code of Ethics for Licensed Practical Nurses*, are based on values that are deemed important for the profession of nursing. An understanding of the values of the nursing profession assists nurses in comprehending and applying these codes, which articulate value statements, principles, and responsibilities that guide the ethical and moral actions of nurses and the profession (Canadian Council for Practical Nurse Regulators, 2013; CNA, 2017; Sellman, 2011). These codes highlight nursing values related to compassion, accountability, trust, and competence.

Nurses' individual values may influence their responses to ethical issues, their decisions, and the care they provide to patients.

Canada comprises a mosaic of cultural and religious perspectives. Thus, nurses care for patients and families whose basic value systems—and, hence, beliefs, rituals, and customs—may differ from their own. Responding appropriately in contexts where the values and rituals of others differ from our own can be challenging if these differences are not understood.

There are values across cultures that are shared, such as the sanctity of life, a belief that human beings have intrinsic worth and should be treated with dignity and respect. Though the value of human life may be shared across cultures, it may be demonstrated in different ways, through customs, traditions, and rituals. For example, respect for persons across many cultures continues after death and influences the treatment of the body and the rituals and behaviours associated with death and dying. With this respect for persons and our shared humanity comes the value of treating persons with compassion. Within the Buddhist tradition, there exists the notion of *karuna*—"compassion"—which is manifest in the custom of continuing to ensure comfort, support, and love to a dying person for as long as there is life. Their belief in an after-life influences end-of-life rituals such as chanting, which they believe helps guide the spirit of the dying person to the higher being (Chan et al., 2011).

Similar values and beliefs about the after-life influence the rituals performed during the dying process in some Indigenous communities. They can include the pipe ceremony, which entails the burning of sacred medicines (e.g., sage, sweetgrass, and cedar) to help purify the dying person; during the ceremony, those present pray for the safe passage of the person's spirit to the after-life. In Catholic and Orthodox Christian religions, rituals, such as a series of prayers and anointing known as *last rites,* are performed to ensure reconciliation with God as one nears death. In Orthodox Judaism and Muslim religions, there are strict rules associated with the care of the person after death.

How might nurses ensure that these culturally significant rituals are respected, whether in the home or in an institutional setting? Respect for the values of persons necessitates that nurses not make assumptions, but seek information about what is most important to the patient and family, and then facilitate the processes that ensure respect for their values and beliefs. Nurses who seek to understand and respect the important values of others strengthen their role as moral agents and enrich their relationships with patients and families (Varcoe et al., 2004).

Nurses interact and collaborate within a broad interprofessional team. The respective professional values of nurses and those in other health care disciplines may influence the perspectives that each offers when discussing ethical issues. As the value of working within interprofessional teams in health care is recognized, so, too, is the necessity to understand and respect the values of each member and their contribution to ethical decision making. Though health care professionals may share similar values, nurses interact with other professionals within the health care setting with whom there may be a conflict in values. Consider nursing leaders who engage with professionals such as accountants, who might value financial constraint as the best means of staying within budget. The nursing leader, with a strong value on quality of care, might argue that investing in more nurses would not only achieve better care but also be cost effective by avoiding costs associated with poor patient outcomes.

Value conflicts may occur when professionals disagree about how a particular ethical situation (e.g., withdrawal of treatment, allocation of resources, use of restraints, discharge planning) should be managed.

The obligation of nurses as professionals and as members of a health care team is to understand and respect the values of others. Because conflict in values can result in moral distress, it is imperative that team members are able to articulate and clarify their values to one another, and to establish processes whereby this can be done.

Value Clarification

Value clarification is a process through which team members, including patients and families, come to understand the values they hold and the relative importance of each of these values. To ensure a shared understanding of each other's values, open and transparent discussions and active listening that builds mutual respect are essential. Reflection on specific situations, stories, or narratives can assist in identifying and clarifying values, and thus result in a shared understanding of differing and shared perspectives.

Frequently, workload challenges limit the opportunity for these important discussions. However, making the time for such dialogue is a worthwhile investment. The rewards include improved communication and collaboration among team members, deeper, more meaningful relationships, prevention of moral distress, and enhanced patient care as ethical problems are addressed and action plans identified.

Relativism

Not all thinkers and philosophers agree that there is a single, correct, and objective framework for morality (Arutyunova et al., 2016; Beauchamp & Walters, 2003; Dwyer, 1999; Grassian, 1992). Some consider individual and group responses to morality to be relative to the norms and values of a particular culture or society, time in history, or to the situation presenting itself. This view is called **cultural relativism** or **normative relativism**.

Relativists consider morality to be more a matter of cultural differences and taste, an arbitrary notion of what one believes or feels, and not based on some deeper set of objectively justifiable principles (Beauchamp & Walters, 2003; Grassian, 1992). Proponents of relativism believe that moral beliefs and principles apply only to individual cultures or persons, and that the values of one culture do not govern the conduct of others. What is morally right or morally wrong varies from place to place; that is, what may be considered moral in one culture may be considered immoral in another. They argue that there are no absolute or universal moral standards that can apply to all persons at all times (Arutyunova et al., 2016; Beauchamp & Walters, 2003; Kitayama & Uskul, 2011; Nisbett et al., 2001) and that concepts of rightness and wrongness are specific to the contexts in which they arise. For example, some societies value democracy as the right way to govern, while others disagree with **political plurality** and endorse authoritarian forms of government, which they believe is the most appropriate or works the best for that particular society.

Relativists note that what is deemed worthy of moral approval or disapproval in one society may differ from standards in other societies, even though they accept that humans possess a moral conscience or general sense of right and wrong. The moral beliefs of individuals, relativists argue, vary according to historical, environmental, and familial differences; therefore, particular actions, motives, and rules that are praised or blamed may vary from culture to culture (Beauchamp & Walters, 2003), and there are no universal norms (Arutyunova et al., 2016; Kitayama & Uskul, 2011; Nisbett et al., 2001). For example, in Western society, female genital mutilation is viewed as an abhorrent practice and a means to control women's sexuality. In cultures where it is practised, it is justified on the basis of issues related to hygiene, religion, modesty, and other factors.

Relativism has also been raised with respect to the judgements of morality related to historical actions, such as with colonialism and the treatment of Indigenous peoples in Canada, as was discussed earlier. It would be difficult to imagine how, at any time in history, regardless of motivation, it would ever be considered moral to take communities of children away from their families.

Opponents of relativism argue that despite apparent differences in conclusions, there is a "universal structure of human nature, or at least a universal set of human needs which leads to the adoption of similar or even identical principles in all cultures" (Beauchamp & Walters, 2003). Individuals or groups may disagree about the ethics of a particular situation or practice, but this does not mean that they hold different fundamental moral standards or principles (Arutyunova

et al., 2016; Beauchamp & Walters, 2003). For example, a principle related to minimizing harm may ground the arguments for and against genital mutilation, and theories of justice could justify various political systems.

Critics of relativism argue that certain core principles underly fundamental moral judgements and that some aspects of moral thinking may be universal across cultures (such as respect for life and the judgement that killing another person is immoral), and that these core principles are part of what it is to be human (Brannigan, 2000; Dwyer, 1999).

Some core principles may influence moral judgements across societies, implying that some core ethical principles are universal, though some sociocultural factors may result in variation (Arutyunova et al., 2016; Dwyer, 1999). Presenting a view different from that of relativists, critics offer that a society may agree on ideals of individual liberty and general happiness, and yet they disagree on whether society has the right to make people happy in spite of themselves. That is, they agree on principles but disagree on their range of application. For example, many in Canadian society support the principles of preventing harm and promoting health, but not all agree with smoking ban legislation or with vaccine mandates.

The golden rule is an example of a moral principle that would seem to be universal, a maxim that is found within most religions and cultures: "do unto others as you would have them do unto you," as a means of governing one's conduct or behaviour. The notion of the golden rule goes back as early as Confucian times, and though perhaps stated differently, the concept is prominent in most major religions and is evident in most ethical traditions and cultures. Consider how this maxim is communicated by the Yoruba, a community in West Africa:

One who is going to take a pointed stick to punch a baby bird should first try it on himself to feel how it hurts. https://en.wikipedia.org/wiki/Golden_Rule

NORMATIVE ETHICAL THEORIES

Ethical theories, developed to answer questions about what is right or wrong, are called *normative*. Normative theories offer a system of principles and concepts to help determine what ought or ought not to be done.

Their goal is to provide evaluative standards to determine the actions or norms that are deemed to be good, or morally justified.

Ethical theories focus not only on moral decision making, but also on the character of the people who make such choices. These theories of morality address questions such as,

- In a particular moral decision-making situation, which is the morally correct choice?
- What are the particular virtues of character that constitute a good person?
- Are there certain human actions that, without exception, are always morally correct or morally incorrect?

The following section introduces the most influential historical approaches to moral thinking and those that offer relevance and application to nursing practice today. Each theory will be used to reflect on My Story (Case Scenario 2.1). Additional scenarios are shared to illustrate each theory.

Traditional Theories of Morality

Virtue Ethics

In virtue ethics, attention focuses on the character of the person, or persons, making moral decisions. This approach asserts that a virtuous person, one whose character is good or morally praiseworthy, is more likely to make the right decision and take the morally correct action (IEP, n.d.).

One of the earliest and most influential contributors to virtue ethics was Aristotle (384–322 BC), who in his work, *Nicomachean Ethics*, considered the question of how one is to live a good life. He offered that a person's character, as judged by the moral virtues they possess, is an indicator of how "good" they are as a person. He was of the opinion that the natural instinct or inclination of humanity is to be a good person, and if persons strive through learning and practice to be the best they can be, they will do the right thing (IEP, n.d.).

A virtue is a characteristic, or a distinguishing trait, that is considered to have moral value and is therefore an indicator of a person who possesses high moral standards. Moral virtues, according to Aristotle, include such traits as "courage, temperance, compassion, generosity, honesty, and justice." He asserted that a person with strong moral virtues would be committed

to making the right choice and choosing the right action (IEP, n.d.).

Virtue ethics is applicable to health care and nursing ethics, as health care professionals have traditionally been expected to possess strong moral characteristics and are relied upon by society to practise morally in both their actions and decision making. Some offer that this approach should supplement other duty-based and utilitarian approaches to ethics (discussed later), which have limitations when solely applied in the health care context (Armstrong, 2006; Scott, 1995).

Virtue Theory: Its Foundation in the Nursing Profession

Virtue theory was fundamental to the historical evolution of nursing's ethical traditions. Early in the profession, great emphasis was placed on the values and moral character of the nurse. First promoted by Florence Nightingale, nursing ethics was built on the premise that the nurse, while caring for patients, ought to be motivated by intrinsic values that seek to achieve high moral standards. She believed that these values should include such traits as honesty, trustworthiness, patience, compassion, honour, moral courage, and devotion (Nightingale, 1882). She asserted that the commitment to these ideals was the distinguishing feature of the profession. While embracing Aristotelian thinking that the character of the person was essential to morality, she focused attention on the traits and moral virtues that make a good nurse. Hence she sought to recruit women of good character, and then through education, experience, and the influence of virtuous role models, develop in them the essential character qualities of the nurse which in her view were fundamental to the moral value of the nurse–patient relationship (Armstrong, 2006; Fowler, 2021; Hoyt, 2010; Scott, 1995; Sellman, 1997, 2011). As Nightingale stated:

> A woman cannot be a good and intelligent nurse without being a good and intelligent woman. (Benjamin & Curtis, 1985, p. 257)

Nightingale offered that the ethical foundation of nursing should be based on the moral character of the nurse and the moral community of practice. This is a framework that, in her view, should determine the knowledge and skills required of a professional nurse. While acknowledging that order, structure, diligence, supervision, and skills are vital to exemplary nursing practice, she claimed it is the moral character of the nurses, and the possession of virtues such as caring and compassion, that influences the nurse's manner and approach to patient care. (Bradshaw, 1999).

Nightingale's attention to the high moral expectations demanded of nurses influenced the advancement of nursing as a profession, as did her many other contributions (Hoyt, 2010; Sellman, 1997, 2011). In 1914, Margaret Fox, an early leader in nursing, wrote:

Is it not, then, important that you should at once begin to realise the responsibilities you have taken upon yourselves in becoming nurses? This sense of responsibility should influence all you say and do, for your words and actions will show what you are. Therefore, as conduct is the outcome of character, so character is more important in a nurse than mere cleverness. How necessary it is then, that such attributes as reverence, gentleness, discretion, and uprightness should enter into every nurse's character, and be continually cultivated by the earnest practice of good habits and patient continuance of well-doing. (Fox, 1914, p. 4)

Some contemporary thinkers in the profession continue to promote virtue theory as the foundation of ethical practice, as it builds on this nursing tradition and highlights the core values of the profession (Bradshaw, 2011). This view is based on the premise that nursing practice should be motivated by internally motivated values, by nurses of strong moral character; and therefore nurses should seek to uphold these traditional, social moral standards as first defined by Nightingale (Nightingale, 1934).

Alan Armstrong (2006) criticizes the dominance of obligation and act-based theories in health care, such as deontology and utilitarianism. Suggesting they are limited, "inadequate," and not grounded in the reality of practice, he offers an alternative approach using virtue ethics as an action-oriented guide to ethical nursing practice. This practice-based approach, he suggests, takes into account the context of the situation and the relationships involved. This pathway to moral decision making in nursing emphasizes three features

(1) exercising the moral virtues such as compassion; (2) using judgement; and (3) using moral wisdom,

understood to include at least moral perception, moral sensitivity, and moral imagination. (Armstrong, 2006, p. 110)

Virtue ethics, Armstrong argues, has merit in nursing practice as it reflects the moral language of nursing, considers the emotional responses of the patient and the nurse, and requires professional judgement and moral wisdom. He suggests that moral wisdom, as acquired through learning and experience, enables ethical nursing practice. (Table 2.1). He agrees with Nightingale that it is possible to enhance virtues through learning and positive role models. Further, this approach aligns with patient-centred care and allows patients to share their narrative or story as a means to identify the morally relevant aspects in the context of the specific situation. Narrative ethics and caring ethics will be highlighted later in this chapter. In relation to patient-centred care and the nurse–patient relationship, Armstrong highlights the virtues of compassion, courage, and respectfulness (Table 2.2).

TABLE 2.1
Elements of Moral Wisdom

Perception	Being aware of moral situations, understanding what is meaningful and relevant in a particular situation or context.
Sensitivity	Being able to identify needs, perceive and understand feelings, and respond in a morally appropriate manner.
Imagination	Putting oneself in another's situation, being empathetic, "how would I feel?"

Source: From Armstrong, A. E. (2006).

TABLE 2.2
Virtues in Patient-Centred Care and the Nurse–Patient Relationship

Compassion	"the moral foundation of the helping relationship between nurse and patient"
Courage	needed by a nurse "to be an advocate for a patient"
Respectfulness	"necessary to empower patients"

Source: From Armstrong, A. E. (2006).

The virtue of compassion will be explored in more detail.

COMPASSION. As the nursing profession evolved, many promoted compassion as fundamental to the helping relationship and hence grounding the morality of the nurse–patient relationship. This virtue, equated with the human quality of kindness, is about the intent and manner of care and can be nurtured and modelled within the culture and ethos of practice. Compassion is not limited to good times and ought not be displaced by other stressors—the greater the challenges, the greater the need for compassion (Bradshaw, 2011). For example, during the COVID-19 pandemic, isolation practices, the requirements for personal protective equipment (PPE), and virtual care, imposed great challenges to the nurse–patient relationship, which, according to Armstrong (2006), "is only achievable if nurses make themselves available to patients, spend sufficient time with patients, and listen attentively to what patients have to say" (p. 112). It was during this time that the need for compassion was the greatest.

Returning to Florence Nightingale, recall her view that the moral nurse was a good person who cultivated a virtuous character, including compassion. Historically, developing the "compassionate character" was the impetus for care; it gave the nursing profession its ethos or culture, and guided its focus on the patient. Patient-centred care is not a modern concept. Nightingale and nursing leaders who followed held that patients should be at the centre of compassionate nursing care. Catherine Wood, the superintendent of Great Ormond Street Hospital for Children, wrote in 1878:

Gentleness of the heart will teach gentleness to the hand and to the manners. I can give no better

rule than to put yourself in your patient's place. (Bradshaw, 2011, p. 13)

The critical importance of compassion in nursing was illustrated by an Indigenous person who described his childhood experience as a patient in an "Indian hospital":

The doctors and nurses were all imported from the south. The ward I was in became very fond of one particular nurse and so did I. She had such a gentle face and nature . . . When she was on duty we behaved for her, her pleasantness kept us pleasant. When she was off duty, we were just the opposite. We wore long faces like the ones that were on duty. We sneaked around behind their backs. We ran to the windows to look out. They treated us like children, so we acted like children. (Lux, 2016, p. 104)

Criticism of Virtue Ethics

Criticisms of virtue ethics include the perceived ambiguity regarding what constitutes good virtues, lack of clarity regarding the motivation of the agent, and lack of practical content to guide actions and decisions. Defenders of virtue ethics view it as an alternative or complementary approach to traditional theories. In that virtue ethics considers the judgement, experience, and insights of the nurse, and it involves the nurse has a greater sensitivity in the context of the moral encounter (Begley, 2005; Hursthouse, 1999). Further, they argue that virtue ethics is action guiding, asserting that the action is right if it is what a person with a virtuous character would do in in these circumstances. The virtuous person, motivated to be good and to act morally, would follow this maxim (Begley, 2005).

CASE SCENARIO 2.2

COMPASSIONATE CARE

While talking with colleagues at the nursing station, J. L. expressed frustration with a patient who was to be discharged home that day. The patient had been on the call bell frequently that morning, complaining of abdominal cramps. "The patient claims to need to have a bowel movement and has been on and off the commode all morning with no success. Now the patient is complaining of nausea and I think is trying to avoid discharge, and I have made all the arrangements for the transfer." J. L. was about to go on break, but prior to leaving asked the unit clerk to call the transport team as the patient's partner had just arrived. When the transport team member arrived, M. S., the

Continued on following page

CASE SCENARIO 2.2 *(Continued)*

nurse covering for J. L., went to assist and found the patient on the commode, vomiting and in tears. M. S. quickly assessed the situation, cancelled the transport, and informed the medical team that the discharge had to be cancelled. M. S. then stayed to comfort and reassure the patient and the patient's partner.

M. S. listened to the patient's story, and heard that the patient had recently been told that an earlier cancer had reoccurred and had spread. Apparently, no further treatment was possible and palliative care was to be provided at home. The patient was worried that they wouldn't be able to manage and that the pain and suffering would get worse. The medical team thanked M. S. for taking action and agreed that more needed to be done to understand and manage these symptoms effectively.

Interpretation

This story illustrates the approach to virtue ethics offered by Armstrong. Clearly, M. S. demonstrated

moral wisdom in this response to the patient. Even without having a previous relationship with the patient, M. S. very quickly perceived that there were issues that needed to be explored further, and that given the symptoms, the patient could not go home. M. S. was sensitive to the emotional and physical distress the patient was experiencing, and by cancelling the discharge, exercised the courage to advocate on the patient's behalf. Further, sensitive to the patient's need for support and understanding, M. S. seemed to "imagine" that if in a similar situation, they would have similar needs to be comforted and listened to. Seeming to understand that there was more to uncover, M. S. responded with compassion, stayed present with the patient, and hence responded in a morally appropriate manner. J. L., on the other hand, seemed not to have compassion or respect for the needs of this patient. Rather, J. L. made assumptions and seemed to be more self-oriented than patient-centred in this situation.

Deontology and Teleology

Two traditional categories of normative moral theory are teleology (derived from the Greek *teleos,* meaning "end") and deontology (derived from the Greek *deontor,* meaning "duty") (Beauchamp & Walters, 2003; Freeman, 1994; IEP, n.d.). *Deontological* theories make explicit the duties and principles that ought to guide our actions, whereas *teleological* theories focus on the principle of **utility**, the ends or outcomes and consequences of decisions and action. When making an ethical choice, teleologists, also known as consequentialists, look ahead to the consequences or outcomes of an action; deontologists look at the nature of the act itself, evaluating it in terms of the moral duties and obligations of persons to oneself and others in society (Begley, 2005; Grassian, 1992; Mandal et al., 2016). The most well-known teleological theory that considers ends, outcomes, and the consequences of decisions and actions is **utilitarianism**; the most prestigious version having been offered by philosopher John Stuart Mill (1806–1873), whose work was based on that of Jeremy Bentham (1748–1832). The most influential deontological theory, known as *Kantian ethics*, was

formulated by Immanuel Kant (1724–1804). At the core of Kantianism is the categorical imperative, which states: "Act only on that maxim whereby you can, at the same time, will that it should become a universal law" (Health Care Ethics, 2022). There are no page numbers it is in the section c. Deontological Theories: Kant. It is considered the fundamental principle of morality (Donaldson, 2017; Health Care Ethics, 2022).

Utilitarian/Consequentialist Theory

In utilitarian theories, there are no absolute principles, moral codes, duties, or rules; rather, there is the assumption that good can be quantified and calculated relative to the benefits or harms that result from moral choices (Beauchamp & Walters, 2003; Begley, 2005; Häyry, 2021; IEP, n.d.). In utilitarianism, the consequences of a given action are the measure of its moral worth.

In order to identify the right and wrong action, the future or potential outcomes or consequences of proposed actions are evaluated and calculated based on some theory of value that varies depending on the particular utilitarian approach. The chosen values might include well-being, welfare, pleasure, happiness, absence from pain, harm, and so on. In practice, then, a person might list the alternative actions available, consider the possible consequences or outcomes of each act, and then evaluate and quantify those consequences in relation to that theory of value (IEP, n.d.). Also, in making this calculation, Utilitarians offer that one acts best by choosing and acting on the option that provides the greatest good and the least harm for the greatest number of people; that is, it maximizes the total utility for all those affected. For example, in a situation where withdrawal of treatment is being considered, the consequences of this action would be evaluated based on the best outcome, as determined by the identified values, not only in relation to the patient in this particular situation but also to the family, the health care professionals involved, and society as a whole. In addition, both immediate and long-term consequences would be considered.

If happiness was identified as the most morally relevant value, then the correct action should lead to the greatest possible balance of happiness, or to the least possible balance of unhappiness, both long term and immediate, for all those concerned (Beauchamp & Walters, 2003; IEP, n.d.). Essentially, the consequences of an act consist of the sum total of differences that act will make in the world, and in utilitarianism this is the standard of morality.

A THEORY OF VALUE. Fundamental to utilitarian theory is the requirement for the identifiable good or value that has the greatest significance or meaning. There is great debate among utilitarians on what outcome has the greatest utility or value—the ultimate intrinsic good or the moral value of an act. The notion of utility depends on a *theory of value*, or what is perceived to be this intrinsic good. The consequences of an act, therefore, are evaluated based on this utilitarian theory of value and, as mentioned earlier, are measured in their totality (the greatest good and the least harm for the greatest number of people).

As mentioned, utilitarians do not always agree on specific goals and values, whose goals count, or why. Pluralistic utilitarians believe that no single goal or state constitutes the good. They accept many values—they consider a range of intrinsic values to be important products of a good action, and they believe

the greatest aggregate good is achieved when these multiple intrinsic goods are considered in the analysis of right and wrong actions. Other utilitarians consider one specific value to constitute the ultimate end (Beauchamp & Walters, 2003).

John Stuart Mill falls within the category of utilitarians who are described as hedonistic, who view utility in terms of the values of pleasure or happiness. (Beauchamp & Walters, 2003).

Mill's Utilitarianism

Mill formulated one of the better-known utilitarian theories, outlined in his text *Utilitarianism* (1861). Fundamental to his theory of value, the principle of utility is viewed in terms of pleasure or happiness. He argued that the ultimate intrinsic good is happiness and that all other goods are instrumental, or a means, toward this end. He offered that the principle of utility is grounded in the pursuit of pleasure and the avoidance of pain, which results in happiness—which he believed to be the main goal of life. For example, if an action results in the elimination of pain and suffering, then this, in effect, results in happiness. The elimination of pain and suffering is not the ultimate end but a means toward a state of happiness.

Hence, in choosing among alternatives, an act is right if, and only if, its utility is higher in terms of happiness than the utility of any other act (Mill, 1948; Mill & Warnock, 2003). Because Mill valued happiness as the ultimate outcome, he offered that the best moral choice is that which results in the greatest happiness for the greatest number of people; actions are right when they promote happiness and wrong when they produce the opposite. He argued that pleasure and freedom from pain can be measured and compared. Thus, the moral value of an action is determined by adding the total happiness produced and subtracting the pain involved (Beauchamp & Walters, 2003; IEP, n.d.).

While arguing that the only intrinsically desirable outcome or end is happiness or pleasure, he noted that there are higher forms of pleasure, such as intellect and moral sentiments, and rejected hedonistic views of pleasure focused on the "self"; he offered that a person's interests count no more than those of others (IEP, n.d.).

In response to those who question pleasure and happiness as the foundation of the principle of utility, Mill responded that these are higher forms of pleasure that are understood and appreciated by human beings. He offered that the calculation of utility is not concerned with individual pleasure or happiness, but instead with the actions that produce the most happiness for society as a whole, even if the action produces less happiness for the individual. The person, engaged in moral decision making therefore is no more, or less, important in the evaluation of options. In fact, he argued that actions have even greater moral significance (and, therefore, a greater calculation of utility) when they have a greater effect on the pleasure or happiness of others (Mill, 1948; Mill & Warnock, 2003; SuperSummary, 2022).

Mill's utilitarianism has both a normative and psychological foundation—normative in the (moral value) principle of utility, and psychological in Mill's views regarding human nature. Vital the psychological foundation of utilitarianism is his understanding of the human conscience, which leads to a person's experience of distress, pain, or remorse when actions break the moral code. He believed that humanity's inclination is to exist as social beings, and as such would desire unity and harmony with one another (Mill, 1948). Also, he believed that humans have a natural instinct to be part of a community and that the nature of persons is to help one another. Based on these assumptions, he concluded that it followed that all rational beings would strive to do their best. Further, he argued that this inclination would lead them to seek the betterment of society as a whole, and therefore would be inclined to follow this moral framework. Mill viewed utilitarianism as a moral framework that would not only guide the moral behaviour of individuals, but also facilitate the achievement of broad social goals (Mill, 1948; Mill & Warnock, 2003).

In summary, Mill argued that because people desire unity and harmony with others, and because their goal is happiness, they can reasonably predict and evaluate what actions would produce the greatest happiness and choose the right action.

Act and Rule Utilitarianism

There are two approaches to utilitarian theory: the evaluation of particular acts in relation to particular circumstances; and the establishment of the rules of conduct that determine what is right or wrong in general. In *act utilitarianism,* the utility of each act

is judged on its consequences, asking what consequences will result directly from *this action in this circumstance?* (Beauchamp & Walters, 2003). In *rule utilitarianism,* the utility of general patterns of behaviour is considered, rather than that of one specific action, asking rather what consequences will result *generally from this sort of action?* (Beauchamp & Walters, 2003).

In rule utilitarianism, even after it is determined that the utilitarian calculation of the ratio of happiness to unhappiness in a particular moral situation identifies an option to be morally correct, an additional calculation must take place to determine whether this option, in similar future cases, would consistently be identified as the appropriate one. A rule is correct provided that more utility would be produced by people following it, rather than any other rule that would apply to the situation or act. (Some argue that this approach is similar to Kant's notion of universality, which is discussed later in this chapter.) The right rule would be the one that, consistently applied, would produce the greatest good or the least harm for the greatest number of people.

Rule utilitarians hold that rules have a central position in morality and cannot be compromised by the demands of a particular situation. The effectiveness of a rule is judged by determining that its observance would, in theory, maximize social utility (Beauchamp & Walters, 2003) better than any possible substitute rule and better than no rule. Theoretically, utilitarian rules are firm and protective of all individuals, independent of factors of social convenience and momentary need (Beauchamp & Walters, 2003).

Critics of rule utilitarianism question how one resolves conflict among moral rules in particular circumstances. They argue that ranking of rules is almost impossible; therefore, in circumstances of conflict, the principle of utility decides, and the theory is reduced to act utilitarianism (Beauchamp & Walters, 2003). Rule utilitarians argue that every moral theory has practical limitations in cases of conflict, when the right choice is not clear, but that in the majority of circumstances, in the long term, the rules make sense.

During the COVID-19 pandemic, many public health requirements, such as wearing of masks, lockdowns, and vaccine mandates, were based on some utilitarian calculation. However, in making that calculation, not all consequences were understood at the time, such as the harms resulting from restricting family presence in long-term care settings. Also, utilitarian considerations informed other discussions related to triage when deciding who would have priority if life-saving technologies became scarce (Savulescu et al., 2020).

Criticism of Utilitarianism

Critics of utilitarianism argue that it is impossible and impractical to use this theory in determining what one ought to do in daily life. They suggest that the model is relatively useless for purposes of objectively quantifying widely different interests (Beauchamp & Walters, 2003). Furthermore, when the focus is on values such as pleasure as the desired end, critics suggest that individuals with morally unacceptable preferences would use these in their calculations. In response, supporters suggest most people are not perverse; if they were, then their actions would result in great unhappiness in society, thus demonstrating the validity of the theory (Beauchamp & Walters, 2003). They also argue that as Mill suggests, humans must rely on common sense and past experiences when quantifying consequences, and that because one need may be only reasonably predictive, it is not possible to always be error-free. Also, as argued by Mill, most humans strive to do their best and seek constant improvement in moral decision making.

Other critics suggest that "good" cannot be measured and comparatively weighed. In response, utilitarians argue that humans make crude, basic comparisons of values every day; what is important is to be morally conscientious and serious in our analysis (Beauchamp & Walters, 2003). Further, as Mill notes, pleasure and freedom from pain can be measured and compared.

One of the more serious judgements against utilitarianism is that it can lead to injustice. Critics argue that the greatest value for the greatest number may bring harm to a minority, thus failing to consider issues of *distributive justice* (Beauchamp & Walters, 2003). Utilitarians respond that considerations regarding justice and social utility are part of the calculations considered in the short- and long-term evaluations of the rightness of a particular act or rule under utilitarian theory. Rule utilitarians deny that single cost–benefit determinations ought to be accepted and believe that general rules of justice should constrain the use of cost–benefit analysis in all cases and ensure that standards of distributive justice are adhered to (Beauchamp & Walters, 2003; Camic, 1979; Gandjour & Lauterback, 2003). In *Utilitarianism* (1861), Mill examined the relationship between utility and justice and offered that justice is instrumental to achieving happiness. Based on his view of humanity's inclination to be part of a community, and to protect self and others, Mill argued that justice is ultimately concerned with the happiness and good of society (SuperSummary, 2022).

CASE SCENARIO 2.3

THE EXPERIENCE OF RACISM

K. K., a nurse, has just accepted a position at a community care agency, located in a rural town, and spent the first day meeting patients in their homes. Overall, it was a good experience, but one patient was somewhat aloof and irritable. K. K. assumed that this was related to the patient's chronic condition, which caused a great deal pain and discomfort.

The next morning, K. K.'s manager received a call from this patient, who requested a different nurse. The manager was puzzled and asked if there was a problem with K. K.'s nursing care, to which the patient responded, "It's not that, I just don't trust those people."

K. K. was born and educated in Canada after K. K.'s parents immigrated from Pakistan. K. K. follows the Muslim faith and has chosen to wear a hijab in recognition of this religious and ethnic identity (Zempi, 2016).

The manager is conflicted and uncertain of what action to take. The manager is aware that autonomy, founded on respect for a patient's choice, is an important principle in health care. They are concerned that the patient's request is based on racism, yet also

Continued on following page

CASE SCENARIO 2.3 *(Continued)*

know that nurses cannot abandon patients in need of care. Further, the manager worries about the emotional distress this knowledge would cause for K. K. and questions whether to protect K. K. from such racism and to ensure the patient receives the needed care, another nurse should be assigned.

Interpretation

From a utilitarian perspective, the manager must consider all of the options available and evaluate the consequences associated with each of them. There are a number of potential consequences associated with this option that must be considered. Though in the short term this approach might seem to resolve the immediate challenge, there are many other possible consequences to consider, including the following:

■ Assuming that the manager's values include respect for all persons, regardless of race, religion, and ethnicity, lack of alignment with these values would risk moral distress, which if unresolved might result in moral residue. Also, this approach would deceive K. K., who would not be afforded due process and respect.

■ Since the demographics of the community are changing, there is the risk that such racist behaviour might increase in frequency, making it a challenge to change assignments on a regular basis.

■ The reasons for the change in assignment may be evident or revealed to K. K. by others, causing distress and feelings of abandonment. Assuming the manager condoned this behaviour, K. K. might lose trust in the manager and consider resigning from this position. This would leave fewer nurses

to care for other patients in need. Further, this might negatively affect the reputation of this setting as a safe and supportive environment, risking future recruitment of nurses.

Racism in the health care environment is unacceptable. This story represents a major challenge faced by leaders in health care who strive to achieve high moral standards and who are guided by values that are both patient-centred and supportive of healthy work environments for staff. There are no easy solutions, but nursing as a profession is addressing these challenges, as discussed in Chapters 10 and 11. In this particular scenario, some strategies that might produce better moral outcomes include:

■ Disclosure to K. K. so the manager can demonstrate support and so they can identify the best option together.

■ An honest and open discussion with the patient (guided by best practices) that might include some form of mediation and knowledge sharing.

■ Education in the community about cultural diversity, and ways of celebrating and welcoming new arrivals.

■ Making it clear that racism and prejudice is never tolerated; through public awareness and by making it explicitly embedded in the rights and responsibilities of the community care agency when new staff are recruited, and when new patients are admitted.

Take the time to reflect on this scenario and consider other options to manage this moral challenge and how it can be prevented in the future.

CASE SCENARIO 2.1A

RELEVANCE TO MY STORY

Utilitarians would certainly be concerned with the short- and long-term consequences of whatever choice I make. If the choice was to allow the wife to be present, the discomfort of team members might distract them from their resuscitation efforts. Such distractions might affect the outcome. If the patient

dies, the wife might feel guilty about interfering, or be angry at the team members, blaming them for not doing enough. The experience may create moral conflict for the team and risk moral distress. Utilitarians would consider the negative consequences of refusing the wife's request. These might include the potential detrimental effect on her short- and

CASE SCENARIO 2.1A *(Continued)*

long-term grieving process, having been denied the opportunity to be with her husband when he died. Perhaps she might take legal action. Even if futile, this action could cause emotional and financial distress for all involved. Utilitarians would also consider the impact this would have on other family members.

However, if her request is granted, perhaps as she promised, she would just sit quietly with her husband and pay no attention to the actions of the team. Perhaps her presence would positively influence the outcome, and resuscitation efforts would be successful. If not, then at least being with her husband when he died might help her through the grieving process.

I might be tempted to honour the wife's request, but as a novice nurse, I was concerned about the consequences if I were to override the wishes of the team. In not following the rules, I might face discipline and disdain from other team members. However, if the family brought their concerns forward to the hospital, I might experience additional distress and guilt for not honouring this request.

These are the types of outcomes a utilitarian would consider. Using the theory, discuss the case in more detail and consider other potential options and outcomes. Would this theory help if you were me?

Deontological Theory

In deontological theory, duties and obligations guide decisions about what is right or wrong, the foundation of which are unchanging or absolute principles derived from universally shared values. Contrary to teleological theory, including utilitarianism, deontologists believe that standards for moral behaviour exist independently of means or ends (Beauchamp & Walters, 2003; Donaldson, 2017). Consequences, they argue, are irrelevant to moral evaluation. An action is right if it satisfies the demands of an overriding principle or principles of duty. Deontologists argue that our duties to each other are complex and vary according to our relationships within society; for example, consider the duties and obligations of a parent to a child or the responsibilities of physicians and nurses to patients (Beauchamp & Walters, 2003; Freeman, 1994; Jameton, 1984; O'Neill, 2013).

Deontological theories identify the foundation of moral standards to make clear the duties and obligations required of moral agents (persons). There are various deontological perspectives on the foundation of duty—for example, the will of God, reason, intuition, universality, or the social contract (Beauchamp & Walters, 2003).

As with utilitarianism, there are two types of deontological theory: act and rule. The *act deontologist* believes that an individual in any situation should grasp immediately what ought to be done without

the need to rely on rules. Act deontologists emphasize the particular and changing features of the moral experience and value the intuitive response to situations or circumstances (Beauchamp & Walters, 2003).

Rule deontologists promote that acts are right or wrong relative to their alignment to one or more principles or rules (Beauchamp & Walters, 2003). There are two types of rule deontologists: pluralistic deontologists, who believe that there are many principles that guide moral conduct, and monistic deontologists, who hold that there is one fundamental principle that provides the foundation from which other more specific moral rules can be derived—one such example being the golden rule, described earlier in this chapter (Beauchamp & Walters, 2003).

Rule deontologists argue that rules facilitate decision making and suggest that act theories present problems for cooperation and trust and reduce morality to "rules of thumb." Moral rules, they say, should be binding (Beauchamp & Walters, 2003).

As noted earlier, philosopher Immanuel Kant formulated the best-known rule-oriented deontological theory.

Kantian Ethics

Central to Kant's philosophy is the notion that morality is based on a fundamental rule or imperative, from which all moral duties and obligations derive. He called this the *categorical imperative,* which he set out in his book *Groundwork of the Metaphysics of Morals* (Kant, 2007; O'Neill, 2013). The categorical imperative denotes an absolute rule or requirement for behaviour that exists in all circumstances.

Kant believed that the uniqueness of humans, and their ability to reason, provides the foundation of morality. He asserted that the rational person should not need guidance in determining right from wrong, and that what is right should be clear to every decent human being (Grassian, 1992). In addition, he offered that as a function of their humanness, persons have the capacity to act autonomously and, hence, should be treated with respect and dignity. The challenge, he believed, is for people to maintain the self-control to do what is right (Eaton, 2004; Grassian, 1992).

Kant rejected the utilitarian notion that the maximization of human desires, such as happiness, was the basis for morality. People, he said, do not derive their dignity or worth from the pursuit of pleasure. Morality, he insisted, must be based on the values derived from rationality and freedom. He argued that one could not be acting morally while justifying one's actions by an appeal to human desires (Grassian, 1992; Wood, 2008). Furthermore, a focus on the principle of utility, he believed, would lead to grave injustices because there was no assurance that the distribution of perceived good outcomes would be fair. Hence, Kant placed great emphasis on justice and individual liberty (Grassian, 1992).

Kant's intent was to establish a comprehensive theory of the nature of morality to explain how morality was both possible and rational. He offered two distinct theories of morality: a theory of moral obligation and a theory of moral value. His theory of moral obligation focused on how persons decide an act is right, whereas the theory of moral value considers the assessment or evaluation of persons moral character (Dean, 2006; Grassian, 1992).

Kant's Theory of Moral Obligation

The theory of moral obligation focuses on how to determine the principles and rules that guide duty. He argued that the foundation for the validity of moral rules was grounded in pure reason, not intuition, conscience, or some notion of utility. Therefore, a theory of morality should offer a rational and universal

framework of principles and moral rules that guide everyone, regardless of other personal goals and self-interests (Beauchamp & Walters, 2003; Zinkin, 2006).

He reasoned that the moral worth of an individual's action depends only on the moral acceptability of the general principle that guides that act. He added that a person's act has moral worth only when performed with the intention of goodwill and in accordance with universally valid moral principles (Beauchamp & Walters, 2003; Wood, 2008). These valid moral and ethical principles, he suggested, are based on an abstract, *a priori* (based on deduction and logic versus observation) foundation that is independent of empirical (observation or experience) reality. Therefore, morality is objectively and universally binding; it is absolute, not flexible. If an act or behaviour is morally right, then it is right in all circumstances and is not dependent on the outcome or consequences of that act (Albert et al., 1975). For example, if telling the truth is morally correct, then one must always tell the truth, regardless of the context of the situation or the consequences (Box 2.2).

Kant believed that we are able to isolate these a priori, or absolute, elements that ground morality through reasoning and that the universal basis of morality lies in an individual's rational nature (Albert et al., 1975). He offered the one supreme principle that

---

BOX 2.2
KANT AND TRUTH: NO EXCEPTIONS

Kant famously offered an example to clarify and support his argument that one should always tell the truth, even when by lying, one hopes to achieve a better outcome. He describes the homeowner, who lies to a potential murderer, denying that the intended victim is hiding there. Kant argues that, because we cannot predict the consequences of that lie, then the lie might indeed result in more harm. For example, if the presence of the potential victim is revealed in some manner, then both the potential victim and the homeowner might be murdered. Kant would say that one ought not to commit the known wrong action, telling a lie, to avoid a potential wrong. If there are harmful consequences, one cannot be held responsible for those consequences, having acted out of the duty to tell the truth. If the duty to tell the truth was ignored, and the person was murdered anyway, then the homeowner could be considered blameworthy. What, if by telling the truth, the home-owner was able to negotiate a resolution to the conflict (Eaton, 2004)?

a law of morality must follow: the **categorical imperative**. This principle is categorical in that Kant admits to no exceptions to the rule (or maxim) that is absolutely binding, and it is imperative in that it gives instructions about how one must act (Albert et al., 1975; O'Neill, 2013; Wood, 2008). According to Kant, a maxim is a personal rule or a general principle that supports a particular action, a rule that tells us what to do in different circumstances. A stated maxim includes the action, and the purpose and specific circumstances under which the action is taken (Kranak, 2022).

Kant set out some guidelines for determining the maxims that guide conduct based on the categorical imperative. Kant characterized the categorical imperative, or moral law, in two significant formulations.

I *I am never to act otherwise than so that I could also will that my maxim should become a universal law. We must be able to will that the maxim of our action should become a universal law. . . . Since you would not want others to behave in the way you propose to behave, you should not behave in that way. (Albert et al., 1975)*

In this first formulation, Kant is asking whether the maxim of the chosen action could be universalized such that all rational beings would be morally justified in taking the same action in similar circumstances. For example, *to ensure my patients are pain-free, when they are prescribed, I will administer pain medications in a timely manner.* This general principle provides guidance by telling a nurse what to do to avoid a patient's pain. If the attempt to universalize the maxim were to result in a contradiction (that is, it would not be appropriate in all circumstances, such as an occasion when it would be inappropriate to administer pain medication in a timely way), such inconsistencies would dictate that the maxim in question cannot be universalized. If the maxim cannot be universalized, then one ought not to commit the action (IEP, n.d.). In this formulation, Kant is suggesting that we must determine the implications of universalizing the rules that guide our actions. For example, would we be able to establish a rule that lying is morally correct? What would happen if everyone lied? Who would we be able to trust? If it were universally acceptable to lie, then no

one would believe anyone, contradicting, then, the assumption of truth. Could we establish a rule that only health care teams can decide on treatment options for patients? What would a society be like if health care professionals made all the decisions about people's health care? A rule must undergo such scrutiny. According to Kant, if it can be applied universally, then it is what we "ought" to do. If not, it is morally wrong.

II *So act as to treat humanity whether in thine own person or in that of any other, in every case as an end withal, never as means only. (Albert et al., 1975)*

In this second formulation of the categorical imperative, Kant is calling on human beings to treat themselves and others as ends and not as means to some other end. Since the existence of humanity has in itself absolute worth, then all human beings are deserving of respect (Grassian, 1992). For example, lying to another person out of self-interest or for personal gain is treating that person as a means to one's own end. Kant argues that all rational beings are capable of displaying a "goodwill," which he claims is the only thing in the universe that has intrinsic value, and since a goodwill can only be found in rational beings, then human beings should always be treated with dignity and respect. Therefore, the principle declares that persons are valuable in and of themselves (they are ends in themselves) and are never merely a means to some other end (All Answers Ltd, 2018; Kant, 2007).

This formulation of the categorical imperative can be applied to the earlier example about truth telling. Kant would also argue that we have a further duty to tell the truth because persons ought to be respected and not used as a means to some other desired end (e.g., keeping the truth from someone to protect our own interests). Even if lying were to produce some desired outcome for the person being lied to, the act would still be disrespectful. Kant did not say that we, as persons, would never be used as a means—for example, for some instrumental good. But if we are used as an instrument toward some other good, we must also be regarded as ends in ourselves. Hence, for example, the notion of informed consent: Kant would probably agree that it is morally acceptable to use persons for research or organ donation, but only if the right to self-determination, through consent, is respected.

To summarize, according to Kant, a maxim is a fundamental moral rule or general principle that guides our action—a rule that tells us what to do in different circumstances. It is an objective moral law grounded in pure, practical reasoning, on which all purely rational moral agents in asserting their humanity would act. Kant identifies rational thought as the unique characteristic of humans, and this characteristic thereby accords them an inherent dignity and worth. Therefore, persons, by virtue of being human, are compelled to follow this universal law—the categorical imperative. By not doing so, they would deny the intrinsic value of their humanness (IEP, n.d.).

KANT'S THEORY OF MORAL VALUE. Kant's theory of moral value questioned how we determine the moral character of a person. According to Kant, it is insufficient to look only at actions and the consequences of those actions without also looking at the person's motives and intentions. Actions alone do not give the complete picture of a person's moral character, because a bad person may do the right thing for the wrong reasons. The only moral motive, a sign of good character, is the motive of conscientiousness (acting out of duty) (Grassian, 1992). For example, a person with goodwill will tell the truth because of the duty to tell the truth, regardless of the consequences (O'Neill, 2013; Wood, 2008).

Fundamental to Kant's theory of moral value is the notion of freedom and rationality. As discussed, Kant viewed persons as rational, moral agents who have the right to make their own choices unless those choices interfere with the freedom of others. He believed that morality presupposed the existence of free will and that persons have the choice to act from goodwill or not (Grassian, 1992; Zinkin, 2006).

Kant placed great emphasis on the fulfillment of duty for its own sake. Although it is possible to engage in right actions for many reasons—for example, fear or self-interest—Kant considered such actions morally praiseworthy only if performed out of duty (Grassian, 1992). Thus, to be moral, persons must demonstrate goodwill or good intention by doing what they ought to do, rather than acting from inclination or self-interest (Albert et al., 1975). If an act and one's motivation to do that act is right, then it is intrinsically good; that is, it is good in and of itself. If an act is intrinsically good, then it has moral value (Albert et al., 1975).

Some actions based on inclination or self-interest may be worthy of praise; they may also happen to be in accordance with duty. However, these actions would not have the same "moral" value (Albert et al., 1975). For example, a rich benefactor may donate millions of dollars to a health care facility to have the facility named in their honour. This act might be praiseworthy, but not in accordance with duty, so it would not have the same moral value. Kant would likely agree that a recently unemployed individual who continues to contribute weekly to a charity would be acting out of a sense of duty, and hence this action would have greater moral worth or value than that of the rich benefactor. Actions with true moral worth, when they are evaluated, stand alone, independent of other motives. An act performed out of duty has moral worth because of the principle guiding that act; the worth does not spring from the act's results or outcomes.

In summary, Kant emphasized duty in accordance with moral law, the essential characteristic of which is universality, as the prominent feature of moral consciousness (Albert et al., 1975).

CASE SCENARIO 2.4

LOYALTY AND COMMITMENTS

A nurse in the emergency department of an acute care hospital was invited to accompany a new friend to a wedding being held the following evening. This would be a great opportunity to meet new friends, and though looking forward to going, this nurse was scheduled to work. Even though it was last minute, the nurse asked the unit manager if the schedule could be changed. The manager responded that this was not possible and that the nurse would have to find a colleague who would be willing to make a schedule change. This attempt failed, and frustrated that no one offered help, the nurse decided to call in sick.

CASE SCENARIO 2.4 *(Continued)*

Interpretation

A deontologist, such as Kant, would invite the nurse to consider whether the maxim of this action, calling in sick to go to a wedding, would state: *Whenever I need a day off to attend an event, I shall deceitfully call in sick as the easiest way to ensure I have the needed time off.* To universalize this maxim, one would need to consider a future where all nurses would routinely act on this same maxim whenever they found themselves in relatively similar circumstances.

The nurse would likely come to realize that this maxim could not be universalized since it would result in a contradiction. For, if such an action were to become a routine practice by all nurses in relatively similar circumstances, then the leaders in these settings would soon realize that nurses are routinely lying to ensure they have the time off, rather than going through more acceptable processes. This would compromise the trust between leaders and staff, and even nurses who were legitimately sick would be suspect. Also, if this became a universal practice, then there would be risks to patient care, a greater workload for the remaining staff, and general disharmony within the workplace. So, because a contradiction results from the attempt to universalize this rule, it cannot be made universal, and the nurse ought not to call in sick.

Consider this story in more detail and further evaluate the action of the manager in not trying to accommodate this request.

CRITICISM OF KANT'S THEORY. There are several criticisms of Kant's theory, particularly in relation to its application in everyday practice. For example, how is duty to be determined when two or more duties are in conflict? What happens if, to protect someone from harm, one must lie or withhold the truth? Kant's view on lying was discussed earlier. However, consider a situation where a nurse, working in a shelter and obligated to protect women from intimate partner violence, encounters the husband of one of the residents who arrives asking about her whereabouts. In this scenario, the nurse would seem to have duties to not only tell the truth, but also respect the resident's confidentiality and prevent emotional and physical harm. Kant's theory demands that all relevant duties be fulfilled. Kant did not provide a means to deal with this type of situation; he indicated only that persons must be true to their duties and moral obligations (Beauchamp & Walters, 2003; O'Neill, 2013; Wood, 2008).

Critics also argue that the categorical imperative is ultimately reduced to a determination of consequences. That is, by evaluating the universal application of an action, one is actually looking at the overall consequences of that act. If the universal performance of a certain type of action is undesirable overall, then it is wrong (Beauchamp & Walters, 2003). In response, Kantians argue that consequences are not totally disregarded, but the features of making something right are not dependent on any outcome alone (Beauchamp & Walters, 2003).

The Deontology of W. D. Ross

W. D. Ross (1877–1971), a British philosopher of the early twentieth century, developed a pluralistic, rule-oriented deontological theory that attempts to resolve the problem of conflict of duties. Ross introduced the notion of **prima facie duties**, those duties that one must always act on unless they conflict with or are overridden by those of equal or stronger obligation (Beauchamp & Walters, 2003; Ross & Stratton-Lake, 2002). The higher duty is determined by an examination of the respective weights of the competing prima facie duties. Ross accepts that prima facie duties are not absolute because they can be overridden. Instead, he argues that they have greater moral significance than mere rules of thumb (Beauchamp & Walters, 2003).

Ross argued that when one is faced with a number of alternatives, the "right" choice or action is the one consistent with all the rules. If a number of alternatives are consistent with the rules, then the choice is one of preference. When each choice is consistent with one rule but in conflict with another, then one attempts to appeal to the higher rule to resolve the conflict. For example, sanctity of life would have priority over the rule of veracity or truth telling. In the situation described above, when one weights the competing duties, the likely conclusion is that the higher-level duty of the nurse would be to protect the resident from harm.

In response to criticisms that it is not always possible to evaluate the respective weights of principles in conflict, Ross reduced his argument to a claim that no moral system is free of conflicts and exceptions (Beauchamp & Walters, 2003; Ross & Stratton-Lake, 2002).

Would a deontological approach assist the nurse in My Story (Case Scenario 2.1) in making the right choice? How? What ethical duties and obligations apply to this scenario? Which ones have greater priority?

Contemporary Theories and Approaches to Morality

Ethical Principles: Principlism

Principle-based ethics is an applied approach frequently used in health care to resolve ethical conflicts and is based on the analysis, balancing, and prioritizing of moral principles derived from moral theory. Presumed to be reflective of commonly held religious and cultural values, prima facie (binding unless in conflict with another) ethical principles serve as rules that guide moral conduct and choices (Beauchamp & Walters, 2003).

Ethical principles provide a framework for ethical decision making and are expressed in many professional codes of ethics, which are discussed in Chapter 3.

This principle-based approach has dominated health care ethics since 1979 (Beauchamp & Childress, 1979; Donaldson, 2017; Engelhardt, 1986; Veatch, 1981), when it was proposed as a framework for ethical reasoning by Beauchamp and Childress in *Principles of Biomedical Ethics,* which has since undergone a number of revisions (see Beauchamp & Childress, 2013). They offered four main principles as most relevant in health care: (1) autonomy—free will or agency, respect for persons; (2) nonmaleficence—prevention or avoidance of harm; (3) beneficence—to do good, taking positive action for the advantage of another; and (4) justice—fairness, social distribution of benefits and burdens.

Beauchamp and Childress asserted that these principles are grounded in a common morality and are relevant to the ethical challenges experienced in health care. They also maintained that the best moral decisions are made when all of these principles align in support of a particular moral position or decision (Beauchamp & Childress, 2001; McCarthy, 2002).

Promoters of principlism argue that from the beginning of recorded history, most moral decision-makers descriptively and prescriptively have considered these four moral principles, arguing that they are integral or compatible with most intellectual, religious, and cultural values and beliefs (DeMarco, 2005).

The ideal alignment of all of these principles in choosing the most ethical option is not always possible.

CASE SCENARIO 2.1B

RELEVANCE TO MY STORY

From a deontological perspective, I have a duty to honour the wishes of my patient and to ensure the well-being of both he and his wife. I also have an an obligation to respect the rights of my team members, who expressed their concern that the presence of the patient's wife might compromise the resuscitation efforts. Is it possible for me to use the categorical imperative to identify the maxim that would guide my action in this situation? Are we able to establish a maxim or rule that can be generalized to similar situations? Is it

possible to establish a universal law that families may choose to be present during emergency interventions whenever they wish? At the same time, can we establish that it is always the health care team that decides who may and may not be present? How would we want to be treated if we were the family member? Is there an option where all obligations can be upheld?

Continue to reflect on this situation from a deontologist's perspective. How does this theory assist your thinking in this case relative to teleological or utilitarian ethical theory?

CASE SCENARIO 2.5

CONFLICTING OBLIGATIONS: MAKING THE RIGHT DECISION

Consider the scenario in which a community patient reveals to a nurse that he frequently fantasizes about children. He states he has never acted on these fantasies and certainly has never been convicted of an offence. Recently, the nurse has heard that the patient just started employment as a janitor in one of the local primary schools. Clearly, this nurse is facing two principles in opposition to each other.

The principle of autonomy, respect for persons, also means granting individuals the right to privacy and confidentiality, especially in the context of the nurse–patient relationship. The principle of nonmaleficence would impose on the nurse the duty to protect children from potential harm. Moral reflection and deliberation would assist this nurse in deciding the best course of action based on the principle that has the most weight in this circumstance—nonmaleficence, that is, protecting children from harm.

However, ethical principles are considered prima facie (discussed earlier relative to Ross's theory); that is, their application may be relative to another principle that may have more weight or priority in a given situation. Therefore, in the course of moral deliberation, engaging in a process of reflection is encouraged so that each principle can be considered, balanced, and evaluated within the context of the specific circumstance.

Some may consider particular principles or values to be a priori (or binding), as are Kant's categorical imperatives. For example, some people advocate sanctity of life in all forms and at all costs, while others believe that autonomy and quality of life may override sanctity of life in some circumstances. The processes of moral deliberation involve the setting up of options that are evaluated, modified, or rejected on the basis of reasoning and experience. Although it is the ideal, it may not always be possible in complex situations to achieve consistency and unity with all the principles applicable to the situation (McCarthy, 2002).

Autonomy

The principle of **autonomy** (*autos,* from Greek meaning "self"; *nomos,* from Greek meaning "rule") asserts that a capable and competent individual is free to determine, and to act in accordance with, a self-chosen plan (Beauchamp & Childress, 2013). Autonomy, founded on respect for persons, is based on the notion that human beings have worth and moral dignity. To respect persons is to recognize them, without conditions, as worthy moral agents who should not be

treated as mere means to any other end (Beauchamp & Childress, 2013). Thus, individuals should be able to determine their own destiny (free will or agency) and be allowed to make their own evaluations, choices, and actions, so long as these do not harm or interfere with the liberty or freedom of others (Beauchamp & Walters, 2003). Respect for autonomy also means granting individuals the right to control information that is important to them, hence the right to privacy and confidentiality. Confidentiality is important in the health care environment, since in order to receive the care they need, patients and families must trust health care professionals to protect the privacy of the information they reveal, unless there is a risk to self or others or unless disclosure is required by law.

This principle aligns with Kant's categorical imperative, that individuals be respected as ends in and of themselves and never as means to some other end, which is based on the belief that humanity itself has absolute worth (Beauchamp & Childress, 2013).

The principle of autonomy is also consistent with Mill's utilitarianism, which states that autonomy maximizes the benefits of all concerned and that social and political control over individual action is legitimate only if it is necessary to prevent harm to others (Beauchamp & Childress, 2013).

Autonomy is the foundation of the legal doctrine of **informed consent** (see Chapter 6), which respects individual rights to the information necessary to make health care decisions. Failure to do so limits a person's autonomy and interferes with these rights.

Further, autonomy underscores the duty of respecting a person's values and choices. It assumes the person is competent; has the ability to decide rationally, rather than impulsively; and has the ability to act upon those decisions and choices (Beauchamp & Childress, 2013). Autonomy also assumes voluntariness, which means having the freedom to make choices and to be free of coercion.

To be autonomous, a person must be free of external control and be able to take action to control their own affairs (Beauchamp & Childress, 2013). Even if it is believed that a person's decision is not in their best interests, if acting on them poses no threat of serious harm to others, then the principle of autonomy presumes that their decision be respected. Autonomy may at times conflict with other principles, such as beneficence—for example, when a patient refuses treatment that the nurse and health care team firmly believe is in the patient's best interests. As nurses know, illness puts limits on individual autonomy. As well, the environment in many health care settings, such as hospitals and long-term care facilities, may influence a person's sense of control. For example, consider how the effects of sleep deprivation (a risk in these settings) on cognition may complicate a person's reasoning process. Further, the biases of the health care team may be readily apparent to the patient or substitute decision maker, leading to subtle forms of coercion. Patients may experience anxiety and stress and even be overwhelmed by uncertainty about their future and prognosis. As moral agents, nurses have a duty to support patients and families through this process, ensuring that they have the information and time required to make the decision most appropriate for them.

Some believe autonomy to be the primary moral principle that takes precedence over all other moral considerations (Beauchamp & Childress, 2013). The challenge for health care professionals is to ensure that the people they care for have the ability to act autonomously, that is, that they are making decisions with a full understanding of the facts, issues, and consequences of those choices. Some persons are unable to act autonomously because of immaturity, incapacity, lack of information, or coercion.

Persons with diminished autonomy, who are unable to choose a plan because of controlled deliberations, may be highly dependent on others. Young children and persons with dementia may fall into this category of individuals whose rights may need to be protected by others. However, it is important not to assume that persons with diminished capacity cannot make any decisions on their own behalf. Consider the 15-year-old patient who was diagnosed at age 8 years with leukemia. Having experienced a series of treatments and their complications for some time, this patient would likely understand the consequences of further interventions. Contrast this with a 15-year-old adolescent who has never been in a hospital, is scared, and refuses to undergo surgery for a ruptured appendix. Also, do not assume that people receiving treatment for a mental illness do not have the capacity to make decisions, including advance directive, regarding their care. Persons with dementia may have varying degrees of mental capacity, and this should be appropriately evaluated and understood in the context of the decision to be made.

Another important principle based on autonomy is **veracity**, the duty to tell the truth. Veracity, or truth telling, is central to ensuring and maintaining trust within the nurse–patient relationship and is linked to respect for persons. Patients should expect that nurses will provide honest responses to their questions and communicate truthfully to them about the nature of their condition and the care they receive.

Conflicts associated with the principle of veracity arise when the truth may result in harm. For example, consider a patient who is terminally ill and dying. How should health care professionals respond to questions associated with the outcome of a particular treatment when the likelihood of success may be poor, but they still wish to communicate some sense of hope? How do nurses respond to an agitated patient with advanced dementia, who is worried that their parents don't know where they are and that they must go home? Do the nurses remind them that their parents died years ago and that they now live in a long-term care home? Or, appreciating the patient's short-term memory loss, do the nurses reassure the patient that their parents know where they are and that they will be arriving shortly? Or do the nurses be present in this person's world and encourage a conversation about the important memories the patient shared with their parents?

How and when to communicate bad news is a critical ethical issue, and one cannot appeal to the principle of veracity as justification for revealing difficult news to a patient without considering the timing and manner of communication and the need for follow-up care and support. For example, when the parents are not present but will be returning shortly, is it appropriate for the team to disclose to a 16-year-old the finding of a potentially fatal lung condition and the need for a transplant, even though the rules of age and consent would allow it? (Nicholas & Keatings, n.d.).

Truth telling is fundamental to the establishment and maintenance of trusting relationships. Vital to the relationship between nurses and patients is the nurse's ability to care, to provide comfort, and to maintain honest and truthful communication while continuing to convey a sense of hope and purpose.

FIDELITY. **Fidelity**, or keeping promises, a principle some consider grounded in autonomy, is the foundation of the nurse–patient relationship. It is fundamental to nursing values such as loyalty, caring, honesty, and commitment to those entrusted to their care. When nurses enter the profession, they promise to uphold these values (through their codes of ethics), and to meet their obligations and duties as professionals (Beauchamp & Childress, 2013; Cooper, 1988). Fidelity guides a nurse's commitment to provide quality care, relieve suffering, and provide comfort and support when needed; and to advocate for their patient's best interests. However, this principle is tested when nurses are placed in situations in which being loyal to a patient compromises their own values, such as through involvement in MAiD or abortions. In these circumstances, nurses with different moral or religious beliefs and values may express conscientious objection and make arrangements with their employer to not participate in these interventions. Taking care that any conscientious objection is not communicated to the patient and being careful not to convey personal moral judgements about the beliefs, lifestyle, identity, or characteristics of others, nurses must take all reasonable steps to ensure that the quality and continuity of care for patients are not compromised.

THE INFLUENCE OF PATERNALISTIC OR MATERNALISTIC ATTITUDES. In the past, some health care professionals, behaved in paternalistic ways ("Father or Mother knows best") toward patients in an effort to protect them from the potentially harmful consequences of their choices (Beauchamp, 2010). That is, out of a desire to be beneficent, they have, at times, allowed their

sense of what they perceive to be in their patient's best interests gain ascendancy over other important ethical principles (autonomy, truth telling).

This approach had the potential to restrict the liberty of individuals and was in conflict with the principle of autonomy. Treatment may have been given or withheld without the patient's consent; the justification for such action was either the prevention of some harm or the achievement of some benefit (Beauchamp & Childress, 2001). Some health care professionals went so far as to withhold information from patients with terminal illnesses to protect them from the distress of knowing that their death was imminent. Others would fail to disclose all of the side effects or consequences of major surgery to secure consent. However, it is important to note that some patients may choose to have information withheld from them in certain circumstances and instruct the health care team to do what is in their best interests. Following through with this request would be respecting their autonomy and choice not to know.

Paternalism is considered justified in some societies today in certain situations, and it influences policy in areas that include the following (Jochelson, 2006):

- Involuntary committal to a mental health facility
- The prevention of suicide
- Denial of unusual, untested, and possibly dangerous treatment
- Requirements to use bike helmets and seat belts
- Immunization against disease (Nelson et al., 2012)

Nonmaleficence

The principle of **nonmaleficence** is associated with the Latin maxim *primum non nocere*: "above all (or first), do no harm." This is expressed in many professional codes of ethics and is highlighted in the Hippocratic oath: "I will use treatment to help the sick according to my ability and judgement, but I will never use it to injure or wrong them." This principle obliges members of society to act in such a way as to prevent or remove harm (Beauchamp & Childress, 2013).

In nursing, professional practice standards express the competencies that nurses must meet to ensure the provision of safe patient care. Some actions of nurses may produce temporary harm (e.g., the administration of medication by injection; limited use of restraints; painful procedures, such as application of dressings or insertion of an intravenous line). This temporary harm is justified if it is a means to producing a good outcome, such as relief of pain, treatment for an illness, and when the principle of autonomy is respected through informed consent.

There are four hierarchical elements related to nonmaleficence based on a priority of obligations (Beauchamp & Childress, 2013). The first three represent adherence to the principle of nonmaleficence, whereas the fourth, the highest standard, relates to the principle of beneficence, described next:

"1. One ought not to inflict evil or harm (what is bad).
2. One ought to prevent evil or harm.
3. One ought to remove evil or harm.
4. One ought to do or promote good." (Frankena
   (1973), p. 47)

Beneficence

The principle of **beneficence** sets a higher standard than nonmaleficence as it requires that one take positive action for the good or benefit for another. It asserts an obligation to assist those in need (Beauchamp & Childress, 2013). Many argue that though the ideal is to be beneficent, we are not morally obliged to meet this standard. In the common law tradition (the Canadian legal system is discussed in Chapter 4), a distinction is drawn between misfeasance and nonfeasance. The term **misfeasance** is used in the sense of active misconduct that causes injury to another, and **nonfeasance** refers to not taking positive steps to help a person. Liability cannot be imposed for inaction, such as a failure to rescue, because in Canadian law (except in Quebec) there is no general legal obligation to help others. Criminal liability in Canada requires a guilty intent, and inaction is not easily brought within this concept. Indeed, the law in Canada, except in Quebec, does not require us to assist others, even in emergencies (Linden, 2016; Linden et al., 2016; Mandhane, 2000). This differs from "good Samaritan" laws in force in some European countries (e.g., Italy, Poland, France, and Denmark). In France, individuals can face criminal charges for failing to help in emergencies; in Quebec, a person who fails to render assistance can be sued by the injured person for such failure (*Gaudreault v. Drapeau*, 1987).

However, health care professionals have a higher duty to act in such a manner that not only protects patients from harm but also produces some good or benefit. Their commitment as professionals is to honour the principle of beneficence. This is fundamental to nursing's professional duties and obligations, as is discussed in Chapters 3 and 5.

At times, the principle of beneficence may conflict with that of autonomy—for example, when a particular intervention is likely to benefit a patient and yet the patient refuses to provide consent. This is often a source of distress for health care professionals. However, making sure that patients are provided with the information, support, and time to make decisions ensures their best interests.

Justice

The principle of **justice** is derived from values such as fairness and equity. Theories of justice focus on how individuals and groups are treated within a society, the distribution of benefits (e.g., health care) and burdens (e.g., taxes) in an equitable way, procedural justice such as fairness in legal proceedings, and compensation for those who have been unfairly burdened or harmed. In health care, justice is fundamental to the allocation of resources and rationing in times of scarcity or diminishing resources. Procedural justice is discussed in Chapter 4. Two forms of justice relevant to health care, distributive justice and compensatory justice, are discussed in the following sections.

DISTRIBUTIVE JUSTICE. **Distributive justice** is the proper distribution of both social benefits and burdens across society (Beauchamp & Childress, 2013). Decisions regarding the equitable distribution of resources may be based on one of several considerations (Beauchamp & Childress, 2013):

To each person:

- An equal share
- According to individual need
- According to that person's rights
- According to individual effort
- According to societal contribution
- According to merit

Determining how to distribute resources equitably is a challenge when resources are scarce, as they increasingly are in health care. Nurses, especially those in leadership roles, participate in discussions and decision-making processes about how financial resources are distributed, which programs are funded, how staff is allocated, how patient assignments are organized, who gets the rare organ for transplantation, and many others. Restructuring in many Canadian health care organizations, both in the hospital and community, has led to the introduction of different models of care that include various levels or categories of care providers. These models add a new dimension to resource allocation from a nursing perspective in that there is a further requirement to evaluate the care needs of patients and to determine the type of provider authorized and competent to provide that care.

Rationing is a method of allocating scarce resources to those who will benefit the most. A well-known example of rationing in health care is in the area of organ donation. Even if Canada's federal and provincial governments have provided all the health care dollars necessary to perform all the transplantations needed, donor organs may be scarce. Thus, transplantation programs must determine how the limited resources will be distributed. Should an organ be given to the person who has waited the longest, to the person with the best chance for survival, to the sickest, to the one with the greatest need, or to the person who "deserves" it the most (e.g., the person who has never consumed alcohol needing a liver transplant, or the one who has never smoked needing a lung transplant)?

Macro-decisions on resource allocation are made at the policy level. Administrators or legislators decide which programs will be funded—for example, whether to increase the number of cardiac surgical procedures performed annually, whether an investment in prevention programs should be made, or whether safe injections sites should be established in the community. Nurses face micro-decisions on resource allocation daily. For example, they decide which patient out of many in pain receives pain medication first, how much home care is provided to a dying patient, and how nursing time is allocated among the eight community patients to be visited that day.

If there is a limit on a particular resource, theories of justice are applied to determine how this scarce resource is allocated. For example, frequent challenges occur when there are global shortages of specific

drugs or agents, such as isotopes, and both macro- and micro-level processes must occur to ensure that the limited resources are provided to those in most need. At the macro-level, policies must be established to determine how these drugs are allocated across health care facilities. At the micro-level, facilities need to put processes in place for triage, which determines which patients or procedures are a priority. For example, how does one determine priorities if there is a shortage of lidocaine hydrochloride, a local anaesthetic agent that is used across the system in hospitals, community clinics, and dental offices (Bodie et al., 2018)? Is the product proportionally distributed across all of these organizations? Is distribution based on patient need and case priority? Is the drug only to be used in emergency contexts? Should elective treatments or surgeries be cancelled?

The Canadian government, in response to the COVID-19 pandemic, faced resource allocation challenges, including the distribution of personal protective equipment and vaccines. In response, resource allocation guidelines and frameworks were developed to support a consistent approach to ethical deliberation and decision making.

Early in the pandemic, the potential for rationing care of specialized equipment, such as ventilators and critical care beds, was identified. In anticipation of such situations where life-saving technology and human resources could become scarce, triage models were created to guide health care facilities and health care professionals to prepare for such an eventuality.

The document "COVID-19 Pandemic Guidance for the Health Care Sector" offered guidance to health care professionals to ensure fair and transparent resource-allocation decision making, giving some assurance to the public. Four key questions were identified to guide these decisions (Government of Canada, 2020):

1. Who is entitled to a given resource?
2. On what grounds ought one person to have priority over another?
3. How should priority-setting decisions be made?
4. Who should make them?

In the document "Public Health Ethics Framework: A Guide for Use in Response to the COVID-19 Pandemic in Canada," the focus was on ethical deliberation and decision-making in the development of policy related to areas such as vaccine distribution, curtailment of individual freedom, and other related issues. The ethical considerations proposed in this framework were offered to "help decision makers identify competing values and interests, weigh relevant considerations, identify options and make well-considered and justifiable decisions" (Government of Canada, 2021b, p. 1). The framework was guided by five values and principles that align with the four main principles proposed by Beauchamp and Childress (2013):

1. Trust (autonomy)
2. Justice (justice)
3. Respect for persons, communities and human rights (autonomy and justice)
4. Promoting well-being (beneficence)
5. Minimizing harm (nonmaleficence) (Government of Canada, 2021b)

COMPENSATORY JUSTICE. **Compensatory justice** requires compensation or payment for harm that has been done to an individual or a group. Compensation may be provided to individuals or groups because of negligence or malpractice (discussed in Chapter 7). For example, federal and provincial governments compensated victims who contracted human immunodeficiency virus (HIV) infection and hepatitis C through transfusions of tainted blood. Also, because the drug had been approved for use, children born with birth defects as a result of their mothers taking the drug thalidomide received multiple rounds of compensation from the federal government. Compensation is sometimes paid when people have suffered, even when there is no clear misconduct. For example, people, including medical personnel, who were quarantined because of the severe acute respiratory syndrome (SARS) outbreak were compensated by the Government of Ontario for lost wages.

In response to the Canadian Human Rights Tribunal's finding that Child and Family Services discriminated against First Nations children by underfunding child services on reserves (requiring their removal from their homes to access services), the Government of Canada agreed to provide compensation. Funding was allocated to both reform the First Nations Child and Family Services program and to compensate the individual children affected (Government of Canada, 2022a).

Criticism of Principlism

Though the initial intent of the principled approach offered by Beauchamp and Childress was to guide moral decision-making, some argue that the unique challenges and complexities in health care limit it as a stand-alone framework. One criticism is that, on occasion, one or more of the principles come into conflict with each other, which restricts their ability to provide guidance on the nuanced and unique moral situations in health care. Of concern to critics, is that this approach can be reduced to a mere checklist of ethical considerations and that the principles are not seen as equal in terms of value. Of note is the superiority placed on autonomy (Agledahl et al., 2011), given the extent it may be misinterpreted or seen as an easy solution to a dilemma (Walker, 2009). The priority given to autonomy, some suggest, has the risk of compromising patient care because attention to the other moral obligations is diminished, limiting options available to navigate nuanced ethical situations. If autonomy is perceived to have the greatest value, then principles such as non-maleficence and beneficence are viewed to have less significant than that of the will of the patient, risking negative outcomes where the patient is ill-informed, lacks a full understanding of the issues, or is influenced by their emotional state and/or physical distress (Fiester, 2007). A focus on principlism alone is limited without simultaneously addressing the uniqueness of each situation and the moral foundation of the relationships between the patient and the health care provider (Walker, 2009).

CASE SCENARIO 2.6

PROMISE KEEPING

R. J., a nurse who works in a general medical unit, is considered by their patients and colleagues to be a compassionate role model. During the COVID-19 pandemic, R. J. struggled with the restrictions that limited family presence, especially for the more vulnerable patients and those nearing end of life. In response, R. J. tried to spend as much time as possible with them, being present and using the technology available to help them communicate with their families. One such patient, M., had been admitted weeks earlier with chronic liver disease. Because their

CASE SCENARIO 2.6 *(Continued)*

husband (Z.) wasn't able to visit, R. J. ensured that the couple were able to chat through Zoom on a regular basis. As R. J. developed a therapeutic relationship with Z., also over Zoom, R. J. promised him that M. would receive the best care possible and committed to keeping Z. up-to-date with M.'s progress. One morning, M. suddenly deteriorated and, afraid to be dying, M. begged to see their Z. In this context, close family members were permitted to be present, and, as promised, R. J. contacted Z. right away to inform them of M.'s change of status and suggested that Z. come right away. R. J. had a busy assignment but was able to reorganize priorities and committed to staying with M. until the husband arrived. Soon after, an emergency situation occurred with another patient; a previously stable patient was experiencing shortness of breath and severe chest pain. Now faced with a serious ethical dilemma, R. J. was torn between the promise to M. and the obligation to this other patient. This presented a conflict between the principles of fidelity (promise keeping) and beneficence. Though principlism would suggest that the principle of beneficence, given the emergency situation, would have priority in this situation, R. J. struggled, knowing this was abandoning the promise and commitment to M. and their husband, Z.

Interpretation

Sadly, this moral situation is not uncommon in nursing. When experienced on a regular basis and when not addressed appropriately, it can lead to moral distress. This story highlights the ethical nuances in care that nurses face, and how, at times, principles and theories, though they may help guide decisions, don't always resolve the moral conflicts and moral residue experienced by nurses.

In Chapter 12, the moral issues associated with leadership and organizations are discussed. The chapter also demonstrates how moral leadership and ethical systems help in preventing this conflict and ensuring that both the principles of beneficence and fidelity can be upheld. For example: An organizational standard demonstrating a commitment to supporting persons at end of life, including ensuring family or staff presence, would require that systems are in place to reallocate resources in these situations. If possible, the charge nurse, knowing this is a priority, could reorganize the assignment to allow R. J. to stay with M. while another nurse responded to the emergency. For situations where this is not possible, this could mean having an organizational commitment to a system or process where other volunteers or staff are made available to help.

CASE SCENARIO 2.1C

RELEVANCE TO MY STORY

Several ethical principles are relevant to My Story. The principle of autonomy would suggest that it is the patient's right to decide who may or may not be present at any time. In my situation, however, the patient was not capable of making such a decision. One would assume, however, that his wife as his substitute decision maker could represent his wishes and values and make this decision on his behalf. Adherence to the principle of beneficence, which requires that health care professionals act to benefit others, might also require that I allow the wife to be with her husband for their mutual comfort. Also, if he were to die, the experience of being pres-

ent at the time of his death might help with her grieving. But based on the principle of nonmaleficence, the team might argue that there is the possibility of harm to both the patient (if the team is distracted) and the wife (if she becomes upset by the resuscitation process). Beyond this situation, the principle of justice would require that the hospital review its policy to ensure fairness to all patients and families.

Continue the discussion in light of these principles, and compare their relevance with that of previous theories. Discuss, too, the value of a policy or guideline regarding family presence during emergencies.

Social Justice

Theories of social justice address the equitable and fair distribution of resources, opportunities, and privileges within a society. This political and philosophical theory focuses on the concept of fairness and equal access to wealth, opportunities, and social privileges. Attention to social justice first emerged in the nineteenth century, when wide disparities in wealth and social standing perpetuated through the social structure of the era. The main principles of social justice are summarized in Table 2.3.

Social justice holds that those most advantaged in society have a particular responsibility to meet the needs of those who are least advantaged. John Rawls, an important political philosopher in the twentieth century, proposed a theory of justice focused on fairness and provided a framework for a society characterized by:

- Free and equal persons
- Political and personal liberties and equal opportunity
- Cooperative arrangements that benefit all citizens, including disadvantaged members such as the poor and marginalized.

Rawls offers two important principles of social justice: (1) the Equal Liberty Principle, that is, all persons have the right to basic liberty; and (2) the Principle of Equal Opportunity, that is, all persons have fair and equal opportunity, with greater benefits provided to the least advantaged (Rawls, 1996).

In his work *A Theory of Justice* (1971), Rawls argued that principles of justice should guide citizens within a society and contended that individuals and groups within a society have intrinsic values, aspirations, and goals that are based on such fairness. He also put forth the difference principle, which requires that social and economic inequalities be addressed to ensure the greatest benefits are given to the least advantaged. He offered that inequalities be arranged to benefit the least advantaged members of society. This reasoning supports affirmative action strategies intended to compensate marginalized members of society who should not be disadvantaged by arbitrary factors such as wealth and position in society. For example, a student from a wealthy family is more likely to be better prepared to do well on an entry exam compared with a student from a poorer family who may not have access to the same preparatory resources ("What Is Rawls's Difference Principle?" 2021).

Furthermore, he reasoned that mutually agreed upon principles of justice are achieved through collaboration and cooperation to ensure that one person or group is not more privileged than another. For example, principles of social justice guide policies and approaches to the acceptance of refugees and asylum seekers who are seen as disadvantaged compared with many in Canadian society. Also, decisions made by the National Advisory Committee on Immunization (NACI) regarding the allocation of vaccines during the COVID-19 pandemic gave priority to vulnerable older persons, especially those living in congregate settings, persons at risk with pre-existing illnesses, and Indigenous people. Indigenous people have had historically poor outcomes during previous outbreaks and have a higher risk of dying from preventable illness. The underlying causes are the disadvantages inflicted on them by colonialism and continuing issues associated with poverty, such as inadequate access to clean water, substandard housing, and overcrowded living conditions. Indigenous people are also less likely to access health care services, even when they are available, due to historical experiences with systemic racism in the health care system (Greenwood & MacDonald, 2021). An historical injustice comparable to residential

---

TABLE 2.3
Five Principles of Social Justice

Access	All socioeconomic groups receive equal access to resources.
Equity	Resources are provided based on needs so that all people in society are equal and can achieve the same outcomes.
Participation	All in society are given an opportunity to give voice to their opinions and concerns and are engaged in decisions that affect their livelihood and standard of living.
Diversity	Diversity and cultural differences are valued and considered in the establishment of social policy.
Human rights	It involves accountability and respect for the civil, economic, political, cultural, and legal rights of individuals and groups within society.

Adapted from CFI Education Inc. (2022, March 16). *Social justice.* https://corporatefinanceinstitute.com/resources/esg/social-justice/

schools was the establishment of "Indian hospitals" (1920–1980s). These hospitals, established across the country, had a number of objectives, including the segregation of "Indians" in order to protect white people from infectious diseases such as tuberculosis (ironically, introduced by European settlers). Infectious diseases are more prevalent in Indigenous communities due to inequities in the social determinants of health, such as poverty and living conditions (Geddes, 2017; Indigenous Corporate Training, 2017; Lux, 2016). The injustices associated with these hospitals is discussed in more detail in Chapter 10.

Many other health care experiences of Indigenous people contribute to their distrust in the health care system. Brian Sinclair, an Indigenous man, died in a Winnipeg hospital of complications of a treatable bladder infection after 34 hours without care, while in the waiting room of the emergency department. A number of system factors contributed to his death, including potentially racist assumptions made that he was drunk and sleeping it off or homeless and needing respite from the cold (Brian Sinclair Working Group, 2017). Also, an inquest held in 2021 to review the 2020 death of Joyce Echaquan, an Atikamekw woman, in a hospital north of Montreal found that racism played a role in her preventable death. Assumptions were made that she was experiencing substance withdrawal when this was not the fact. Joyce recorded a Facebook video of herself screaming in distress as health care providers yelled racist and abusive comments at her (Friesen, 2020; Kamel, 2021). Her story is discussed further in Chapter 5.

During the COVID-19 pandemic, concerns related to social justice led the World Health Organization (WHO) to encourage nations to work together and contribute to the international sharing of vaccines as a means of protecting all global citizens and those most disadvantaged (WHO, 2021b).

Views of social justice have shifted toward a stronger emphasis on human rights and improving the lives of those who have historically faced discrimination in society. A commitment to social justice guides strategies to redistribute wealth to the underprivileged by providing them with income, employment, and education support and other opportunities. There is a greater focus on diversity, inclusion, and equity in health care organizations across the country, leading to the development of strategies to address this issue.

Social Justice: The Influence of Nursing

Since Nightingale, nurses have advocated for social justice and equality. Many of her writings encourage nurses to consider the influence of social issues on health and well-being (Selanders & Crane, 2012). The CNA *Code of Ethics* (CNA, 2017), described in Chapter 3, places a strong emphasis on the role of nurses to advocate for strategies that address the societal issues that affect the health and well-being of persons. The code stresses that nurses should "endeavour to maintain an awareness of the aspects of social justice that affect the social determinants of health and well-being and to advocate for improvements" (CNA, 2017, p. 3). It emphasizes the role of nursing in improving systems and societal structures that will create greater equity for all by "individually and collectively" maintaining current awareness of the issues and by being "strong advocates for fair policies and practices" (CNA, 2017, p. 18).

Social justice is an important consideration for nurses in all domains of practice, notably in public health, the community, and isolated settings across the country (Hines-Martin & Nash, 2017). Although the *Canada Health Act* guarantees equity in health care, this is not always achievable. The health of individuals and communities is very much influenced by the social determinants of health and by inequity and disparities across the country (Commission on the Social Determinants of Health, 2008). Many factors, including income, lack of housing, and disability, contribute to these disparities.

Equitable access to health care, or health equity, means that the social and health care structures and processes are in place to ensure access to care for all persons in a fair and timely way. Health equity cannot be achieved without addressing health disparities, historical injustices, prejudices, and the needs of vulnerable populations.

Frequently, nurses who work in the community—in clinics or public health settings—are guided by the social determinants of health, which are key to influencing positive health outcomes and quality of life. Research demonstrates that those less affluent, less educated, and marginalized have a lower life expectancy and are more vulnerable to substance dependencies, food insecurity, violence and abuse, mental health issues, suicide, and homelessness (Acevedo-Garcia, et al., 2014). Nurses are in a strong position to add voice to these issues and, through their leadership, to influence the root causes of these inequities. There are many challenges across Canadian communities related to the social determinants of health and their impact on vulnerable populations, including the homeless, persons from diverse cultural backgrounds, those living in poverty, and Indigenous people.

The COVID-19 pandemic provided living evidence of the influence of the social determinants of health on outcomes. The pandemic revealed the extent of differences across social groups and the impact of these inequities on outcomes such as morbidity and mortality (Marmot et al., 2020; WHO, 2021a). Advocates for social justice and fairness offer that social determinants should guide strategies for future pandemic prevention, preparedness, and response (WHO, 2021a).

Social justice, as articulated in the CNA *Code of Ethics*, is fundamental to the strategies and approach to many issues discussed in this book. These include the rights of Indigenous peoples in Canada, the Two-Spirit, Lesbian, Gay, Bisexual, Transgender, Queer, Intersex, Plus (2SLGBTQI+) community, and the mentally ill, as well as issues related to poverty and frail older persons, and others.

Social Justice in Policy and Legislation

Social justice is a driver of policy and legislation that attempts to address these many challenging issues. For example, this principle is the foundation for government approaches and polices related to welfare, support for the homeless, persons with disabilities, and other related issues.

Jordan's Principle is a *child-first principle* that was unanimously approved by the House of Commons in 2007 and was promoted to ensure that Indigenous children in Canada receive the health care and services they need (Government of Canada, 2022a).

This legal principle honours the memory Jordan River Anderson, a First Nations child from a Cree Nation in Manitoba.

Disputes between governments over such funding for Indigenous children were common. The creation of the child-first principle, in Jordan's name, was to ensure First Nations children could access the services they needed immediately, in advance of any jurisdictional debates regarding funding. The intent was to help the child "now" and sort out the responsibility for funding later. This includes funding for a broad range of services: health, social, and educational needs, including the unique needs of those with disabilities and 2SLGBTQI+ children and youth.

However, in the beginning, the application of this principle was so restrictive that few First Nations children qualified. In 2016, the Canadian Human Rights Tribunal (CHRT), finding these restrictions discriminatory, ordered the government to implement the full scope of the principle; failing to comply after 3 months, the government was met with a noncompliance order. After judicial reviews and appeals, in 2021, the federal court upheld orders by the CHRT regarding eligibility for products and services under Jordan's Principle. In 2022, the government and the parties to two federal court class actions announced agreements-in-principle, which included:

- Compensation for First Nations children on reserves and in the Yukon who were removed from their homes, and those impacted by the government's narrow definition of Jordan's Principle, including their parents and caregivers
- Long-term reform of the First Nations Child and Family Services program and a renewed approach to Jordan's Principle, in order to eliminate

---

CASE SCENARIO 2.7

JORDON'S STORY

Jordan was born with complex medical needs and spent more than 2 years in hospital, waiting to go home, during which time the federal and provincial governments debated jurisdictional issues regarding who should fund the home care he needed. Any other child with similar needs, would have had the care provided immediately through provincial funding. At 5 years of age Jordan died in the hospital still waiting to go home.

discrimination, prevent recurrence, and reform Indigenous Services Canada (Government of Canada, 2023)

The Canadian government, offered that the principle of "substantive equality" guided their decision and actions. This recognized the existing disadvantages and past mistreatment of First Nations in Canada, and that to achieve equity and ensure that First Nations children have opportunities equal to all children in Canada, they required extra assistance when needed (Box 2.3)

Social justice is emerging as a major theme in our society, and in health care. The inequities across the system are becoming more apparent, and this requires that the nursing profession embrace a strong leadership role. Nurses, already strong role models across the system with a focus on the social determinants of health, are in a strong position to add voice to these issues and influence the root causes of these inequities. The values associated with social justice have been embedded in the profession for decades, so nursing is situated to influence and foster a deeper understanding of the social determinants of health in order to ensure the equitable and fair distribution of resources and opportunities in society.

Feminist and Feminine Perspectives on Ethics

Feminine and feminist perspectives on ethics offer alternatives to traditional ethical theories, which place a strong emphasis on rationality and notions of justice. Feminine and feminist approaches challenge those theories as limiting because they were developed by men and are based on male views, standards, biases, and experiences (Baier, 1985). If, as Carol Gilligan's study of moral development demonstrates, the moral development of women differs from that of men, then these approaches may be problematic for women (Gilligan, 1982, 1995a, 1995b; Gilligan and Attanucci, 1996). Gilligan, a feminist, ethicist, and psychologist, challenged the notion that there is one superior way to think about moral problems—that is, in terms of abstract and general notions of duty, justice, and rights. Feminine and feminist thinkers would propose alternative models to guide moral action that have merit in health care, where the challenges involve not only complex situations but also complex human relationships that are further complicated by the milieu of politics and power.

Feminine and feminist theorists resist rationalistic ethics, believing that ethical analysis must make sense and be applicable in the real world (Sherwin, 1992). They offer that there is more to understanding what is right or wrong than just through abstract reasoning: the context of the situation, the nature of the relationships, and the unique interests of all the individuals involved all play a part.

Feminine and feminist theorists argue that traditional theories that search for structured frameworks with a focus on arguments and justifications for morality, and what rules should be followed, may not fit the moral experience and intuitions of many women and therefore fail to address their unique moral perspective (Downie & Sherwin, 2013; Sherwin, 1989, 1992, 1998). The different experiences of women, they argue, are ignored or downplayed in traditional theories, suggesting that reason and justice offer little help, for example, in explaining women's moral duties to children, the ill, or other vulnerable people who have traditionally been cared for by women rather than men.

BOX 2.3
SUBSTANTIVE EQUALITY

Substantive equality is a legal principle that refers to the achievement of true equality in outcomes. It is achieved through equal access, equal opportunity and, most importantly, the provision of services and benefits in a manner and according to standards that meet any unique needs and circumstances, such as cultural, social, economic and historical disadvantage.

First Nations children have experienced historical disadvantage due to Canada's repeated failure to take into account their best interest as well as their historical, geographical and cultural needs and circumstances. For this reason, substantive equality for First Nations children will require that government policies, practices and procedures impacting them take account of their historical, geographical and cultural needs and circumstances and aim to safeguard the best interest of the child as articulated in the United Nations Committee on the Rights of the Child General Comment 11.

Source: From Government of Canada. (2019). Jordan's Principle: Substantive equality principles. What is substantive equality? https://sac-isc.gc.ca/eng/1568396042341/1568396159824#chp02

The term *feminist ethics* refers to a wide range of feminist-related moral issues. The goal of feminist ethics is to create a path, or ideology, that will end the social and political oppression of women. Feminists believe there is a unique female perspective of the world that can be shaped into an important and relevant theory of morality (Reich, 1995). Requisite to an appreciation of feminist ethics is an understanding of how it is grounded in feminist theory.

Feminist Theory

To provide a context for understanding feminine and feminist approaches to ethics, two premises associated with feminist thinking should be understood (L. Shanner, personal communication, March 28, 1995):

- Female and male experiences, bodies, and socialization are not identical.
- Male perspectives are dominant, and female perspectives are often marginalized, muted, or simply unrecognized.

A feminist is described as anyone who acts to give voice to these different female perspectives, attempts to balance or integrate male and female thinking, or promotes feminine views over masculine views. Feminist work considers gender and sex to be important analytical categories and seeks to understand their operation in the world. The major focus is on the effort to change the distribution and use of power and to stop the oppression of women (Wolf, 1996). Although all feminists agree that women have been historically oppressed and that oppression is wrong, various feminists characterize oppression differently and offer different approaches to overcoming it (Cudd & Andreasen, 2005).

Liberal Feminism

This branch of feminism is concerned with the equality of women and the equitable distribution of wealth, position, and power. Although not critical of the traditional roles of woman as wife and mother, liberal feminists are concerned with the social, political, and economic forces that channel women into these roles. Liberal feminists affirm individual choice and urge equal rights for women and the reform of systems to ensure their inclusion (Reich, 1995). The liberal tradition emphasizes rights and

freedoms and seeks to replace patriarchal protection of male freedoms and limitations with equal rights for women. For example, because men can father children well into their later years, a liberal feminist might argue that women should have rights to access postmenopausal infertility treatment (Chokr, 1992; L. Shanner, personal communication, March 28, 1995; Throsby, 2004).

The liberal feminist agenda, then, is to influence the social and political forces that overcome oppression and provide women with the same rights and opportunities as those of men. Some of the strategies they propose include providing greater educational opportunities for women, ensuring women have access to male-dominated professions (e.g., medicine, engineering, and politics), and implementing legislation that ensures equality for women (Valentine, 1994). For example, in 2017 and 2018, the federal government made a commitment to engage in a process of gender-based analysis of the budget. The thinking is that some budget expenditures have a disproportionate impact on women than on men (Government of Canada, 2022b).

In the 2021 budget, the federal government proposed investments to support women's health, and it offered a feminist plan to expand employment and career opportunities for women. Noting the disproportionate effect of COVID-19 on women, the budget outlined a recovery plan to advance the ability of women to fully participate in the Canadian economy. It included investment in the Canada-Wide Early Learning and Child Care System, which is intended to drive economic growth, increase women's participation in the workforce, and offer each child the best start in life (Government of Canada, 2021a).

From the liberal feminist perspective, the notion of the autonomous agent might be acceptable, but both women and men should be able to act as free, rational agents unless their actions constrain the equal rights of others. The concern of the liberal feminist is that women's freedoms are unfairly constrained (Sherwin, 1998).

Social Feminism

Social feminists examine the cultural institutions that contribute to the oppression of women and the relationship between the private sphere of the home and the public domain of productive work. They focus primarily on the role of economic oppression in women's lives (Reich, 1995). Of major concern to them are poverty, the challenges of lone parenthood, and the influence of the social determinants of health on women and children. They argue that equity will not be attained until changes are made to social structures such as the patriarchal family, motherhood, housework, and consumerism because these structures influence the distribution of power, wealth, and privilege. Furthermore, they believe that social and political structures must change so that women's responsibilities within the home and in traditionally female professions, such as nursing, are valued to the same extent as those professions traditionally dominated by men (Valentine, 1994).

To help distinguish between social feminism and liberal feminism, consider the different reactions of the two groups to the provision of in vitro fertilization (IVF)—which, could involve the freezing of ova—to fertile women in their twenties so they can complete their education, launch careers, and choose to have children later in life with reduced risks. A social feminist would respond that the educational and business institutions are not structured in ways that allow women to work and have families at the healthiest time in their life cycle and that the institutions should, therefore, be restructured. The liberal feminist is more likely to assert the right of women to having both (Dawson & Singer, 1988; Valentine, 1994).

Radical Feminism

Radical feminists view women-centred perspectives as the only or primary ones, thus inverting, not just challenging, patriarchy. They argue that women's oppression is the crucial problem and challenge the concepts and frameworks of traditional philosophical and scientific inquiry. This perspective challenges the patriarchal underpinnings of society because radical feminists seek to analyze and value women's experiences from the perspective of female rather than male standards and biases (Valentine, 1994).

The focus of radical feminism is the development of women-defined thought, culture, and systems. For these to evolve, they believe that gender discrimination and sexual stereotyping need to be eliminated. Although the child-bearing role of women and values

such as nurturance are considered important, radical feminists also see them as the historical basis of the oppression of women. There is a greater (not universal) tendency in radical feminism to blame men for oppressing women, not merely to acknowledge that structures in a society are problematic (L. Shanner, personal communication, March 28, 1995). An implicit, or explicit, recommendation is that men should be removed from their position of dominance and replaced by women. Thus, they argue that the liberal feminist goal of economic and political equality with men is perceived as aiming too low (Shanner, 1995).

Although the role of child-bearing and child rearing in the oppression of women may be a concern within all forms of feminism, for the radical feminist, this role is central. All feminists tend to want women, not men, to control the means of reproduction and to have at least an equal voice in reproductive policies. They may also argue that women's voices should dominate because women are more greatly affected by pregnancy and reproductive interventions than men. The liberal feminist wants greater reproductive liberty and, thus, is more likely to want minimal restrictions on surrogacy, selling ova, and other aspects of reproductive choice. The social feminist not only wants to change the institutions that limit women's choices so that women can decide whether or not to have families but also challenges the values placed on reproduction and family life. (Thus, social feminists may wish to reject some practices, such as surrogacy or selling ova, as exploitative of women and children.) Radical feminists are more likely to characterize a reproductive intervention as a plot to control the bodies of women (Shanner, 1995).

Although these three perspectives embrace a broad range of feminist thought and practice, all share the following themes:

- Recognition of the oppression of women
- Support for equal rights and opportunities for women
- An orientation to initiating change (Adamson et al., 1988)

Feminist theory is complex, as are the ethical perspectives it raises. Nurses can benefit through increased awareness of, and interest in, the ethical views that feminist theory offers.

Feminist Ethics

Feminist approaches to ethics have historically challenged the ways in which health care practices contribute to the oppression of women. Challenging the paradigms of traditional bioethical thinking, feminists reject liberal views regarding the primacy of autonomy (Reich, 1995), arguing that humans are fundamentally relational, and this in itself is morally significant (Reich, 1995). Of key interest to feminists in the area of bioethics are the debates over abortion, reproductive technologies, maternal–fetal relations, medical conditions affecting women that have historically been ignored (Tashjian, 2017), and health equity.

The feminist movement empowered women's knowledge regarding their health and challenged paternalistic, oppressive practices and systems within health care. The impact of inequities within society on women's lives and health is also a concern in feminist ethics, specifically the effects of gender-related violence, race, ethnic conflicts, poverty, and immigration. Some offer the integration of feminist thinking into health care action and social policy as one solution to improving the condition of women in society (Shai et al., 2021).

As discussed earlier, health inequities are a dominant influence on the health and well-being of persons and groups within a society. Feminists are concerned with the effect of such inequities on women and are concerned about the relationships between gender, disadvantage, and health. In addition, they question the distribution of power and this differential on policy-making and program delivery (Rogers, 2006).

Feminist thinkers noted concerns related to some of the policies introduced during the COVID-19 pandemic and the unique challenges that had the potential to disadvantage women, especially in relation to reproductive outcomes, protocols for deferral of elective surgery, the prevention and treatment of COVID-19 in pregnancy, maternal health outcomes, and restrictions in mobility that increased the risk of violence toward women (Bruno et al., 2021).

In feminist ethics, the oppression of women—the issue of utmost moral concern—"is seen to be morally and politically unacceptable" (Sherwin, 1992); therefore, the main moral imperative is "eliminating the subordination of women" (Sherwin, 1992). Within the context of feminist ethical thinking, the predominant question asked is, "What does this mean for women?" The focus is on changing the status quo, empowering women, and eliminating oppression (Sherwin, 1992). Without such changes, feminists believe a truly ethical reality is not possible.

CASE SCENARIO 2.8

THE COMPLEX WORLD OF NURSING ON THE STREET

A street nurse working with the homeless in one of Canada's biggest cities is the case manager for a 30-year-old woman addicted to fentanyl who left an abusive relationship 2 years earlier but did not have the resources to retain custody of her two young children, ages 4 and 6 years old. Her husband would not allow her access to them, leaving her depressed and vulnerable to substance abuse. She hopes to get well, find employment, and gain access to her children. All her attempts at rehabilitation have failed so far.

One morning, the nurse finds her in the usual location, still high after a night of alcohol and drug use. She has sustained a severe gash on her left leg, but doesn't remember what happened. The wound is still bleeding, and the nurse, worried about the risk of infection, suggests they go to the nearby emergency department. The woman refuses. She doesn't trust hospitals and is worried that someone might inform her husband and then may never see her children again.

The nurse is overwhelmed by these challenges and questions what is behind the woman's reluctance to go to the hospital—is there more to this story? The nurse worries about long-term effects on the children if their mother does not get well and dies alone and homeless. Further, she wonders whether the woman's present impairment is influencing her judgement?

Interpretation

This story reveals the many complex ethical issues and challenges faced regularly by nurses in such roles and raises a number of ethical questions. Where

CASE SCENARIO 2.8 *(Continued)*

were the supports this woman needed when she was forced to escape an abusive relationship? What were the factors that led to her being denied access to her children? What are the reasons behind her mistrust of hospitals? What was her past experience with the health care system? This nurse is faced with the competing principles of beneficence and autonomy. Aware of the risks associated with the injury, the nurse also knows this woman cannot be forced to seek medical attention against her will. These are system-wide challenges that individual nurses are challenged to resolve. Many of the solutions lie in policy, legislation, and program design and implementation.

From a feminist perspective, this story highlights the power differential between women and men. It also reveals the disadvantages women experience when, based on circumstances and due to social

structures and systemic gender inequalities, they are dependent on men and less likely to have full-time employment. Feminists would note the social factors that influence these dependencies and the role of women as the primary caregiver. One example of policy that intends to address this challenge is the federal-provincial child care agreements that promote and facilitate career opportunities for women (Government of Canada, 2021a).

Further, they would criticize the inadequate system response to violence against women and argue for targeted interventions such as access to safe havens and counselling. Intimate partner violence continues to be a worldwide problem that tends to be viewed as an individual rather than a collective social problem, rooted in social norms and notions about male masculinity and power (UN Women, 2022).

CASE SCENARIO 2.1D

RELEVANCE TO MY STORY

A feminist reflecting on this story would be concerned about the interests of the patient's wife. A feminist might ask questions related to whether rules or policies excluding this woman from her husband's bedside were established primarily by men who might dominate the hospital hierarchy. One might also ask,

if the situation were reversed and the husband wanted to be present, would his request be granted? A feminist might also raise questions regarding the power differential and the authority or power the nurse, if a woman, would have if the resuscitation team was dominated by men. Reflect on whether you think feminist ethics would assist me with my dilemma.

Feminine Ethics

Feminine ethics as posited by Carol Gilligan (1982) suggests that women and men make ethical choices based on different sets of values, perceptions, and concerns. Feminine views give greater significance to the nature of the relationships within a particular ethical context without the political nature of feministic thinking (Tong, 1995).

Gilligan argues that when faced with a moral issue, women use an empathetic form of reasoning (Reich, 1995) and tend to seek out innovative solutions to ensure that the needs of all parties are met, whereas men tend to seek the dominant rule, even when someone's

interests are sacrificed (Sherwin, 1989, 1992, 1998). An example might be the various approaches to visiting hour rules in hospitals. One could treat all visitors the same, imposing strict time limits, or recognize the special needs of individual patients and families, allowing a more open, patient-directed approach. Family presence emerged as a major concern as a result of public health restrictions during COVID-19 (Johnston et al., 2022).

Those with a feminine view of ethics argue that traditional theories are overly concerned with rational and objective thinking. In contrast, the feminine view places greater emphasis on values, feelings, and desires.

There is more significance given to being present, listening, taking feelings seriously, searching for meaning, and seeing the person and the world from a more holistic perspective (Lind et al., 1986). In contrast to Kantian thinking, in which emotion is considered to have no role in morality, in feminine ethics emotion and intuition are viewed as key indicators of right action. Consider the work of Patricia Benner, who described the expert nurse's ability to detect the changing condition of a patient without apparent changes in physiological status. She proposed that this is based on the nurse's intuition, which, she offers, is refined through experience in assessing the needs, worries, and concerns of patients and families. Benner proposed that within any complex social interaction, emotions are central to perception and can signal preference, danger, attraction, and so on. Within any situation or context, emotions have significance; they influence responses, such as compassion and fear, and provide insights into the meaning of human interactions and relationships (Benner, 1990, 2000; Benner & Wrubel, 1989). When nurses reflect on these experiences and understand their responses and reactions to situations and events, they may gain insight into their moral selves (Malmsten, 2000).

Feminine thinkers assert that more than one dimension needs to be considered to understand the moral issues and principles that prevail. The study of feminine ethics is, therefore, essential to understanding and clarifying ethics as it relates to the complex practice and values of nursing and the context and relationships within which care is given.

An Ethic of Care

Feminine thinkers, such as Gilligan, critical of the dominance of principles and of the historical preference in traditional theories for abstract rules that reinforce a deductive reasoning process, argue instead for an inductive process in which the starting point is the individual's circumstances or personal story (Reich, 1995). This approach, they suggest, more accurately depicts real life and ensures that all dimensions of the situation are addressed (Larrabee, 2016; Wolf, 1996).

Reasoning from abstract rules and principles governed by requirements for universality and impartiality, they argue, overlooks the importance of partiality, context, and relationships. An "ethic of care," formulated by

Gilligan, is instead relational, contextual, and empathetic, as opposed to the abstract, universalized, and principled approach of an ethic of justice (Mahon & Robinson, 2011; Peter, 2001; Sherwin, 1998; Wolf, 1996). An ethic of care offers an approach to ethical thinking that values feelings, emotions, empathy, and care—all important components of our ethical responses (Scott, 2000). Furthermore, it recognizes the nuances of relationships and the uniqueness and context of particular situations.

Using the experience of women as the foundation of a model of ethical theory, an ethic of care encourages spontaneous caring for others as appropriate to each unique circumstance and experience. Feminine ethical decision making is based on the desire to respond to the unique needs of each person with the focus on caring, rather than on justice or principled approaches. A caring approach recognizes the nature of complex relationships and the challenges people face in life. For example, rather than treating all people alike in the name of fairness, an ethic of care recognizes that some people need and want to be treated differently. Out of interest and concern for each individual's personal context, a focus on caring requires an examination of all of the dynamics of a particular situation. From this perspective, nurses enter another's world to see things as that person sees them; thus, they can better understand the values, beliefs, and experiences of others (Crowley, 1989). In doing so, the ethical issues become clearer and are understood from the experience of empathy, an enhanced awareness of the morally relevant features and responsibilities of the relationships involved, and the uniqueness of the situation (Mahon & Robinson, 2011; Sherwin, 1992, 1998).

In care ethics, the emphasis is on the process of self-awareness and understanding. The sharing of unique perspectives facilitates a clearer picture of the dynamics of a situation and therefore provides greater insights that can guide choices. This open approach, similar to value clarification discussed earlier, enhances the nurse's relationship with the patient and is also a means of understanding and respecting the various views and life experiences of all members of the health care team (Baker & Diekelmann, 1994).

Not all feminine thinkers agree that caring should supplant all principles; some worry that it is a "compassion trap" that will keep women in their traditional roles (Reich, 1995). Some radical feminists express concerns about an emphasis on caring, which they view as a gender trait and a survival skill of a historically oppressed group (Sherwin, 1992). Too much concern about the welfare of others, they believe, can drain the resources and energy of women. These feminists do not reject the relevance of caring but, instead, attempt to identify criteria for determining when it is relevant and when it is not. Social feminists would agree that emotions play a role in ethical decision making but that these need to be balanced with the need for social justice (Sherwin, 1992).

Others suggest that caring, which women take more into consideration because of their traditional role within the family, is the only moral consideration (Noddings, 1992; Sherwin, 1992). This position has been criticized because it suggests the exclusion of not only women who do not have children but also men from the possibility of such caring and nurturing (Condon, 1992). Noddings (1992) argued that an ethic of care is a quest for new virtues based on traditional women's practices and that the traditional female role as nurturer can be shaped into an ethic of care (Brilowski & Wendler, 2005; Crowley, 1994).

CASE SCENARIO 2.9

COMPASSIONATE AUTONOMY

A nurse on a general medical unit is caring for a 75-year-old patient admitted with anemia of unknown cause. Preliminary investigations have identified hydronephrosis of the left kidney caused by a stricture of the ureter, a complication of chronic infections related to an ileal conduit established 30 years ago. The nurse was present when the urology resident came by to share the results with the patient. The resident advised that the patient's only option was to have their ureter dilated under the guidance of ultrasonography. The patient became very upset and stated that they did not want to undergo the procedure. The resident explained that if they refused, their condition would deteriorate, their ureter would become infected, and they could die. However, the resident stated that this was the patient's choice; his responsibility was only to inform the patient of the options and the risks associated with having or not having the procedure.

Two years earlier, the patient had experienced the same problem. Not only was the procedure extremely painful, but the patient became septic and was seriously ill for 2 weeks. Just as they were recovering, a nurse accidentally removed the stent (in place to ensure the ureter remained dilated), and the procedure needed to be repeated.

The nurse is not aware of this history but is concerned about this interaction, and she believes there is a story behind the patient's emotional response.

Interpretation

The nurse's concerns are justified. This nurse clearly understands that what happened was not right. The resident, devoid of caring and compassion, seemed to think that by following all the rules regarding informed consent, the right action was taken. This story highlights the nuances of ethical situations. It also demonstrates why those who promote a care and relationship orientation toward ethics have concerns with the focus on autonomy without reflecting on other moral considerations. As well, it shows the value of understanding a person's story and those experiences that might influence ethical considerations.

The nurse now has a challenge to resolve and an ethical standard to meet. Because context is important, first, the patient needs time to settle and relax. Second, suspecting something triggered this very emotional reaction, the nurse needs to engage the patient in conversation to understand their story. The nurse might explore whether they want to have a family member of her family present to provide support them. The patient needs time to decide, and once there is an understanding of their past experience, the nurse will be in a better position to consider next steps.

The nurse can also play a role in educating the resident to better understand how sharing bad news is more than giving information, and that the context of the person's situation needs to be understood. It is important to listen, to communicate compassionately, and to appreciate that as health care professionals, the caring role must consider other important value perspectives.

Caring Ethics in Nursing

Theories in nursing have focused on understanding and clarifying the concept of care. Nursing theorist Jean Watson (2008) offered the "Philosophy and Science of Caring" as an alternative to traditional models of health–illness and science, which she found inadequate for understanding the lived world of patients and the lived caring–healing experiences of nurses. Watson argued that caring avoids the moral objectification of persons and introduces new healing possibilities. Caring ensures the preservation of human dignity and relationship equality within the context of illness and suffering. As a moral ideal, caring is not only a standard that demonstrates commitment to patients but also an end in and of itself. Essentially, it is both the process and goal of nursing (Watson, 1985, 1988, 1989).

Given the importance of the notion of care and caring in the nursing profession, it is not surprising that care-based approaches are highly relevant to nursing ethics. They emphasize the moral imperative of reducing human suffering as well as the relational aspect of nursing and the nurse–patient relationship (Austin, 2007; Brilowski & Wendler, 2005; Cloyes, 2002; Crowley, 1994; Mahon & Robinson, 2011; Peter & Gallop, 1994).

These approaches are seen as more meaningful alternatives to principle-based options. Theorists pose that the moral experience of nurses cannot be limited to principles alone. Rather than serving as tools to facilitate ethical decisions, principles can become an excuse to defend personal biases and to pass them off as absolutes. Some thinkers note that moral conflicts arise precisely because moral rules and principles cannot be applied to every situation clearly and without contradiction, and that this demonstrates the limitations of this type of reasoning. Furthermore, the role of the nurse as a moral agent may be compromised if a focus on rules leads the nurse to become more detached from the situation—and the person—becoming more of a "distant observer" rather than seeking to understand the situation within the context of the caring relationship (Parker, 1990).

Others argue that models based solely on care have limitations in that without moral obligation to principles, such as justice, caring relationships can be exploitative or unfairly partial (Peter & Morgan, 2001).

Believing that the heart, or emotions, and the mind , or rationality, need not be adversaries in moral reflection, and that principles such as justice and caring are not mutually exclusive (Olsen, 1992), they promote a combination of an ethic of care and an orientation toward principles that would address injustice while maintaining a more connected sense of social relationships. Researchers studying the guiding ethical framework of nurses have found that both a caring orientation and a justice orientation were frequently present as part of their reflection on moral issues (Millette, 1994). Nurses are often found to be committed to both the principles of patient rights and autonomy and their duty to the patient while at the same time obligated to the caring relationship with the person. The relationship with a patient informs the nurse's moral responses (Cooper, 1991), as engagement facilitates recognition of what autonomy, justice, and so on mean for that person at that time.

Consider the stories of critical care nurses when caring for patients receiving aggressive treatment that causes pain and suffering while offering only a slim chance of survival. It may be that the family supports such treatment or that the patient at an earlier time completed an advance directive agreeing to such measures. However, in the reality of the moment and the current experience of the patient, the nurse may, through the caring relationship, intuitively perceive that the patient's views may now be quite different. The nurse, by being present with patients, experiences their expressions of pain and suffering (Benner & Tanner, 1987). A focus on principles such as autonomy and quality of life alone in this circumstance would not alleviate the moral distress of the nurse. If only principles are used to justify care, without any connection to the nurse–patient relationship or the human experience, the nurse may become disengaged.

Care ethics organizes social and moral theory around care and the connections that bring us in touch with others through the nurse–patient relationship (Parker, 1990). Care is seen as a relational response to a fundamental human need, central to nursing practice, not only as a therapeutic interaction but also as a moral imperative. As the deliverers of care, nurses then become moral agents. Care is also seen as a means of being ethical and, therefore, a normative moral concept of that which is good (Benner, 1990, 2000, 2009; Benner & Tanner, 1987). As moral agents, then, nurses nurture those they care for and demonstrate caring attributes of compassion, competence, confidence, commitment, conscience, communication, concern, and courage (Cloyes, 2002).

Essential to an ethical nurse–patient relationship is trust (Peter & Morgan, 2001). Trust is significant in that, frequently, the nurse is in the position of power, especially when caring for those most vulnerable. To trust is to make oneself or let oneself be more vulnerable to the power of others and to be confident that one will be cared for and protected from harm (Baier, 1985). Trust is especially relevant to challenges related to the need for basic care. For example, patients who lose the ability to control bodily functions essentially give control over their bodies to another, trusting their capacity to meet or facilitate their physical, social, emotional, and spiritual needs.

Some theorists propose that it is difficult to separate the ethic of care from the notion of the "good nurse." Two positions are put forth: some see caring ethics as a distinct approach to ethics, whereas others see it as the way virtues are acted out within specific relationships (Izumi et al., 2006; Watson, 1992). The characteristics of nurses are relevant to their status as moral agents (Catlett & Lovan, 2011). As discussed earlier, virtue ethics considers the character of the person, or persons, making moral decisions. The normative standard is that a virtuous person, one whose character is good or morally praiseworthy, will want to do what is good in all circumstances (Armstrong, 2006; Fowler, 2021; Hoyt, 2010; Pellegrino, 1995; Scott, 1995; Sellman, 1997, 2011) For example, a nurse may provide care that follows policy or protocol, but unless the nurse is also motivated to care about the person, the therapeutic intervention would not be considered caring and ethical (Izumi et al., 2006). Without the commitment to care and to do what is best for that patient in that circumstance, the nurse simply completes a task. It is suggested that there are four qualities that support a caring relationship: being a good person, presenting as a good person, being interested in the other person (patient) as a person, and caring for the other person (patient) (Izumi et al., 2006).

CASE SCENARIO 2.10

A CARING RELATIONSHIP?

A nurse who works in a rehabilitation setting and is responsible for the care of four older males who are recovering from orthopedic surgery is attentive to protocol, well organized, and focused on the task at hand. The norm in this setting is to address older males as "Papa." The nurse is particularly concerned about one of the men who has diabetes and is not eating well. Dutifully, the nurse checks his blood sugar and finds that it is very low and proceeds to scold him for not eating and asks him to drink a glass of orange juice with added sugar. He refuses. Frustrated by his "noncompliant behaviour," the nurse leaves to alert his physician. A visitor, also a nurse and the son of one of the other patients, observes the exchange. This visitor has become acquainted with the patients in the room and is aware that they are highly competent men with prestigious professional backgrounds. The visitor has noted their responses to various caregivers and has observed them "bristle" when they are addressed as "Papa." The patient with diabetes is a senior accountant at a local bank and misses his partner, who is taking time during his convalescence to visit family. The visitor hears his frustrations about how he is being treated and then kindly encourages him to drink the orange juice, which he does. This patient is well aware of how to manage his diabetes and knows the importance of raising his blood sugar level.

Interpretation

The nurse caring for these patients has failed to meet the standards of a moral agent within the moral framework of the nurse–patient relationship. Clearly, this nurse has not invested in developing these relationships and has not taken the time to get to know the patients. This lack of respect, amplified by the discourtesy demonstrated by addressing them as "Papa," also suggests ageism, which diminishes trust and compromises cooperation and collaboration.

CASE SCENARIO 2.1E

RELEVANCE TO MY STORY

Those who have a caring-oriented perspective on ethics would try to understand the context of the dilemma I was facing. They would be interested in the nature of the relationship I had with the patient and his wife. How long had I cared for him? How well did I know their story and understand their values? They would note and take seriously the wife's reactions and my intuitive and emotional reaction to the situation. From a relational perspective, they might highlight the long and loving relationship between the patient and his wife and the chance that he might not survive the resuscitation efforts. Putting themselves in the wife's place, they might ask the question, "If we had the option, would we want to be present when those we love are dying? They would also consider the effect on the wife if denied the opportunity to say goodbye and support her husband during his final moments and how this would influence her grieving process. They would ask me about my my inclination at this time and if I believed that I was acting as a caring moral agent, wanting to do what is right.

Narrative Ethics: Revealing the Story

Storytelling has a long tradition in our history. It is how many children learn to understand the world, the nature of relationships, what is right or wrong, and how to behave. The experience of nursing is rich in stories that are deep in emotion, sadness, joy, confusion, guilt, stories that make nurses proud, stories where they wish more could have been done. Nurses share these stories with one another every day. Some stories remain in their memory for years.

Narrative ethics encourages the sharing of these stories with the goal of gaining a clearer understanding of the ethical issues and challenges embedded in them, which is attained through questioning, challenging, and information seeking. Reflecting on and discussing narratives with others uncovers the moral dimensions of the experience and enables learning that becomes entrenched in memory more so than that of theory alone (Benner, 1994, 1996; Parker, 1990; Sherwin, 1989).

Sharing an experience through a story uncovers the respective values and perspectives of those involved. Stories can be shared from a personal or a universal view. Each person or profession may see the situation through a different lens. All of what is seen has meaning, and through the conversation, each team member will become aware of what is important both to self and to others. One's understanding of the situation may sometimes be altered. In this way, learning occurs as the team reviews what happened, what can be gained from the experience, and how this experience will influence future practices and behaviour. Storytelling, hence, offers the opportunity to identify both excellence and how things could have been better (Adams, 2008; Benner, 1994).

Benner (1996) identified the dominant ethical themes that emerge in many of the stories nurses share: "care, responsiveness to the other, and responsibility" (p. 233). These themes align with an ethic of care, which can be appreciated through the sharing of stories of lived experiences. Learning occurs as themes are revealed and one is able to recognize the important ethical issues that arise in various circumstances. Because each situation is different and because the nature of relationships vary, the nurse's ethical thinking may change based on understanding the person's story and experience. As different perspectives are shared, and the person's story unfolds, it should become clearer what the right action is in each situation. And as numerous stories emerge and are shared over time, it may become evident that not all rules apply in all situations—each circumstance is unique.

Narratives differ from case studies. Case studies are often used to encourage debate and to illustrate ethical theory or principles. Narratives are real situations and encourage an inductive process in which one is able to examine the notions of morality that are embedded in the story, rather than starting with the theory or principles. This process of sharing the story reveals the extent to which nurses come to know and understand a person's stressful and vulnerable circumstances. As stories progress, relationships deepen, caring evolves, and wisdom is acquired. The narrative provides the background for understanding the ethical components, issues are identified, and innovation becomes much more possible (Benner, 1996, p. 235). Consider the story of an 80-year-old patient with Alzheimer's disease living in a long-term care community, who is confused and agitated most of the time. Frequently they pace, call out for their dad, and shout, "Go away, go away!" The staff have a very difficult time "managing" this responsive behaviour. Knowing this patient's story by learning more about their past would possibly have helped the staff find empathy and a greater understanding of the care and the comfort they need to ease their fear. What would the difference be if the staff knew that when they were about 4 years old, they were alone one day when a strange man approached their house. Frightened, they hid under the porch and waited for a long time before their dad found them. The patient constantly reliving what, for them, was a very frightening experience. Understanding this background and the issues behind their agitation would deepen the therapeutic relationship and reveal more ethical, creative, and innovative approaches to this patient's care.

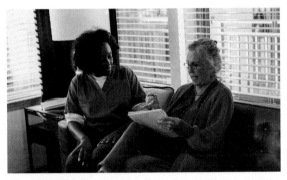

Storytelling uncovers the moral dimensions of the experience and enables learning to a larger degree than theory alone. *Source: iStock.com/kali9.*

The ethical issues and principles are better understood in the context of everyday practice and relationships, making them more meaningful and understandable. Narrative accounts of practice help nurses recognize needs and patterns. This understanding aids the nurse in responding to the concerns, needs, preferences, and inclinations of patients and families. Stories reveal what is good and what is important in relationships, and provide a clearer picture of the context and defining elements of the situation. They help to further one's understanding of the patient and others (Benner, 1996).

Through the sharing of stories, the moral engagement of the nurse advances (Benner, 1996). Stories of practice uncover moral concerns and notions of good. As the storyteller reports feelings, thoughts, and experiential knowledge, the actual ethical dimensions can be identified and examined: "We need to listen to our stories of practice to examine distinctions of worth, competing goods, and the relational ethics of care, responsiveness, and responsibility" (Benner, 1994, p. 410).

Leaders in all contexts play a significant role in enabling these stories to be heard. Through the learning resulting from discourse, the stories advance the moral agency of the nurse and the moral culture of the environment.

CASE SCENARIO 2.1F

RELEVANCE TO MY STORY

Understanding the personal stories of patients and families deepens the nurse's understanding of their values and perspectives. This understanding begins with the nurse's first encounter with the patient and deepens throughout the therapeutic moral relationship. Knowing their story would reveal the nature and meaning of the relationship between the patient and his wife. I needed to make a quick assessment, based on the reaction of the patient's wife, and needed to take immediate action. I didn't have the time to discover their story or consult with others. However, by being present with the wife in those moments, I was able to understand the depth and meaning of their relationship and gain some sense of what she valued most.

Also, after the fact, sharing my story and the consequences of whatever action I did take would reveal the issues, the relationships involved, and help the team reach a shared understanding of the moral complexities of this situation.

Sharing the story and discussing the consequences of my action would give the team a clearer view of what did happen, what should have happened, and how practice can be improved through this learning experience. Reflecting on and discussing narratives with others uncovers the moral dimensions of the experience and enables learning.

REFLECTIONS ON THE MORAL PERSPECTIVES OF INDIGENOUS PEOPLES IN CANADA

Matters of culture, beliefs, and values have been discussed within the context of complex ethical issues and challenges. Five common threads found in Indigenous world views are noted by Bob Joseph and Cynthia Joseph in their book *Indigenous Relations: Insights, Tips and Suggestions to Make Reconciliation a Reality* (2019) (Box 2.4). Bob Joseph, a hereditary chief in the Gayaxala clan of the Gwawaenuk Nation, was an associate professor at Royal Roads University, and is the author of several books on Indigenous issues. Joseph and Joseph offer that Indigenous world views, "a way of knowing, seeing, explaining and living in the world," (p. 25) are grounded in harmony and a nonhierarchical holistic view that depicts all living elements as equals, with the Creator at the centre.

The experience of Indigenous peoples in Canada carries a legacy of oppression and colonization. The devastating impacts of residential schools, Indian hospitals, the child welfare system, and other colonial experiences have created deep losses for Indigenous peoples. Nurses must be aware of this history and, given Indigenous peoples' position in Canada, understand and respect their values, culture, and moral traditions.

It is important to appreciate that not all Indigenous communities hold to one philosophical view, religious belief, or moral code. There are differences in moral and ethical value systems across and within First Nations, Inuit, and Métis communities, just as there are across other societies and cultures across the world (Joseph & Joseph, 2019). Many Indigenous communities have a unique language, culture, and social system. For example, some communities trace their lineage, families, and clans through the male parent (patriarchy), whereas others are matriarchal and track their heritage through the female parent (Aboriginal Justice Implementation Commission [AJIC], 1999, Ch. 2).

With each therapeutic encounter, nurses must consider the particular circumstance, beliefs, and values of that person and their community. As with all cultures, nurses cannot assume that a common moral view is shared by all individuals and within all communities (AJIC, 1999, Ch. 2).

Guiding Moral Behaviour

While there is much diversity among Indigenous peoples and communities, Indigenous ethics resonates with the values of honour, trust, honesty, and humility; these values reflect a commitment to the collective and embodying a respectful relationship with the land (Biin et al., 2021). Two approaches that offer guidance for moral behaviour are described next.

Shared Values

Dr. Clare Brant, a Mohawk man who was Canada's first Indigenous psychiatrist (Petten, 2017), offered that there are some shared commonalities with respect to morality, guiding principles, and rules of behaviour (Brant, 1990) across Indigenous communities, many similar to those described throughout this chapter. They include traditionally held values such as wisdom, love, respect, autonomy and noninterference, bravery, honesty, freedom, integrity, and collaboration. Of note is the strong focus on harmony within interpersonal relationships and the value of collective well-being.

Brant described four major ethical principles or rules of behaviour that are fundamental to the moral framework and social structure of Indigenous communities: noninterference, noncompetitiveness, emotional restraint, and sharing (Brant, 1990) (Box 2.5).

These principles align with many of the moral principles and theories previously discussed. They emphasize autonomy, underscore the importance of social justice, and highlight the significance of having a worthy character and personal integrity.

The Seven Sacred Teachings of White Buffalo Calf Woman

In *The Seven Sacred Teachings of White Buffalo Calf Woman*, Bouchard and Martin (2009) provide an illustration of universally shared Indigenous teachings that guide "life's journey." Also known as, *the Seven*

BOX 2.4
FIVE COMMON THREADS

- Holistic perspective
- Unified vision
- All life is sacred
- All forms of life are interconnected
- Humans are not above or below others (Joseph & Joseph, 2019, p. 26)

> **BOX 2.5**
> ## INDIGENOUS PRINCIPLES FOR ETHICAL BEHAVIOUR
>
> **NONINTERFERENCE**
>
> This principle promotes positive interpersonal relationships and discourages coercion of any kind—physical, verbal or psychological. It is based on respect for each person's independence and personal freedom.
>
> **NONCOMPETITIVENESS**
>
> This rule discourages competition, considered to be a source of internal conflict within a group and, instead, advocates for a more cooperative approach, rather than one that enforces the dominant person's view or one that results in the success of one individual to the disadvantage of the group.
>
> **EMOTIONAL RESTRAINT**
>
> This principle calls for control of emotions that could cause conflict and tension within the community and within the family.
>
> **SHARING**
>
> This principle is enshrined in social behaviours that emphasize equality within the community. Sharing guarantees equality so that no one becomes too rich or too powerful and no one is too poor or too powerless. The intent is to limit the manifestation of greed, arrogance, envy, and pride within the community.

Grandfather Teachings, they are based on values of caring for each other, collective decision making, and sustainability. These teachings resonate in most Indigenous cultures and foster respect, courage, honesty, humility, truth, wisdom, and love. These principles are associated with sacred animals, and plant and tree life, each having a special gift to help people understand and to maintain a connection to the land and to each other (Table 2.4). These teachings align with Indigenous culture and traditions and the goal of living in peace and harmony.

The values embodied in the teachings coupled with storytelling, and articulated through Indigenous language, reinforce Indigenous ways of being and doing. In other words, fortifying ethical thinking lends itself to ethical practice (Bouchard & Martin, 2009).

The Oral Tradition of Indigenous Peoples in Canada

The importance of these principles in guiding behaviour is understood through the oral tradition of Indigenous communities. When counsel is given, it is usually in the form of a story that allegorically describes the situation and possible approaches to a resolution. The use of narrative to uncover the complexity of moral issues in nursing clearly aligns with Indigenous traditions and cultures. In fact, understanding the oral tradition of Indigenous peoples enables a better appreciation for the power of the narrative in nursing. Although the approach may vary across Indigenous communities, there is a rich oral culture that has transcended centuries through storytelling. Through stories, shared from generation to generation, they have created a strong system of knowledge and mythology that guides moral thinking and actions and affirms relationships with the earth and with one another (Canada, 1996, pp. 37–40; Castellano, 2000). As nurses listen to the stories shared by Indigenous patients, families, and community Elders, they gain a better understanding of Indigenous culture, learn about what Indigenous people value most, become more sensitive to Indigenous patients' needs and preferences, and strengthen the therapeutic relationship.

Traditionally, in Indigenous communities, the process of ethical thinking begins early in a child's development with storytelling as the primary learning process. Stories are used to provide children with guidance on moral responsibility and behaviour, and to encourage engagement with the family and community. The community articulates and embraces its shared valued system through storytelling. It also lays out its ethical thinking through its customs, teachings, and ideals (Biin et al., 2021).

The Role of Elders

Elders play a prominent role in Indigenous cultures and are largely responsible for retaining and sharing the knowledge of cultural and moral traditions.

The role of Elders varies but generally involves helping the people and the community to appreciate their history, traditions, customs, values, and beliefs and to assist them in maintaining their well-being and health. They are called upon to advise people and guide the community on what to do in difficult situations. They are valued for the wisdom and knowledge they gain from following their cultural beliefs and by walking the traditional path (Taylor, 2019). Elders link the ancient traditions and beliefs of the people to modern-day influences (AJIC, 1999). It would not be unusual for an

TABLE 2.4
Seven Sacred Teachings

Teaching	Animal	Quotes
Humility	**Wolf/*Ma'iingan*** "The wolf does not live for himself but for the pack."	"Become humble." Can you not sense there is something much stronger than you out here?"
Honesty	**Raven/*Kitchi-Sabe*** The Raven "does not seek the power, speed or beauty of others."	"Be honest with yourself as well as with others. When you speak, speak truthfully."
Respect	**Buffalo/*Bashkode-bizhiki*** The buffalo "offers himself to sustain you, does not make his life any less than yours . . ."	"And treat others as you would have them treat you, respectfully."
Courage	**Bear/*Makwa*** "Just as courage sleeps in Makwa through long winter months, it is dormant within you. It needs only be awakened."	"To do what is right is not easy. It takes courage."
Wisdom	**Beaver/*Amik*** "Amik uses his gift wisely to thrive and so must you."	"To live your life based on your unique gifts is to live wisely."
Truth	**Turtle/*Miskwaadesii*** Slow-moving Miskwaadesii understands, as you should, that the journey of life is as important as the destination."	"Truth is to know all these Teachings."
Love	**Eagle/*Migizi*** "Migizi flies high above the earth and sees all that is true. Look to her as one who represents and models love."	"Look within yourself for Love. Love yourself, and then love others."

Bouchard, D., & Martin, J. (2009). *The seven sacred teachings of White Buffalo Calf Woman.* More Than Words Publishers. http://www.btgwinnipeg.ca/uploads/5/2/4/1/52412159/the_seven_sacred_teachings_.pdf

Indigenous patient to embrace both traditional and contemporary approaches to the treatment of a disease.

The prominent role that Elders play explains the preference of an Indigenous person or family to engage the broader community, usually represented by Elders, in health care decision making and for guidance when moral challenges are faced. As moral agents, it is important that nurses respect this approach and facilitate it.

Resources related to Indigenous culture, ethical values, and philosophies are available on the websites of universities who offer Indigenous programs of study and provide additional insights into Indigenous ways of knowing, morality, and world views. One example is the website of First Nations and Indigenous Studies at the University of British Columbia (https://indigenousfoundations.arts.ubc.ca).

CASE SCENARIO 2.11

A LIFE AT RISK

Edith, a member of a Mohawk First Nation in Quebec and named after Edith Monture, the first Indigenous woman to become a registered nurse in Canada, works as a community mental health nurse in an urban Alberta setting (Canadian Women's Foundation, 2021). She has been assigned to manage the care of a 15-year-old member of a Métis community in northern Alberta, C. K., who was transferred to the

care of foster parents at the age of 10, when C. K.'s parents were deemed unfit. The parents, both children of residential school survivors, suffer from substance abuse, and a violent incident involving C. K. led to the decision made by social services. C. K.'s non-Indigenous foster parents tried their best to provide support but could not prevent the bullying C. K. experienced at school, or deal with the depression resulting from C. K.'s loss of family and community.

CASE SCENARIO 2.11 *(Continued)*

C. K. has attempted suicide twice and was recently discharged from a mental health facility. Edith understands all too well the challenges faced by Indigenous children in these circumstances. She has a plan to help move C. K. back home and hopes she has the courage to carry this through.

Interpretation

Suicide rates are highest among Indigenous peoples in Canada (Statistics Canada, 2019), and the highest cause of death in youth. These rates are influenced by the historical, and existing, injustices and harms resulting from colonization, residential schools, and the removal of children from their families and communities during the "Sixties scoop." Many consequences associated with these actions have influenced these suicide rates, including marginalization, exposure to traumatic events, and the breakdown of families (and they would have had an impact on C. K. in this story). The location of these communities also makes a difference. Remote communities may have higher rates of suicide due to lack of services such as community substance abuse and mental health supports. But as there is diversity across Indigenous communities, there is diversity associated with these rates: some communities have high suicide rates and others have none (Chandler et al., 2004).

This story illustrates the very complex challenge faced by nurses in these circumstances, whether they practise at the direct care, system, or policy level.

Many of the *Seven Sacred Teachings* have relevance to this story, including truth, respect, courage, and love. Regarding *truth*, that as a society we must acknowledge the harms of the past, and at all levels implement the 94 Calls to Action of the Truth and Reconciliation Commission of Canada. Regarding

respect, as individuals and as a society we should treat others as we ourselves would like to be treated and therefore remedy and not repeat the harms of the past. With respect to C. K.'s story, imagine what we, as nurses, would want if we were in the same circumstance. Regarding *courage*, as a society we must stay committed to carrying through on these Calls to Action, and it is hoped that Edith has the courage to advocate on C. K.'s behalf and do what is right. Finally, *love*, can help C. K., who needs to be loved by others and self to heal.

Early in life, C. K. would have been influenced by the values, traditions, and culture of the community, founded on values such as sharing, harmony, and collective well-being. Canadian society has come to realize the need for children such as C. K. to remain in their own community where they can be supported by others and guided by the wisdom and best practices of their Elders (Chandler et al., 2004, 2019). Saving C. K. is more complicated. More than simply a move back to the community, the right resources need to be in place to facilitate the transition to the community and to repair the harm and support the healing journey. Resources, developed by Indigenous people and founded on their values and traditions, are available to provide such support (Waniskahk, 2020).

Nurses like Edith would have always known the right thing to do, but now systems and processes are being introduced, including federal legislation introduced in 2020, which affirm the rights of Indigenous communities to exercise jurisdiction over child and family services (*An Act Respecting First Nations, Inuit and Métis children, Youth and Families,* 2019) to ensure this happens.

CASE SCENARIO 2.1G

RELEVANCE TO MY STORY

Though there are diverse beliefs and practices related to spirituality and death and dying across Indigenous communities, there are commonalities in values and traditions. The *Seven Sacred Teachings* would serve as a useful guide for me as I face this dilemma.

The teachings of humility, respect, wisdom, courage, and love are worth considering.

Humility is the recognition that the relationship between the wife and her husband is stronger than the power of the team. Respect would encourage the team

Continued on following page

CASE SCENARIO 2.1G *(Continued)*

to reflect on what their wishes would be if they were in the position of the wife and her husband. Wisdom would guide me in recognizing the knowledge I have acquired as a nurse and my understanding of the impact on family members when not present during important transitions. Courage would guide me to do the right thing. Finally, love is at the heart of the compassionate nurse–patient relationship.

CASE SCENARIO 2.1H

CONCLUSION: MY CHOICE

What action did I actually take? I was profoundly influenced by the comment the wife made to me: "He is my husband, not yours. I need to be with him if he dies."

Sensing the strong bond between the patient and his wife, I was concerned about the wife's well-being if he were to die alone, without her presence. At the same time, I was worried about the team's response if I were to bring the wife into the room. However, I had a strong conviction that the right thing to do was to allow the wife to be present, and I was convinced that she would stay focused on her husband. I also thought that this would be in the best interests of the patient, who might be aware of his wife's presence. I also believed that if the patient died, which at the time seemed likely, his wife would be better able to accept his death if she had been present, and less so if she was denied entry. On reflection, I believe I demonstrated moral courage by advocating for the wife and announcing that I would be bringing her into the room. I was prepared to defend my action and accept all responsibility for the consequences of this decision. I guided the wife into the room and prepared a space for her to sit beside her husband. She sat quietly beside her husband and whispered words of comfort and love as she caressed and comforted him. She paid absolutely no attention to the team. She was at peace as he died.

The implications for this one moral action were profound for me and the team and influenced my view on the moral value of person-centred care. As a team, we were comforted that although the efforts at resuscitation were not successful, in the end, by allowing the wife to be present, we were acting as caring moral agents. I had listened to the wife and understood what was most important to her. I thought about how I would feel if I was in a similar position and was denied being present with a loved one who was dying. I realized this was the wife's right, and this was their relationship. This story was shared with the hospital leaders, and, as a result, practice changes were introduced to facilitate, when requested, family presence in such circumstances.

SUMMARY

In this chapter, traditional theories, principles, codes, and decision frameworks that can guide ethical decision making were introduced. In recent decades, as the field of ethics has advanced and the role of the nurse has become more complex, ethical challenges have intensified. Recognizing that traditional theories have limitations when dealing with the complex reality of nursing practice and moral relationships with others, nursing theorists have offered alternative ethical approaches that consider the art of nursing and emphasize values of caring and compassion. They posit that through understanding the person's story, the moral dimensions of the situation and the respective values of all involved are best understood.

Nurses' commitment and loyalty to the individuals they serve may, at times, be in conflict with their own values and the interests of others, and this conflict may emerge in many everyday practical decisions that nurses have to make. Ethical challenges and decisions may relate to standards of care, to quality of life, and, indeed, to the very ethic of caring within the nursing profession and the health care system. These issues have multiplied in recent years as the COVID-19 pandemic magnified the ethical issues embedded in nursing and health care. Further, societal values were challenged as human rights violations were identified, especially those of Indigenous peoples in Canada, and the legacy of colonialism revealed significant issues of racism and discrimination. The need to address these issues is further amplified as we welcome more culturally diverse communities into this country. These factors and others have made more urgent the role of nursing in promoting a more respectful and just society.

Nurses not only must stay focused on the everyday issues they face but also must be in a position to influence such issues as poverty, inequity, and the changing role of society. At the same time, nursing leaders must ensure a safe environment for nurses and the patients and patients they serve.

Nurses require knowledge of ethics and of the various approaches to understanding morality to be able to recognize ethical issues, communicate with others about them, make good choices, and evaluate how to provide not only the best but also the most ethical nursing care. This understanding is essential to ensuring the moral agency of the nurse and to advance the important caring relationships nurses have with their patients and one another.

The material covered in this chapter provides nurses with a solid foundation in ethics and, thus, launches a lifelong learning process.

CRITICAL THINKING

Discussion Points

1. Do the approaches described in this chapter guide discussions of ethical issues in your practice environment?
2. Do these theories have limitations when applied to practice?
3. Compare and contrast utilitarian and deontological approaches. Although feminists are critical of these traditional approaches, do these approaches share any similarities with feminism?
4. Is there a theory that is most consistent with your values? In what way?
5. Do you think it is possible to develop a perfect ethical theory that will assist in resolving the major ethical issues faced in health care and nursing?
6. Does using a theory to resolve an issue necessarily lead to consensus on the solution? Why, or why not?
7. What approaches best guide your nursing practice?
8. What personal narratives can you share with your colleagues to create shared understanding of your respective values?
9. Will the theories presented in this chapter influence your nursing practice and assist you in ethical reflection?

Narratives for Ethical Reflection

The following scenarios are presented to provide you with the opportunity to evaluate the various ethical perspectives outlined in this chapter, to facilitate self-reflection, and to be the focus of team discussions.

CASE SCENARIO 2.12

AN ETHIC OF RULES

It is a busy evening in the critical care unit of a major city hospital where a 27-year-old patient is dying, having sustained major head injuries in a motor vehicle accident.

Members of their family have just arrived from out of town and wish to see them. On this unit, only two visitors at a time are permitted for 10 minutes of every hour. That maximum has already been met, yet two brothers and two sisters are still waiting. The patient's nurse is involved in preparing for a new admission and informs the family about the rules, adding that it is "just too busy" to have visitors at this time. The family complains to the charge nurse, who sympathizes, especially because it is likely the patient will not survive the shift.

Continued on following page

CASE SCENARIO 2.12 *(Continued)*

Another patient, who received a lung transplant earlier in the day, has just had a cardiac arrest. The nurses are preparing for an admission from the emergency department, and it is dinnertime, so nurses are covering for one another's patients.

When approached by the charge nurse, the nurses cite unit policy and suggest that their priority is helping the new patient, who still has a chance to live. How can they do their job effectively if this family is in the way? Before this issue can be resolved by the charge nurse, the 27-year-old dies.

Questions:

1. What are the moral dimensions of this story?
2. On what grounds would the hospital have based its visiting policy? Are these grounds justified?
3. What position would you take in this circumstance?
4. What are the relevant ethical considerations for deciding on a course of action?

CASE SCENARIO 2.13

YOUNG ENOUGH TO CHOOSE

A 16-year-old patient, diagnosed with sarcoma in their right foot 2 years previously, had received aggressive chemotherapy and had their foot amputated. They have done well since, although they have been unable to participate in the contact sports they love. Now the cancer has recurred in the right tibia. The planned treatment involves an above-the-knee amputation and more chemotherapy.

Since the previous chemotherapy, treatments have advanced and outcomes have improved dramatically. However, now the patient is refusing to have further treatment. They do not accept the optimistic projections and state that they cannot go through chemotherapy again and do not want to lose their leg. The patient maintain their refusal even when informed of its consequences and the pain they will likely experience without the surgery.

The patient's parents are very distressed. They ask if their child can be forced to accept the treatment.

Questions:

1. What are the moral dimensions of this story?
2. What position would you take in this circumstance?
3. What are the relevant ethical considerations for deciding on a course of action?

CASE SCENARIO 2.14

GENDER EXPECTATIONS

A 40-year-old single woman who works as an accountant with a major consulting firm lives in Halifax, and sometimes has to travel for work. She has two brothers who moved to Vancouver some years ago.

Her mother died about a year ago; her 82-year-old father continues to live alone in the family home. He has done well but recently was admitted to hospital with pneumonia. He is recovering, and the hospital team would like to discharge him with home care. Home care resources are limited, so she is told that he will need the family to provide him 24-hour assistance for at least 2 to 3 weeks. She has already taken her vacation for the year, and this is audit time for her clients.

Questions:

1. What are the moral dimensions of this story?
2. What position would you take in this circumstance?
3. What are the relevant ethical considerations for deciding on a course of action?

REFERENCES

Statutes and Court Decisions

An Act Respecting First Nations, Inuit and Métis Children, Youth and Families, S.C. 2019, c. 24.

Canada Health Act, R.S.C. 1985, c. C-6, as amended.

Gaudreault v. Drapeau, 1987 RJQ 2286.

Texts and Articles

Aboriginal Justice Implementation Commission. (1999). *The justice system and Aboriginal people* (Ch. 2). http:// www.ajic.mb.ca

Acevedo-Garcia, D., McArdle, N., Hardy, E. F., et al. (2014). The Child Opportunity Index: Improving collaboration between community development and public health. *Health Affairs, 33*(11), 1948–1957.

Adams, T. E. (2008). A review of narrative ethics. *Qualitative Inquiry, 14*(2), 175–194.

Adamson, N., Briskin, L., & McPhail, M. (1988). *Feminists organizing for change: The contemporary women's movement in Canada.* Oxford University Press.

Agledahl, K. M., Forde, R., & Wifstad, A. (2011). Choice is not the issue. The misrepresentation of healthcare in bioethical discourse. *Journal of Medical Ethics, 37*(4), 212–215.

Albert, E., Denise, T., & Peterfreund, S. (1975). *Great traditions in ethics* (pp 210–212). Van Nostrand.

All Answers Ltd. (2018, November). *Applying Kants ethical theory to nursing.* https://nursinganswers.net/essays/applying-kants-ethical-theory-to-nursing-ethics-nursing-essay.php?vref51

Almond, B. (1995). *Introducing applied ethics.* Wiley-Blackwell.

Amer, A. B. (2019). The health care ethics: Overview of the basics. *Open Journal of Nursing, 9*(2), 183–187.

Armstrong, A. E. (2006). Towards a strong virtue ethics for nursing practice. *Nursing Philosophy, 7*(3), 110–124.

Arutyunova, K. R., Alexandrov, Y. I., & Hauser M. D. (2016). Sociocultural Influences on Moral Judgments: East-West, male-female, and young-old. *Frontiers in Psychology, 7*, 1334.

Austin, W. (2007). The ethics of everyday practice. Healthcare environments as moral communities. *Advances in Nursing Science, 30*(1), 81–88.

Baier, A. (1985). What do women want in a moral theory? *Nous, 19*, 53–65.

Baker, C., & Diekelmann, N. (1994). Connecting conversations of caring: Recalling the narrative to clinical practice. *Nursing Outlook, 42*, 65–70.

Batho, D., & Pitton, C. (2018). *What is moral distress? Experiences and responses.* The University of Essex. https://powerlessness.essex.ac.uk/wp-content/uploads/2018/02/MoralDistressGreenPaper1.pdf

BBC. (2014). *Ethics: A general introduction.* https://www.bbc.co.uk/ethics/introduction/intro_1.shtml

Beauchamp T. L. (2007). History and theory in "applied ethics." *Kennedy Institute of Ethics Journal, 17*(1), 55–64.

Beauchamp, T. L., (2010). The concept of paternalism in biomedical ethics. *Jahrbuch für Wissenschaft und Ethik, 14*, 77–92.

Beauchamp, T. L., & Childress, J. F. (1979). *Principles of biomedical ethics.* Oxford University Press.

Beauchamp, T. L., & Childress, J. F. (2001). *Principles of biomedical ethics* (4th ed.). Oxford University Press.

Beauchamp, T. L., & Childress, J. F. (2013). *Principles of biomedical ethics* (7th ed.). Oxford University Press.

Beauchamp, T. L., & Walters, L. (2003). *Contemporary issues in bioethics* (6th ed.). Wadsworth-Thompson Learning.

Begley, A. M. (2005). Practising virtue: A challenge to the view that a virtue centred approach to ethics lacks practical content. *Nursing Ethics, 12*(6), 622–637.

Beliso-De Jesús, A., & Pierre, J. (2020). Anthropology of white supremacy. *American Anthropologist, 122*(1), 65–75.

Benjamin, M., & Curtis, J. (1985). Virtue and the practice of nursing. In E. E. Shelp (Ed.), *Virtue and medicine: Explorations in the practice of nursing: Vol. 17.* Springer-Dortrecht.

Benner, P. (1990). The moral dimensions of caring. In J. S. Stevenson & T. Tripp-Reimer (Eds.), *Knowledge about care and caring: State of the art and future developments* (pp. 5–17). Academy of Nursing.

Benner, P. (1994). Discovering challenges to ethical theory in experience-based narratives of nurses' everyday ethical comportment. In J. F. Monagle & D. C. Thomasma (Eds.), *Health care ethics: Critical issues* (pp. 401–411). Aspen Publishers.

Benner, P. (1996). The primacy of caring and the role of experience, narrative, and community in clinical and ethical expertise. In P. Benner, C. A. Tanner, & C. A. Chesla (Eds.), *Expertise in nursing practice: Caring, clinical judgment, and ethics* (pp. 232–237). Springer Publishing Company.

Benner, P. (2000). The roles of embodiment, emotion and life world for rationality and agency in nursing practice. *Nursing Philosophy, 1*(1), 5–19.

Benner, P. (2009). Expertise in nursing practice, caring, clinical judgement & ethics (2nd ed.). Springer Publishing.

Benner, P., & Tanner, C. (1987). Clinical judgment: How expert nurses use intuition. *The American Journal of Nursing, 87*(1), 23–31.

Benner, P., & Wrubel, J. (1989). *The primacy of caring. Stress and coping in health and illness.* Addison-Wesley.

Biin, D., Canada, D., Chenowith, J., et al. (2021). *Pulling together: A guide for researchers, Hitk'ala.* (sec. 3). https://opentextbc.ca/indigenizationresearchers/chapter/indigenous-ethics-and-mindset/

Bodie, B., Brodell, R. T., & Helm, S. (2018). Shortages of lidocaine with epinephrine: Causes and solutions. *Journal of the American Academy of Dermatology, 79*(2), 322–393.

Bouchard, D., & Martin, J. (2009). *The seven sacred teachings of White Buffalo Calf Woman.* More Than Words Publishers. http://www.btgwinnipeg.ca/uploads/5/2/4/1/52412159/the_seven_sacred_teachings_.pdf

Bradshaw, A. (2011). Compassion: What history teaches us. *Nursing Times, 107*(19/20), 12–14.

Bradshaw, A. R. (1999). The virtue of nursing: the covenant of care. *Journal of Medical Ethics 25*, 477–481

Brannigan, M. (2000). Cultural diversity and the case against ethical relativism. *Health Care Analysis, 8*(3), 321–327.

Brant, C. (1990). Native ethics and rules of behaviour. *The Canadian Journal of Psychiatry, 35*(6), 534–539.

Brian Sinclair Working Group. (2017). *Out of Sight.* https://www.dropbox.com/s/wxf3v5uh2pun0pf/Out%20of%20Sight%20Final.pdf?d=0

Brilowski, G. A., & Wendler, M. C. (2005). An evolutionary concept analysis of caring. *Journal of Advanced Nursing, 50*(6), 641–650.

Brown, M. B., & Gilligan, C. (1992). Meeting at the crossroads: Women's psychology and girls' development. *Feminism & Psychology, 3*(1), 11–35.

Bruno, B., Shalowitz, D. I., & Arora, K. S. (2021). Ethical challenges for women's healthcare highlighted by the COVID-19 pandemic. *Journal of Medical Ethics, 47*(2), 69–72.

Bufacchi, V. (2017). Colonialism, injustice, and arbitrariness. *Journal of Social Philosophy, 48*(2), 197–211.

Burston, M., & Tuckett. (2013). Moral distress in nursing: Contributing factors, outcomes and interventions. *Health Education Journal, 20*(3), 312–324.

Camic, C. (1979). The utilitarians revisited. *American Journal of Sociology, 85*(3).

Canada, Royal Commission on Indigenous Peoples. (1996). *Report of the Royal Commission on Aboriginal Peoples. Volume 1: Looking forward, looking back* (Ch. 10). Supply and Services Canada.

Canadian Council for Practical Nurse Regulators (2013). *Code of ethics for licensed practical nurses in Canada.*

Canadian Nurses Association. (2017). *Code of ethics for registered nurses.*

Canadian Women's Foundation (2021). *Indigenous firsts: 14 Indigenous women to know on National Indigenous Peoples Day.* https://canadianwomen.org/blog/indigenous-firsts-14-indigenous-women-to-know-on-national-indigenous-peoples-day/

Castellano, M. B. (2000). Updating Aboriginal traditions of knowledge. In G. J. Sefa Dei, B. L. Hall, & D. G. Rosenberg (Eds.), *Indigenous knowledge in global contexts: Multiple readings of our world.* University of Toronto Press.

Catlett, S., & Lovan, S. R. (2011). Being a good nurse doing the right thing: A replication study. *Nursing Ethics, 18*(1), 54–63.

CFI Education Inc. (2022, March 16). *Social justice.* https://corporatefinanceinstitute.com/resources/knowledge/other/social-justice/

Cha, M., Haddadi, H., Benevenuto, F., et al. (2010). Measuring user influence in Twitter: The million follower fallacy. *Proceedings of the Fourth International Conference on Weblogs and Social Media, 4*(1), 10–17.

Chan, T. W., Poon, E., & Hegney, D. G. (2011). What nurses need to know about Buddhist perspectives of end-of-life care and dying. *Progress in Palliative Care, 19*(2), 61–65.

Chandler, M. J., & Lalonde, C. E. (2004). Transferring whose knowledge? Exchanging whose best practices? On knowing about Indigenous knowledge and Aboriginal suicide. *Aboriginal Policy Research Consortium International, 144*(2), 111–123.

Chandler, M. J., & Lalonde, C. E. (2019). Cultural continuity and Indigenous youth suicide. In *Suicide and Social Justice* (pp. 53–70). Routledge.

Chokr, N. (1992). Feminist perspectives on reproductive technologies: The politics of motherhood. *Technology in society, 14,* 317–333.

Cloyes, K. G. (2002). Agonizing care: Care ethics, agonistic feminism and a political theory of care. *Nursing Inquiry, 9*(3), 301–314.

Commission on the Social Determinants of Health. (2008). Closing the gap in a generation: *Achieving health equity through action on the social determinants of health.* World Health Organization.

Condon, E. H. (1992). Nursing and the caring metaphor: Gender and political influences on an ethic of care. *Nursing Outlook, 40*(1), 14–19.

Cooper, M. C. (1988). Covenantal relationships: Grounding for the nursing ethic. *Advances in nursing science, 10*(4), 48–59.

Cooper, M. C. (1991). Principle-oriented ethics and the ethic of care: A creative tension. *Advances in Nursing Science, 4,* 22–31.

Copp, D. (2007). Introduction: Metaethics and normative ethics. In *The Oxford Handbook of Ethical Theory.* Oxford University Press.

Correctional Services Canada. (2021). *Indigenous healing lodges.* https://www.csc-scc.gc.ca/002/003/002003-2000-en.shtml

Crowley, M. A. (1989). Feminist pedagogy: Nurturing the ethical ideal. *Advances in Nursing Science, 11*(3), 53–61.

Crowley, M. A. (1994). The relevance of Noddings' ethics of care to the moral education of nurses. *Journal of Nursing Education, 33*(2), 74–80.

Cudd, A., & Andreasen, R. (2005). *Feminist theory: A philosophical anthology.* Wiley-Blackwell.

Dawson, K., & Singer, P. (1988). Australian developments in reproductive technology. *Hastings Center Report, 18*(2), 4.

Dean, R. (2006). *The value of humanity in Kant's moral theory.* Clarendon Press.

DeMarco, J. P. (2005). Principlism and moral dilemmas: A new principle. *Journal of Medical Ethics, 31,* 101–105.

Donaldson, C. M. (2017). Using Kantian ethics in medical ethics education. *Medical Science Editor, 27,* 841–845.

Downie, J., & Sherwin, S. (2013) Feminist health care ethics consultation. *Research Papers, Working Papers, Conference Papers.* 18. https://digitalcommons.schulichlaw.dal.ca/working_papers/18

Dwyer, S. (1999). Moral competence. In K. Murasugi & R. Stainton (Eds.), *Philosophy and Linguistics*, (pp. 169–190). Westview Press.

Eaton, M. (2004). *Ethics and the business of bioscience.* Stanford University Press.

Engelhardt, H. T. (1986). *The foundations of bioethics.* Oxford University Press.

Epstein, E., & Delgado, S. (2010). Understanding and addressing moral distress. *The Online Journal of Issues in Nursing, 15*(3), Manuscript 1.

Fiester, A. (2007). Why the clinical ethics we teach fails patients. *Academic Medicine Journals, 82*(7), 684–689.

Fowler, M. D. (2021). The nightingale still sings: Ten ethical themes in early nursing in the United Kingdom, 1888–1989. *The Online Journal of Issues in Nursing, 26*(2).

Fox, E. M. (1914). *First lines in nursing.* Scientific Press.

Frankena, W. (1973). *Ethics* 2nd ed. Prentice-Hall N.J. p. 47.

Frederiksen, C. S., & Nielsen, M. E. J. (2013). Ethical theories. In S. O. Idowu, N. Capaldi, I. Zu, et al. (Eds.), *Encyclopedia of Corporate Social Responsibility.* Springer. https://doi.org/10.1007/978-3-642-28036-8_613

Freeman, S. (1994). Utilitarianism, deontology, and the priority of right. *Philosophy of Public Affairs, 23*(4), 313–349.

Friesen, P. (2020). Trust in health care after the death of Joyce Exhaquan. *Impact Ethics: Making a Difference in Bioethics.* https://

impactethics.ca/2020/11/09/trust-in-health-care-after-the-death-of-joyce-echaquan/

Fry, S. T. (1989). Toward a theory of nursing ethics. *Advances in Nursing Science, 11*(4), 9–22. https://doi.org/10.1097/00012272-198907000-00005

Gandjour, A., & Lauterback, K. W. (2003). Utilitarian theories reconsidered: Common misconceptions, more recent developments, and health policy implications. *Health Care Analysis, 11*(3), 220–244.

Geddes, G. (2017). *Medicine unbundled: A journey through the minefields of Indigenous health care.* Heritage House.

Gilligan, C. (1982). *In a different voice. Psychological theory and women's development.* Harvard University Press.

Gilligan, C. (1995a). Hearing the difference: Theorizing connection. *Hypatia, 10*(2), 120–127.

Gilligan, C. (1995b). Moral orientation and moral development. In C. Held (Ed.), *Justice and care: Essential readings in feminist ethics* (Ch. 2). Westview Press.

Gilligan, C., & Attanucci, J. (1996). The moral principles of care. In *Introducing psychological research.* Palgrave Publishing.

Government of Canada. (2019). *Jordan's Principle: Substantive equality principles. What is substantive equality?* https://sac-isc.gc.ca/eng/1568396042341/1568396159824#chp02

Government of Canada. (2020). *COVID-19 pandemic guidance for the health care sector.* https://www.canada.ca/en/public-health/services/diseases/2019-novel-coronavirus-infection/health-professionals/covid-19-pandemic-guidance-health-care-sector.html

Government of Canada (2021a). *Budget 2021: Supporting Woman. Department of Finance Canada.* https://www.canada.ca/en/department-finance/news/2021/04/budget-2021-supporting-women.html#:~:text=Establishing%20A%20Canada-Wide%20Early%20Learning%20and%20Child%20Care%20System

Government of Canada (2021b). *Public health ethics framework: A guide for use in response to the COVID-19 pandemic in Canada.* https://www.canada.ca/en/public-health/services/diseases/2019-novel-coronavirus-infection/canadas-reponse/ethics-framework-guide-use-response-covid-19-pandemic.html

Government of Canada. (2022a, January 24). *Agreements-in-principle reached on compensation and long-term reform of First Nations Child and Family Services and Jordan's Principle* [Press release]. https://www.canada.ca/en/indigenous-services-canada/news/2022/01/agreements-in-principle-reached-on-compensation-andlong-term-reform-of-first-nations-child-and-family-service-sand-jordans-principle.html

Government of Canada, (2022b). Federal gender equality laws in Canada. https://www.international.gc.ca

Government of Canada. (2023, March 6). *Jordan's Principle: About Jordan's Principle.* https://sac-isc.gc.ca/eng/1568396042341/1568396159824#chp02

Grassian, V. (1992). Moral reasoning: Ethical theory and some contemporary moral problems. Prentice-Hall.

Greenwood, M., & MacDonald, N. (2021). *Vaccine mistrust: A legacy of colonialism* (RSC COVID-19 Series, Publication #102). https://rsc-src.ca/en/voices/vaccine-mistrust-legacy-colonialism

Hanson, E., Gamez, D., & Manuel, A. (2020, September). The residential school system. *Indigenous Foundations.* https://indigenousfoundations.arts.ubc.ca/residential-school-system-2020/

Haslam-Larmer, L., Grigorovich, A., Quirt, H., et al. (2022). Prevalence, causes, and consequences of moral distress in healthcare providers caring for people living with dementia in long-term care during a pandemic. *Dementia, 22*(1), 5–270(0).

Häyry, M. (2021). Just better utilitarianism. *Cambridge Quarterly of Healthcare Ethics, 30*(2), 343–367.

Hines-Martin, V., & Nash, W., (2017). Social justice, social determinants of health, interprofessional practice and community engagement as formative elements of a nurse practitioner managed health center. *International Journal of Nursing and Clinical Practice, 4*, 218–223.

Holtz, H., Heinze, K., & Rushton, C. (2018). Interprofessionals' definitions of moral resilience. *Journal of Clinical Nursing, 27*(3-4), e488–e494.

Hoyt S. J (2010). Florence Nightingale's contribution to contemporary nursing ethics. *Holistic Nursing, 4*, 331–332.

Hursthouse, R. (1999). *On virtue ethics.* Oxford University Press.

Indigenous Corporate Training. (2017). *A brief look at Indian hospitals in Canada.* https://www.ictinc.ca/blog/a-brief-look-at-indian-hospitals-in-canada-0

Inglehart, R. (1977). *The silent revolution: Changing values and political styles among Western publics.* Princeton University Press.

Institute for Patient and Family-Centered Care. (2021). *Family presence during a pandemic: Guidance for decision makers.* https://www.ipfcc.org/events/IPFCC_Family_Presence.pdf

Internet Encyclopedia of Philosophy. (n.d.). Health care ethics. https://iep.utm.edu/h-c-ethi/#SH2a

Izumi, S., Konishi, E., Yahiro, M., et al. (2006). Japanese patients' descriptions of "the good nurse": Personal involvement and professionalism. *Advances in Nursing Science, 29*(2), E14–E26.

Jameton, A. (1984). *Nursing practice: The ethical issues.* Prentice-Hall.

Jochelson, K. (2006). Nanny or steward? The role of government in public health. *Public Health, 120*(12), 1149–1155.

Johnston, P., Keatings, M., & Monk, A. (2022) Experiences of essential care partners during the COVID-19 pandemic [Special issue]. *Healthcare Quarterly, 25*, 41–47.

Joseph, B., & Joseph C. F. (2019). *Indigenous relations: Insights, tips and suggestions to make reconciliation a reality.* Indigenous Relations Press.

Kamel, G. (2021). Investigation report: Law on the investigation of the causes and circumstances of death for the protection of human of life concerning the death of Joyce Echaquan, 2020–00275. https://www.coroner.gouv.qc.ca/fileadmin/Enquetes_publiques/2020-06375-40_002__1__sans_logo_anglais.pdf

Kant, I. (2007). *Groundwork of the metaphysics of morals.* (P. Guyer, Ed.). Continuum International Publishing Group. (Original work published 1785).

Keller, D. (2009). *A brief overview of basic ethical theory.* SelectedWorks.

Kitayama, S., & Uskul, A. K. (2011). Culture, mind, and the brain: Current evidence and future directions. *Annual Reviews of Psychoogy, 62*, 419–449.

Kranak, J. (2022). Kantian deontology. In Matthews, G. (Ed.), *Introduction to philosophy: Ethics* (Ch. 6). Rebus. https://press.rebus.community/intro-to-phil-ethics/

Lamiani, G., & Borghi, J. (2017). When health care professionals cannot do the right thing: A systematic review of moral distress and its correlates. *Journal of Health Psychology, 22*(1), 56–57.

Landauer, J., & Rowlands, J. (2001). *Importance of philosophy.* http://www.importanceofphilosophy.com/Ethics_Rationality.html

Larrabee, M. J. (2016). An ethic of care: Feminist and interdisciplinary perspectives. Routledge.

Lind, A., Wilburn, S., & Pate, E. (1986). Power from within: Feminism and the ethical decision-making process in nursing. *Nursing Administration Quarterly, 10*(3), 50–57.

Linden, A. (2016). Toward tort liability for bad Samaritans. *Alberta Law Review, 53*(4), 837.

Linden, A. M., Feldthusen, B. P., Hall, M. I., et al. (2018). *Canadian tort law* (11th ed.). LexisNexis Canada.

Lux, M. K. (2016). *Separate beds: A history of Indian hospitals in Canada, 1920s–1980s.* University of Toronto Press.

Mahon, R., & Robinson, F. (2011). *Feminist ethics and social policy: Towards a new global political economy of care.* UBC Press.

Malmsten, K. (2000). Basic care, bodily knowledge and feminist ethics. *Medicine & Law, 19*(3), 613–622.

Mandal, J., Ponnambath, D. K., & Parija, S. C. (2016). Utilitarian and deontological ethics in medicine. *Tropical Parasitology, 6*(1), 5–7.

Mandhane, R. (2000). Duty to rescue through the lens of multiple-party sexual assault. *Dalhousie Journal of Legal Studies, 9*(1), 1–35.

Marmot, M., Allen, J., Goldblatt, P., et al. (2020). *Build back fairer: The COVID-19 Marmot review. The pandemic, socioeconomic and health inequalities in England.* Institute of Health Equity. https://www.instituteofhealthequity.org/resources-reports/build-back-fairer-the-covid-19-marmot-review

McCarthy, J. (2002). Principlism or narrative ethics: Must we choose between them? *Medical Humanities, 29*(2), 65–71.

Mill, J. S. (1948). *On liberty and considerations on representative government.* B. Blackwell.

Mill, J. S., & Warnock, M. (2003). *Utilitarianism and on liberty: Including "Essay on Bentham" and selections from the writings of Jeremy Bentham and John Austin.* B Blackwell.

Millette, B. E. (1994). Using Gilligan's framework to analyze nurses' stories of moral choices. *Western Journal of Nursing Research, 16*(6), 660–674.

Nelson, A., Parra, M. T., Kim-Farley, R., et al. (2012). Ethical issues concerning vaccination requirements. *Public Health Reviews, 34*(14), 1–20.

Nicholas, D., & Keatings M. (Eds.). (n.d.) *Inter-professional collaboration in family-centred care.* Manuscript in progress.

Nightingale, F. (1882). Nursing the sick. In R. Quain (Ed.), *A dictionary of medicine* (pp. 1043–1049). Longmans, Green, and Co.

Nightingale, F. (1934). Profession with vocation. *The Nursing Times, 30*(1518), 528–529.

Nisbett, R., Peng, K., Choi, I., et al. (2001). Culture and systems of thought: Holistic versus analytic cognition. *Psychology Reviews, 108*(2), 291–310.

Noddings, N. (1984). *Caring: A feminine approach to ethics and moral education.* University of California Press.

Noddings, N. (1992). In defense of caring. *Journal of Clinical Ethics, 3*(1), 15–18.

Norlock, K. (2019, May 27). Feminist ethics. In *The Stanford encyclopedia of philosophy.* https://plato.stanford.edu/entries/feminism-ethics/

Oddi, L., Cassidy, V., & Fisher, C. (2016). Nurses' sensitivity to the ethical aspects of clinical practice, *Nursing Ethics, 2*(3), 197–209.

Olsen, D. (1992). Controversies in nursing ethics: A historical review. *Journal of Advanced Nursing, 17*, 1020–1027.

O'Neill, O. (2013). *Acting on principle: An essay on Kantian ethics* (2nd ed.). Cambridge University Press.

Parker, R. S. (1990). Nurses' stories: The search for a relational ethic of care. *Advances in Nursing Science, 13*(1), 31–40.

Pellegrino, E. D. (1995). Toward a virtue-based normative ethics for the health professions. *Kennedy Institute of Ethics Journal, 5*(3), 253–277.

Peter, E., & Gallop, R. (1994). The ethic of care: A comparison of nursing and medical students. *Journal of Nursing Scholarship, 26*(1), 47–52.

Peter, E. (2013). Advancing the concept of moral distress. *Journal of Bioethical Inquiry, 10*(3), 293–295.

Peter, E., & Morgan, K. P. (2001). Explorations of a trust approach for nursing ethics. *Nursing Inquiry, 8*(1), 3–10.

Petten, C. (2017). *Clare Clifton Brant: Mohawk man and doctor used his gifts well.* https://windspeaker.com/news/footprints/clare-clifton-brant-mohawk-man-and-doctor-used-his-gifts-well/

Rawls, J. (1971). *A theory of justice.* Harvard University Press.

Rawls, J. (1996). *Political liberalism.* Columbia University Press.

Reich, W. T. (Ed.). (1995). *Encyclopedia of bioethics.* Simon & Schuster/Macmillan.

Rodney, P. A. (2017). What we know about moral distress. *The American Journal of Nursing, 117*(2), S7–S10.

Rogers W. A. (2006). Feminism and public health ethics. *Journal of Medical Ethics, 32*(6), 351–354.

Ross, D., & Stratton-Lake, P. (Eds.). (2002). *The right and the good.* Clarendon Press.

Rushton, C. H. (2008). Defining and addressing moral distress: Tools for critical care nursing leaders. *AACN Advanced Critical Care, 17*(2), 161–168.

Rushton, C. H., Schoonover-Shoffner, K., & Kennedy, M. S. (2017). A collaborative state of the Science Initiative: Transforming moral distress into moral resilience in nursing. *American Journal of Nursing, 117*(2), S2–S6. doi:10.1097/01.NAJ.0000512203.08844.1d

Salwin, M. B., & Dupagne, M. B. (1999). The third-person effect: Perceptions of the media's influence and immoral consequences. *Communication Research, 26*(5), 523–549.

Savulescu, J., Persson, I., & Wilkinson, D. (2020). Utilitarianism and the pandemic. *Bioethics, 34*(6), 620–632.

Scott P. A. (1995). Aristotle, nursing and health care ethics. *Nursing Ethics. 2*(4), 279–285. doi:10.1177/096973309500200402

Scott, P. A. (2000). Emotion, moral perception, and nursing. *Nursing Philosophy, 1*(2), 123–133.

Selanders, L. C., & Crane, P. C. (2012) The voice of Florence Nightingale on advocacy. *Online Journal of Issues in Nursing, 17*(1), 1.

Sellman, D. (1997). The virtues in the moral education of nurses: Florence Nightingale revisited. *Nursing Ethics, 4*(1), 3–11.

Sellman, D. (2011). Professional values and nursing. *Medicine, Health Care and Philosophy, 14*(2), 203–208.

Shai, A., Koffler, S., & Hashiloni-Dolev, Y. (2021). Feminism, gender medicine and beyond: A feminist analysis of "gender medicine." *International Journal of Equity in Health, 20*(1), 177.

Sherwin, S. (1989). Feminist and medical ethics: Two different approaches to contextual ethics. *Hypatia, 4*(2), 57–72.

Sherwin, S. (1992). *No longer patient.* Temple University Press.

Sherwin, S. (1998). A relationship to autonomy in health care. In *The Feminist Health Care Ethics Research Network, The politics of women's health: Exploring agency and autonomy* (Ch. 2). Temple University Press.

Singer, P. (2011). *Practical ethics.* Cambridge University Press.

Statistics Canada. (2019). *Suicide among First Nations people, Métis and Inuit (2011–2016): Findings from the 2011 Canadian Census Health and Environment Cohort (CanCHEC).* https://www150. statcan.gc.ca/n1/pub/99-011-x/99-011-x2019001-eng.htm

SuperSummary. (2022). *Utilitarianism.* https://www.supersummary. com/utilitarianism/summary/

Tashjian, A. (2017). The ethical implications of the medical community's failure to differentiate sex- and gender-based medicine from women's health. *Frontiers in Women's Health, 2*(2), 1–4.

Taylor, C. (2019). Personal communication, March 25, 2019.

Throsby, K. (2004). *When IVF fails.* Palgrave Macmillan. https://doi. org/10.1057/9780230505704_2

Tiwari, S., & Agarwal, L. (2020, June 23). Flogging as criminal punishment in the 21st century. *JURIST.* https://www.jurist.org/ commentary/2020/06/tiwari-agarwal-flogging-punishment/

Tong, R. (1995). Feminine and feminist ethics. *Social Philosophy Today, 10*, 183–205.

UN Women. (2022). *Ending violence against women.* https://www. unwomen.org/en/about-us

Valentine, P. E. (1994). A female profession: A feminist management perspective. In J. M. Hibberd & M. E. Kyle (Eds.), *Nursing management in Canada* (pp. 372–390). W. B. Saunders.

Varcoe, C., Doane, G., Pauly, B., et al. (2004). Ethical practice in nursing: Working the in-betweens. *Journal of Advanced Nursing, 45*(3), 316–325.

Veatch, R. (1981). *A theory of medical ethics.* Basic Books.

Walker, T. (2009). What principlism misses. *Journal of Medical Ethics,* 35, 229–231.

Wallis, L. (2015). Moral distress in nursing. *The American Journal of Nursing, 115*(3), 19–20.

Waniskahk. (2020). *Waniskahk—Time to rise up* [App].

Watson, J. (1985). *Nursing: Human science and human care.* Appleton-Century-Crofts.

Watson, J. (1989). Transformative thinking and a caring curriculum. In E. U. Bevis & J. Watson (Eds.), *Toward a caring curriculum: A new pedagogy for nursing.* National League for Nursing.

Watson, J. (1992). Response to "caring, virtue theory, and a foundation for nursing ethics." *Scholarly Inquiry for Nursing Practice, 6*(2), 169–171.

Watson, J. (2008). *Nursing, the philosophy and science of caring* (Rev. ed.). University Press of Colorado.

Watson, M. J. (1988). New dimensions of human caring theory. *Nursing Science Quarterly, 1*(4), 175–181.

What is Rawls's difference principle? (2021, February 25). *eNotes Editorial.* https://www.enotes.com/homework-help/what-is-rawls-s-difference-principle-268116

White, E. M., Wetle, T. F., Reddy, A., et al. (2021). Front-line nursing home staff experiences during the COVID-19 pandemic. *Journal of the American Medical Directors Association, 22*(1), 199–203.

Wilson, B. (Ed.). (1970). *Rationality.* Wiley-Blackwell.

Wolf, S. M. (Ed.). (1996). *Feminism and bioethics: Beyond reproduction.* Oxford University Press.

Wood, A. W. (2008). *Kantian ethics.* Cambridge University Press.

World Health Organization (2021a). *COVID-19 and the social determinants of health and health equity: Evidence brief.* https://www. instituteofhealthequity.org/resources-reports/covid-19-the-social-determinants-of-health-and-health-equity-—-whoevidence-brief

World Health Organization. (2021b). *Vaccine equity.* https://www. who.int/campaigns/vaccine-equity

Zempi, I. (2016). "It's a part of me, I feel naked without it": Choice, agency and identity for Muslim women who wear the niqab. *Ethnic and Racial Studies, 39*(10), 1738–1754.

Zinkin, M. (2006). Respect for the law and the use of dynamical terms in Kant's theory of moral motivation. *De Gruyter, 88*(1), 31–53.

3 GUIDING ETHICAL DECISION MAKING: RESOURCES FOR NURSES

LEARNING OBJECTIVES

The purpose of this chapter is to enable you to understand:

- The historical development of *codes of ethics* and their influence on the nursing profession
- The application of the International Council of Nurses (ICN) *Code of Ethics for Nurses* and the Canadian Nurses Association *Code of Ethics for Registered Nurses* in ensuring ethical nursing care, guiding moral decision making, and clarifying the ethical obligations and responsibilities of nurses
- The interplay between professional standards and the ethical and legal principles that guide nursing practice
- The way professional practice guidelines support nurses in meeting the standards and values embedded in nursing codes of ethics
- The role of clinical ethics committees and clinical ethicists, and the resources they offer to nurses
- The value of using frameworks to guide ethical reflection and decision making

INTRODUCTION

Professional nurses are expected to think and act ethically within the context of trusting and respectful therapeutic relationships, while adapting to an ever changing sophisticated and complex health care system. As the fabric of society evolves, global challenges emerge, and new health policies and legislation are introduced, the complexity of the issues faced by nurses grows. Nurses are challenged to respond while continuing to provide safe, compassionate care to those most vulnerable.

In this chapter, the International Council of Nurses (ICN) *Code of Ethics for Nurses* and the Canadian Nurses Association (CNA) *Code of Ethics for Registered Nurses* are highlighted. These codes are founded on the theories, concepts, and principles described in Chapter 2 and emphasize the responsibilities and accountabilities of the professional nurse. In order to meet the ethical standards made explicit in these codes, frameworks and guidelines based on ethical theories and principles have been developed to guide ethical practice, assist nurses in meeting their moral duties and obligations, and facilitate the resolution of challenging ethical problems. To facilitate the application of these codes and ethical frameworks, case scenarios are provided to encourage discussion about the everyday ethical challenges nurses face. In addition, expert resources, such as ethics committees, Best Practice Guidelines, and ethicists are described.

CODES OF ETHICS

Standards for the ethical practice of professionals are expressed in codes of ethics. Historically, professions were created to serve the public interest and the common good. As part of its contract with society, a profession commits to the duties and obligations embedded in its role, mission, and ethical foundation (Jennings et al., 1987). The possession of such a code is regarded as a key characteristic of a profession and is a public declaration of the societal mission, values, commitments, and responsibilities of that profession

(Wall, 1995). As members of a professional body, nurses have a duty to their individual patients, but at a societal level, the profession influences policy on many issues, such as population health and social equity. In nursing, ethical codes offer standards that guide and support ethical practice across all domains and settings (Epstein & Turner, 2015).

Professional codes of ethics are grounded in moral theory and values. Because values and priorities shift over time, codes are reviewed regularly and are informed by members of the profession who seek to clarify the challenges they face and understand the ethical standards they must meet. Codes integrate such concepts as duty, virtue, and justice and are frequently based on ethical principles such as autonomy, beneficence, nonmaleficence, and fidelity.

Nursing codes of ethics are not only grounded in theories and principles but also highlight nursing theory and the values and concepts related to:

- Relationships
- Leadership
- Compassion and caring
- Communication
- Collaboration
- Social justice (CNA, 2017; Olsen & Stokes, 2016)

Having a code of ethics protects the integrity of a profession; it conveys the profession's commitment to the public and in doing so earns trust and respect. The public trusts that professionals will apply their knowledge and skills in the best interests of the individuals and communities they serve. To maintain this trust, it is essential that professionals maintain scrupulous standards of conduct and be accountable to the public (Epstein & Turner, 2015; Jennings et al., 1987). To that end, a profession's code articulates its ethical standards and obligations to the people it serves and to society as a whole (Jennings et al., 1987). The code defines acceptable and unacceptable behaviours, rules of conduct, and professional values and responsibilities. A profession's code conveys and clarifies the principles that guide an individual member's decisions and actions.

Nursing codes of ethics not only outline the values, duties, and responsibilities of the nurse but also place emphasis on the role of the nurse as a **moral agent**. As moral agents, nurses identify moral issues or challenges, make moral choices, and take steps toward their resolution. Acting as a moral agent can be challenging within the complex realities of health care, so codes of ethics offer guidance in meeting this responsibility (Fortier & Malloy, 2019; Grace, 2018).

Codes also provide a standard against which a nurse is evaluated if disciplinary action is taken by a regulatory body (Chapter 5) or legal action is brought against the nurse in the courts (CNA, 2017, p. 2; Chapter 7).

THE HISTORY OF CODES OF ETHICS

Codes of ethics have a long tradition and history as illustrated by the examples of codes that follow. Their foundational principles have been consistent over time, but the interpretation and application of these principles have changed as cultures and their values have evolved (Boxes 3.1, 3.2, and 3.3).

THE HISTORY OF NURSING CODES OF ETHICS

As noted, a key characteristic of a profession is having a code of ethics that makes clear the obligations and responsibilities of that profession to society. The evolution of codes of ethics in nursing mirrors the growth of nursing as a profession (Viens, 1989). Early nursing

---

BOX 3.1
THE HISTORY OF THE CODE OF HAMMURABI (1780 B.C.E.)

The first recorded collection of laws or codes in history was established in the Babylonian empire by King Hammurabi (1795–1750 B.C.E.), who stated his intent "to bring about the rule of righteousness in the land, to destroy the wicked and the evil-doers; so that the strong should not harm the weak; so that I should . . . enlighten the land, to further the well-being of mankind." Though the code established important legal standards for trade and social relationships, it is an illustration of the cultural values of the time. For example, while the code calls for fairness in society, it also includes the idea of retribution as a form of justice, is paternalistic in nature, and reflects the class distinctions of Babylonia at the time.

Babylonians. (n.d.). http://home.cfl.rr.com/crossland/AncientCivilizations/Middle_East_Civilizations/Babylonians/babylonians.html; Hooker, R. (1996). *Mesopotamia: The Code of Hammurabi* (L. W. King, Trans.). Washington State University; Horne, C. F., & Johns, C. H. W. (1911). Ancient history sourcebook: Code of Hammurabi, c. 1780 BCE. In *The Encyclopaedia Britannica* (11th ed.). Britannica Books.

BOX 3.2
THE HIPPOCRATIC OATH (400 B.C.E.)

This oath, traditionally taken by physicians, is believed to have been written in the fourth century B.C.E. by Hippocrates, who is considered to be the father of medicine. The oath integrates various ancient texts that speak to the expected behaviour of physicians and their relationships with patients. The key components, values, and laws of the original oath are consistent with the principles included in many contemporary codes. The following summary illustrates how elements of the oath relate to contemporary ethical principles.

BENEFICENCE AND NONMALEFICENCE

"I will use those dietary regimens which will benefit my patients according to my greatest ability and judgement, and I will do no harm or injustice to them."

SANCTITY OF LIFE

"I will not give a lethal drug to anyone if I am asked, nor will I advise such a plan; and similarly, I will not give a woman a pessary to cause an abortion. In purity and according to divine law will I carry out my life and my art."

COMPETENCE

"I will not use the knife, even upon those suffering from stones, but I will leave this to those who are trained in this craft."

PROFESSIONAL INTEGRITY

"Into whatever homes I go, I will enter them for the benefit of the sick, avoiding any voluntary act of impropriety or corruption, including the seduction of women or men, whether they are free men or slaves."

PRIVACY AND CONFIDENTIALITY

"Whatever I see or hear in the lives of my patients, whether in connection with my professional practice or not, which ought not to be spoken of outside, I will keep secret, as considering all such things to be private."

National Library of Medicine. (2002). *The Hippocratic oath* (M. North, Trans.). http://www.nlm.nih.gov/hmd/greek/greek_oath.html

BOX 3.3
THE NUREMBERG CODE (1947)

In the aftermath of World War II, Nazi officials, accused of unethical human experimentation, were tried at Nuremberg. At the time, there were no existing rules or laws to guide research on human subjects. Hence, the *Nuremberg Code* was established in 1947 to address issues such as informed consent, the competence of the investigator, and the balance of harm and benefit to the research subject. This code continues to be the ethical foundation for research on human subjects today. The following excerpts from the code clarify the relationship of its elements to key ethical principles.

PRINCIPLE OF INFORMED CONSENT
(AUTONOMY, RESPECT FOR PERSONS)

"The duty and responsibility for ascertaining the quality of the consent rests upon each individual who initiates, directs, or engages in the experiment. The human subject must:
- Give voluntary consent
- Have the legal capacity to give consent
- Be able to exercise free power of choice, without the intervention of any element of force, fraud, deceit, duress, overreaching, or other ulterior form of constraint or coercion
- Have sufficient knowledge and comprehension of the elements of the subject matter involved to understand and make an enlightened decision
- Understand the nature, duration, and purpose of the experiment; the method and means by which it is to be

conducted; all inconveniences and hazards reasonably to be expected; and the effects upon his health or person which may possibly come from his participation in the experiment
- Be at liberty to bring the experiment to an end if he has reached the physical or mental state where continuation of the experiment seems to him to be impossible"

CONTRIBUTE TO THE GREATER GOOD
(BENEFICENCE)

"The experiment should:
- Yield fruitful results for the good of society, unprocurable by other methods or means of study, and not random and unnecessary in nature
- Be designed and based on the results of animal experimentation and a knowledge of the natural history of the disease or other problem under study that the anticipated results will justify the performance of the experiment"

DO NO HARM (NONMALEFICENCE)

"The experiment should:
- Be conducted as to avoid all unnecessary physical and mental suffering and injury
- Not be conducted where there is an *a priori* reason to believe that death or disabling injury will occur, except, perhaps, in those experiments where the experimental physicians also serve as subjects

BOX 3.3—cont'd
THE NUREMBERG CODE (1947)

■ Ensure that proper preparations should be made and adequate facilities provided to protect the experimental subject against even remote possibilities of injury, disability, or death"

RISK BENEFIT (BENEFICENCE VERSUS NONMALEFICENCE)
"The researcher should ensure that:
■ The degree of risk to be taken should never exceed that determined by the humanitarian importance of the problem to be solved by the experiment
■ The experiment be conducted by scientifically qualified persons

■ The research be terminated at any stage if there is probable cause to believe that a continuation of the experiment is likely to result in injury, disability, or death to the experimental subject"

Canadian Institutes of Health Research, Natural Sciences and Engineering Research Council of Canada, & Social Sciences and Humanities Research Council of Canada (2014). *Tri-council policy statement: Ethical conduct for research involving humans*; The Nuremberg Code (1947). (1996). *British Medical Journal, 313*, 1448. https://www.bmj.com/content/313/7070/1448.1

codes and curriculum in nursing schools focused on the character and behaviour of the nurse and had a strong foundation in Christian morality.

Recognized as the founder of nursing as a profession, Florence Nightingale's view of nursing ethics was grounded in this Christian tradition. She saw nursing as a calling from God and promoted a moral education of nurses, based on Aristotelian thinking (Sellman, 1997). Aristotle placed a strong emphasis on virtue, character, perception, and emotion in moral decision making, which, some argue, continues to have relevance for nursing ethics today (Scott, 1995). Subscribing to this Aristotelian tradition, early in the profession, great emphasis was based on the virtues, values, and moral character of the nurse. Nightingale's virtue-based nursing ethics was built on the premise that the nurse, while caring for patients, should be motivated by intrinsic values that seek to meet high moral standards. She believed that these values ought to include such traits as honesty, trustworthiness, patience, compassion, honour, moral courage, and devotion (Nightingale, 1882). She promoted that commitment to these ideals was the distinguishing feature of the profession and fundamental to the moral value of the nurse–patient relationship (Armstrong, 2006; Fowler, 2021; Hoyt, 2010; Scott, 1995; Sellman, 1997).

Nightingale's approach to ethics also included attention to etiquette, the rules and standards of behaviour. The rules applied to how student nurses behaved not only in the hospital wards but also in their residences and in public (Levine, 1999). Nurses were expected to be role models in the community, and as such needed to exhibit strong virtuous behaviour and character at all times (Aikens, 1926).

Nightingale not only had a strong belief in the importance of caring in nursing but also was an early leader in quality management (Meyer & Bishop, 2007). As well, she promoted ongoing learning toward the achievement of high standards of practice. When offering advice to nursing students in 1873, Nightingale made the following remarks:

Nursing is most truly said to be a high calling, an honourable calling. But what does the honour lie in? In working hard during your training to learn and to do all things perfectly? The honour does not lie in putting on Nursing like your uniform. Honour lies in loving perfection, consistency and in working hard for it: in being ready to work patiently: ready to say not "how clever I am!" but "I am not yet worthy; and I will live to deserve to be a Trained Nurse." (Sellman, 1997)

She is viewed as a forerunner in influencing policy related to societal health and social equity and an early proponent of the importance of the social determinants of health (Falk-Rafael, 2005; Selanders & Crane, 2012). The CNA *Code of Ethics*, discussed later in this chapter, addresses these important concepts of caring and compassion, social justice, and equity. Social justice is explored in more detail in Chapter 2.

Her philosophy is embedded in the **Nightingale Pledge**. This pledge was written by a committee chaired by Lystra Gretter, a nursing instructor at Harper Hospital in Detroit, Michigan, and was first used by its graduating class in the spring of 1893. It was, in fact, an adaptation of the Hippocratic oath taken by physicians (Nightingale, n.d.), see Fig. 3.1.

THE FLORENCE NIGHTINGALE PLEDGE

~ ~

I SOLEMNLY PLEDGE MYSELF BEFORE GOD AND IN THE PRESENCE OF THIS ASSEMBLY TO PASS MY LIFE IN PURITY AND TO PRACTICE MY PROFESSION FAITHFULLY. I WILL ABSTAIN FROM WHATEVER IS DELETERIOUS AND MISCHIEVOUS, AND WILL NOT TAKE OR KNOWINGLY ADMINISTER ANY HARMFUL DRUG.

I WILL DO ALL IN MY POWER TO MAINTAIN AND ELEVATE THE STANDARD OF MY PROFESSION, AND WILL HOLD IN CONFIDENCE ALL PERSONAL MATTERS COMMITTED TO MY KEEPING, AND ALL FAMILY AFFAIRS COMING TO MY KNOWLEDGE IN THE PRACTICE OF MY CALLING.

WITH LOYALTY WILL I ENDEAVOR TO AID THE PHYSICIAN IN HIS WORK, AND DEVOTE MYSELF TO THE WELFARE OF THOSE COMMITTED TO MY CARE.

Fig. 3.1 ■ The pledge card was presented to early graduates at Toronto's Women's College Hospital, School of Nursing by Clara Dixon, the hospital's first nurse. The Nightingale Pledge, often recited at graduation ceremonies. *Source: The Miss Margaret Robins Archives of Women's College Hospital, School of Nursing fonds, K1-10.*

Other nursing leaders continued this philosophical tradition. **Isabel Robb (1860–1910)**, also an early influencer in the nursing profession, contributed to the advancement of nursing theory and education, specifically related to the establishment of standards and the evaluation of students' abilities and qualifications. In her book *Nursing Ethics for Hospital and Private Use* (Robb, 1900), she also emphasized the conduct and behaviour of nurses. The following excerpt from Robb's book illustrates this approach and how the nurse is expected . . .

To always yield a cheerful and prompt obedience to those in authority and to give up one's own will; . . . to keep up pleasant relations with other nurses, some of whom may be uncongenial, . . . to render a ready compliance to the many little and seemingly capricious demands of patients, especially when they come at the end of a long day's work, when her own back is aching and her feet are tired, or when she may not be feeling well herself, all these must be looked upon as affording opportunities for self-control and self-discipline. The true nurses must be "all things to all men." (Robb, 1900)

This moral tradition focused not only on the key duties and principles that guide the ethical care and well-being of patients, but also the importance of the nurse's strong commitment to God and religion, the expectation that would live a pure and virtuous life. For much of the early part of the 1900s, the moral education of the nurse continued to focus on obedience, compliance with rules, and etiquette rather than judgement, reflection, and critical thinking (Kelly, 1981). The nurse was also expected to be loyal and deferential to the physician, who was considered the leader. This is in contrast to today's environment, where the physician and nurse are collaborators within a broader health care team.

Charlotte Aikens, an American nursing leader, wrote in her 1926 text *"Studies in Ethics for Nurses"*:

Loyalty to the physician is one of the duties demanded of every nurse, not solely because the physician is her superior officer, but chiefly because the confidence of the patient in his physician is one of the important elements in the management of his illness, and nothing should be said or done that would weaken this faith or create doubts as to the character or ability or methods of the physician on whom he is depending. (Aikens, 1926, p. 2)

THE INTERNATIONAL COUNCIL OF NURSES

The ICN is a federation of more than 130 national nurses' associations and represents more than 27 million nurses worldwide. Founded in 1899 as the world's first international organization for health care professionals, its roots were based on movements associated with women's rights, social progressivism, and health care reform. In 1899, the forward-thinking nurses who founded ICN held their first provisional committee meeting at St. Bartholomew's Hospital, London, and by 1900 had developed and approved its constitution (ICN, 2022c).

The ICN advances the nursing profession and global health through its leadership, advocacy, policies, partnerships, networks, congresses, and special projects. A voluntary organization, nurses worldwide secure membership when they join their national nursing group. Governed by nurses, the organization influences nursing, global health, and social policy, and it establishes standards for the profession across the globe. It takes a leadership role internationally to ensure that nursing's voice is heard, and that care meets the highest possible standards through the advancement of knowledge and ensuring competent and engaged nurses (ICN, 2022d).

The ICN has strong alliances with international, national, and regional nursing and non-nursing organizations. It strives to build positive relationships with these stakeholders to position the organization and the profession to influence nursing and health across the globe now and into the future. The ICN engages with the United Nations, the World Health Organization (WHO), and other important agencies, such as the International Labour Organization and the World Bank. In addition, it works closely with a range of international nongovernmental organizations (ICN, 2022b).

Assuming an important leadership role, the ICN launched a major initiative to raise awareness and support for the achievement of the United Nations' Sustainable Development Goals (SDGs). The ICN has focused on raising awareness within the nursing profession of the SDGs and nurses' role in achieving them. For example, it recognizes the role of nurses in promoting good health and well-being; reducing inequalities within and between nations; and recognizing the influence on health of social factors such as education, income, sexual orientation, and ethnicity. The ICN has also wanted to ensure that the historical role of nursing in addressing these issues was recognized by leaders and international organizations (ICN, 2018).

The ICN, as the global voice for nurses, played an advocacy and leadership role during the COVID-19 pandemic. For example, in 2022, the ICN released a policy statement, *"A Statement by the International Council of Nurses on COVID-19 Vaccination,"* which acknowledged the efficacy of COVID-19 vaccinations; encouraged nurses, as trusted role models, to play a role in promoting the uptake of vaccinations; advocated for equitable global access to vaccines; and encouraged governments across the globe to enact any legislation necessary to protect health care workers involved both with immunization and the care of patients with COVID-19 (ICN, 2022a).

The *ICN Code of Ethics for Nurses*

It is significant that nursing has a professional code of ethics with a global reach. An international code of ethics was first adopted by the ICN in 1953 and has been revised many times since, most recently in 2021. The code (the *ICN Code of Ethics for Nurses*) informs other nursing codes across the world, ensuring consistency in the values and standards for nurses everywhere (Tisdale & Symenuk, 2020).

The code summarizes the ethical values, responsibilities, and professional accountabilities of the profession across all settings and domains of nursing practice. It guides the roles, responsibilities, behaviours, judgements, and relationships of nurses, and it offers a framework for ethical decision making. It affirms that the need for nursing is universal and that

> *inherent in nursing is a respect for human rights, including cultural rights, the right to life and choice, the right to dignity and to be treated with respect. Nursing care is respectful of and unrestricted by considerations of age, colour, culture, ethnicity, disability or illness, gender, sexual orientation, nationality, politics, language, race, religious or spiritual beliefs, legal, economic or social status. (ICN, 2021, p. 2)*

The code acknowledges that from the beginning, the profession has given voice to the "traditions and practices of equity and inclusion" and that nurses continue to be leaders in promoting these values across the world while preventing illness, restoring health, alleviating suffering, and advocating for a dignified death.

The code is organized around four principal elements, with a focus on the conduct, duties, and values of nurses in all domains of practice. The code includes examples to assist in the application of these standards. The elements summarized in Fig. 3.2 provide a visual representation of the code.

1. Nurses and Patients or Other People Requiring Care or Services

This element clarifies the nurse's primary responsibility to the people needing care and emphasizes the value of safe patient- and family-centred care. It highlights nursing's role in protecting human rights and respecting the values, beliefs, and culture of the individual, the family, and the community. A strong emphasis is placed on informed consent, transparency, confidentiality, advocacy, social justice, and integrity. In addition, it reinforces the value of human relationships within the context of a more complex technology-driven system, and the imperative of nurses living and demonstrating the core values of the profession.

2. Nurses and Practice

This element emphasizes the responsibility and accountability of nurses for competent and safe practice, exercising professional judgement, and for their own personal health. Central to this element is ensuring public confidence through personal conduct and ethical behaviours.

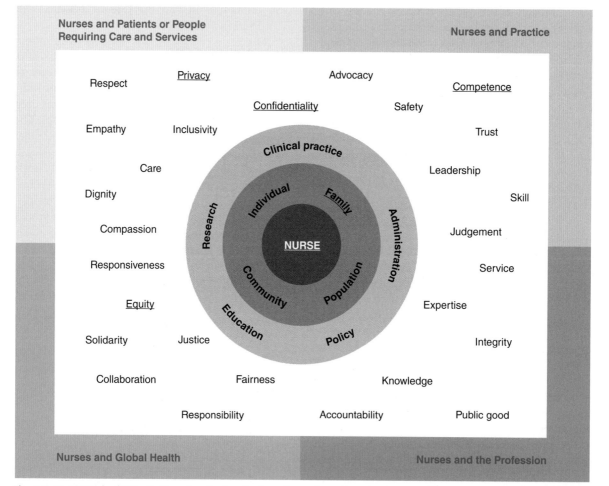

Fig. 3.2 ■ *ICN Code of Ethics for Nurses'* professional values. *Source: https://www.icn.ch/system/files/2021-10/ICN_Code-of-Ethics_EN_ Web_0.pdf, p. 21.*

It addresses the nurse's responsibilities for mentoring and guiding others, their role in advocacy and their accountabilities regarding conscientious objection.

- Responsibilities
- Role
- Accountabilities

3. Nurses and the Profession

This element focuses on nursing's accountability for meeting acceptable standards of clinical practice, management, research, education, and evidence-informed practice. It clarifies expectations that nurses participate in creating positive and ethical practice environments and maintain safe, equitable social and economic working conditions. Highlighted is nursing's role in preparing for and responding to "emergencies, disasters, conflicts, epidemics, pandemics, social crises, and conditions of scarce resources" (ICN, 2021, p. 15).

4. Nurses and Global Health

This element reinforces that nurses should also sustain collaborative and respectful relationships with other disciplines. It addresses values such as respect for the rights, dignity, freedom, and worth of all human beings, and the rejection of all forms of human exploitation. It states that nurses must contribute to the development of health policy and the advancement of population health (with a focus on the social determinants of health, advocacy for universal access to health care, and the achievement of the United Nations' SDGs). Also, given global concerns regarding climate change, it states that they must participate in the preservation, sustainability, and protection of the natural environment, as well as the prevention and mitigation of the potential health consequences of environmental issues.

THE CANADIAN NURSES ASSOCIATION

Founded in 1908, the CNA is a national nursing organization with links to provincial and territorial associations, which collectively represent more than 450,000 professional nurses in Canada (CNA, 2023a). With the mission "To unify and empower the voices of specialized nurses in Canada, in partnership with the Canadian Nurses Association, such that the specialized knowledge and skills of Canadian nurses become a vital component of all aspects of evidence-informed clinical, educational,

policy and political decision-making, as well as research, at the local, provincial/territorial and national levels". (CNA, 2023b.). CNA is the collective voice for nurses. Canadian nurses become members of the CNA when they join some provincial nursing associations or other nursing or student networks. Membership is not obligatory but nurses can also become members directly. The CNA is not a regulator of nursing. Instead, its role is one of advocacy and persuasion.

The CNA assists and supports the development of standards of nursing practice, education, and ethical conduct. It influences legislation, government programs, and national and international health policy. The CNA establishes and supports research priorities, facilitates information sharing, and represents the profession to health groups, government bodies, and the public (Box 3.4).

The priorities of CNA respond to current national and international challenges in health care. In 2022, some of these advocacy priorities included COVID-19, aging and seniors care, Indigenous health, Medical Assistance in Dying, mental health, and racism in health care.

BOX 3.4
CNA'S PURPOSE AND GOALS

With a focus on the public interest, CNA's purpose is as follows:
- To act in the public interest for Canadian nursing and nurses, providing national and international leadership in nursing and health
- To advocate in the public interest for a publicly funded, not-for-profit health system
- To advance nursing excellence and positive health outcomes in the public interest
- To promote profession-led regulation in the public interest

CNA's goals are as follows:
- To promote and enhance the role of nurses to strengthen nursing and the Canadian health system
- To shape and advocate for healthy public policy provincially/territorially, nationally and internationally
- To advance nursing leadership for nursing and for health
- To broadly engage a diverse representation of nursing to advance the nursing profession and the health of individuals living in Canada

Source: Adapted from *Canadian Nurses Association Strategic Plan 2023–2026*, p. 3. https://hl-prod-ca-oc-download.s3-ca-central-1.amazonaws.com/CNA/2f975e7e-4a40-45ca-863c-5ebf0a138d5e/UploadedImages/documents/Public_CNA_Strategic_Plan_2023-2026.pdf

THE CNA *CODE OF ETHICS FOR REGISTERED NURSES*

The CNA *Code of Ethics for Registered Nurses* offers Canadian nurses standards and values to guide ethical practice. The code affirms that each nurse must accept responsibility, not only for individual patients and families, but also for society and must participate in activities that contribute to the community as a whole.

The code, first introduced in 1980, has been revised several times, most recently in 2017. Modifications occur in response to changing societal and health care contexts that significantly influence the practice and work environment of nurses. For example, before the 2008 revision, Canadian nurses encountered the outbreak of severe acute respiratory syndrome (SARS), the Canadian military became engaged in the Afghanistan conflict, and worries about pandemics emerged. Since then, the need for healthy work environments was identified and Medical Assistance in Dying (MAiD) legislation was enacted. There is growing national and international attention to social and health equity, amplified by the COVID-19 pandemic and access to vaccines. The position of refugees and asylum seekers has become more critical due to wars and environmental disasters across the globe. Increased attention is being given to the rights of Indigenous peoples in Canada, and remedies for some historical harms against them are being introduced. The Truth and Reconciliation Commission of Canada, the Missing and Murdered Indigenous Women and Girls (MMIWG) Commission, and the discovery of unmarked graves on the grounds of former Indian residential schools have all served to increase the profile of Indigenous issues and move the agenda forward. These issues not only inform future revisions to the code, but also reinforce the critical importance of such a code in guiding "nurses in all contexts and domains of nursing practice and at all levels of decision-making" (CNA, 2017, p. 2).

The code provides a framework for the integration of ethical theory and concepts to guide ethical reflection and action. It is both aspirational (because it seeks to advance the aims of the profession) and regulatory (because it outlines the standards nurses must meet and guides the evaluation of professional practice in regulatory as well as legal contexts).

There are two parts to the code. Part I focuses on "Nursing Values and Ethical Responsibilities," and Part II, "Ethical Endeavours," outlines the approaches nurses may take to address social inequality. As well as outlining the ethical responsibilities of nurses and their accountability to "individuals, families, groups, populations, communities, and colleagues," the code addresses the "broad societal issues" that influence health and well-being and encourages nurses to "maintain awareness of aspects of social justice that affect health and well-being and to advocate for change" (CNA, 2017, p. 3). This is significant because the social context of Canada is one of great diversity.

The following sections highlight the key values and responsibilities included in the code.

Part I: Nursing Values and Ethical Responsibilities

Part I of the *Code of Ethics for Registered Nurses* is organized around seven primary values. Following the summary of each value, a case scenario is provided to illustrate its application.

Providing Safe, Compassionate, Competent, and Ethical Care

This value highlights nurses' accountability for person-centred care and their responsibilities for meeting safe ethical practice standards, individually and as members of the health care team. It calls attention to values of honesty and compassion, and reinforces the importance of having trusting relationships and meaningful communications with patients, families, and colleagues. There is a clear focus on ensuring competence and the requirement for a nurse to seek assistance when necessary, and hence the obligation to minimize harm and promote patient safety. This value clarifies nurses' accountability during job actions, natural and human disasters, and when rationing of resources is required. It reinforces the need for research to advance the profession and for nursing's role in advocacy. Finally, it speaks to safe work environments and collaborative approaches to conflict resolution (CNA, 2017, pp. 8–9).

CASE SCENARIO 3.1

A WORRIED DAUGHTER; A FATHER AT RISK

L. K., a nurse, receives a call from her aunt to hear that her 89-year-old father, P. K., fell and was taken to the local community hospital. Arriving at the emergency department, L. K. finds P. K. in the observation area and notes that it is reasonably staffed, with three nurses caring for eight patients who appear to be in relatively stable condition. The area is designed to ensure maximum visibility of patients.

Apparently, P. K. fell on his right hip and is unable to move his leg. An X-ray has not been taken, and it is not known which nurse is caring for him.

Shortly after L. K. arrives, P. K. asks to go to the bathroom, so L. K. approaches one of the nurses for assistance. The nurse asks if P. K. is able to stand by the side of the stretcher to use a urinal. Already very anxious about her father, L. K. becomes more upset and asks whether a nurse has undertaken an assessment, noting that he had been there more than 3 hours. The nurse responds by handing L. K. a urinal and walks away. Subsequently, L. K. is approached by another nurse, who gives her the business card for the hospital's Patient Relations office and suggests she take her concerns there.

Discussion

A number of practice and system issues are influencing this potentially unsafe situation. From a system/organization perspective, it appears that there are no processes or protocols in place to guide/fast-track the process for patients at risk, such as older persons presenting with a possible fractured hip. Older persons who sustain such injuries are at risk for many complications when the appropriate evidence-informed interventions are not initiated in a timely way. The patient was in the emergency department for over 3 hours, and proper assessments and diagnostics had not been initiated. Current evidence demonstrates that older persons experiencing pain and anxiety in confusing surroundings are at risk for delirium, which can result in further complications and challenges. In order to uphold the principles of beneficence and nonmaleficence, it is the moral obligation of

organizational leaders to ensure that evidence-informed structures and processes to facilitate the best care and to protect persons from harm are in place.

Because best practices and processes were not in place, this left the responsibility with the staff nurses, who did not appear to meet important clinical and ethical standards of care. Clearly, the patient had not been appropriately assessed in a timely way, placing him at a greater risk for harm, such as another fall. (Negligence is discussed in Chapter 7.)

By asking whether the patient could stand, the nurse added to L. K.'s anxiety by demonstrating a lack of knowledge of his condition and any potential risks. It was probable that there was a fracture of the hip and possibly pelvis. Thus, therefore standing could have resulted in extreme pain, serious consequences for the existing fracture, and possibly precipitated another fall. Further the nurses demonstrated a lack of respect for the patient's privacy and dignity when L. K. was asked to assist him with a personal and private function.

The encounter between the nurses and L. K. did little to build a trusting therapeutic relationship. In fact, the opposite occurred, as the daughter became more concerned about the safety and well-being of her father. In addition, the response from the nurses increased the potential for the situation to escalate further.

It is important for organizations to have structures in place to address patient and family concerns, for example, patient relations departments, when conflicts are not easily resolved. However, this does not eliminate nurses' accountability for responding to these issues at the time, by listening and responding to the worries and fears of families. Rather than handing over a business card, the other nurse could have listened to L. K.'s concerns and discussed a plan in place to ensure P. K. would be safe.

This scenario highlights the value of safe, compassionate, competent, and ethical care and the significance of meaningful communication in establishing trusting and collaborative relationships with patients and families.

Promoting Health and Well-Being

In conveying this value, there is recognition that central to nursing is the health and well-being of the person and acknowledgement that nurses work in collaboration with interprofessional teams and other key stakeholders. It is noted that interprofessional practice models have responded to the growing need for greater flexibility from professionals so they can respond more effectively to complex and evolving health care needs. These models challenge the exclusivity of knowledge and recognize that by respecting the knowledge, skills, and perspectives of team members, nurses are better able to respond to the growing complexity and diversity of the patient, community, and society. This value clearly points to the profession's obligation to consider the influence of the social determinants of health, while addressing the social, economic, and geographical factors that lead to inequities. Further, nurses are expected to safeguard the integrity of the profession by addressing patterns of care and behaviours that erode the supportive environment essential to safe and quality care (CNA, 2017, p. 10).

CASE SCENARIO 3.2

CHALLENGES TO CARING

A nurse is working in a pediatric critical care unit and has been a 7-year-old's primary nurse since the child's admission 3 months earlier. The patient has cerebral palsy, the consequence of a traumatic birth, and the parents are not able to visit as frequently as they would like because they have four other young children. This nurse and the young patient spend a lot of time together and have developed a strong bond. Though ventilator-dependent, the patient is doing well in spite of many developmental challenges. The plan under discussion is to transfer the patient to a youth-oriented long-term care facility. The team, including the physician, the social worker, the physiotherapist, and the occupational therapist, is meeting to discuss the plan and the transition. The primary nurse has a busy assignment and is unable to attend the meeting. The team goes ahead with the meeting without the primary nurse who knows and understands the patient the best.

Discussion

Not being able to attend patient-focused meetings is a frequent concern for nurses and one that could be remedied with the introduction of structures and processes that would facilitate nursing participation in these very important discussions. The structures associated with nursing care delivery are such that nurses do not have the same flexibility as do other members of the team. Of course, there are times when it is impossible for nurses to leave their patients to attend such meetings. However, leaders acting ethically and doing what is best for the individual nurse, the team, and, most importantly, the patients should consider this a priority and organize assignments, scheduling, and coverage to make it possible. The interprofessional team should understand these challenges and accommodate their schedule to ensure the presence of nurses who have a significant role in the well-being and safety of the patient being discussed.

There has been a long-standing recognition of the need for teamwork in clinical practice, and finding new ways to ensure delivery of interprofessional care has been raised as an imperative for best practice.

The plan was compromised because the professional who knew and understood the patient better than anyone else was not present. This scenario demonstrates a lack of respect for the nurse–patient relationship and how the primary nurse would be best suited to represent the patient in the development of the plan. Also, when good nurses are unable to act on the interests of their patients, they are at higher risk for moral distress and compassion fatigue. It is also not clear whether any attempts were made to encourage family participation. If the parents couldn't be present in person, technology such as video conference could have been used to engage them in the discussion. This value embodies the expectation that nurses are to safeguard the integrity of the profession by addressing patterns of care and behaviours that erode the supportive environment essential to safe and high-quality care. It is a moral imperative that these patterns that prevent nurses' involvement in important planning processes be addressed.

Promoting and Respecting Informed Decision Making

This value clearly articulates the expectation that nurses ensure respect for persons by promoting informed decision making. Whether written, verbal, or simply implied, a valid consent is one that must be (1) based on the relevant and accurate information required to make that choice, (2) free from coercion and be open and transparent, and (3) made by someone capable of making this level of decision. The process also allows for a person to refuse consent or to withdraw it after it has been given. This value makes clear that nurses must understand the law related to assessing capacity (Canadian Nurses Protective Society [CNPS], 2004). A patient may be able to make decisions about activities of daily living and yet may not be competent to decide whether surgery is in their best interests. The challenge for the nurse and the team is to assess the patient's competence to make decisions and to ensure that choices are made in a noncoercive environment. If a person is deemed incapable of making such decisions, then it needs to be determined whether there is a substitute decision maker and/or an advance directive.

Decisions about health care interventions are not always easy. Therefore, nurses have an obligation to ensure, as much as is possible, that their patients have the time and opportunity to reflect and consider their options and to make the choice they think is best for them. Though other professionals, such as physicians, have an obligation to secure consent for medical procedures, nurses have a responsibility to raise concerns when the appropriate

---

CASE SCENARIO 3.3

DISCOVERING THE PATIENT'S STORY

R. S. is community nurse who has been caring for an older woman, M. M., in her home for several months. They have developed a strong relationship, and M. M. has shared many life experiences with R. S. Born outside of Canada, M. M. lived through the Depression, married at age 16, and gave birth to three children. She left her abusive husband and immigrated to Canada when she was in her mid-30s. Successful professionally and personally, in her own words, she has "had a great life." Now in the terminal phase of lung disease, she is ready for—and even welcomes—death. Her one wish is to die at home surrounded by the people she loves.

One weekend, while R. S. is off duty, M. M. experiences severe respiratory distress. The family panics and calls 911. M. M. is subsequently admitted to the critical care unit (CCU), placed on a ventilator, and started on an aggressive treatment plan. Returning to work the following Monday, R. S. discovers this and visits M. M. in the hospital. R. S. learns that, though it is unlikely M. M. will survive, her family and the team have agreed that life support will continue.

Discussion

This story illustrates the challenges with communication and team collaboration within a fragmented and compartmentalized health care system. The community nurse knows the patient's story and wishes, but the system does not facilitate interprofessional collaboration across practice settings.

This scenario raises numerous questions about how the patient and family were prepared for the complications and symptoms that might arise as the disease progressed and whether an effective plan was in place for care at home. It is unclear why the family agreed to the aggressive treatment, and whether they knew of her wishes. If they did, this raises questions regarding the power differential and perhaps the family's reluctance to challenge the medical team. It is also possible that, though her death was anticipated, they might not be ready to let go. Would it be appropriate for R. S. to discuss the situation with the family and recommend a team meeting with all stakeholders, including the family, to discuss a plan to ensure the patient's wishes to die with dignity are respected? Would R. S. be supported in doing this? Nurse leaders play a role in ensuring such collaboration and in ensuring that the circle of care includes team members who are associated with that person across all settings where care is delivered.

standards for obtaining consent have not been met. Nurses must also be aware of their accountability for obtaining consent, whether implied or direct, for nursing interventions. Nurses must be aware of the power differential that exists between the patient and the team and ensure that this does not influence decision making. Nurses are also expected to understand the differences that exist across individuals, families, and cultures. A person may choose to have others consent on their behalf, perhaps a family member, or in the case of an Indigenous person, a community elder. However, nurses must be aware of the ways the person's choices may be controlled by other factors and persons and be prepared to engage in an advocacy role.

This value also makes clear the expectation that nurses respect others regardless of lifestyle choices, respect patients' decisions, and provide care without judgement (CNA, 2017, pp. 11–12).

Honouring Dignity

The expression of this value makes explicit that nursing is guided by consideration for the dignity and integrity of persons and their right to be treated with respect and compassion. Disrespectful communication, disregard for patient privacy, or failure to involve patients in discussions that relate to their health care violates this moral responsibility. People need nursing care during difficult and meaningful periods in their lives, from birth to death. Respect for dignity is especially essential when nurses care for persons at the end of life, ensuring that the journey is peaceful and that the emotional, psychological, and physical needs of the patient, the family, and significant others are met. Issues related to end of life are discussed in Chapter 8. Nurses are obligated to provide optimal patient comfort and pain management. They are also obligated to deal compassionately with situations where treatment is withdrawn and upon request for MAiD. Nurses can also advocate for a person's

---

CASE SCENARIO 3.4

DIGNITY AFTER DEATH?

A family has just been informed that their son and sibling, F. K., has been killed in a motor vehicle accident. F. K.'s identity has been confirmed, but the family wants to make sure. When they arrive at the emergency department, the staff say little to them other than that they have called the supervisor to assist them. They wait in the corridor for about 20 minutes until the supervisor arrives to offer them condolences and shares that the team worked very hard to save their family member. They are taken to the hospital morgue with a number of drawers containing deceased persons. When the supervisor opens the drawer, they find F. K. wrapped in plastic, their hands bound tightly with string, and covered in blood.

Discussion

Nurses' obligations to respect the dignity of persons continues after their death. Deceased persons are the responsibility of nurses until they are transitioned from their care, and of the organization until they leave that facility. The nurses in the emergency department did not meet their obligation to provide compassionate care to the family who clearly would have been devastated. Rather than leaving them in the hallway to wait, alternative accommodation

could have been provided, such as for them to wait in a private office or meeting room, where they could have been offered support and solace. Empathetic nurses place themselves in another's situation, and hence act with others in such a way that they themselves would want to be treated.

The morgue, as described, was not a suitable environment for this bereaved family to view their sibling and child. Most facilities have viewing rooms, designed to offer a warm and comfortable setting for this important experience. Leaders in nursing should ensure that such settings are in place, as this is important not only for the family but also for the nurses who usually accompany them.

Standards regarding the care of a person after death require that they are prepared in such a manner that would be acceptable to family members. The experience of a family seeing a loved one in this state could have long-term consequences, especially for their grieving process. The nurses in the emergency department had an obligation to treat the deceased person with dignity, and to ensure appropriate care after death. The supervisor had the responsibility to ensure this in advance of the family presence. The family also had the right to be treated with dignity, respect, and compassion.

choice to die at home, when possible. This occurs in the context of an open, trusting relationship of mutual respect, where nurses communicate effectively and listen to what is important to the person and the family. At the same time, professional therapeutic relationships are maintained, and nurses ensure that the boundaries of these relationships remain intact. Nurses also take into account the diversity of people living in Canada and consider each people unique culture, values, and beliefs.

On the basis of this value, it would be the moral obligation of the nurse to ensure, for example, that everything possible is done so that a patient does not die alone, unless he or she expresses the wish to do so. Nurses should ensure that families are notified in a timely manner if a patient's condition changes; and, if this is not possible, then the same priority should be given to these situations as that provided to emergencies. Assignments can be reorganized and help can be requested so that someone is present with the person if that is what is desired.

The expression of dignity also recognizes the importance of maintaining professional relationships within the team and to treat each other with dignity and respect (CNA, 2017, pp. 12–13).

Maintaining Privacy and Confidentiality

This value clarifies that fundamental to a trusting therapeutic relationship is the nurse's obligation to protect patient confidentiality and privacy. Thus, the patient can fully disclose information essential to achieving the goals of care, trusting that this information will not be revealed. Nurses ensure that all forms of communication, whether it be in the form of team discussions, online, or documentation, focus only on what is necessary with regard to care and that they take the necessary measures to protect privacy. Social media should not be used as a vehicle for sharing confidential patient information; even when names are not used, often the circumstances can identify that person. Consent must be obtained before the release of information and if photography of any kind involves patients or families directly or indirectly.

Overriding of this obligation, however, is justified if harm to the patient or to others might result if confidentiality were maintained. Also, from a legal perspective, there are situations where legislation requires disclosure (e.g., reporting child abuse or notifying police about patients with gunshot wounds) (*Child, Youth and Family Services Act*, 2017; *Gunshot and Stab Wounds Mandatory Reporting Act*, 2007).

Nurses also facilitate a person's access to his or her own health record and take the necessary steps to ensure the information is understood accurately (CNA, 2017, pp. 14–15).

CASE SCENARIO 3.5

CONFIDENTIALITY—A SACRED TRUST?

A public health nurse has been visiting a young patient, L. D., who recently gave birth to a second child. Recently separated, L. D. is now on welfare. L. D.'s relatives live in other provinces. To become more self-reliant, L. D. plans to return to school on a part-time basis. The nurse admires this patient, and they have developed a sound professional relationship.

The nurse has observed the patient's strong parenting skills and the care provided to the children. One day, during a home visit, the nurse observes that one of the children has a black eye. Before the nurse asks about the injury, L. D. starts to cry and reveals that the child had an outburst while L. D. was trying to settle the baby. The baby had been sleeping poorly, so being very tired and frustrated, L. D. lashed out and struck the child who would not stop yelling.

L. D. says that she has never done this before and will never do it again, and she asks the nurse to keep this conversation confidential; if L. D.'s ex-partner was to find out, the incident would be raised during custody disputes.

This nurse knows that L. D. loves her children and would not intentionally do anything to harm them, and the nurse has not seen any evidence of harm before this. Furthermore, L. D. was open and transparent about what happened.

Discussion

This is clearly a dilemma for this nurse, who has developed a therapeutic professional relationship with

Continued on following page

CASE SCENARIO 3.5 *(Continued)*

this patient, and respects her for how she has faced the many challenges in her life so far. At the same time, what are this nurse's legal responsibilities? Must this information be reported to Children's Aid? Would that cause further distress and have consequences for the custody issue?

As a lone parent on welfare, L. D. is under a great deal of stress. How can this nurse do what is best for L. D., while also ensuring that the children are not at risk of harm? Are there resources to support this nurse with this dilemma?

Nurses should not have to manage these distressing situations alone. If a nurse has reasonable grounds to believe that a child has suffered harm, then it is the nurse's duty to protect the child by reaching out to the appropriate child protection agency because it offers the knowledge, skills, and resources to investigate the situation further (Government of Alberta, 2018; Information & Privacy Commission of Ontario & Provincial Advocate for Children & Youth, 2018). This nurse should not assume that the outcome will be a negative one for the patient because child protection agencies can offer help and assistance to parents in crisis. This nurse should be open and transparent with the patient about nurses' legal and ethical responsibility to engage child protection agencies and should also reassure this patient that the care and support needed will be provided.

Every jurisdiction in Canada has legislation requiring the reporting of suspected child abuse. The precise wording varies from province to province, and nurses should refer to the specific provincial legislation. Before reporting, nurses can consult with colleagues and supervisors, the relevant college, the Children's Aid Society (CAS), or an equivalent organization, and the CNPS. For example, current legislation in Ontario requires reporting in 13 situations including the one in the Case Scenario.

Duty to report child in need of protection
125 (1) Despite the provisions of any other Act, if a person, including a person who performs professional or

official duties with respect to children, has reasonable grounds to suspect one of the following, the person shall immediately report the suspicion and the information on which it is based to a society:
1. *The child has suffered physical harm inflicted by the person having charge of the child or caused by or resulting from that person's,*
   i. *failure to adequately care for, provide for, supervise or protect the child, or*
   ii. *pattern of neglect in caring for, providing for, supervising or protecting the child.*

In Prince Edward Island, the *Child Protection Act* (1988) outlines mandatory reporting requirements:

10. Mandatory reporting
(1) Notwithstanding any other Act, every person who has knowledge, or has reasonable grounds to suspect that a child is in need of protection shall (a) without delay, report or cause to be reported the circumstances to the Director, or to a peace officer who shall report the information to the Director; and (b) provide to the Director such additional information as is known or available to the person.

On its face, there appears to be no discretion regarding not reporting when a nurse knows of an injury being caused by a parent.

The following recommendations are included in a guideline "Recognizing & Responding Safely to Family Violence," developed by the VEGA (Violence, Evidence, Guidance, Action) Project, which was funded by the Public Health Agency of Canada:

Immediate response to the disclosure should:
- *Respond to maltreatment disclosures with care and compassion; affirm the child's experiences.*
- *If unsure whether the case is reportable, consult with colleagues/CPA first (taking care to maintain the confidentiality of the child/family).*
- *Remind the child/family of your role as a reporter. Discuss how you will file a report and potential child welfare agency response.*
- *Ensure that the child and, in the case of IPV (intimate partner violence) exposure, the nonoffending caregiver, are safe during the reporting process. (McTavish et al., 2016)*

Promoting Justice

This value makes explicit that the principles of justice and equity establish the right to health care for every individual in Canadian society. If the values of the *Canada Health Act* are to be upheld, then issues related to equal access to health care must be constantly addressed by nurses and other health care professionals. There is a strong focus on resource allocation, including having appropriate staffing and resources. This value also focuses on issues of fairness—that nurses treat persons of all cultures, ethnicities, and religions respectfully without judging, labelling, stigmatization, any form of discrimination, and so on. There is recognition of the unique history and rights of the Indigenous peoples in Canada.

Recognizing that global issues, such as terrorism and war, can affect nurses, there is explicit caution against torture and engagement in the punishment of others (CNA, 2017, pp. 15–16).

CASE SCENARIO 3.6

RESPECT FOR PERSONS

An Indigenous family is driving from Thunder Bay to Toronto when their 14-year-old child becomes violently ill. They go to the nearest emergency department of a local community hospital they find along their route. Their child is admitted to a medical unit and undergoes diagnostic testing. The family, concerned about the child's well-being, begins a smudging ceremony, a purification rite that involves the burning of sacred medicines, including sweetgrass, sage, and tobacco. The staff members are not familiar with these rituals. As a result, when the nurses observe the process, they worry about the risk of fire and ask the family to stop the practice immediately. The nurse caring for the child asks the family about the ritual and looks it up online. This nurse does not find a policy in this hospital that pertains to traditional healing practices. However, this nurse, appreciating the family's distress and their cultural values, allows the ceremony to proceed against the wishes of other colleagues. The next day, the nurse is called by a manager and is asked to account for these actions.

Discussion

Health care organizations should have policies and programs in place that ensure respect for diversity and cultural sensitivity. These policies and programs should guide nurses in advocating for the rights of all communities and supporting the values and beliefs of all individuals in Canadian society.

Nurses must sometimes take risks to do what is right and respectful for patients and families. Of course, the risks and benefits need to be thoughtfully evaluated and the law needs to be followed, and nobody should be at risk of harm. In the present situation, there is minimal risk of fire, and steps could have been taken to mitigate even minimal risks. For example, could the ritual have taken place outside on the grounds of the hospital? Could the ceremonies take place in a conference or meeting room so that other patients and families would not be disturbed? Was there a supervisor or manager on call that the nurse could have consulted? Nurses and organizations that facilitate the practice of Indigenous ceremonies can potentially reduce barriers to care, enable trusting relationships, contribute to the healing process, and ensure culturally safe care (Toronto Central Regional Cancer Program, 2016).

In this situation, it would be important for the nurse to maintain constant communication with the family to reassure them that attempts were being made to find a solution, so that they would understand the concerns of the nurses and appreciate their willingness to find a solution.

Having allowed the ritual to proceed, it would be prudent for the nurse to communicate this action with the manager, explaining what happened and the reasons behind the decision. In meeting their responsibility for advocacy, the nurse and the manager together could then take a leadership role in facilitating positive change in this setting for the future benefit of persons from diverse communities and cultures.

Being Accountable

This value articulates the duty of nurses to protect patients from harm. For example, when a nurse is aware of another's incompetence and neglects to take action, then that nurse also assumes responsibility for harm that may result from such incompetence.

In non-emergencies requiring specialized skills that the nurse does not have, or in situations where the care required conflicts with the nurse's moral beliefs (e.g., abortion, MAiD), the nurse is required to refer the patient to another nurse. In cases of conscientious objection, nurses should alert their employers in advance so that, where possible, accommodations that respect their beliefs can be made. In emergencies or in situations where alternative resources are not available, any nurse may be called on to provide care.

This does not include situations where a patient's values and behaviours do not align with those of the nurse, such as providing care to a person who has just committed a serious crime or is a member of a radical group. The care required would not, in itself, conflict with a nurse's moral beliefs as would be the case in relation to abortion and MAiD.

When delegating responsibility to others (e.g., students, the family, personal support workers), nurses must be assured that all the requirements with regard to appropriateness and competence are met.

Nurses advocate for health equity across the system, with special consideration for those with mental health issues and those most vulnerable due to social and health inequities.

Nurses must act with honesty and integrity and disclose conflicts of interest if they arise. Nurses mentoring students and novice nurses must treat them with respect while meeting their learning needs. Nurses represent themselves appropriately to patients by providing their name, role, title, and so on (CNA, 2017, pp. 16–17).

CASE SCENARIO 3.7

WHAT MAKES A NURSE?

A nursing faculty member at a renowned Canadian university is assigned to be a mentor for a nursing student in the final year. The student's academic performance is remarkable, having the best grade point average (GPA) in the class. However, the faculty member is concerned that the student rarely attends class and has expressed that this form of learning is boring. Most disturbing are the comments the faculty member hears from clinical preceptors, who find the student lacking in caring and compassion. The student rarely interacts with the team and patients and is described by family members as "cold, aloof, and lacking in kindness."

The faculty member does not believe the student will make a good nurse and has to decide whether failing the student based on these evaluations is the best option. There would likely be an appeal at the university, especially in the context of the student's amazing academic performance.

Discussion

There are many important values and responsibilities related to accountability that are relevant to this scenario. As stated in this value, nurses have the responsibility to mentor and support students and one another. At the same time, there is shared accountability to ensure that nurses and students are competent and able to provide safe patient care. It would appear that the student has the knowledge and skills to provide nursing care. Yet, they do not seem to have the right characteristics (e.g., empathy and compassion) and the skills to build relationships to work effectively within a team and provide safe and high-quality care to patients.

However, have the teachers and preceptors attempted to understand the root cause of the student's reluctance to engage both in the classroom and in the clinical area? Has feedback been provided? Are there emotional or psychological issues that the student is experiencing that need to be addressed through counselling or other interventions? Is the student experiencing anxiety and discomfort in situations where they must relate to and interact with others? Is there any special support or education that could be provided to help them?

Is nursing perhaps not the right fit for this person? What made nursing a career option in the first place? The student's grades are good, so if the

CASE SCENARIO 3.7 *(Continued)*

core issues regarding approach cannot be resolved, is there an opportunity to counsel this student to reflect on other career options that are better aligned with their interests? These considerations would be more respectful than simply failing this student.

This value requires that we provide support, mentoring, and the right opportunities to students. It also expresses nurses' accountability for competent and safe care to themselves and to others. Professional nurses must be competent and able to provide high-quality, compassionate, and ethical care.

Part II: Ethical Endeavours

Part II of the code highlights the significant role the nursing profession plays in advocating for social justice and the health of people living in Canada. Moreover, the code challenges the profession to be responsive to the factors that influence the health and well-being of the world's population and to play a strong role in addressing issues of poverty, homelessness, vulnerability, and globalization. Noting that nurses are citizens of the world, they must collectively work with others to address and resolve these rising challenges in the international arena of health care.

The code reflects the diversity and complexity of the nursing profession. Nurses work with the homeless. They also serve in the military, caring not only for military personnel but also for those in crisis across Canada, such as residents in long-term care facilities during the COVID-19 pandemic. Nurses play a role in developing policy for all levels of government and contribute to programs related to health care, human resources, poverty, transitioning new immigrants into Canadian society, and more.

As people are displaced as a result of war, ethnic conflicts, and climate change, Canada is playing a leading role in welcoming refugees and asylum seekers, and offering permanent or temporary homes to them. Canadian nurses play an important role in addressing not only new immigrants' physical health but also their psychological, emotional, and social needs.

The code draws attention to those who are vulnerable in society, including children, older persons, the mentally ill, visible minorities, Indigenous peoples, and the homeless. Reducing health disparities among these vulnerable groups is critical, both for those whose opportunities in life might otherwise be compromised and for society, which has a responsibility to nurture a social environment where all persons living in Canada can sustain health and realize their potential for academic success, economic independence, and constructive interactions with others. It is a matter of fairness and social justice that every person in Canada has the opportunity to be healthy and have a good quality of life.

The data suggest that there are significant health disparities among the population with regard to functional health, early childhood tooth decay, emotional and behavioural problems, obesity, respiratory conditions, readiness to learn at school entry, abuse, injury, and so on. Disparities are evident among those who live below the poverty line, especially in lone-parent households (McKeown, 2007; McNeill, 2008a, 2008b). Poverty is increasingly being defined along ethnoracial lines, and there are indications that systemic barriers confront visible minorities (Access Alliance Multicultural Community Health Centre, 2005).

Consider the extent to which ethical endeavours influence the responsibilities of the nurse and nursing in the case scenarios that follow.

CASE SCENARIO 3.8

DOES MY LIFE MATTER?

A 30-year-old, L. B., has moved back in with their parents, who live in an urban community. L. B. has a university degree and was a successful accountant for a couple of years before an injury and subsequent personal challenges resulted in a dependency on

narcotics. L. B. lost their job and was homeless prior to being convinced to return home. L. B. had entered a substance abuse program, but the rehabilitation was not going well. Feeling frustrated and hopeless one evening, L. B. overdoses on fentanyl, and even though high, regrets doing so. L. B. calls their parents

Continued on following page

CASE SCENARIO 3.8 *(Continued)*

for help. Concerned about L. B.'s level of conscious-ness, the parents take L. B. to the closest emergency department, where they refuse to assess L. B. who is then sent away to seek other resources in the com-munity. Observing this, a novice nurse on orientation is distressed.

Discussion

The staff in the emergency department ignored their responsibilities to provide care and ensure the safety of this vulnerable person. The nurse was right to be distressed. It is also a moral imperative that more re-sources be made available in the community to support persons with substance abuse challenges. Often, they have nowhere to go but to the emergency department.

The issue of the system's inability to manage drug and alcohol problems is frequently the subject of widespread media discussion. As required by the code, nursing professional groups, both nationally and provincially, are engaged in collaboration with

other groups to address these great needs and very challenging issues.

For example, in 2017, the CNA, the Canadian Association of Schools of Nursing (CASN), and the Canadian Council of Registered Nurse Regulators (CCRNR) participated in an emergency summit called by the federal government to identify solu-tions to the opioid crisis, which resulted in a joint statement of action (Jaimet, 2017). In 2019, the CNA received a grant of $1.3 million from Health Canada's Substance Use and Addictions Program (SUAP) to develop a national nursing framework in response to the legalization of Cannabis in 2018 (CNA, 2018). This funding acknowledges the im-portant position of nursing in Canada to contrib-ute to the education of the population regarding best practices. In 2022, CNA released its publi-cation *Non-Medical Cannabis: A Nursing Framework* (CNA, 2022).

CASE SCENARIO 3.9

A GLOBAL RESPONSIBILITY?

A young woman, M. M., recently gained asylum status in Canada and is now pregnant. M. M. has been diagnosed with the human immunodeficiency virus (HIV) and is concerned about the impact this will have on the unborn child. M. M. was a politi-cal prisoner and was raped while in prison. From the prison, M. M. was abducted to another country and was forced to work in the sex trade. Fortunately, M. M. managed to escape to Canada. Although M. M. demonstrates considerable resilience in spite of these terrible experiences and has a positive attitude toward the unborn child, M. M. is also experienc-ing panic attacks, problems sleeping, and feelings of depression and hopelessness.

Discussion

This story is not unusual. Refugees and asylum seekers are particularly susceptible to mental health and emo-tional issues (Mental Health Commission of Canada,

2016). This is not surprising because many refugees have faced war, persecution, and torture, and they have left their families and their culture behind.

A commitment to social justice influences nursing's approach to refugees and asylum seekers. When the patient and the future child in this story are assessed on the basis of the social determinants of health, it is clear that they are potentially at a greater risk of emotional and physical harm. Given their complex needs, it is critical that they be referred to an expert team of health care professionals in the community, and to those programs that could combine their knowledge to mobilize the resources needed. Nurs-ing can play a significant role in helping this patient navigate a system that can be both overwhelming and complicated.

Fortunately, the CNA and provincial nursing or-ganizations provide resources and toolkits for nurses caring for such vulnerable populations (CNA, 2018).

Additional case scenarios are available on the Evolve website. They are intended to facilitate reflection and discussion, using the code as a guiding framework. While reflecting on and discussing these scenarios, consider the following questions:

1. What are the key moral issues raised by the scenario?
2. Does the CNA *Code of Ethics for Registered Nurses* assist you in identifying these issues?
3. Does the *Code of Ethics for Registered Nurses* clarify the responsibilities of the nurse?
4. Do any of the theories presented in Chapter 2 assist in clarifying your thinking?
5. Does the *ICN Code of Ethics for Nurses* assist in the discussion?

ALIGNMENT OF POLICY AND BEST PRACTICE GUIDELINES WITH THE CNA *CODE OF ETHICS*

There are many examples of how policy and programs align with and support nurses in meeting the standards of the code. One significant example is the Best Practice Guideline (BPG) program of the Registered Nurses, Association of Ontario (RNAO, 2022). This multiyear program, funded by the Ontario Ministry of Health and Long-Term Care (MOHLTC), is intended to support nurses by providing them with evidence-informed BPGs for several areas, including practice and healthy work environments. There are over 50 published guidelines, as well as toolkits and educational resources to support their implementation. These guidelines were developed by teams of nursing experts from across Canada, an illustration of nursing collaboration throughout the country. Many of these publications are available in French and other languages. They are updated regularly and have been implemented not only in Canada but also around the globe (see http://rnao.ca/bpg).

Best Practice Guidelines

Best Practice Guidelines (BPGs) are comprehensive documents intended to guide evidence-informed best practices to enhance practice and facilitate decision making. They are designed to assist nurses and the interprofessional team, in partnership with patients and their families, to make decisions about health care

services and to advance the standards and the quality of health care. The guidelines are relevant to all practice settings and domains, including clinical, research, education, and administration. Recommendations in the guidelines apply to practice, education, organization, and policy (Grinspun et al., 2002; RNAO, 2002, 2005). Guidelines relevant to ethics and the law include *Professionalism in Nursing* (RNAO, 2007b) and *Promoting 2SLGBTQI+ Health Equity* (RNAO, 2021).

These clinical guidelines support many elements of the CNA *Code of Ethics* and speak to values such as competence, health and well-being, collaborative and informed decision making, and respect for dignity, privacy, and accountability.

Healthy Work Environment Best Practice Guidelines

With funding from the Ontario MOHLTC, the RNAO partnered with Health Canada's Office of Nursing Policy to develop guidelines to promote healthy work environments. This initiative was in response to priorities identified by provincial and countrywide nursing committees and task forces. The initiative identified major concerns and challenges in the recruitment and retention of nurses across the country. The necessity to build healthier environments for the practice of nursing emerged from major studies included in the report *Ensuring the care will be there: Report on nursing recruitment and retention in Ontario* (RNAO & Registered Practical Nurses Association of Ontario [WeRPN], 2000). Additional reports and publications reinforced these challenges (Baumann et al., 2001; Canadian Nursing Advisory Committee, 2002). These challenges were magnified through the COVID-19 pandemic and drew additional attention to the work environment and the ethical and emotional challenges faced by nurses.

The RNAO Healthy Work Environment Best Practice Guidelines (HWE BPGs) contribute to a better understanding of the relationships among nurses' work environments, patient outcomes, and organizational and system performance. In addition to improved nursing engagement and better quality of care, the evidence shows that having a healthy work environment results in financial benefits to the organization in terms of reduced absenteeism, improved productivity, lower organizational and health care costs, and lower expenses associated with adverse patient outcomes (Cho et al., 2003; Person et al., 2004; Sasichay-Akkadechanunt et al., 2003;

Sovie & Jawad, 2001; Tourangeau et al., 2002). "Healthy work environments for nurses are defined as practice settings that maximize the health and well-being of the nurse, quality patient outcomes, organizational performance, and societal outcomes" (RNAO, 2009, p. 24). Guidelines relevant to ethics and the law include *Embracing Cultural Diversity in Health Care: Developing Cultural Competence* (RNAO, 2007a).

Many aspects of the CNA code focus on the environments within which nurses practice. There are values and standards associated with the behaviour of a professional nurse, including respect for cultural differences, collaboration and teamwork, and having the right models and resources necessary to support quality care.

The BPG initiative is an important example of where nursing values and standards are enabled through government policy and collaboration among nursing leaders across the country who take action based on the best evidence and a strong commitment to the profession.

ETHICAL DECISION-MAKING MODELS

The CNA *Code of Ethics for Registered Nurses* "points to the need for nurses to engage in ethical reflection and discussion" (CNA, 2017, p. 28). Ethical frameworks or models assist nurses and the interprofessional team in addressing ethical problems and concerns. They provide a guide to facilitate communication and discussion of the issues and can serve as useful tools to "guide nurses in their thinking about a particular issue or question" (CNA, 2017, p. 28).

The CNA has provided examples of guidelines that assist in ethical reflection and decision making (CNA, 2017, pp. 28–32).

Decision-making frameworks provide a process or approach to help nurses focus on relevant questions and issues and to guide them in ethical decision making (Table 3.1 and Fig. 3.3).

TABLE 3.1	
An Ethical Decision-Making Framework	
Steps	**Process**
(1) Identify problem or issue statement.	■ Clarify and expand further.
(2) Decide who should be involved in the discussion.	■ Determine whether the patient is able or willing to participate. ■ Identify the interprofessional team members most involved (e.g., primary nurse). ■ As appropriate, engage family, substitute decision maker, community Elders, or clergy. ■ Consider engaging other advisors, (e.g., ethicist, ethics committee, patient relations. risk management).
(3) Describe the issue in detail.	■ Confirm who brought the concern forward. ■ Clarify the ethical concerns. ■ Determine whether there is a clear ethical or legal violation. ■ Assess whether there are gaps in the care process, such as serious communication issues.
(4) Share preliminary perspectives on the issue.	■ Listen to the views of the participants. ■ Identify existing or potential conflicts within the team, the family, or between the team and the patient or family.
(5) Share the person's story and undertake a comprehensive assessment and analysis of the situation.	■ Share the personal story of the patient/family. ■ Invite the participants to share their perspectives, emotions, and reactions to this story. ■ Examine whether the situation is influencing the patient's care and address this, if necessary. ■ Review the person's diagnosis, prognosis, and abilities. ■ Determine whether the patient is competent to make decisions. Ascertain whether there is a power of attorney for personal care, an advance directive, or if a substitute decision maker or guardian has been appointed. ■ Assess whether the patient's values, culture, or religion is relevant to the issue. ■ Determine the key relationships important to the patient, and if they are engaged. ■ Identify the members of the health care team with the most significant relationships with the patient and family. ■ Consider other complexities or stakeholders external to the team and family (e.g., child welfare groups) that may be a factor.

TABLE 3.1

An Ethical Decision-Making Framework *(Continued)*

Steps	Process
(6) Explore relevant legal factors.	■ Investigate whether there are any legal rules that govern this situation (e.g., release of confidential information, Medical Assistance in Dying).
(7) Share values.	■ Clarify the values of the patient, the family, and team members, and consider whether there are significant conflicts.
(8) Clarify ethical principles.	■ Identify the ethical principles that apply. ■ Evaluate whether these principles apply consistently to the issue or whether any are in conflict. ■ Determine whether one principle (or more) has priority over the others.
(9) Select applicable ethical theories.	■ Evaluate which ethical theories are relevant and helpful in clarifying the issues and guiding the conversation.
(10) Identify alternatives or options available.	■ Summarize any options or alternatives. ■ Determine whether there is a clear choice, ethically and legally. ■ Examine whether the participants have an emotional reaction about what should be done, even though they cannot articulate their reasons.
(11) Deliberate and agree on the potential alternatives.	■ Weigh each option in relation to ethical theories or principles. ■ Consider the potential consequences of each alternative. ■ Determine what rules or principles apply and whether they are in conflict.
(12) Choose a course of action.	■ Identify the course of action most consistent with the ethical theories, principles, and rules. ■ Consider whether this choice is consistent with the values and beliefs of the participants and whether there is consensus. ■ Evaluate the emotional reactions to this choice. Confirm the extent to which the participants can accept accountability for this decision.
(13) Develop an action plan.	■ Decide on an action plan, including how it will be communicated to others. ■ Identify who will be involved and the responsibilities of the patient, the family, the nurse, and the team.
(14) Evaluate the plan.	■ Evaluate the outcomes and make modifications, as necessary. ■ Consider, in retrospect, if there is continued confidence in the decision, whether anything should have been done differently, and how the process could be improved in the future. ■ Consider whether anything in this process should be incorporated into a guideline to help others deal with similar situations in the future. ■ Assess for any residual moral distress over the situation.

The framework outlined in Table 3.1 and Fig. 3.3 integrates the key concepts, theories, and principles introduced in this book. The framework ensures the proper collection of information that is relevant to a sound ethical decision-making process and encourages consideration of all aspects of the situation. This framework may be used to guide discussion and reflection on the case scenarios presented throughout this book and on the Evolve website.

EXPERT RESOURCES

Most ethical problems are resolved, and moral decisions are made, in collaboration with the patient, family, and the health care team. However, at times the team may need support from those with expert knowledge of ethics (and perhaps the law). Today's ethical challenges are often extremely complex, nuanced, and not easily resolved, or they may have larger implications for the health care facility, community, and society. Consider the media stories, for example, of parents who want life-sustaining treatment for their child to be continued when the health care team disagrees and considers any intervention to be futile. Many of these disputes are resolved within the health care organization, but when they are not, they become high-profile legal challenges.

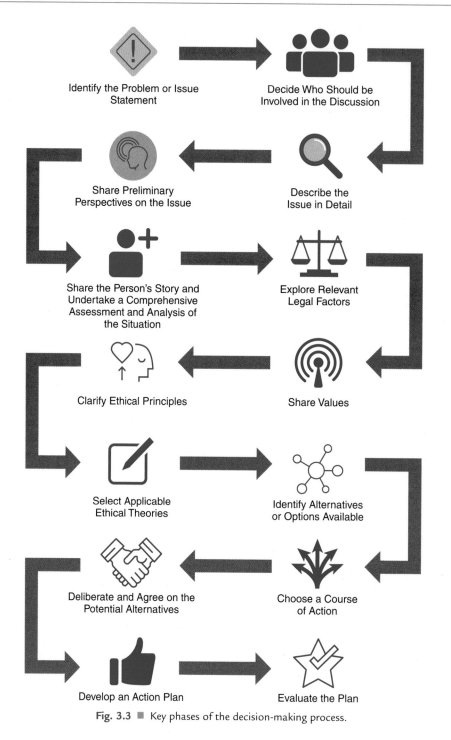

Fig. 3.3 ■ Key phases of the decision-making process.

Structures and Roles Providing Ethics Consultation and Support

Clinical Ethics Committees

These committees focus primarily on ethical issues related to patient care (Storch et al., 1990), unlike research ethics committees, which have the function of reviewing the ethical aspects of research proposals. They can take a passive role and wait for issues to be brought to them where they can offer advice and guidance in response to an ethical challenge, or they can take an active role in influencing practice across an organization or clinical setting (Piette et al., 2002). The latter is done, for example, by building ethics into organizational processes, making the ethics committee visible through the establishment of educational programs, and presenting at rounds.

Ethics committees are a resource accessible to nurses in some settings and regions across Canada and may be composed of nurses, physicians, patient/family advisors, community members, chaplains, lawyers, administrators, social workers, and other members of the interprofessional team with a strong interest in and commitment to ethics. The voices of the patients and family are heard when they are invited to discussions pertaining to them. Many organizations, recognizing the value of person-centred care, engage patient and family representation, ensuring their voices are heard. There is value when the committee includes various perspectives that represent the cultural diversity of the community, therefore having multiple "lenses" looking at the issues being discussed.

The roles of clinical ethics committees vary and may include one or more of the following functions.

Consultation

Clinical ethics committees may offer advice to patients, families, nurses, the broader team and leaders about how a situation may be approached, or they may guide them through the decision-making process. Essentially, it is the patient, the family, and the caregivers who decide and take action, but they can ask for input and guidance from ethics committees.

Education

Many ethics committees play a role in the education of staff. A more knowledgeable team may be able to prevent the escalation of a difficult issue if the concern is addressed early on.

Policy

Ethics committees may contribute to the establishment of policies or guidelines to assist staff in dealing with complex issues or to help clarify the ethical values and duties within an organization. These may include policies on confidentiality and guidelines about resuscitation, withdrawal of treatment, Medical Assistance in Dying (MAiD), and informed consent. Guidelines can also serve as educational tools for the staff if the ethical rules and principles involved in developing the guidelines are clear.

Research

Ethics committees may also undertake research on ethical issues and processes. For example, a committee may conduct surveys to identify the extent of ethical problems that caregivers face and the decision processes they use.

Organizational Ethics

Ethics committees may also be invited to engage in discussions regarding organizational ethics, which is discussed in Chapter 12. As quality improvement in most settings has become a priority, there is interest in integrating ethics into existing leadership and quality processes (Piette et al., 2002), such as an organization's approach to disclosure of adverse events, organizational practices regarding human resources, and allocation of limited resources (Singer et al., 2001).

Clinical Ethicists

Over the past few decades, the role of clinical ethicists has evolved. In some settings, clinical ethicists are shared across organizations. When available, they serve as an expert resource for the health care team, patients, and patients' families to support and facilitate ethical decision making. Usually, through graduate studies, clinical ethicists acquire knowledge of ethical theory and consultative methods, and gain clinical experience and the skills to manage conflict and facilitate decision making (Chidwick et al., 2004).

Clinical ethicists may do the following:

- Offer support to the team (at rounds or targeted meetings) or individual team members, patients, families, and students
- Provide advice or assistance in understanding the components of various types of ethical problems

- Facilitate case discussions and decision making by guiding discussions, posing meaningful questions, helping the team understand the principles involved in contributing to an ethical plan of care
- Aid in value clarification and ensuring each perspective or voice is heard
- Deliver ethics education
- Be involved in organizational issues such as challenges related to resource allocation, supporting staff experiencing ethical conflict and ethical distress, and providing input into a key strategic ethical challenge, such as:
  - How to disclose to multiple patients the potential for harm from exposure to an infectious agent (Gibson, 2008) or findings that inappropriate care was provided.

Implications for Nurses

Nurses, more than any other health care professionals, have prolonged interaction with the patient. Consequently, they are more likely than any other member of the health care team to understand the patient's situation and perspective. This knowledge is critical when making ethical decisions. Furthermore, nurses are involved in the implementation of decisions and the proposed plan of care.

Nurses are aware of the extent of ethical problems and violations because they face them daily. Therefore, they must be represented in ethics committees. Involvement in these processes is essential so that the voices of nurses directly facing these challenges are heard.

Leaders should ensure that nurses are aware that these resources are available to them. As professionals who are held accountable for their practice, nurses have the right (and often the responsibility) to go directly to ethics committees for advice and consultation. This action is supported in the values of the CNA *Code of Ethics* (CNA, 2017, p. 8).

Other Resources Available to Nurses

Guidelines, tools, and resources are available through most provincial regulatory colleges and associations. Regulatory colleges also have practice consultants available as confidential resources for nurses facing ethical and professional challenges. Many faith groups and cultural organizations also provide information to assist in clarifying their various values and beliefs. These resources can usually be accessed through their respective websites.

SUMMARY

This chapter provided historical context to the evolution of codes of ethics and offered an overview of the many resources and supports available to nurses dealing with everyday ethical issues and complex ethical challenges. The *ICN Code of Ethics for Nurses* and the CNA *Code of Ethics for Registered Nurses* highlight the fundamental values and responsibilities of professional nurses, provide guidance to the nurse as a moral agent, and offer models to support ethical nursing practice. Case scenarios that reflect nursing challenges were presented to facilitate a deeper understanding of the CNA *Code of Ethics*, to encourage ethical dialogue and reflection, and therefore foster an understanding of the moral issues nurses face. To guide these discussions, an ethical decision-making framework was offered.

Additional resources available to nurses, such as access to Best Practice Guidelines, clinical ethics committees, and clinical ethicists, were described. Because all of these resources are not available in all settings, nurses are encouraged to explore the resources available through professional associations, regulatory colleges, and cultural and faith organizations. It is hoped that enhanced awareness of these resources will help guide the ethical practice of the nurse.

CRITICAL THINKING

Discussion Points

1. As you review the history of ethical codes, consider to what extent do you think we have evolved as a society? To what extent have professional nursing codes progressed?
2. What are the differences and similarities between The *ICN Code of Ethics for Nurses* and the CNA *Code of Ethics for Registered Nurses*? Do you have a preference? What aspects of that code align with your way of thinking ethically?
3. Have you had experiences with ethical challenges in the past? Would these codes have helped you in addressing these challenges?
4. As you review the codes, are any of the theories presented in Chapter 2 evident to you? Take one of those theories and analyze it relative to the codes.
5. In your setting, organize a simulated ethics committee. Does the discussion among team members help to identify the issues and preferred option?

Does using an ethical decision-making framework assist you? Do individual team members offer various/unique perspectives?

6. What ethical resources are available to you through your own provincial or territorial college or association?

REFERENCES

Statutes

Child Protection Act, RSPEI 1988, c. C-5.1 (Prince Edward Island).

Child, Youth and Family Services Act, 2017, S.O. 2017, c. 14, Sch. 1 (Ontario).

Gunshot and Stab Wounds Mandatory Reporting Act, S.S. 2007, c. G-9.1. (Saskatchewan)

Texts and Articles

Access Alliance Multicultural Community Health Centre. (2005). *Racialised groups and health status: A literature review exploring poverty, housing, race-based discrimination and access to health care as determinants of health for racialised groups.* https://www.toronto.ca/legdocs/mmis/2007/hl/bgrd/backgroundfile-1734.pdf

Aikens, C. A. (1926). *Studies in ethics for nurses* (2nd ed.). W.B. Saunders Company.

Armstrong, A. E. (2006). Towards a strong virtue ethics for nursing practice. *Nursing Philosophy 7*(3), 110–124.

Babylonians. (n.d.). http://home.cfl.rr.com/crossland/Ancient Civilizations/Middle_East_Civilizations/Babylonians/babylonians.html

Baumann, A., O'Brien-Pallas, L., Armstrong-Stassen, M., et al. (2001). *Commitment and care: The benefits of a healthy workplace for nurses, their patients and the system—A policy synthesis.* Canadian Health Services Research Foundation and The Change Foundation.

Canadian Institutes of Health Research, Natural Sciences and Engineering Research Council of Canada, & Social Sciences and Humanities Research Council of Canada. (2014). *Tri-council policy statement: Ethical conduct for research involving humans.*

Canadian Nurses Association. (n.d.). *Strategic plan: 2023–2026.* https://hl-prod-ca-oc-download.s3-ca-central-1.amazonaws.com/CNA/2f975e7e-4a40-45ca-863c-5ebf0a138d5e/UploadedImages/documents/Public_CNA_Strategic_Plan_2023-2026.pdf

Canadian Nurses Association. (2017). *Code of ethics for registered nurses.*

Canadian Nurses Association. (2018). *Cannabis. CNA Health Canada SUAP project.* https://www.cna-aiic.ca/en/policy-advocacy/advocacy-priorities/cannabis

Canadian Nurses Association. (2022). *Non-medical cannabis: A nursing framework.* https://hl-prod-ca-oc-download.s3-ca-central-1.amazonaws.com/CNA/2f975e7e-4a40-45ca-863c-5ebf0a138d5e/UploadedImages/documents/Non_Medical_Cannabis_-_A_nursing_framework.pdf

Canadian Nurses Association. (2023a). *Who we are.* https://www.cna-aiic.ca/en/about-us/who-we-are

Canadian Nurses Association (2023b). vision Mission Objectives and Priorities. p. 1. https://www.cna-aiic.ca/en/membership/canadian-network-of-nursing-specialties/who-we-are-and-how-to-join/vision-mission-priorities

Canadian Nurses Protective Society. (2004). Consent of the incapable adult. *InfoLaw, 13*(3), 1–2.

Canadian Nursing Advisory Committee. (2002). *Our health, our future: Creating quality workplaces for Canadian nurses.* Advisory Committee on Health Human Resources.

Chidwick, P., Faith, K., Godkin, D., et al. (2004). Clinical education of ethicists: The role of a clinical ethics fellowship. *BMC Medical Ethics, 5*, 6.

Cho, S., Ketefian, S., Barkauskas, V., et al. (2003). The effects of nurse staffing on adverse events, morbidity, mortality and medical costs. *Nursing Research, 52*(2), 71–79.

Epstein, B., & Turner, M. (2015). The nursing code of ethics: Its value, its history. *Online Journal of Issues in Nursing, 20*(2), 4.

Falk-Rafael, A. (2005). Speaking truth to power: Nursing's legacy and moral imperative. *Advances in Nursing Science, 28*(3), 212–223.

Fortier, E., & Malloy, D. (2019). Moral agency, bureaucracy and nurses: A qualitative study. *Canadian Journal of Practical Philosophy, 3*(1), 1–14.

Fowler, M. D. (2021). The Nightingale still sings: Ten ethical themes in early nursing in the United Kingdom, 1888–1989. *The Online Journal of Issues in Nursing, 26*(2), 1–12.

Gibson, J. L. (2008). Clinical ethicists' perspectives on organizational ethics in healthcare organizations. *Journal of Medical Ethics, 34*, 320–323.

Government of Alberta. (2018). *Child intervention fact sheets.* https://alignab.ca/government-alberta-child-intervention-fact-sheets-february-1-2018/

Grace, P. (2018). Enhancing nurse moral agency: The leadership promise of Doctor of Nursing Practice preparation. *The Online Journal of Issues in Nursing, 23*(1), 4.

Grinspun, D., Virani, T., & Bajnok, I. (2002). Nursing best practice guidelines: The RNAO (Registered Nurses' Association of Ontario) project. *Hospital Quarterly, 5*(2), 56–60.

Hooker, R. (1996). *Mesopotamia: The Code of Hammurabi.* (L. W. King, Trans.). Washington State University.

Horne, C. F., & Johns, C. H. W. (1911). Ancient history sourcebook: Code of Hammurabi, c. 1780 BCE. In *The Encyclopaedia Britannica* (11th ed.). Britannica Books.

Hoyt, S. J. (2010). Florence Nightingale's contribution to contemporary nursing ethics. *Journal of Holistic Nursing, 28*(4), 331–332.

Information & Privacy Commission of Ontario, & Provincial Advocate for Children and Youth. (2018). *Yes, you can: Dispelling the myths about sharing information with Children's Aid Societies.* https://www.oacas.org/wp-content/uploads/2016/11/7798OPACYMyths-Booklayout-Web.pdf

International Council of Nurses. (2018). *Nurses' role in achieving the sustainable development goals.* http://www.dgnm.gov.bd/cmsfiles/files/ICN_AVoiceToLead_guidancePack_EN_Lowres.pdf

International Council of Nurses. (2021). *The ICN Code of Ethics for Nurses.*

International Council of Nurses. (2022a). *A statement by the International Council of Nurses on COVID-19 vaccination.* https://www.icn.ch/system/files/documents/2022-02/ICN%20Statement%20COVID-19%20Vaccination%20%E2%80%93%20Nurses%20lead%20the%20way_ENG_2.0.pdf?msclkid59ecab7fccf0611ec9d206daf8a067e55

International Council of Nurses. (2022b). *Strategic priorities.* https://www.icn.ch/sites/default/files/inline-files/Strategic%20plan.pdf

International Council of Nurses. (2022c). *Twelve decades of the International Council of Nurses.* https://icntimeline.org/page/0001.html

International Council of Nurses. (2022d). *Who we are.* http://www.icn.ch/who-we-are/who-we-are/

Jaimet, K. (2017). The fentanyl crisis. *Canadian Nurse, 113*(1), 23–25.

Jennings, B., Callahan, D., & Wolf, S. (1987). The professions: Public interest and common good. *Hastings Center Report, 17*(1), 3–10.

Kelly, L. Y. (1981). *Dimensions of professional nursing* (4th ed.). Macmillan.

Levine, M. E. (1999). On the humanities in nursing. *Canadian Journal of Nursing Research, 30*(4), 213–217.

McKeown, D. (2007). *The health of Toronto's young children. Toronto Public Health Report.* http://www.toronto.ca/health/hsi/hsi_young_children.htm

McNeill, T. (2008a, May 22–25). *Children, poverty and health* [Report presentation]. Social Work National Conference, Session 92, Toronto, ON.

McNeill, T. (2008b). *Children, poverty and health care utilization: Research and implications.* Canadian Public Health Association.

McTavish, J. R., MacMillan, H. L., & Wathen, C. N. (2016). *Briefing note: Mandatory reporting of child maltreatment.* VEGA Project and PreVAiL Research Network, 2016.

Mental Health Commission of Canada. (2016). *Supporting the Mental Health of Refugees to Canada.* https://www.mentalhealthcommission.ca/wp-content/uploads/drupal/2016-01-25_refugee_mental_health_backgrounder_0.pdf

Meyer, B. C., & Bishop, D. S. (2007). Florence Nightingale: Nineteenth century apostle of quality. *Journal of Management History, 13*(3), 240–254.

National Library of Medicine. (2002). *The Hippocratic oath* (M. North, Trans.). http://www.nlm.nih.gov/hmd/greek/greek_oath.html

Nightingale, F. (n.d.). *The "Nightingale pledge."* http://www.country-joe.com/nightingale/pledge.htm

Nightingale, F. (1882). Nursing the sick. In R. Quain (Ed.), *A dictionary of medicine* (pp. 1043–1049). Longmans, Green, and Co.

The Nuremberg Code (1947). (1996). *British Medical Journal,* 313, 1448. https://www.bmj.com/content/313/7070/1448.1

Olsen, L. L., & Stokes, F. (2016). *The ANA Code of Ethics for Nurses with interpretive statements.*

Person, S., Allison, J., Kiefe, C., et al. (2004). Nurse staffing and mortality for Medicare patients with acute myocardial infarction. *Medical Care, 42*(1), 4–12.

Piette, M., Ellis, J. L., St. Denis, P., et al. (2002). Integrating ethics and quality improvement: Practical implementation in the transitional/extended care setting. *Journal of Nursing Care Quality, 17*(1), 35–42.

Registered Nurses' Association of Ontario. (2002). *Toolkit: Implementation of clinical practice guidelines.*

Registered Nurses' Association of Ontario. (2005). *Educator's resource: Integration of Best Practice Guidelines.*

Registered Nurses Association of Ontario, (2007). Embracing Cultural Diversity in Health Care. Healthy Work Environments Best Practice Guidelines. Toronto, ON: Author.

Registered Nurses Association of Ontario, (2007). Professionalism in Nursing. Healthy Work Environments Best Practice Guidelines. Toronto, ON: Author.

Registered Nurses' Association of Ontario. (2007a). *Embracing cultural diversity in health care: developing cultural competence.* https://rnao.ca/bpg/guidelines/embracing-cultural-diversity-health-care-developing-cultural-competence

Registered Nurses' Association of Ontario. (2007b). *Professionalism in nursing.* https://rnao.ca/bpg/guidelines/professionalism-nursing?_ga=2.184872557.518739584.1683212156-1688993547.1680547001

Registered Nurses' Association of Ontario. (2009). *Preventing and managing violence in the workplace. Healthy work environments best practice guidelines.*

Registered Nurses' Association of Ontario. (2021). *Promoting 2SLG-BTQI+ health equity.* https://rnao.ca/bpg/guidelines/promoting-2slgbtqi-health-equity

Registered Nurses Association of Ontario, (2021). Promoting 2SLGBTQI+ Health Equity. Equity, diversity and inclusion (EDI), Population health. *Best Practice Guidelines.* Toronto, ON: Author.

Registered Nurses' Association of Ontario. (2022). *Guidelines.* Retrieved from https://rnao.ca/bpg/guidelines

Registered Nurses' Association of Ontario, & Registered Practical Nurses Association of Ontario. (2000). *Ensuring the care will be there: Report on nursing recruitment and retention in Ontario.*

Robb, I. H. (1900). *Nursing ethics for hospital and private use.* E. C. Koeckert. https://ia801408.us.archive.org/14/items/nursingethicsfo00robbgoog/nursingethicsfo00robbgoog.pdf

Sasichay-Akkadechanunt, T., Scalzi, C., & Jawad, A. (2003). The relationship between nurse staffing and patient outcomes. *Journal of Nursing Administration, 33*(9), 478–485.

Scott, P. A. (1995). Aristotle, nursing and health care ethics. *Nursing Ethics, 2*(4), 279–285.

Selanders, L. C., & Crane, P. C. (2012). The voice of Florence Nightingale on advocacy. *Online Journal of Issues in Nursing, 17*(1), 1.

Sellman, D. (1997). The virtues in the moral education of nurses: Florence Nightingale revisited. *Nursing Ethics, 4*(1), 3–11.

Singer, P., Pellegrino, E. P., & Siegler, M. (2001). Clinical ethics revisited. *BMC Medical Ethics, 2,* 1.

Sovie, M., & Jawad, A. (2001). Hospital restructuring and its impact on outcomes: Nursing staff regulations are premature. *Journal of Nursing Administration, 31*(12), 588–600.

Storch, J. L., Griener, G. G., Marshall, A., et al. (1990). Ethics committees in Canadian hospitals: Report of the 1989 survey. *Healthcare Management Forum, 3*(4), 3–8.

Tisdale, D., & Symenuk, P. M. (2020). Human rights and nursing codes of ethics in Canada 1953–2017. *Nursing Ethics, 27*(4), 1077–1088.

Toronto Central Regional Cancer Care Program. (2016). *Supporting & enabling Indigenous ceremonial practices within healthcare institutions: A wise practices guideline—Toronto Regional Indigenous Cancer Program.* https://www.trcp.ca/en/indigenous-cancer-program/Documents/CWP_Guideline.pdf

Tourangeau, A., Giovannetti, P., Tu, J., et al. (2002). Nursing-related determinants of 30-day mortality for hospitalized patients. *Canadian Journal of Nursing Research, 33*(4), 71–88.

Viens, D. C. (1989). A history of nursing's code of ethics. *Nursing Outlook, 37*(1), 45–48.

Wall, A. (1995). Health management guide. Ethics and probidity. *Health Service Journal, 105*(5451), Suppl. 1–12.

4 THE CANADIAN LEGAL SYSTEM

LEARNING OBJECTIVES

The purpose of this chapter is to enable you to understand:

- The basics of Indigenous law and the two primary legal systems in Canada—French civil law and English common law—and their historical foundations
- How these systems of law are applied in practice
- The division of powers between the federal and provincial governments
- The legislative process
- The difference between civil responsibility and criminal responsibility
- The structure and responsibilities of the court system
- The Constitution and the *Canadian Charter of Rights and Freedoms*
- Some of the basic elements of the relationship between Indigenous people and the Canadian legal environment

INTRODUCTION

The legal system is viewed by many as a complicated institution with its own language and rituals, shrouded in mystery. The law is often misunderstood or only partly understood. It is believed by many to be infallible; it is not. As a creation of the human mind, the law is never perfect because human circumstances are seldom black and white or as cut and dried as the representations in popular culture. Very often, an absolute solution to a problem is elusive, and legal rules and principles yield imperfect compromise solutions. Nevertheless, a good understanding of the law's basic machinery is essential for nurses. The legal and social interrelationships between individuals and institutions are complex. The law influences most aspects of the nursing profession, including nurses' everyday actions and decisions. Thus, nurses with a working knowledge of the legal system are better able to understand and work within the myriad rules and regulations that govern their profession, their relationships with other health care practitioners, and the health care system. This is important for their own self-protection and to ensure they exercise prudence in their practice.

Also, to ensure that the interests of their patients are represented, nurses must understand patient rights as well as their own professional obligations to protect and respect these rights. Like all Canadians, under the *Canadian Charter of Rights and Freedoms* (1982), nurses have the right to privacy and respect, and to freedom of expression. At the same time, they are subject to certain limitations related to the right to say, write, or otherwise act in accordance with their beliefs.

Society holds nurses to high standards of professional, moral, and ethical competence, but it also affords them certain rights and privileges. The law strives to keep these competing interests in balance.

The law influences many aspects of the professional practice of nurses. For example, the law:

- Regulates the education and licensing of nurses.
- Clarifies nurses' duty toward patients, the public, and one another.
- Provides a forum for resolving disputes and conflicts
- Clarifies processes related to compensatory justice when individuals suffer injury as a result of

99

the negligence of a nurse who fails to meet an accepted standard of care
- Establishes legislation related to the rights of patients, including consent, confidentiality, Medical Assistance in Dying (MAiD), reproductive technologies, and organ donation
- Outlines the civil and criminal consequences that can flow from the nurse–patient relationship

NATURAL JUSTICE AND PROCEDURAL FAIRNESS

During the Enlightenment of the mid-eighteenth century, thinkers and philosophers refined the concept of a "higher law"—a set of overarching principles that govern human society and relationships. This higher law, usually called "natural law," is viewed as being either divinely ordained or derived from nature, depending on one's philosophical or spiritual perspective. The idea was appealing during the Enlightenment as a response to the theory of the divine right of kings. Because human beings reason and think, they can use this ability to discern the natural and universal rules according to which they govern themselves, their societies, and their relationships with others. Therefore, as discussed in Chapter 2, humans use reason to discern what is "good," "just," and "morally right" behaviour.

One of the main principles of natural law is that all human beings must be treated fairly and consistently. Thus, for example, the rules of natural justice require that before being subjected to any moral or legal punishment for alleged wrongdoing, people must be given an opportunity to defend themselves and to have their "side of the story" considered or heard by the persons or body charged with reviewing or adjudicating upon their conduct. As we shall see in Chapter 5, this natural justice gives rise to certain procedural rights to fairness in both disciplinary and legal proceedings. These rights include the right to be informed of the allegations of misconduct, to be informed of the time and place at which that conduct will be reviewed, to be given an adequate opportunity to prepare and present evidence and raise arguments in defence of one's actions, and to have one's case heard before an impartial and objective decision-making adjudicator.

Consider Case Scenario 4.1.

CASE SCENARIO 4.1

THE RIGHTS OF NURSES TO LEGAL PROCESSES

P. W. is a registered nurse working in the pediatric unit of a hospital in a small prairie town. One morning, before commencing a work, they are called into their supervisor's office and told that serious allegations of sexual misconduct have been made against them in connection with a 6-year-old child with diabetes receiving dialysis treatment in the unit. These allegations, P. W. is informed, were made by a colleague, who learned of P. W.'s actions from the child's parent. P. W. is further told that the matter has been reported to the local police, that their employment at the hospital is being terminated immediately, and that the regulatory college, which governs nurses in that province, has been informed of their conduct.

In such a case, to which requirements of procedural fairness would P. W. be entitled?

P. W. should:
- Be given details of the allegations them and provided detailed disclosure of the evidence in support of those allegations
- Be advised of the date, time, and place of any disciplinary hearing and the procedures that will be followed
- Be given the opportunity to consult with a lawyer, not only in connection with the disciplinary proceedings, but also for advice on any criminal proceedings that may ensue
- Also consult an employment lawyer with respect to any possible claim for wrongful dismissal that they may exist against the hospital have against their employer
- Be heard by an unbiased and impartial disciplinary decision-making body. This should not include anyone personally connected with the case or anyone P. W. reports to

DUE PROCESS AND RULE OF LAW

Flowing from the concept of natural justice are the principles of due process and rule of law. These are common to both common law and civil law in Canada. As in other democratic countries with highly developed legal systems, these principles permeate the legal system and give it legitimacy. In Case Scenario 4.1, this guarantees P. W. the right to know the procedures that will be followed in any disciplinary proceedings before the professional college and to know that those procedures will be followed in letter and spirit. In terms of any legal proceedings, P. W. is entitled to due process and to have their legal rights under the *Canadian Charter of Rights and Freedoms* respected and enforced. These rights are discussed in more detail later in this chapter.

Due process is a feature of justice that encompasses the notion that all people are equal before the law and are entitled to the same rights and benefits arising from the law. In the past, the applicability of rules and laws was often determined by a person's social status, ancestry, religion, race, or wealth. A basic tenet of the current Canadian legal system is that any person, no matter how rich, poor, powerful, famous, or unknown, and regardless of that person's race, gender, sexual orientation, physical or mental disability, religion or creed, is entitled to be treated by the law in exactly the same manner as any other person. For example, if the adult child of a government minister were arrested for impaired driving, they should and would receive no special or preferential treatment by the criminal justice system simply because their parent is a member of the government. *Due process* refers to more than just consistent treatment under the law; it also encompasses the concept that the state (usually referred to as the **Crown** in Canada) will strictly follow the law, affording every person the same opportunity to know the evidence against them and the case they have to meet. Due process is the concept underlying such judicial rulings as the exclusion of improperly obtained evidence or the dismissal of criminal trials where the Crown has failed to disclose potentially relevant evidence to the defence.

The rule of law means that those who are charged with administering and enforcing laws are obligated to behave in accordance with them, that they will not overstep or act beyond their legal authority, and that their decisions will be respected and complied with by members of society and persons in positions of authority. This gives a court order or judgement its finality and authority, or the decision of a government official (e.g., a judge, tribunal officer, or minister of the Crown) its force. If it were otherwise, while a society might have the best written law, chaos and disorder would ensue. Acceptance of the rule of law ensures that contracts are enforceable, for example, and encourages a stable, democratic society and a prosperous economy.

FOUNDATIONS OF CANADA'S LEGAL SYSTEM

The geographical territory that is now Canada was occupied by Indigenous peoples, long before the first Europeans arrived in North America. Current Indigenous peoples in Canada are the descendants of the original inhabitants of North America, and, as described in Chapter 1, include First Nations, Inuit, and Métis. As there are cultural differences across Indigenous communities historically, there are also variations in their legal systems, though there are some commonalities.

Often ignoring the rights of the original inhabitants, the British and the French colonizers competed to claim eastern North America, and the country of Canada was formed from these origins. As a nation-state, Canada began as a confederation of former British and French colonies and territories. French and British settlers brought with them not only their languages, religions, and culture, but also the legal structures, rules, and principles of their countries of origin.

Legal Traditions of Indigenous Peoples in Canada

European and Indigenous concepts of law and justice come from different world views. Europeans had trouble recognizing or accepting that Indigenous peoples had social or legal systems for dealing with relationships, crime, and rights. The European legal systems relied on documented laws with a major oversight role for the state. "Regardless of whether the laws of Aboriginal societies conformed to the preconceptions of Europeans, there were laws and a system of sanctions that allowed Aboriginal people to function in a coherent and orderly fashion" (Aboriginal Justice Implementation Commission [AJIC], 1999, V. 1, c. 2 Aboriginal Concepts of Law). For example, sophisticated trade and diplomatic relationships existed between Indigenous nations across North America.

Legal systems differed widely across Indigenous communities, but concepts of law had some common features and usually relied on oral traditions supported by knowledgeable Elders. Elders, considered the knowledge keepers, were responsible for teaching, history, customs, values, and beliefs. As leaders, they were instrumental in the resolution of disputes and issues of concern. Because most communities were small and included extended kinship groups and people who knew each other well, moral suasion was often a powerful tool to ensure good conduct and conformity to generally accepted social rules. Further, survival in a harsh environment often depended on mutual cooperation. As such, social harmony was frequently an important goal in Indigenous societies. Within this context, the "underlying philosophy in Aboriginal societies in dealing with crime was the resolution of disputes, the healing of wounds and the restoration of social harmony" (AJIC, 1999, Ch. 2). Much of the law was focused on the personal interactions between individuals and did not involve a concept of a central authority (such as a monarch) that required conformity.

Ultimately the Canadian legal system has little recognition of Indigenous legal traditions and is primarily based on English and French concepts of law and justice. Therefore, the historical and cultural traditions of Indigenous peoples may make their contacts with the criminal justice system complicated and unfair. "[T]he daily, systemic cultural discrimination inflicted upon Aboriginal people by the justice system, however unintentional, demeans and diminishes the importance and relevance of their cultures, languages and beliefs" (AJIC, Introduction, 1999, Ch. 2).

Indigenous law is an important issue in the evolution of Canada, and although its significance in our legal system has varied, it must be taken into account in the administration of justice and in understanding our laws, culture, and traditions.

French Civil Law

What today is Quebec was governed exclusively under French civil law until the French colonies in the St. Lawrence Valley (New France) were ceded by France to Great Britain in 1763 under the Treaty of Paris, the peace treaty that concluded the Seven Years' War. French civil law was based on the Roman civil law system, which is still prevalent in Western Europe and many other countries around the world. In Roman civil law systems, legal rules and principles that establish the rights and responsibilities of individuals, including the various principles governing land ownership, contracts, civil wrongs (called *delicts*), marriage laws, the laws of inheritance, and so forth, are formally written—or, as lawyers say, **codified**—in a single document known as a **civil code**. Lawyers and judges view this code as the chief source of all rules and principles necessary to resolve disputes or legal issues.

In New France, the civil codes of the French monarchy served as the sole legal tradition. After 1763, the British tried to enforce their laws within the territory but frequently had to adapt to the existing French legal traditions. In 1774, the British granted their French-speaking colonies in Canada the right to follow French legal traditions in civil (noncriminal) law.

English Common Law

Unlike civil law systems, the majority of common law is not the product of a formal set of principles. Historically, the term **common law** describes a system based on rules, principles, and doctrine developed by English judges over time and which was meant to be applicable to all the English and Welsh people. These legal rules and principles emerged from the decisions of courts over centuries. The law was contained in a large collection of judgements, or "case law," derived from these judicial rulings. There were laws enacted by the state, but these were usually quite limited. The relevant decisions in past cases (referred to as *case law* or *precedent*) are reviewed and considered to identify the principles at the core of those decisions and applicable to the current dispute.

The judges who made these rules and principles over the centuries did not claim to be making law—because that was the exclusive purview of, first, the sovereign, and, later, the sovereign and Parliament—but, rather, claimed that they were interpreting the law from the ancient body of unwritten principles that existed throughout the English legal tradition and from the wisdom of past judges.

These legal principles and rules are often derived from common sense and ethical principles. For example, the law holds that touching a person without the consent of that person is a civil wrong (battery) and potentially a criminal offence (assault). The need for consent is based on the principle of autonomy, in which a person's independence and sense of personhood encompasses the right to control their body and to determine their own destiny. The law prohibiting touching another person without consent is also derived from the principle of nonmaleficence—that one should do no harm.

All jurisdictions in Canada, except Quebec, rely on the English common law tradition as the basis of their legal system. Quebec has continued to use the traditions of the French civil law system in many areas of the law. In areas of federal jurisdiction, such as criminal law or aviation, common law approaches are used in Quebec. In areas of provincial responsibility, such as health and education, the Quebec civil code and the French civil law traditions are used.

FUNDAMENTALS OF COMMON LAW

In both French civil law and British common law traditions, the courts also apply statute laws. **Statute law** is a formal written set of rules passed by a legislative body to regulate a particular area, such as those acts that regulate nursing in provinces across the country. Statute law has greatly expanded in the last two centuries, and statutes (also called *legislation*) are a major part of the law today. Canadian courts, except those in Quebec, have the task of interpreting statute law and applying common law precedents to resolve disputes. Quebec courts have similar statutes to consider within the framework of the civil code.

Statute law is a way for the legislature to change common law: to shape the law to achieve desirable consequences. For example, a law requiring children to be given certain vaccinations before they attend school improves public health outcomes and reduces the burden of diseases for families and the health care system. The court can interpret the statute but cannot change it.

The *Canadian Charter of Rights and Freedoms* (1982), part of the Constitution, is a statement of principles guaranteeing rights and freedoms for everyone, subject only to such limits as are reasonable in a free and democratic society. The Charter supersedes all precedent and all statute law unless the strict tests in the Charter are met. For example, in *Vriend v. Alberta*

(1998), the Supreme Court of Canada was asked to consider an Alberta human rights law that prohibited discrimination on several grounds, including, race, religious beliefs, colour, gender, physical disability, mental disability, age, ancestry, and place of origin. The issue of sexual orientation was not included as a prohibited ground of discrimination in the statute and had been deliberately left out. Vriend, employed in a private college, had been terminated on the basis of his failure to comply with the college policy on homosexual practice. Vriend tried to file a human rights complaint with the Alberta Human Rights Commission but was advised that the commission had no jurisdiction to act because sexual orientation was not a prohibited ground of discrimination in the statute.

Vriend challenged the constitutionality of the statute on the ground that in excluding sexual orientation as a prohibited ground of discrimination, the statute violated his Charter section 15 rights to equal treatment before the law. The Supreme Court agreed that Vriend's section 15 rights had been violated and that the omission in the statute was not a reasonable limit on Charter rights. The court held that sexual orientation as a prohibited ground of discrimination should be treated as though it was listed in the statute. Vriend was permitted to proceed with his complaint.

A secondary source of law is found in textbooks and journals written by legal scholars and experts. These experts may address specific topics, such as contracts or property law, and the scope may be narrow or broad. Although invaluable to common law scholarship and legal education, this scholarly writing, or doctrine, is not binding on common law courts, and it is subordinate to statute and case law. For example, one of the most influential texts on Canadian constitutional law for many years was Peter W. Hogg's (1997) *Constitutional Law of Canada*. Professor Hogg's analysis and ideas were often discussed by courts in Constitution-related cases, but only as a possible interpretation of the legislation and case law. As discussed further below, in Quebec's civil code legal system, doctrine, highly respected by the courts in their judicial decision making, is often considered authoritative.

Custom constitutes another, less prominent source of law in common law systems. As its name suggests, *custom* means that in the absence of specific and applicable legal principles in case law, statutes, or doctrine, the courts will be guided by the long-standing practices of a particular industry, trade, or other endeavour. In nursing, this might include codes of ethics, policies, standards of practice, curriculum, and so on.

Table 4.1 lists the four major sources of common law.

Case Law (Precedent)

Case law refers to judges' decisions rendered over centuries of judicial consideration and refinement. Case law is found in many nations—including Canada, the United States, Australia, and New Zealand—that have embraced English common law. In each case, a judge applies legal principles to resolve a legal issue arising in a situation that is considered similar to that of a past case on the basis of the presence of similar or identical facts. These principles are usually derived from ethical concepts.

For example, one particular legal principle holds that a person suing another for negligence must prove three things: (1) that they have suffered **damages** (i.e., either physical or mental injury to the person suing or damage or loss to that person's property); (2) that the other person owed them a duty of care (in other words, owed a specific responsibility—e.g., a nurse toward a

patient or a teacher toward a pupil); and (3) that the damages suffered were caused by the other's breach of duty, or failure to perform that duty. This rule evolved from early cases in which someone was harmed as a result of another person's carelessness. The courts sought to generally protect people from carelessness while not imposing unreasonable restrictions. Therefore, they developed the requirement to show the existence of these three elements to prove negligence in law. The principles of negligence are discussed in more detail in Chapter 7.

Civil Lawsuits

The use of precedent and case law can be illustrated in the example of a lawsuit. When an action, or claim, is brought forward to the court, each party (litigant) to the suit (usually represented by a lawyer) presents evidence to the court in support of their position. The person making the claim (the plaintiff) is the first to introduce evidence through witnesses with direct personal knowledge of the facts and expert witnesses with specialized knowledge. Each witness is questioned by the person or persons being sued (the defendant or defendants) or their lawyer. Then, the defendants

TABLE 4.1	
Sources of Common Law (in Decreasing Order of Authority)	
Source and Degree of Authority	**Definition and Characteristics**
Statute Law and Regulations Most authoritative; overrides case law in court.	Formal written laws and regulations passed by legislature or under legislative authority that set forth rules and principles governing a particular subject.
Case Law Very authoritative; depends on level of court that rendered the decision and its relationship to the court considering the precedent.	Individual court decisions constitute a body of precedent in which rules, definitions of legal concepts, and legal principles have been fashioned by judges over centuries. Applied in similar-fact situations.
Doctrine Seldom seen as authoritative by common law judges; depends on the respect accorded to, and the stature of, the author of the work by the legal community and, in particular, by judges.	Articles, texts, treatises, and other materials by legal scholars and academics elucidating a particular area of law. Authors comment on statute and case law, and elaborate on and interpret the legal principles found in these sources.
Custom Least authoritative; must be a complete absence of guidance from other sources before courts will resort to custom. Rarely invoked.	Principles and rules of a particular trade or relationship. The courts will elevate accepted practice in a particular trade or relationship to a rule of law when statutes and common law are silent on a particular issue.

present their evidence, which can also be tested by the plaintiff. After all of the evidence has been submitted to the court, each side has the opportunity to make its final argument, summing up the relevant facts and citing case law containing facts similar to the case at hand. Each litigant relies on cases containing a principle or rule of law that, if applied in this case, yields a result favourable to them. If the person bringing the suit cannot present enough **evidence** that they suffered any damages, the case would, following precedent, be dismissed. If damages are proven, case law might be used to establish the amount of compensation. For example, the law might place a higher value of damages in the case of a child who suffered brain damage than in the case of an adult who lost a limb as a result of the same negligence.

The court must select from among precedents or case law those that are most relevant and most authoritative or binding. The principles stated in the precedents are then applied to the facts of the case before it. The court may elaborate or expand upon the principles derived from previous cases, thus further developing the law. In this sense, common law is fashioned by judges, who have to observe established legal rules in developing it. The decision itself then becomes a further precedent, which serves to bolster or undermine a future litigant's case. For example, in the Ontario Superior Court decision of *Latin v. Hospital for Sick Children et al.* (2007), discussed in detail in Chapter 7, the court considered a case involving an infant who suffered severe brain damage following a series of seizures experienced while she was in the hospital's emergency department. In this action, the mother of the child alleged that when she brought her daughter—who was suffering from a high fever and "jerking" episodes—into the hospital and the charge nurse on duty that day had negligently classified the infant as an "urgent" case, rather than as an "emergent" one. The plaintiff claimed that the child's brain damage had been caused by oxygen deprivation and that if she had been classified as an "emergent" case, a physician would have seen her sooner, recognized signs of early shock, and taken appropriate measures to prevent status epilepticus. The plaintiff in this case was the child, through her parents and family. Their claim essentially was that if not for the delay in examining the child, she would not have suffered the brain damage. They claimed that the

charge nurse owed the child a duty to carry out an appropriate assessment, and had failed to do so.

In considering the standard of care owed by the nurse to the child, the court applied the legal principles (case law) in a previous decision of the Supreme Court of Canada: *Wilson v. Swanson* (1956). In that case, the Supreme Court held that although the law does not require a standard of perfection, it does require the exercise of such care and skill that would be reasonably expected of a prudent and careful hospital and a prudent and careful nurse in the same circumstances. In *Latin v. Hospital for Sick Children et al.*, the court ultimately ruled that the actions of the hospital and the nurses involved (who were also defendants in the action) met the prudent and careful standard, and they were not responsible for the infant's brain damage. In the context of nursing, the court would consider the standards expected of nurses by the regulatory body, as well as those standards (usually higher) set within their particular organization, to establish what can be expected of a prudent and careful nurse. An example would be those higher standards expected of nurses working in a critical care environment.

In common law, when any applicable existing precedent of a **superior court** exists, an **inferior court** is bound to decide cases by using the same legal principles and rules pronounced by the superior court in cases with similar circumstances. This is called the doctrine of **stare decisis**. *Stare decisis* is a Latin phrase that means "to abide by the decision" (Stuart, 1982, p. 7). Because an inferior court (usually a trial court) is judicially subordinate to an appellate (appeal) court in the hierarchical court structure, it is bound to follow the decisions and precedents of that higher court. Litigation begins in trial level courts (sometimes called **courts of first instance**). Decisions of the trial level courts can be appealed to higher courts. The exact path of appeal depends on where the original case started (provincial court, federal court, specialized tribunal), what the subject matter was (special courts exist for family law, tax cases, wills, shipwrecks, military cases), and the type of claim (some courts are limited to specific dollar amounts or to granting certain types of relief).

The decision of an appeal court is binding on a trial level court and, as a corollary, the decisions of an appeal court are bound by the decisions of a higher-level appeal court. So, for example, the trial level court in each province or territory, is bound to follow the decisions of the Court of Appeal for that province or territory when the previous decision is relevant and involves similar facts. All trial level courts and the Courts of Appeal in each jurisdiction are bound to follow the decisions of the Supreme Court of Canada in the same way. However, the trial level court in a specific province or territory is not bound by the decisions of other trial level courts or territories or by the decisions of appeal courts in other provinces. The Supreme Court of Canada is not bound by its previous decisions, although in practice the court will not ignore a previous decision lightly.

The application of precedent in English common law is designed to achieve two primary objectives. First, the law strives to be as consistent as possible. Review of relevant case law is necessary to determine which judicial pronouncements have the force of law and which have been overruled by subsequent decisions by higher courts. Consistency is achieved by applying the same legal principles in similar circumstances in a similar manner over time. Consequently, a degree of certainty is a characteristic of the common law system.

For example, in *Latin v. Hospital for Sick Children et al.* (2007), the plaintiff claimed that the defendant nurse had failed to meet the standard of care owed to the plaintiff. The test of the standard of care owed by nurses to the patients in the emergency department had been established in the Supreme Court of Canada decision *Wilson v. Swanson* (1956). As the facts were similar, the trial court applied the duty of care test from *Wilson* to the evidence before it in *Latin* and determined that the nurse had satisfied the duty of care owed the plaintiff. If the facts had been different, the trial court would have had to consider the differences and decide whether the test should be changed from the one used in *Wilson*.

Second, common law strives to be as predictable as possible. If lower courts were not bound to follow the decisions and precedents of higher courts, then the outcome of a given case would be unpredictable. A court would be free to decide the case on the basis of any principle of its own choosing, regardless of existing legal principles and rules previously found and applied in case law in similar-fact situations. This would defeat the requirement of consistency, as we would never know which principles would be applied in a given situation.

In the common law tradition, predictability and consistency of the law are seen as conducive to a well-ordered society in which people know their rights and obligations toward one another. For example, A can enter into a **contract** with B because A knows that the law will compensate A if B fails to perform the contract. This certainty follows from a primary legal principle established in case law that people who freely enter into contracts should and will be bound to perform their obligations or pay compensation unless the contract is contrary to existing law or public policy or was obtained through misrepresentation or fraud. Within such a legal framework, a society flourishes both politically and economically because people can predict the likely legal consequences of their activities, which lends greater stability to their social and economic endeavours.

This body of precedents spans roughly nine centuries and has become quite large and comprehensive. Over time, case law has developed and adapted, albeit slowly, to changing social, moral, and economic conditions and situations. For example, previously, a person who was harmed by a defective product could not sue the manufacturer unless they had a direct contract with the manufacturer. In contract law, the purchaser from the manufacturer could expect that a good was fit for its intended purpose. A purchaser from a shop had no claim as the shop had not been negligent in the manufacture of the good and the purchaser had no contract with the negligent manufacturer. The law changed in the 1930s when a person bought a bottle of ginger beer from a shop and found a mouse in it. At the time, he had no valid claim against the producer of the drink because he had no contract with the manufacturer; his only contract was with the shop owner. However, he sued, and the law changed when a decision was made by the highest British appeal court (at the time, also the highest appeal court for Canada) that the maker of the ginger beer, regardless of a contract being present or not, owed a duty of care to the ultimate consumers of the ginger beer. Thus, an extension of the law of negligence was created (*Donoghue v. Stevenson,* 1932). With this requirement established, the duty of care was considered to have been breached because the person who found the mouse inside the bottle of ginger beer suffered mental distress.

In some areas of law, case law developed by judges, is no longer acceptable to society. The state can correct this situation by passing a statute that replaces the judge-made law with a set of rules more in keeping with the desires of society. An example of this is the concept of contributory negligence. A principle of common law established by judges was that if a plaintiff was even 1% responsible for the injuries that they suffered and another person was 99% responsible, the plaintiff was disqualified from receiving any compensation because of their contributory negligence. For example, a pedestrian struck by a speeding car while jaywalking was not entitled to any compensation for their injuries because they were partly at fault. The legislatures in nearly every jurisdiction have passed a law that allows a court to award damages to a plaintiff who was partly responsible for the injuries they suffered in proportion to their responsibility. So, in the example of the pedestrian, the person would be awarded damages for their injuries, and then the amount of those damages would be reduced to reflect the degree of their own responsibility (see, for example, the *Ontario/ Negligence Act,* 1990).

Statutes and Regulations

Case law can be a rather slow means of altering and fashioning the law to meet changing social and economic conditions. Yet, the impact of court decisions on society is significant and far reaching. In some cases, like those involving abortion, same-sex marriage, and Medical Assistance in Dying (MAiD), the courts have moved ahead of the government and, perhaps, society.

Courts, by nature, tend to be conservative institutions. Traditionally, they have defined their role as interpreting and applying an existing body of laws and regulations, rather than creating law from abstract principles. The court, as the impartial arbiter of societal conflicts, is usually loath to infringe on Parliament's power to make the nation's laws. In more recent years, however, courts have occasionally taken a more activist role in interpreting and applying the law—for example, in cases concerning the rights of same-sex couples and the parental roles in blended families. This has been particularly true since the Charter came into force. The Charter places courts in a position to do more than just interpret legislation.

Perhaps the best example of this is found in laws dealing with **abortion** and **assisted suicide**. Until recently, the courts upheld laws that prohibited abortions, except in special cases. The *Criminal Code* (1985) made it an offence for anyone to perform such a procedure unless it was intended to preserve the life of the mother and was deemed necessary by a hospital committee. In a legal challenge of the provision within the *Criminal Code* prohibition, the Supreme Court of Canada, in *R. v. Morgentaler* (1988), ruled the law unconstitutional and a violation of a woman's right to life and personal security. The federal government tried to fashion a new criminal law in relation to abortion but ultimately chose not to take any action. Abortion is, therefore, regulated by provincial health legislation and no longer prohibited through federal criminal law.

With respect to the controversial issue of assisted suicide, the *Criminal Code* (1985) provided that it was an offence for anyone to assist a person to take his or her own life. Counselling a person to die by suicide remains a crime. The decision of the Supreme Court of Canada in the case of Sue Rodriguez (described more fully in Chapter 8) illustrates the court's reluctance to strike down statutory provisions respecting assisted suicide (*Rodriguez v. British Columbia (Attorney General),* 1993). In 2015, the Supreme Court of Canada was asked to reconsider the issues raised in *Rodriguez.* In *Carter v. Canada (Attorney General)* (2015), the Supreme Court of Canada ruled that sections 14 and 241(b) of the *Criminal Code* were invalid in relation to the prohibition of "physician-assisted death for a competent adult person who (1) clearly consents to the termination of life; and (2) has a grievous and irremediable medical condition (including an illness, disease, or disability) that causes enduring suffering that is intolerable to the individual in the circumstances of his or her condition" (para. 147). The court found that a less restrictive approach than the *Criminal Code* wording would allow persons to have assistance in dying in circumstances that avoided concerns about patient competence and voluntariness and that coercion, undue influence, and ambivalence could all be reliably assessed as part of that process. This legal decision forced the federal government to try to structure a MAiD law that complied with the legal principles and the Charter.

FUNDAMENTALS OF THE *CIVIL CODE OF QUÉBEC*

Despite some similarities with English common law, Quebec civil law is sufficiently different that it deserves a separate discussion. It has many features and characteristics that are unique to civil law. Although Quebec's legal system is principally derived from the French legal system, it has also been influenced (to some degree) by English common law for historical, social, and geographical reasons.

In the Quebec system, the primary source of law is the *Civil Code of Québec* (1991): a lengthy, detailed, and comprehensive statute that sets out a variety of legal rules and principles dealing with matters that include contracts; civil wrongs or "delicts" (e.g., trespassing, slander, assault); negligence; family relations; children's rights; marriage; property rights; wills and the laws of inheritance; corporate law; and insurance law. Quebec's legal system, like that of the common law provinces, has a body of decided case law called **jurisprudence**. In the Quebec legal system, however, jurisprudence is subordinate to the Civil Code. Jurisprudence is merely evidence of how previous courts have treated a particular provision of the Code; it is not binding on a subsequent court because the doctrine of *stare decisis* does not apply in the Quebec civil law system.

Quebec also has a body of statute law, but the Civil Code takes precedence unless the relevant statute expressly states otherwise. Ultimately, the principles set out in the Code, derived and developed from doctrinal writings of legal scholars, common sense, and ethical principles, are the primary source of law to resolve civil disputes. As the Civil Code preamble states:

> *The Civil Code comprises a body of rules which, in all matters within the letter, spirit or object of its provisions, lays down the jus commune [the law that applies to all of Quebec], expressly or by implication. In these matters, the Code is the foundation of all other laws, although other laws may complement the Code or make exceptions to it. (Civil Code of Québec, 1991, Chapter CCQ-1991, Preliminary Provision)*

Doctrine, or the scholarly writings of law experts, is another guide that has the force of law for the civil court. It takes precedence over even the jurisprudence of a higher court in helping a judge to interpret a provision of the Civil Code and to apply it in a particular situation. Doctrine may take the form of law review articles, textbooks, or, frequently, multivolume treatises on various areas of civil law. The more respected the author, the more respected, relevant, and authoritative that author's works will be in the eyes of the court.

Although a Quebec civil court is not strictly bound by the decisions of a higher court, this does not mean that it can ignore jurisprudence. A court in Quebec is still required to treat such decisions with utmost respect and must have a sound reason—in the Code itself, in accepted doctrine, or in earlier decisions—for departing from a precedent. This is a requirement more so in Quebec than in other civil law jurisdictions because of the influence of English common law on Quebec's judicial traditions. An added consequence of the nonbinding nature of civil law jurisprudence is that the courts have somewhat greater leeway in applying the Code's various provisions to new situations. Because of this, civil law has often been said to have greater flexibility and adaptability compared with common law.

Table 4.2 lists the three major sources of civil law in Quebec.

An interesting illustration of the court's deliberative process is found in the controversial decision of the Quebec Superior Court in *Nancy B. v. Hôtel-Dieu de Québec* (1992). This case involved a young woman, age 25 years, stricken with Guillain-Barré syndrome, a rare and sometimes incurable neurological disease, which, in its final stages, leaves a person completely paralyzed and dependent on a respirator. Patients can survive for years; however, they are incapable of physical activity. Nancy's life was limited to lying in bed and watching television. Her mental faculties were keen, and yet she felt trapped in a useless body, an existence that she found unbearable. She expressed her wish to die a natural death and requested that her intravenous feedings be discontinued and her respirator turned off. The physician and hospital involved in her care had difficulty complying with her request and took the matter to court.

Nancy retained a lawyer and brought an application to the Quebec Superior Court for an **injunction** (a court order) directing the hospital and physicians to cease all treatment, nourishment, and use of the respirator so that

TABLE 4.2

Sources of Civil Law (in Decreasing Order of Authority)

Source and Degree of Authority	Definition and Characteristics
Civil Code of Québec, Statutes, and Regulations Binding on all courts, the Code is often used as an aid in interpreting statutes and takes precedence, unless the statute says otherwise.	The Code embodies rules, definitions, and legal principles regulating many areas of provincial law. Other statutes and regulations supplement the Code and usually regulate a specific area (e.g., highways).
Doctrine Usually given wide deference and seen as persuasive and authoritative in civil law courts.	Articles, books, treatises, and other written materials by legal scholars; used by courts as an aid to interpreting ambiguous provisions of the Code or statutes.
Jurisprudence Persuasive but not binding; accorded less authority in some cases than doctrine; seen as evidence of how courts have interpreted and applied law in past cases.	Resembles common law case law (see Table 4.1) but is not strictly binding on civil law courts. Doctrine of *stare decisis* does not apply in Quebec.

she might die. The court considered a provision of the Civil Code then in effect (Article 19.1, *Civil Code of Lower Canada,* no longer in force), which stipulated that without obtaining consent, no one could be made to undergo medical treatment of any kind. The court held that this provision applied to this case, and thus, it was determined that Nancy had the right to refuse further treatment. The court also considered certain doctrine that held that, in the absence of a threat to the rights of others or a threat to public order, the right to refuse consent was effectively absolute. As an example of how Quebec courts use doctrine, Justice Dufour, J. said (translated from French to English):

> [37] *Professor Jean-Louis Beaudoin, now a justice of the Quebec Court of Appeal, also considered this subject. In a seminar entitled "Le droit de refuser d'être traité" (The right to refuse to be treated) and given under the auspices of the Canadian Institute for the Administration of Justice, he advanced the following [translation]:*
> *"For a competent person of the age of majority, the making of his own decisions with respect to his own body is the legal expression of the principle of personal autonomy and of the right to self-determination."*
> [38] *Further on:*
> *The ability to consent is not however absolute, but rather subject to two limitations. First, the*

corresponding rights of others. Accordingly, an individual may not use his body in a manner which may have the effect of putting in jeopardy the life or health of others. Second, public order (policy). The law sometimes imposes limits on the right to freely do what one wishes with one's body. Accordingly, it does not allow a person to dispose inter vivos of a part of his body which is not capable of regeneration or, a vital organ. Subject to these two limits however, one may consider that the right to autonomy and self-determination is absolute. (Nancy B. v. Hôtel-Dieu de Quebec, 1992).

To supplement the Code, the court relied on further doctrine stating that the act of placing a person on a respirator constituted medical treatment and, thus, fell within the meaning of the provision of the Code requiring consent.

In dealing with the argument that to remove Nancy from the respirator would be a violation of the *Criminal Code* (insofar as the physician and hospital would be assisting her in committing suicide or could arguably be committing murder), the court stated that the discontinuation of treatment would merely allow natural death to occur. It noted, referring as well to US case law, that natural death is a consequence of neither murder nor suicide. Thus, the removal of the respirator could not be classified as assisted suicide or murder.

The court further reasoned that these particular provisions of the *Criminal Code* could not reasonably be interpreted in such a way as to make removal of the respirator an offence. To interpret it so would hamper the medical profession in that any course of treatment, no matter how ineffective, could never be discontinued once undertaken. This, the court held, could not have been the intent of Parliament in enacting these provisions. Thus, it ruled that Nancy had the right to withhold consent to her treatment and accordingly granted her the injunction. Once the time for an appeal of the decision had lapsed, the respirator was disconnected, and Nancy died shortly thereafter.

This example, in which doctrine was used to uphold a patient's right to autonomy, demonstrates the Quebec court's use of doctrine and case law from another jurisdiction in interpreting a crucial provision of the Civil Code and illustrates how the courts of Quebec tend to value doctrine to a far greater extent than do their common law counterparts. Examples of how a common law court might have resolved the issue are found in the Supreme Court of Canada decisions of *Rodriguez v. British Columbia (Attorney General)* (1993) and *Carter v. Canada (Attorney General)* (2015) (which will be discussed in greater detail in Chapter 8).

In 1992, the Civil Code was revised in its entirety. The new Code came into force on January 1, 1994.

The new Code has added provisions dealing with areas of law unforeseen in the nineteenth century when the former Code was enacted. It includes explicit provisions for the patient's right to consent to medical treatment, enshrines the right to refuse treatment, expands children's rights to have a say in their treatment, and introduces a host of other new provisions dealing with mentally incompetent or terminally ill persons, organ donation, substitute decision making, and so on.

THE LEGISLATIVE PROCESS

The slower pace of life in the preindustrial era may have been well suited to the gradual and incremental work of common law courts. However, a modern and swiftly changing society demands more rapid response, which our legal institutions have sometimes struggled to provide.

Canada's government comprises three branches: (1) the judicial branch, or the courts that apply the law impartially to resolve disputes between individuals or an individual and the state; (2) the executive branch, or the King and his ministers, who enforce the law; and (3) the legislative branch, which consists of Parliament. Fig. 4.1 illustrates the three branches of government in Canada.

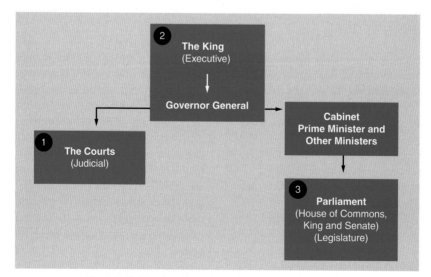

Fig. 4.1 ■ The three branches of government in Canada.

In Canada, the power to make laws (or pass legislation) rests with Parliament or, in the case of a province or territory, the **legislative assembly**. Parliament and the provincial and territorial legislatures make laws, which are also called *acts* or *statutes*. These take priority over common law and may confirm, clarify, alter, limit, or rescind common law as determined by the courts. Further, Parliament and the legislatures can adopt urgently needed laws more quickly and comprehensively than can the courts if sufficient political will exists and is brought to bear. When this does not happen, however, judges sometimes will take on the task of developing precedents to deal with new situations, as happened in *Vriend v. Alberta* (1998). The legislatures may also create laws in areas in which the courts have not yet pronounced, thereby preempting judicial "law-making" that might steer the law in a direction other than that desired by elected lawmakers. Or they may formalize into legislation rules developed by the courts through common law. For example, the common law principle that one must consent to being touched has been formally codified in the health consent statutes now in force in many provinces and territories.

Cabinet ministers, including the prime minister, who is the head of the government, are usually elected members of the political party that holds the majority of seats in the House of Commons. Ministers can also be chosen from the Senate, but this is a rare occurrence. By unwritten **constitutional convention** (a practice that is not part of the **Constitution** and yet is followed by tradition derived from British parliamentary practice), such members are entitled to form a government because with their majority in Parliament, they are considered to command the confidence of the House. With minority governments, when the government is formed by a party that does not hold a majority of the seats in the legislature, there is a risk that the government will no longer command that confidence. A confidence motion occurs when members of the House of Commons are asked to vote on the Speech from the Throne, financial matters such as the budget, or if the government declares that a specific bill will be a confidence motion. The opposition can also put forward a motion during opposition days to ask for a vote on the confidence of the government. If the majority of the members of Parliament do not support the government during such votes, then there is nonconfidence in the government's ability to lead. In such circumstances the prime minister is required to recommend to the Governor General that Parliament be dissolved and that a general election be called.

The Governor General has the power to accept this recommendation or to invite the other members or parties in Parliament to work together to form their own majority. Where it is unlikely that any parties could put together a majority, an election will usually be called.

Government ministers and the prime minister are formally appointed and chosen to form a government by the Governor General. Provincial and territorial governments are formed in the same way; however, the provincial Lieutenant Governor or territorial commissioner, the King's representative in that province or territory, makes the formal appointment.

Before it can become law, a statute must pass the scrutiny of Parliament or, in the case of a provincial law, the legislative assembly. The draft version of a proposed law, called a **bill**, is usually prepared by a legislative committee made up of members of Parliament to address a specific area of concern to the government, special interest groups, constituents of a particular geographical region, or the general public. It can deal with any subject within the **jurisdiction** of the assembly in which it is to be proposed—criminal law, taxation and government spending, agricultural policy, health care, education, foreign policy, defence, or a host of other areas of concern to various sectors of society. The subject matter of the proposed legislation will depend on whether it comes within an area of federal or provincial/territorial jurisdiction, according to the Constitution.

The procedure followed in Parliament (Dawson, 1970, pp. 356–357) and in the provincial and territorial legislatures when passing a bill into law is essentially the same, with a few variations across provincial and territorial boundaries.

The bill is first introduced in the legislature and given a formal reading. If approved in principle, the bill is then sent to a committee of the legislature for detailed study. Public consultation and hearings may be held, at which witnesses—private individuals, special interest groups, and others—may provide information or suggest changes, deletions, or additions. On second reading, a bill is again taken to a vote, through which the legislature may approve it in principle. After further debate and refinement, the bill is then put to a third reading, at which time the legislature considers the committee's report. Usually, each of the bill's provisions is debated until the bill is put to a third and final vote. If passed, the bill is then submitted to the Lieutenant Governor for royal assent in the case of provincial legislation. A bill of the House of Commons would be laid before the Senate, where it would proceed in the same fashion. If passed by the Senate, the bill is then submitted to the Governor General for royal assent.

Fig. 4.2 illustrates the process by which a bill becomes law in Canada.

A bill becomes law—an act of Parliament or of the provincial legislature—on proclamation or on a specific date after it receives royal assent. In many cases, an act has the force of law upon proclamation and publication in an official government publication.

At this point, all citizens are deemed to know the law and to be governed by it. As unreasonable as this may

seem, the purpose of this rule is to ensure the efficient and impartial enforcement of the law. Otherwise, ignorance would be used as a defence, the law would be unenforceable, and chaos would ensue. Thus, the rule that "ignorance of the law is no excuse" is fundamental to any society's ability to govern itself and maintain order.

Statutes usually contain a short title—for example, the *Regulated Health Professions Act* (1991). They may have a preamble that briefly states why the act was passed and its purpose. The act will also contain one or more numbered and detailed sections or clauses setting forth definitions, conditions, and prohibitions that are to be regulated by the act. Even though such provisions may seem comprehensive, they cannot provide for every situation that the government wants to regulate. Additional legislative details may be set forth in written regulations created under the authority of the act.

Regulations, also known as *subordinate legislation*, have the same force of law as statutes but are inferior to the act from which they flow. The statute establishes

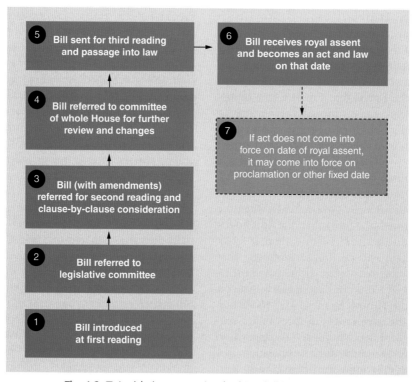

Fig. 4.2 ■ Legislative process involved in a bill becoming law.

the legal scope of the power. Regulations are formulated by the government to carry out the intent of the legislation. So, for example, a statute may empower police officers to take a person to a hospital for a mental health assessment. The procedure and the forms to be used are detailed in the regulations to the statute. In the event that a regulation goes beyond the authority granted in the statute, a court may strike down such a regulation and refuse to enforce it. The government of the day, therefore, must always ensure that any regulations passed are consistent with the act that gives it the authority to make such regulations. As regulations do not go through the legislative process, they can be altered and updated quickly to respond to changing situations and unfavourable judgements.

Because the legislative branch of the government has the ultimate power to make law (subject, of course, to any restrictions contained in the Constitution), it follows that statute law will take precedence over common (i.e., judge-made) law. If there is a conflict or contradiction between a principle of common law and a provision found in a statute of Parliament or of a provincial or territorial legislature, then a court is bound to apply the statute. The court presumes that it was the intent of the legislature to alter common law by enacting the statutory provision. For example, before the passage of the **negligence** statutes by the legislatures of the common law provinces, common law held that a person suing another for negligence could not recover any damages whatsoever regardless of fault if the person claiming the damages (the **plaintiff**) had in any way, however slight, contributed to the accident or occurrence that caused his or her injury or damage. Thus, even if the **defendant** (the person being sued) was 99% to blame for the plaintiff's injuries, the claim would fail because the plaintiff was 1% at fault. This was found to be manifestly unjust, and yet the courts continued to uphold the common law rule. It took the passage of negligence statutes in the provinces early in the twentieth century to change it. Section three of Ontario's *Negligence Act* (1990), for example, provides that:

In any action for damages that is founded upon the fault or negligence of the defendant if fault or negligence is found on the part of the plaintiff that contributed to the damages, the court shall apportion the damages in proportion to the degree of fault or negligence found against the parties respectively.

So, a plaintiff who is, for example, 20% responsible for their injuries is still entitled to recover 80% of their losses from the defendant (provided the defendant has been found liable to that extent). If there is more than one defendant, the court will apportion **liability** among the various defendants (and the plaintiff, if liable) to the extent to which each is responsible for the occurrence.

Division of Legislative Powers

The division of federal and provincial responsibilities (due to the *British North America Act* and *Constitution Act*) has created a permanent tension between the federal government, which collects the largest proportion of taxes, and provincial/territorial governments, which are responsible for a growing number of social programs and costs each year.

The federal government plays an active role in health care through its funding activities, transfer payments to the provinces, and federal–provincial arrangements. A major federal law in this area is the *Canada Health Act* (1985). Health care, however, is largely an area of provincial responsibility under the Constitution (*Constitution Act, 1867*, s. 92(7)). (Specific provincial legislation regulating the nursing profession is discussed in Chapter 5.) The provinces, through their ministries of health, administer and regulate health care systems within their boundaries. This includes matters such as the establishment, administration, and funding of hospitals and clinics; regulations governing public hospitals and private health care institutions, such as long-term care facilities; and public health insurance. The provinces also regulate health care professionals and professional self-governing bodies through their powers to make laws governing property, civil rights, and hospitals.

Due to the *British North America Act* and *Constitution Act*, there are only three ways the federal government can influence policy in areas of provincial/territorial jurisdiction:

- They can change the Constitution for a specific program they wish to introduce (very difficult).

- They can offer cost-sharing programs as they did in the 1940s, and as has been done in the provision of subsidized day care and other social programs.
- They can set national standards with penalties for lack of adherence to the *Canada Health Act* (Storch, 2014, p. 24). For example, see *Cambie Surgeries Corporation v. British Columbia (Attorney General)* (2020).

The division of powers between federal and provincial governments in health care responsibilities has been a constant source of conflict. Leading up to Confederation, the subject of health could not be expected to have an important place in the discussions: "the Fathers of Confederation could not have foreseen the pervasive growth and range of health care needs of a large industrialized urban society, the advances of medical sciences, nor the public expenditures required to maintain high quality health care." (Lalonde, M., 1981, p. 43)

APPLICATION OF THE LAW

Civil Law as Distinct from Criminal Law

The term *civil law* has several distinct meanings to lawyers and judges. In one sense, it describes a legal system based on Roman law, such as Quebec's, in which legal principles and rules are codified and form the primary source of law.

In common law jurisdictions, like the provinces and territories of Canada, excluding Quebec, *Droit Civil* refers to a branch of law distinct from **criminal law**. In this context, *civil law* refers to the body of rules and legal principles that govern relations, rights, and obligations among individuals, corporations, or other institutions. It is separate and distinct from criminal law, which is chiefly concerned with relations between the individual and the state and the breach of the *Criminal Code*. Civil law includes law related to contracts, property, family, marriage and divorce, tort and negligence, health, wills and inheritance, the creation and administration of business and nonprofit corporations or partnerships, insurance, copyright, trademarks and patents, employment, and labour.

To give a simple example of civil law relationships in a nursing setting, suppose that a nurse is called upon one night to administer an antibiotic to a patient suffering

from acute appendicitis. In error, the nurse administers the wrong antibiotic. Furthermore, it is noted on the chart that this patient is allergic to that particular antibiotic. The patient consequently suffers an anaphylactic reaction that results in brain damage. The patient emerges from a coma 2 weeks later, at which time it is determined that they have suffered partial paralysis of the left side. The brain damage is later shown to be permanent and irreversible. In such a case, the patient and their family would have the right to sue the nurse individually, in her capacity as an employee of the hospital, and the hospital for negligence. In the civil system, the laws governing an intentional or nonintentional wrongful act that causes damage or injury to another's person, reputation, or property are called *tort laws.*

This case is essentially a private dispute between two sets of individuals seeking redress in the courts. The state (or, more specifically, society) is not directly interested in the outcome of the case. Because the court's decision may later be applied in similar cases, however, society is, indeed, indirectly interested in the outcome, which may form the impetus for amending or creating legislation to regulate the particular nursing action that gave rise to the negligence. In addition, there is a societal interest in the existence of a viable dispute resolution process.

Another distinction between civil law and criminal law is that of substantive and procedural laws. **Substantive laws** create rights and obligations between individuals—for example, laws governing the creation of a contract, the rights of a spouse within a marriage, an employee's rights versus an employer's, or the creation and governance of a corporation. **Procedural laws**, however, regulate how those rights are preserved and enforced in the courts. Procedural laws include the rules of court governing how a lawsuit is started, when it may be started, what documents must be filed, and to which court the suit pertains.

Civil Law

What Is a Lawsuit?

This area of law has perhaps the greatest significance for nurses. Tort law affects the nursing process directly insofar as nurses are professionals whose conduct must meet a standard of care. As mentioned, a **tort** is a civil wrong (as opposed to a criminal wrong) committed by one person or persons against another; it includes negligence, assault, defamation (e.g., spreading false gossip about a person so as to damage their reputation in the community), or conversion (i.e., the civil law equivalent of theft). The person who is wronged can bring a claim against the offending party or parties for damages to restore the injured party to the position they would have been in had the tort not occurred.

In health care, patients sometimes experience poor outcomes. In such cases, the patients and their families may believe that the health care practitioners involved in the case let them down and that had they acted "better," been more knowledgeable, more experienced, or more careful, the patient would have avoided the poor outcome. Patients who suffer poor outcomes may initiate a legal claim against the persons who are believed to be responsible.

Individual rights are adjudicated and enforced by means of the court **action**. In Canada, a **lawsuit** is not usually the first step in an attempt to resolve a dispute. When harm is done as a result of error on a health care professional's part, then often timely disclosure to the patient or family and an apology may prevent legal action. Otherwise, informal attempts to resolve the problem may include discussions between the parties through mediation or arbitration or other complaint mechanisms. Lawyers should be engaged in the early stages to resolve the dispute without resorting to the courts. If this fails, a court action may be started by the aggrieved party.

The Action (Lawsuit) and Pleadings

The process for starting a lawsuit is similar in all provinces. A lawsuit is initiated by filing a **statement of claim** or similar document, in the appropriate court. This document, which is usually filed by a lawyer acting on behalf of the plaintiff, is also referred to as an **originating process** because it starts the action. It sets out, in a summary manner, the plaintiff's version of the facts, the duties or responsibilities relied on, and the damages suffered or expected, which support the claim made against the defendant(s). (See, for example, rule 25.06(1) of the *Ontario Rules of Civil Procedure*.) A copy of the statement of claim must then be served on (given personally to) the defendant(s) within a specified period.

If a nurse receives a copy of a statement of claim involving patient care or scope of practice, they should

immediately notify the employer and, if working in an agency that is not run by the employer, the agency as well. It is in the nurse's best interests to hire a lawyer, immediately, to ensure appropriate representation. Usually, the employer will have insurance against negligence claims and will have access to law firms who will represent the organization and its employees. Many provincial regulatory bodies now require nurses to have their own insurance, Personal Liability Protection (PLP), beyond that of their employer. Nurses may also have legal representation as part of their benefits as members of a union or professional association. Nurses should also notify the PLP insurer to ensure that their interests will be represented.

After the delivery of the statement of claim, the defendant has the obligation to file a **statement of defence** to the plaintiff's claim within a very short time period. The statement of defence sets out, in a summary fashion, the facts and principles of law relied on to dispute the claim. Failure to file the statement of defence promptly may mean that the defendant will lose all opportunity to defend the action. The statements of claim and defence are collectively known as **pleadings**.

The Examination for Discovery

Following the exchange of pleadings, the parties must produce the relevant documents in their possession under oath. Failure to produce the appropriate documentation may lead to sanctions later on. Sanctions could include legal expense awards, exclusion of documents or evidence, and, in extreme cases, immediate judgement. Frequently, in medical malpractice cases, this phase can be very complex because documents may have to be retrieved from several locations and often involve years of records. As nurses generally do not maintain their own records, the burden will usually be on the employer, the various services, and the physicians. Typically, all of the nursing documentation will be produced and reviewed.

Documentary discovery is designed to eliminate the element of surprise in litigation. If the parties know the quality of the evidence against them, settlement becomes more likely. During or after the documentary discovery phase, each party to the litigation *attends* an interview under oath (**examination for discovery**). The lawyers for the other parties to the litigation can ask any relevant questions and obtain a written transcript that the parties to the litigation can rely on at any trial. The answers given at the examination enable each party to know the other's position and the kind of testimony that the other is likely to give at trial. They can also be used to test the credibility of a party whose answers at discovery differ from those given at the trial.

Before trial, there is a mandatory **pretrial conference**, where the parties review their cases with a trial judge or court appointed mediator and try to settle the action. If a settlement is still not achieved, the parties proceed with the trial.

The Trial

Civil actions may be tried by a judge alone or by a judge and a **jury**. However, certain types of actions, because of their nature or complexity, may only be tried by a judge alone. A civil trial jury is composed of fewer **jurors** than the 12 required in a criminal trial; however, the number of jurors varies from province to province. For example, Ontario requires no more than six persons, whereas Newfoundland and Labrador requires nine. Civil jury trials were abolished in Quebec several years ago.

During the trial, the **burden of proof** is on the plaintiff. It is not up to the defendant to prove that they are not liable. The plaintiff must present enough evidence to show that the injury or harm was caused, on a balance of probabilities, by the defendant. If the plaintiff has failed to prove their case at the end of the trial, or the evidence is at best inconclusive, the defendant will be found not liable, and the action will be dismissed. In a criminal trial, there is a higher standard of proof (the prosecution must satisfy the trier of fact [judge or jury] that the accused is guilty beyond a reasonable doubt).

If the plaintiff wins, the court grants a *judgement,* a court order stating that the defendant must do, or refrain from doing, something or pay compensation to the plaintiff. Damages—monetary compensation for the harm incurred by a plaintiff as a result of the defendant's negligence, willful tort, or breach of contract—are one of the remedies the court may award. Money damages are classed as "general" damages or "special" damages. Special damages are amounts paid to the plaintiff to compensate them for a specific out-of-pocket loss, for example, lost income, medical

expenses, costs of modifying a home to accommodate a disability, or cost of repairing or replacing a car. These damages represent actual amounts that can be calculated, and the expenses may have already been incurred by the plaintiff. General damages are not tied to a specific expense imposed on the plaintiff by the defendant's actions. General damages are granted for intangible injuries to the plaintiff. For example, a plaintiff who has been injured in a car accident can claim general damages for "pain and suffering." Damages can be quite substantial in some cases (e.g., sexual assault) and quite limited in others. There are also some specialized damages that are granted with the intention to punish defendants for reprehensible conduct ("aggravated," "punitive," and "exemplary" damages).

The court may also issue an injunction, an order directing the defendant to do or to refrain from doing something that is causing damage to the plaintiff. Generally speaking, courts do not like making orders that have to be supervised to ensure the parties are meeting the terms of the judgement. Where monetary compensation can compensate a plaintiff, the court will not make an order that the defendant do or refrain from doing something. For example, if a company has agreed to return a leased property to its owner in the same condition as it was when the lease began, the court will not order the defendant to restore the property; it will only order the defendant to pay the plaintiff a reasonable amount of money to restore the property.

Criminal Law

Thus far, we have been discussing court actions involving one or more individuals asserting private claims. These are part of civil law. Other cases—those that involve a breach of fundamental values and rules that threaten the peace, stability, order, and well-being of all citizens—concern society collectively and are the focus of criminal law.

Most criminal law is contained in the *Criminal Code* (1985), which was originally enacted by Parliament in 1892. It is a lengthy statute containing a comprehensive and detailed list of criminal offences and a code of criminal procedure. The *Criminal Code* has been amended and revised many times.

Classes of Criminal Offences

There are three classes of criminal offences in the *Criminal Code* (1985):

- Indictable offences
- Summary conviction offences
- Dual procedure (or hybrid) offences

Indictable offences are generally the most serious type of offence. These include murder, manslaughter, attempted murder, **criminal negligence** causing death, robbery, theft of property having a value of over $5,000, treason, and conspiracy to commit an indictable offence.

Given the serious nature of indictable offences, the procedure for trying them is more complex than that for summary conviction offences. With indictable offences, the accused usually has a preliminary inquiry and is tried by a court composed of a judge and a jury. The jury is composed of 12 Canadian citizens over 18 years of age. In many cases, the trial can be before a judge alone.

The purpose of the preliminary inquiry is to determine whether the Crown has sufficient evidence such that a reasonable jury, reasonably instructed in the law, could (not would) convict the accused of the offence. It is not a trial. If the evidence is deficient, the accused will be discharged. During the preliminary inquiry, the prosecution will present evidence, and the accused will have the opportunity to cross-examine the prosecution's witnesses. The accused does not have to present any evidence during the preliminary inquiry.

Generally, an accused person cannot be charged with and tried for the same criminal offence more than once. If after a preliminary inquiry, however, the Crown obtains additional evidence that suggests that a separate and different offence was committed, the accused can be charged again with the offence or with a new offence. If the Crown's new evidence is insufficient, the charge may be dismissed as an abuse of the court's process. Or the charge may be dismissed because laying it violates the accused's rights under the *Canadian Charter of Rights and Freedoms,* as discussed later in the chapter.

Summary conviction offences are relatively less serious in nature. They include offences such as causing a disturbance, discharging a firearm in a public place, loitering, trespassing at night, and vagrancy. Such offences are tried before a provincial court judge without a jury and involve lower penalties.

The third class of offence under the Code is that of **dual procedure offences** or **hybrid offences**. They are hybrid in that the Crown may choose to try the accused summarily or indictably. Until the Crown attorney prosecuting the case makes the choice, the offence will be deemed indictable. (See *Interpretation Act,* 1985, s. 34(1)(a).) If the Crown elects to proceed summarily, the accused will be tried by a provincial court judge alone.

The Presumption of Innocence

In Canada, as in most common law–based democracies, an accused person is considered innocent until proven guilty. Not only is this principle enshrined in the *Criminal Code* (1985, s. 6(1)(a)), but more significantly, it is also a fundamental right guaranteed in the *Canadian Charter of Rights and Freedoms* (1982). Section 11(d) of the Charter reads:

11. Any person charged with an offence has the right: . . . (d) to be presumed innocent until proven guilty according to law in a fair and public hearing by an independent and impartial tribunal.

The *Canadian Charter of Rights and Freedoms* has been an integral part of the Constitution since 1982. It sets forth the basic legal, mobility, language, equality, and democratic rights of citizens, rights that the state cannot abridge (limit), violate, or infringe upon without breaching the Constitution. (The Constitution and the *Charter* are discussed more fully later in this chapter.)

Two consequences flow from the **presumption of innocence**. First, the Crown must prove all the essential elements of a criminal offence. It is up to the Crown to prove the offence and not for the accused person to disprove the charge against them. This is known as the *burden of proof.* The degree of proof that the Crown must meet to secure a conviction is proof beyond a **reasonable doubt**. Second, although the accused may choose not to present any evidence, frequently, the focus of the defence is to establish a reasonable doubt in the mind of either the judge or the jury, depending on the mode of trial. This means that the Crown (the prosecution) must satisfy the judge or the jury that the accused committed the alleged offence they are giving sufficient *evidence* such that no real or logically compelling reason exists in the trier's mind that the accused did not commit such act.

Elements of a Criminal Offence

Most criminal offences have two main elements: a *physical element* and a *mental element.* The physical element is known in law by the Latin term **actus reus**. Thus, for example, in the offence of assault, the actual physical conduct of striking the victim constitutes the *actus reus.* The mental component, known by the Latin term **mens rea**, is the element of *intent.* In most cases, a person must intend to commit the act which they are charged with. Thus, in an assault, the *mens rea* is the perpetrator's intention to strike the victim. The perpetrator's willful direction of their body to commit the actual physical act is the *actus reus.*

The link between these two elements, insofar as proving the offence is concerned, is that a conscious, rational person, thinking rationally, always intends the consequences of their physical conduct. This means that a sane person, acting voluntarily and rationally, who is seen physically striking another, is presumed to have intended the consequences of that action. In other words, such conduct is the product of a conscious mind acting voluntarily. The two elements of the offence must, therefore, both be present (see *Fowler v. Padget,* 1798; see also *R. v. Bernard,* 1961).

For example, suppose that A suffers a head injury in an automobile accident. They are released from the hospital a few weeks later, seemingly recovered from their injuries. One night A gets out of bed, proceeds to the kitchen, and obtains a carving knife, which A uses to stab their sleeping spouse repeatedly. The spouse dies. A discovers the murder the next day and, to their horror, concludes from the physical evidence at the scene that they committed the deed. However, A has absolutely no recollection of it. A and their spouse loved each other. A had no motive or wish to see their spouse dead and cannot fathom how they could have done such a thing. It may be that the head injury caused A to act involuntarily—that is, their actions were not the product of a *conscious* mind but merely the automatic movement of their body resulting from the brain injury. In such a case, the accused could not be found guilty of murder because they clearly were

not aware of the circumstances; A was not conscious, and was not acting voluntarily. This defence is known in law as the *defence of automatism* (Stuart, 1982, pp. 77–91). It has been accepted in Canadian courts as a legitimate defence since the Supreme Court of Canada's decision in *R. v. Rabey* (1980). In *R. v. Rabey,* the accused was convicted of assaulting a woman he was infatuated with and who had rebuffed him. He had no recollection of the assault. The Supreme Court of Canada recognized (in a split decision) that a person might suffer a psychological blow that could cause them to act unconsciously. This decision seems less strange, however, when one considers the basic principle that persons should be held responsible only for intentional acts that are the product of a rational mind acting voluntarily.

In our example of the case of A with the head injury, if the accused had been conscious, they would not have voluntarily committed the act, would have been fully capable of discerning right from wrong, and would have been aware of the consequences of their actions. An insane person is afflicted with a disease of the mind and is not legally capable of appreciating the nature and quality of their actions and the consequences. Such a person, therefore, is incapable of formulating the necessary intent or *mens rea.* Because one of the elements necessary to prove guilt is absent, such a person would be acquitted (found not guilty). Specifically, this situation would attract a verdict of not guilty by reason of insanity, as provided in sections 16(1) and (2) of the *Criminal Code* (1985):

16. (1) No person shall be convicted of an offence in respect of an act or omission on his part while that person was insane.
(2) For the purposes of this section, a person is insane when the person is in a state of natural imbecility or has disease of the mind to an extent that renders the person incapable of appreciating the nature and quality of an act or omission or of knowing that an act or omission is wrong.

In the *Criminal Code* (1985), breach of criminal law through **malfeasance** (doing something that is one's duty to do, but doing it poorly) or **nonfeasance** (failure to act altogether when a duty to do so exists) can result in charges that could include criminal negligence causing death (s. 220). Also, a parent who fails to provide the necessities of life for their child (s. 215) is also punishable. For example, suppose an accused was driving a car at excessive speed on a residential street and struck and killed a child. The accused's behaviour was clearly out of step with the standard of reasonable behaviour. This negligent departure from that standard is the mental element required to prove the offence. In other words, the driver was aware that they were driving at excessive speed, and knew or ought to have known that injury could result from this carelessness. The law would punish such reckless behaviour in the interest of protecting the public from such gross carelessness.

THE CONSTITUTION OF CANADA

History of the Constitution

Unlike the United States and several other countries with colonial histories, Canada became an independent and sovereign nation by evolution, not revolution.

Canada's Constitution was originally passed by the British Parliament in 1867 as the *British North America Act* (1867). At that time, and until well into the twentieth century, Canada was a self-governing colony of the United Kingdom. Britain, however, possessed ultimate legislative power over Canada, so it alone could provide supreme legislation, which all colonial parliaments in British North America (and later the Parliament of Canada) were subject to.

With the enactment of the *Canada Act 1982* by the Parliament of the United Kingdom, Canada was given the power to amend its own Constitution.

Supremacy of the Constitution

It is a fundamental requirement of any democracy that its government and institutions be subject to a higher law. The constitution of a country is essentially a set of supreme laws that define and regulate the various branches of government, their powers, and restrictions on those powers. Canada's Constitution includes the *Canadian Charter of Rights and Freedoms,* which sets forth the basic legal and democratic rights of Canadians. These are rights that the government cannot infringe upon unless it has a justifiable reason. Any governmental action or law that breaches the Constitution or a person's constitutional rights is itself illegal and invalid. A government is neither

above the law nor immune from the law's reach. It must always act legally. This is an adjunct to the principle of the rule of law and of due process, discussed above.

The *Canadian Charter of Rights and Freedoms*

Fundamental Rights

The *Canadian Charter of Rights and Freedoms* (1982) is an entrenched (integral) part of the Constitution. It codifies as constitutional law many of the **fundamental rights** and freedoms enjoyed by everyone in Canadian society, including freedom of religion and conscience (s. 2(a)); freedom of thought, expression, and the press (s. 2(b)); freedom of peaceful assembly (s. 2(c)); and freedom of association (s. 2(d)).

Democratic Rights

The Charter also protects **democratic rights**, such as the right of citizens (i.e., noncitizens are not entitled to these particular rights) to vote (s. 3); the provision that no Parliament or provincial legislature may continue for more than 5 years from the date of the last election (s. 4(1)); and the requirement that Parliament or a provincial or territorial legislature sit at least once every 12 months (s. 5). These particular rights are meant to ensure that governments remain responsible and accountable to the electors and do not become tyrannical.

Mobility Rights

As well, the Charter provides that Canadian citizens have the right to enter, remain in, and leave Canada, as well as to move and to take up residence in any province to pursue a livelihood (subject to laws providing for reasonable residency requirements in that province) (s. 6). These are called **mobility rights**.

Legal Rights

Perhaps the most important rights enshrined in the Charter are **legal rights**. These rights are guaranteed to all persons in Canada, regardless of citizenship. They include the right to life, liberty, and security of the person (s. 7); the right to be secure against unreasonable search and seizure (s. 8); and the right not to be arbitrarily detained or imprisoned (s. 9). Thus, for example, the police in Canada do not have the right to arrest a person because they do not agree with that person's political views or fear that such person may engage in behaviour that is not illegal but which the police, other government officials, or politicians might find objectionable or offensive. Likewise, the authorities do not have the right (as they do in many totalitarian countries) to apprehend a person and hold them in prison for an indefinite period without a trial or specific criminal charges being laid.

In 2017, the Canadian government settled a lawsuit with Omar Khadr for an amount in excess of $10 million. As a child and Canadian citizen, Mr. Khadr had been taken to Afghanistan by his father and spent several years with insurgent forces. As a 15-year-old, he was severely wounded during a firefight with US forces. His father and others were killed in the skirmish. Khadr was arrested and charged with killing a US army medic during the firefight. He was detained by the US government at the prison in Guantanamo Bay, Cuba, without due process for several years. He was convicted and eventually returned to Canada to serve his sentence. He was released from prison as his conviction had been unconstitutional under Canadian law. The Supreme Court of Canada held several times that the government had violated Mr. Khadr's section 7 Charter rights. Despite the repeated Supreme Court rulings of Charter violations, the government had taken no steps to obtain Khadr's release from American military custody or to correct the Charter violations. When the settlement was reached with Khadr, the government indicated that the settlement was necessary because of the clear violations of Khadr's Charter rights by Canadian officials. Despite what may or may not have happened when Mr. Khadr was in Afghanistan (as a 15-year-old), the actions and decisions of the government against Khadr after he was captured and detained were clearly in violation of the Charter.

According to the Charter, any person in Canada who has been arrested or **detained** (held in police custody) has the right to be informed of the reasons for the arrest (s. 10(a)); to speak with a lawyer without delay and be informed of that right (s. 10(b)); and to have the validity or lawfulness of the detention determined by a court and be released if the detention is unlawful (s. 10(c)).

In the Charter, rights accorded to all accused persons in a criminal trial or other proceeding include the right to be informed without delay of the specific offence (s. 11(a)); to be tried within a reasonable time (s. 11(b)); not to be forced to give testimony against themselves (s. 11(c)); to be presumed innocent until and unless proven guilty (s. 11(d)); to be granted reasonable bail (s. 11(e)); and to be tried by a jury if the punishment for the offence is imprisonment for 5 years or more (s. 11(f)).

The Charter also states that if tried and acquitted of an offence, a resident of Canada has the right not to be tried for the same offence again. If found guilty and punished, persons have the right not to be punished a second time for the same offence (s. 11(h)); not to be subjected to cruel and unusual punishment (s. 12); not to have evidence given as a witness in a proceeding subsequently used against them in another proceeding (s. 13); and to have the services of an interpreter if they do not understand or speak the language in which the proceedings are being conducted or is deaf (s. 14).

Equality Rights

Finally, the Charter sets out that all persons in Canada are equal before the law, regardless of race, gender, national or ethnic origin, colour, religion, age, and mental or physical disability (s. 15(1)). The Supreme Court of Canada has also held that discrimination on the basis of a person's sexual orientation is prohibited under this section of the Charter. In *Vriend v. Alberta* (1998), the majority of the Supreme Court described the effects of discrimination on the basis of sexual orientation in the context of the appellant's termination of his employment because of his homosexuality. The majority agreed that Vriend's section 15 rights had been violated through the omission of sexual orientation as a prohibited ground of discrimination in the Alberta human rights legislation.

Section 15 of the Charter is subject to the enactment of laws implementing affirmative action programs for the benefit of disadvantaged groups in society (s. 15(2)).

It is important to note that the absence of any right from those specifically enshrined as **equality rights** in the Charter does not mean that such unwritten right does not exist and is not otherwise enforceable.

Language Rights

The Charter also contains minority language education rights and states that French and English are the official languages of Canada (s. 16(1)).

Supremacy of the Charter

Because the Charter is part of the Constitution (s. 52(2)), and the Constitution is the supreme law of Canada (s. 52(1)), any law that is inconsistent with that supreme law has no force or effect. This means that any such law is nonexistent, as if it had never been passed, and any action taken pursuant to it may be declared illegal by the court that rules on its constitutionality. However, all laws are presumed to be constitutionally valid until the law is determined to be invalid by a court.

The Notwithstanding Clause

Although any statute law enacted in Canada is subject to the Charter, it is possible for Parliament or a provincial or territorial legislature to override the Charter by invoking the *notwithstanding clause* of the Constitution. This clause provides that a law, even one contravening the Charter, may apply for up to 5 years. The 5-year limitation is designed to ensure that rights are not permanently infringed (violated) by a law. After 5 years, the notwithstanding clause expires insofar as it applies to that particular law, unless it is invoked again. The use of the clause is often threatened by provincial governments but rarely used. Only Quebec, Ontario, Alberta, Saskatchewan, and the Yukon have passed legislation including the clause, and the Yukon law never came into force. In 2019, the clause was used by Quebec to protect Bill 21, the prohibition on wearing religious symbols. In 2021, Quebec used the clause again with respect to a restrictive language law, and Ontario used it to protect a controversial campaign finance law that limited pre-election spending by groups such as unions. In 2022, Ontario tried to use the clause in relation to labour laws but withdrew the legislation.

The Constitution and the Indigenous Peoples in Canada

Background: The Indian Act

The federal government has had oversight over Indigenous affairs since Confederation. The *Indian Act*, first enacted in 1867 but amended a number of times since, is the primary law used by the government to administer many aspects of Indigenous life. This paternalistic legislation gave the government oversight over the First Nations people (it excluded Métis and Inuit) in relation to issues such as status, land, administration, resources, and education. It was designed to "civilize" and facilitate the assimilation of First Nations people into Canadian society. The focus of the government at that time was to carry out this responsibility by acting as a "guardian" until assimilation was realized (Government of Canada, 2017).

Because the goal of the Act was to facilitate assimilation of the First Nations people, certain traditional practices were banned, and women who married non-status men lost their status (as an Indian) and, therefore, the rights associated with that status. The Act "has been the main mechanism for controlling the lives and destinies of [status] Indians in Canada, and throughout the life of the act, amendments have been made to the original document to fine-tune this control" (King, 2012, p. 70). Some provisions of the *Indian Act*, however, were designed to protect the interests of Indigenous peoples, such as land which was reserved or protected for their use (Lawrence, 2016).

Background: Treaty Rights

As the early settlers populated eastern North America, they used different approaches when interacting with Indigenous communities. In some cases, force was used to displace the existing inhabitants. In other cases, the local population was recognized as sovereign, and treaties between Indigenous peoples and the Crown were established. The purpose of the treaties varied, some addressing land rights, confirming peaceful relationships, or providing assurances of military protection against other Indigenous communities and European nations. Some lands belonging to Indigenous peoples in Canada were surrendered (ceded) to the Crown through treaties, whereas other unceded territories have never been surrendered through treaty or otherwise. This approach has led to a patchwork of treaties affirming different rights and relationships. These treaties were viewed differently by each side. The colonial administrators considered the treaties useful tools to manage relations with the Indigenous communities but did not abide by them when the treaties did not serve their interests. Indigenous people usually assert that treaties were intended to be agreements between sovereign states, between those with ancient ties to the land and those whose roots are from elsewhere, and that they are binding under international law. This disconnect in the way that treaty rights were established and viewed has influenced the complex and fractious relationship between Canada and Indigenous peoples today. Despite centuries of contact and active repression, with a focus on assimilation, distinct Indigenous cultural entities have endured.

The Canadian Constitution and Indigenous Rights

When the Constitution, including the Charter, was repatriated in 1982, it initially excluded specific Indigenous and treaty rights. However, after extensive lobbying by First Nations, Inuit, and Métis organizations, section 35 was added to the Constitution to recognize Indigenous and treaty rights:

(1) *The existing aboriginal and treaty rights of the aboriginal peoples of Canada are hereby recognized and affirmed.*

(2) *In this Act, "aboriginal peoples of Canada" includes the Indian, Inuit, and Métis peoples of Canada.*

(3) *For greater certainty, in subsection (1) "treaty rights" includes rights that now exist by way of land claims agreements or may be so acquired.*

(4) *Notwithstanding any other provision of this Act, the aboriginal and treaty rights referred to in subsection (1) are guaranteed equally to male and female persons. (Constitution Act, 1982)*

There was lack of consensus on the definition of these rights; hence, the responsibility to define, interpret, and protect them has been left to the courts.

THE COURT SYSTEM

The Constitution also provides for the establishment of a court system to adjudicate on criminal and civil matters and to interpret the laws (*Constitution Act, 1867*, ss. 92(14) and ss. 96–101). The Canadian court system is organized primarily at the provincial level, where the bulk of litigation occurs. The Constitution gives the provinces the power to establish and maintain provincial civil and criminal courts and to set the rules of civil procedure in these courts. (Recall that criminal procedure is set out in the federally enacted *Criminal Code*.) The specific court structure varies somewhat from province to province; however, there are fundamental similarities, which are discussed next.

Provincial and Superior Courts

Each province and territory except for Nunavut have three levels of court: two types of trial courts: a provincial/territorial court (to hear minor cases) and a superior trial court and an appellate (appeals) level court. The organizational structure of trial courts varies among provinces, but their jurisdiction (i.e., the types of matters they can hear and the orders and judgements they can make) is much the same. Nunavut has only a single level of trial court.

Administrative Tribunals

Canada and the provinces have established administrative boards and commissions, which, although not courts in the strict sense, nevertheless **adjudicate** on the respective rights and obligations of the parties who come before them. Examples of such boards or commissions, known as **administrative tribunals**, include the various provincial human rights commissions, labour boards, energy boards, provincial securities commissions, municipal boards, assessment review boards, and **health disciplines boards** (which regulate and govern nurses and other health care professionals).

For example, the health disciplines boards of the provinces and territories (discussed in greater detail in Chapter 5) establish and enforce minimum standards of competence for health care professionals. These boards have the power to grant permission to individuals to practise a given profession or use a professional title (e.g., registered nurse) within the province or territory and to discipline members who breach the standards or ethical rules of that profession. Thus, they operate like a court, in that they have a duty to decide on such matters fairly and impartially and to give the parties before them a full opportunity to be heard and to present their case.

Fig. 4.3 illustrates the structure of the Canadian court system.

Roles of Trial Courts and Appellate Courts

A **trial court** hears matters as a court of **original jurisdiction** or a **court of first instance**. This means that it is the first court to hear a case. Once a trial court makes a decision or renders a verdict, that decision or verdict may be appealed to an **appellate court**, which reviews the proceedings of the lower trial court to ensure that no procedural, evidentiary, or other rules of law were breached or misapplied, that the trial court acted

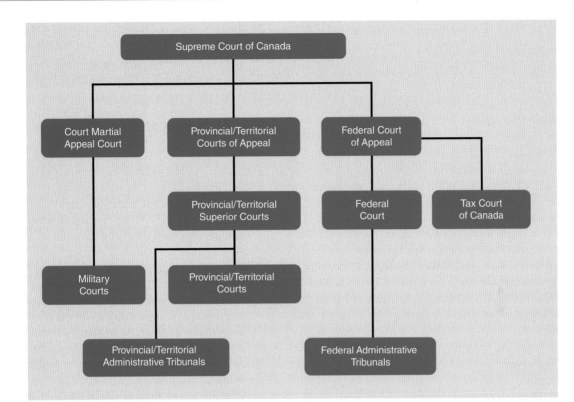

Fig. 4.3 ■ Canadian judicial structure. Actions or proceedings can be started in (1) a provincial/territorial civil court; (2) a provincial/territorial criminal court; (3) an administrative board or tribunal; (4) a superior trial court; and (5) the Federal Court of Canada. Appeals from these various starting points can go to (1) a superior trial court; (2) an appeal branch of superior court (Divisional court); (3) directly to a court of appeal; and (4) to an appeal-level board or tribunal in some cases. Where appeals go varies from jurisdiction to jurisdiction and depends on such factors as the amount of money in dispute, the type of remedy sought, special statutory provisions, and so on. Also, some appeals require permission to be obtained before they can proceed. Generally, appeals from superior trial courts, if available, go to the court of appeal for that jurisdiction. *Source: Government of Canada. (2017). The judicial structure. http://www.justice.gc.ca/eng/csj-sjc/just/07.html.*

within its powers or jurisdiction, and that the accused's constitutional rights were not violated (especially in the case of a criminal trial).

An appeal is not a new trial. There are no witnesses, and new evidence is seldom heard. It is simply a review of the trial proceedings to ensure that no errors of law were made and that **findings of fact** are based on properly admitted evidence. Appeal courts review the decisions of trial courts if a party to the case appeals the decision believing the decision is unsound in law or unsupported by the evidence at trial.

The Supreme Court of Canada

Under the Constitution, the Parliament of Canada may establish courts for the administration of the laws of

Canada—that is, laws made specifically by Parliament or matters over which the federal government has constitutional authority (except matters governed by the *Criminal Code*), not provincial laws. Under this provision, the federal government has established the Federal Court of Canada (*Federal Courts Act,* 1985), which is divided into a trial and an appellate division. The Federal Court hears cases involving tax; shipping; trademarks, patents, and copyrights; and other matters within the jurisdiction of the federal government.

The Supreme Court of Canada, established in 1875, is Canada's highest court and the final interpreter of the meaning and scope of the Constitution and the Charter. The Supreme Court hears appeals from all provincial and territorial appellate courts and from the

Federal Court of Appeal (*Supreme Court Act*, 1985). Its decisions are final until and unless the law is changed by Parliament or the Constitution is amended to reverse the court's interpretation of one of its provisions. Furthermore, all decisions of the Supreme Court are binding on all lower courts. This is in accordance with the principle of *stare decisis*, as discussed earlier.

The Supreme Court is made up of nine judges, who serve until age 75 years and are appointed by the Governor General on the advice of the prime minister. They, like all other federally appointed judges, may be removed from office only by resolution of Parliament. In this way, their independence is assured. They need not fear removal if they do not rule on matters as the government of the day might wish. However, they may be removed if they have broken the law. No federally appointed judge has ever been removed in this fashion since Confederation, although a few judges have resigned after controversies impugning their integrity or impartiality.

SUMMARY

In this chapter, the basic principles and mechanisms of the Canadian legal system were introduced. The foundation of the Canadian legal system, based on English and French traditions is described and though, as a consequence of colonialism were not considered, the legal traditions of the Indigenous Peoples in Canada are also explored. English common law and French civil law—were described, and the distinctions between civil law and criminal law were discussed. Actual cases provided insights into how the law is applied in practice, and where possible, the examples provided were relevant to nursing and health care.

This chapter also reviewed the structure of the provincial and federal court systems and described how existing law is interpreted and how new law is introduced through the legislative process. The significant implications of the Constitution and the *Canadian Charter of Rights and Freedoms*, as well as Indigenous legal concepts were highlighted and examined.

This overview provides insights into how the law influences many aspects of the nursing profession, including nurses' everyday actions and decisions, demonstrating why it is critical that nurses be familiar with the law and have a basic understanding of the Canadian legal system.

As discussed, society holds nurses to high standards of professional, moral, and ethical competence, but it also affords them certain rights and privileges. The law strives to keep these competing interests in constant balance.

CRITICAL THINKING

Discussion Points

1. Compare and contrast the key elements of English common law and French civil law.
2. Describe the concept of due process and the rule of law in Canada. Discuss the benefits and advantages of due process and the rule of law in modern society.
3. What are the implications of a lawsuit for nurses? How would such actions be presented?
4. What values are apparent in Canada's Constitution? Does the Constitution address all of the values that are important to you?
5. Apply the principles of the *Canadian Charter of Rights and Freedoms* to a nursing or health care setting.
6. What aspects of the law in Canada are important to nursing practice? Why should nurses understand the law?

REFERENCES

Statutes

British North America Act, 1867, 30 & 31 Vict., c. 3, now known as The Constitution Act, 1867 (UK).

Canada Act 1982 (1982), c. 11 (UK).

Canada Health Act, R.S.C. 1985, c. C-6 (Canada).

Canadian Charter of Rights and Freedoms, Part I of the *Constitution Act, 1982*, being Schedule B to the *Canada Act 1982* (UK), 1982, c. 11.

Civil Code of Québec, CQLR c. CCQ-1991 (Quebec).

Constitution Act, 1867, 30 & 31 Vict., c. 3 (UK).

Constitution Act, 1982, Schedule B to the Canada Act 1982 (UK), 1982, c. 11.

Criminal Code, R.S.C. 1985, c. C-46 (Canada).

Federal Courts Act, R.S.C. 1985, c. F-7 (Canada).

Interpretation Act, R.S.C. 1985, c. I-21 (Canada).

Lalonde, M. (1981) *A new perspective on the health of Canadians: A working document.* Supply and Services Canada

Negligence Act, R.S.O. 1990, c. N.1 (Ontario).

Ontario Rules of Civil Procedure, R.R.O. 1990, Regulation 194, as amended (Ontario).

Regulated Health Professions Act, 1991, S.O. 1991, c. 18, as amended (Ontario).

Supreme Court Act, R.S.C. 1985, c. S-26, as amended (Canada).

Case Law

Cambie Surgeries Corporation v. British Columbia (Attorney General) [2020] BCSC 1310, para. 347–348 (CanLII).

Carter v. Canada (Attorney General) [2015] SCC 5, 1 S.C.R. 331.

Donoghue v. Stevenson [1932], AC 562 [HL].

Fowler v. Padget [1798], 7 TR 509; 4 RR 511; 101 ER 1103 (KB).

Latin v. Hospital for Sick Children et al. [2007] CanLII 34 (ON S.C.).

Nancy B. v. Hôtel-Dieu de Québec [1992] RJQ 361; (1992), 86 DLR (4th) 385; (1992), 69 CCC (3d) 450 (SC). 1992 CanLII 8511 (QC CS).

R. v. Bernard [1961], 130 CCC 165; 47 MPR 10 (NBCA).

R. v. Morgentaler [1988] 1 SCR 30.

R. v. Rabey [1980] 2 SCR 513.

Rodriguez v. British Columbia (Attorney General) [1993] 3 SCR 519, 1993 CanLII 75 (SCC) [1993] BCWLD 347; (1992), 18 WCB (2d) 279 (SC), aff'd. (1993), 76 BCLR (2d) 145; 22 BCAC 266; 38 WAC 266; 14 CRR (2d) 34; 79 CCC (3d) 1; [1993] 3 WWR 553, aff'd. [1993] 3 SCR 519.

Vriend v. Alberta [1998] 1 S.C.R. 493.

Wilson v. Swanson [1956] CanLII 1 (S.C.C.), [1956] S.C.R. 804.

Texts and Articles

Aboriginal Justice Implementation Commission. (1999). *Report of the Aboriginal Justice Inquiry of Manitoba.* http://www.ajic.mb.ca/reports/final_toc.html

Dawson, R. (1970). In N. Ward (Ed.), *The Government of Canada* (5th ed.). University of Toronto Press.

Dawson, R. M., Dawson, W. F., Ward, N., & Dawson, W. F. (William F. (1989). *Democratic government in Canada* (5th ed.). University of Toronto Press.

Government of Canada. (2017). *First Nations in Canada.* https://www.rcaanc-cirnac.gc.ca/eng/1307460755710/1536862806124

Hogg, P. W. (1997). *Constitutional law of Canada.* Carswell.

King, T. (2012). *The inconvenient Indian.* Anchor Canada.

Lawrence, B. (2016). Enslavement of Indigenous people in Canada. *The Canadian Encyclopedia.* https://www.thecanadianencyclopedia.ca/en/article/slavery-of-indigenous-people-in-canada

Storch, J. L. (2014). Canadian healthcare. In M. McIntyre & C. McDonald (Eds.) *Realities of Canadian nursing: professional, practice, and power issues* (4th ed., pp 17–39). Wolters Kluwer Health.

Stuart, D. (1982). *Canadian criminal law.* Carswell.

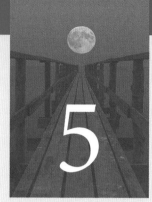

5 REGULATION OF THE NURSING PROFESSION

LEARNING OBJECTIVES

The purpose of this chapter is to enable you to understand:

- The laws, procedures, and structures regulating the nursing profession in Canada
- The role and function of self-regulating bodies and how they protect the public, including managing entry to practice, ongoing competence, and professionalism of nurses
- The processes and procedures used by regulatory bodies to ensure quality, to respond to complaints, and to enforce the ethical, clinical, and professional standards expected of nurses

INTRODUCTION

Earlier chapters discussed the significant influence both ethics and the law have on nursing as a profession. This interplay of ethics and the law is manifest in the legislation and regulations that govern the profession of nursing in Canada. Along with other Canadian health professionals, nurses are held to a high standard of accountability for decisions and actions in providing safe, effective, and ethical practice. These accountabilities must be met within the context of a complex system where nurses face many challenging issues. Structures and mechanisms have been introduced to ensure the nursing profession meets its duty to provide competent and safe nursing in all domains of practice. Professional regulatory bodies, guided by legislation and regulation, exist to develop and enforce standards of behaviour, practice, education, research, and leadership. The primary purpose of health

professional regulatory bodies is to promote and ensure the welfare of the public. This is accomplished through a legal framework intended to protect the public from incompetent, unqualified, or unethical health care professionals and through the establishment and enforcement of professional and practice standards and codes of ethics against which nursing care is measured.

In Canada, nursing is a self-regulated profession. Self-regulation is a privilege, *not a right,* granted, through legislation, by the provincial or territorial government to a profession (e.g., nursing, medicine, dentistry, law, accounting). This privilege allows a profession the autonomy to govern its own members, set standards and processes for entry into the profession, establish and monitor standards of practice, deliver quality assurance programs, receive and investigate complaints, and enforce these standards, when necessary, through disciplinary processes. Having the authority to self-regulate reflects the trust and confidence the public has in these professions (Narrative Research, 2021).

All provinces and territories belong to the Canadian Council of Registered Nurse Regulators (CCRNR), a national collaborative for regulators of registered nurses for interprovincial/interterritorial, national, and international regulatory matters. CCRNR's focus is to support Canada's regulators on such issues as registration, policy, practice, education program approval, professional conduct, and quality assurance/competence.

In some countries, professions are regulated by government departments and managed by civil servants; nonmembers of the profession are essentially responsible for regulation and oversight. Many believe

126

that these approaches result in a loss of professional autonomy. There has been a long-standing preference in Canada for self-regulation and a requirement that these bodies govern their professions with the public interest as their priority. Otherwise, they run the risk of losing the public's trust and the privilege of self-regulation.

Each province and territory has a legislative framework that guides the practice of nursing. Some provinces are directed by legislation that covers several health care professions with specific regulations for groups such as licensed practical nurses (LPNs), registered nurses (RNs), nurse practitioners (NPs), and registered psychiatric nurses where they practice. In other provinces, specific legislation for individual health professions is used instead. Because legislation adapts to changes over time, refer to the Evolve table titled *Overview of Provincial Legislation and Regulatory Bodies and the Category of Nurses Represented* for a current summary of the legislation regulating nursing across Canada.

Whatever form the legislation takes, it provides a legal definition of nursing, summarized in the Evolve table *Definitions of Nursing Across Canada*. In New Brunswick, for example, section 2(1) of the *Nurses Act* (1984) notes that nursing practice "includes the nursing assessment and treatment of human responses to actual or potential health problems and the nursing supervision thereof." In Quebec, section 36 of the *Nurses Act* (RSQ, c I-8) provides that "the practice of nursing consists in assessing health, determining and carrying out the nursing care and treatment plan, providing nursing and medical care and treatment in order to maintain and restore the health of a person in interaction with his environment and prevent illness, and providing palliative care."

In addition, legislation defines the scope of nursing practice, provides the legal authority for use of the title "nurse," and mandates the regulatory or governing body, usually called a college, association, or council, to protect the public interest by managing entry to the profession, establishing and supporting practice standards, overseeing ongoing competence, and enforcing appropriate practice and behaviour.

Nurses should be aware of the basic organization of the self-regulatory bodies overseeing the nursing profession in their respective province or territory. Knowledge of the role of regulatory bodies and the legislative framework is a component of the jurisprudence examination that nurses must take to demonstrate their knowledge of the laws, regulations, and regulatory processes related to nursing.

In the provinces and territories other than British Columbia, Ontario, and Nova Scotia, separate categories of nurses are regulated by different regulatory bodies. In jurisdictions with divided regulatory bodies, separate bodies govern registered nurses (including nurse practitioners), and discrete colleges exist for the other categories of licensed practical nurses/registered practical nurses and registered psychiatric nurses in provinces where they practice. Although the structure of regulatory bodies varies across the country, their shared objectives are to be accountable, responsible, flexible, and adaptable to rapid changes in the evolution of nursing, while remaining focused on the safety and well-being of the public. For a summary of regulatory bodies and the categories of nurses they represent, go to the Evolve site to view the table titled *Overview of Provincial Legislation and Regulatory Bodies and the Category of Nurses Represented.*

There is a distinction between regulatory bodies and other groups that represent nursing, notably professional associations and unions. Although all three have high-quality health care as a priority, their emphasis differs. Professional associations focus on the well-being and advancement of the profession, whereas the mandate of regulatory bodies is the protection of the public. In addition, professional associations are active in advocacy for the profession. They play a role in shaping public policy and in ensuring nurses have a role in influencing government decisions that affect them and the overall health care system (Registered Nurses' Association of Ontario [RNAO], 2023; College of Registered Nurses of Saskatchewan [CRNS], 2023). In most provinces, the regulatory arm and the professional arm are combined under one organization. In Ontario, British Columbia and Alberta, the regulator (College of Nurses of Ontario [CNO] and College of Registered Nurses of Alberta [CRNA], respectively) and the association (RNAO, Nurses and Nurse Practitioners of British Columbia and the Alberta Association of Nurses [AAN], respectively) are distinct organizations. Many professional associations are linked to the Canadian Nurses Association (CNA), as discussed in Chapter 3.

Unions focus on the interests of their members and serve as collective bargaining agents for the various health care facilities where their members are employed. Also, nurses' unions engage in advocacy for the profession as part of their responsibilities to their members. Again, their structure varies across the provinces and territories. The Canadian Federation of Nurses Unions (CFNU) is an organization that represents nurses' unions in eight provinces: Alberta, Saskatchewan, Manitoba, Ontario, New Brunswick, Nova Scotia, Prince Edward Island, and Newfoundland and Labrador. Not all unions representing nurses are nursing specific; they may also represent the interests of other categories of workers. (Labour issues, as they relate to nurses, are discussed more fully in Chapter 11.)

This chapter will summarize the structures, systems, and processes of the regulatory bodies governing the nursing profession in Canada. This will include the legislation that provides a framework for self-regulation and grants qualified nurses the legal authority to practise. The organizational structures and accountabilities of the regulatory bodies that assume responsibility for that mandate will also be discussed. It is not possible to describe each regulatory body in detail, so examples from various colleges or associations will be highlighted to illustrate how their mandate is met. For clarity, the terms *regulatory body* and *college* will be used interchangeably throughout this chapter to represent these organizations.

THE HISTORY OF NURSING REGULATION IN CANADA

The profession of nursing in Canada has been regulated since around the time of World War I. In some provinces—for example, British Columbia (1918), Manitoba (1913), and Prince Edward Island (1922)—the profession has always been self-regulated, whereas in others, government regulation gradually gave way to self-regulation. In Ontario, for example, nursing has been a self-regulated profession only since 1963. In Quebec, until the 1960s, regulation of the nursing profession was primarily within the purview of the Catholic Church because most nurses were members of religious orders. The secularization of the profession came in the early 1970s with the establishment of the Ordre des infirmières et infirmiers du Québec.

LEGISLATIVE FRAMEWORK GUIDING THE REGULATION OF NURSING IN CANADA

Provincial/territorial legislation and regulations are in place to grant qualified nurses the legal authority to practice. Legislation defines the scope of practice of health care professionals, including nurses; describes areas of overlap in practice across health disciplines; and authorizes the performance of controlled acts or interventions that could be harmful if performed by unqualified persons.

Through legislation, nursing regulatory bodies are held accountable for the protection of the public by ensuring safe, competent, compassionate, and ethical practice of the profession. The laws regulating nursing in the provinces and territories of Canada are broadly similar in their purpose and objectives. They seek to establish an orderly and well-regulated process for entry into the nursing profession, develop and communicating standards of practice, ensure nursing competence, and enforce standards through a fair and thorough complaints procedure and disciplinary process. Their mandate is to protect the public from professional misconduct and poor-quality nursing care and from incompetent, unethical, or unprofessional behaviour by its members. The legislation requires that the regulator ensure its members are properly educated and able to meet the standards required to practice nursing.

It is the duty of these regulatory bodies, as servants and protectors of the public, to regulate the nursing profession and to discharge their responsibilities consistent with the public interest, while balancing the need for autonomy in the functioning of the profession.

Definitions of Nursing

Within their respective statutes, most provinces and territories have enacted legal definitions of the term *nursing*. The purpose of such definitions is to describe the nature and scope of nursing by delimiting those acts and procedures that constitute nursing practice. This provides a framework to determine whether certain actions comprise the practice of nursing and allows a distinction to be drawn between nursing and other health care professions. The definition also aids the courts in interpreting other sections of the respective provincial and territorial statutes. The legal definition also provides a framework for findings of professional misconduct. Consider the nurse who was found guilty of professional misconduct for diagnosing, prescribing, and injecting two patients with Botox (botulinum toxin) for the treatment of hyperhydrosis (excessive sweating) in a private setting. This act was not delegated to this nurse, nor was the treatment administered under the supervision of a qualified physician. The definition of nursing did not include the authority to diagnose, prescribe drugs, or administer drugs without a physician's order, so her actions constituted professional misconduct (*College of Nurses of Ontario v. Cecilioni*, 2008). Refer to the Evolve site for the definitions or descriptions of nursing established by each province and territory.

Scope of Practice

The term *scope of practice* describes those activities that nurses are authorized, taught, and competent to perform. Nursing's scope of practice is authorized in provincial/territorial legislation and regulations and is guided by standards, guidelines, policy positions, and ethical codes established by the authorized nursing regulatory bodies. This legislation describes the overall scope and boundaries of practice; other factors, such as patient need, the practice environment, and the policies and standards of the employer, are also relevant. The nurse's level of knowledge and competence are essential factors (CNA, 2015); for example, a nurse working in a psychiatric unit in a hospital may not have the knowledge and competence to work in a critical care unit, and vice versa.

Regulation of Distinct Classes of Nurses

In Canada, there are four regulated designations of nurses: registered nurses (RNs), nurse practitioners (NPs), licensed and Registered Practical Nurses (LPNs in the rest of Canada and RPNs in Ontario), and registered psychiatric nurses (only in British Columbia, Alberta, Manitoba, and Saskatchewan). Although the titles differ, the nature of practice undertaken by LPNs and RPNs is very similar across Canada, though the exact scope of practice may differ. The scope of practice is reviewed often in response to changes in the nursing environment and in response to improvements in education. The process is complicated by the need to coordinate the

scope of practice between the regulated nursing categories. Since the scope of practice of nurses is reviewed regularly, more current definitions are found in the websites of regulatory bodies across the country. For clarity, in this book, the title "LPN" includes RPNs in Ontario.

Registered Nurses and Licensed Practical Nurses

RNs and LPNs share the same body of nursing knowledge and are autonomous professionals in their own right. RNs and LPNs are accountable for their actions and decisions and are expected to collaborate and consult with other professionals and one another to ensure safe practice and the highest quality of care (Canadian Council of Practical Nurse Regulators [CCPNR], 2013; CNO, 2014).

However, because RNs are prepared at the baccalaureate level and have a more extensive program of study, their foundational knowledge is deeper than that of LPNs, who usually complete a 2-year diploma program at the community college level. Given their expanded foundational knowledge base, RNs are expected to have a stronger focus on critical thinking, decision making, critical analysis and evaluation of research findings, and management of complexity (College of Registered Nurses of Alberta. (2023).; CNA, 2015). RNs not only attend to the individual patient but also engage with families, communities, and populations. They work across the continuum, through all stages of life, providing and coordinating care to achieve the best possible outcomes for patients throughout the system. RNs are also prepared to provide leadership in practice, education, administration, research, and policy development (CNA, 2015; CNO, 2014, 2018).

RNs can assume specialized roles in areas such as pediatrics, critical care, psychiatry, research, and leadership. In addition, RNs have opportunities to acquire the expertise and knowledge to undertake advanced nursing roles. Advanced practice nurses (APNs), through graduate educational preparation, expand their knowledge and clinical competencies and assume roles in areas of specialized nursing practice (CNA, 2009; International Council of Nurses [ICN], 2020). In meeting the health needs of individuals, families, groups, communities, and populations, APNs in these advanced roles are involved in the analysis and

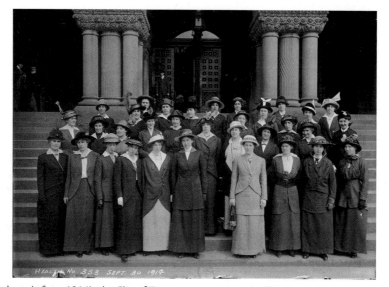

In many years (this photo is from 1914), the City of Toronto commissioned official photographs of its Public Health Nurses, in front of Toronto City Hall, recognizing their important role in maintaining a healthy population. *Source: City of Toronto Archives, Fonds 200, Series 372, Subseries 32, Item 353.*

synthesis of knowledge, the application and interpretation of nursing theory and research, and the development and advancement of nursing knowledge and the profession as a whole (CNA, 2009). These roles are involved in direct patient care, research, education, consultation, collaboration, and leadership activities (DiCenso et al., 2010). They include the roles of clinical nurse specialists (CNSs) and NPs, which are discussed in the next section.

CNSs have expertise in a clinical nursing specialty and focus on specialized and complex practice, consultation, collaboration, education, research, and leadership. By engaging in nursing research, they contribute to the advancement of nursing knowledge and evidence-informed practice (CNA, 2009). CNSs specialize in a specific area of practice that may be defined in terms of a population, setting, disease, medical subspecialty, type of care, or type of problem, such as geriatrics and wound care.

Specialization and leadership opportunities are also available to LPNs, in such areas as perioperative nursing, critical care, and long-term care, when there is stability and flexibility in the care environment. The scope of practice of RNs and that of LPNs differs in that LPNs are intended to care for less complex and more predictable patient populations. However, their level of independence and practice is dependent on variables such as the dynamics of the environment, the complexity of patient needs, access to other nursing resources, and the knowledge and experience of the individual LPN (CCPNR, 2019; CNO, 2018; College of Registered Nurses of Nova Scotia [CRNNS] & College of Licensed Practical Nurses of Nova Scotia [CLPNNS], 2013). The assessment of the complexity and predictability of patients is evaluated in that context.

Regulators across the country have established guidelines to assist nurses and leaders in making decisions regarding the most appropriate category of nurse or nurses to meet the needs of individuals or groups of patients. Elements considered in matching nurses to patient needs include those described earlier: the predictability and complexity of the patient's condition, the depth of knowledge required to provide competent and safe care, access to resources (e.g., other nurses and the interprofessional team), and the nature of the environment in which care is being delivered. Collaboration and consultation are of key importance when the needs of a patient are beyond an individual nurse's knowledge and competence. When the needs of patients change, nurses are accountable to communicate with other health care team members for safe and effective client care and as needed, escalate to an appropriate health care provider (e.g., from an LPN to an RN, or a novice RN to one with more experience) (CNO, 2018; CRNNS & CLPNNS, 2013).

As the complexity and unpredictability of a patient's needs grow, so does the necessity for the RN to provide the full range of care. RNs and LPNs are expected to collaborate in monitoring patient and environmental changes and circumstances, and to reestablish priorities, alter assignments, and seek additional resources when necessary (CNO, 2018). Organizations must ensure that policies and guidelines are in place to facilitate decisions regarding how the appropriate category of nurse is determined. Also, when leaders design and implement the appropriate care delivery model for the care setting, these factors and the flexibility to respond to change need to be considered.

Nurse Practitioners

The RN category includes advanced roles, including extended-class RNs and NPs. NPs have an expanded scope of practice that gives them the authority (within legislation) to autonomously diagnose; prescribe treatments and medication; perform procedures; and order and interpret diagnostic tests. They include primary health care nurse practitioner (PHCNP), acute care nurse practitioner (ACNP), and blended CNS and NP roles. Across Canada, additional legislation and regulation defines these roles and clarifies their scope of practice (DiCenso et al., 2010; *Registered Nurses Act,* 2006; *Registered Nurses Profession Act,* 2002).

NPs usually have extensive clinical experience and are educated, through a graduate or postgraduate program, where they are taught both advanced nursing theory and medical knowledge and prepared with the skills that equip them to function in the role (CNA, 2016). They specialize in many areas, including family health, geriatrics, pediatric and neonatal specialties, and anaesthesia. They work with individuals, families, groups, communities, and diverse populations across the continuum of care.

The title "nurse practitioner" is protected in all jurisdictions (refer to legislation summarized in the Evolve table titled *Overview of Provincial Legislation and Regulatory Bodies and the Category of Nurses Represented*).

Although the NP role is primarily clinical, it also incorporates leadership and research competencies. NPs are also authorized to provide Medical Assistance in Dying (MAiD) under the *Criminal Code* amendments, where that role is consistent with their provincially authorized scope of practice.

PHCNPs usually practise in the community, within primary health care teams and in long-term care settings. They focus on health promotion, preventive care, the diagnosis and treatment of acute minor illnesses and injuries, and the management of stable chronic diseases. ACNPs practice in collaboration with the medical team and provide advanced nursing care in specialized hospital settings for patients who are acutely, critically, or chronically ill (CNA, 2016; DiCenso et al., 2010).

Nursing regulatory bodies are responsible for setting entry-to-practice competencies, standards of practice, and licensure requirements; approving entry-to-practice educational programs; and establishing continuing competence requirements for NPs in Canada (Canadian Council of Registered Nurse Regulators [CCRNR], 2018). However, variation continues to exist across jurisdictions. Most provinces recognizes the NP designation in 3 or 4 categories (streams) including some combination of Family/All Ages, Adult, Child/Neonatal. Pediatric, and Primary Care. In Manitoba, the College of Registered Nurses of Manitoba (CRNM) recognizes the NP designation, which is synonymous with the title of RN (Extended Class [EC]), a formulation that was previously used in other provinces but has been replaced with the NP designation.

For example, to become an NP in British Columbia, an RN must have successfully completed a master's level NP program and met BCCNM registration requirements. There are three specialty certificates available to NPs: Family, Pediatrics, and Adult. Once nurses successfully complete the NP examination and are registered as NPs, they are authorized to practice with an extended scope, perform additional controlled acts within their specialty, and are permitted to call themselves *nurse practitioners*. In acute care, NPs are employees and, as such, are responsible for functioning within the standards set by both the employer and the regulator. In most acute care settings, additional activities beyond their authorized scope are assumed by NPs through the use of medical directives (an authorizing mechanism). However, as the scope of practice of NPs is evolving, reliance on medical directives is decreasing. Employers must have internal processes and systems set up to ensure that NPs are enabled to apply their scope of practice; are approved to use authorizing mechanisms, where needed; and are engaged in performance review processes to ensure safe delivery of care.

Registered Psychiatric Nurses

Registered psychiatric nurses practise in the four western provinces—British Columbia, Alberta, Saskatchewan, and Manitoba—and in the Yukon. They provide care for patients with complex psychosocial, mental health, and physical needs in a variety of health care settings and collaborate with a variety of health care professionals.

Registered psychiatric nurses complete a 2.5- to 4-year psychiatric nursing education program at a college or university. This specialized program includes theory and clinical instruction in psychiatric and general nursing, focusing on behavioural and social sciences, psychiatric nursing theory, and interventions and therapeutic relationships (Registered Psychiatric Nurse Regulators of Canada [RPNRC], 2018).

As autonomous professionals, registered psychiatric nurses work collaboratively with patients and other health care team members. They focus on mental health development, mental illness, and addictions, while integrating physical health care and psychosocial models, thus ensuring a holistic approach to care. As with other nursing groups, psychiatric nursing occurs within the domains of practice, education, administration, and research.

The assessment of emotion, behaviour, and cognition is a major focus of the registered psychiatric nurse's practice. Through therapeutic communication and a therapeutic relationship with the patient, this nurse performs psychotherapeutic interventions that focus on prevention, health promotion, the maintenance of optimal health, rehabilitation, and recovery (RPNRC, 2018).

Controlled Acts

One of the distinctive features of the regulation systems of health professions in several provinces and territories is that the law defines specific medical actions and procedures that may be performed and which professional groups may perform and delegate

them. For example, a province may identify 13 controlled acts, and nurses may be authorized to perform a specific number of those 13 controlled acts. This allows the province to define a single set of controlled acts and then identify which health care professionals can perform those specific acts. The terminology for these acts varies across the country. They may be known as "restricted activities" (*Nurses (Registered) and Nurse Practitioners Regulation*, 2008, s. 8), "controlled acts," "restricted acts," or "reserved acts." Any act within the definition and scope of nursing practice may be performed by an RN or LPN unless it is specifically designated as an act that may be performed only when authorized by legislation.

In Ontario, the *Regulated Health Professions Act (RHPA)* strictly regulates controlled acts (*RHPA*, 1991, s. 27) and identifies which profession may perform and delegate them. The *RHPA* lists 14 controlled acts that may be performed only by members of a professional college who are authorized by the college's governing statute and regulations (see *Nursing Act*, 1991, s. 4) to perform the controlled act (*RHPA*, 1991, s. 27(1)(a)). Five "authorized acts" may be performed by nurses in accordance with the *Nursing Act* (1991). If the particular act is to be delegated, it may be delegated only by an authorized member and only in conformity with the college's statutes and regulations. For example, if RNs are authorized to administer a particular substance via injection (a controlled act under *RHPA*, 1991, s. 27(2), para. 5), then they may delegate the act to an LPN, provided that the regulations under the *Nursing Act* allow such **delegation** and that all procedures for delegation set out in the regulations are followed.

The five authorized acts are:

- Performing a procedure below the dermis, surface of the mucous membrane, the cornea, or in or below the surface of teeth (including scaling teeth)
- Administering a substance by injection or inhalation
- Putting an instrument, hand, or finger beyond the external ear canal, the point in the nasal passages where they normally narrow, the larynx, the urethral opening, the labia majora, the anal verge, or into an artificial opening into the body
- Treating, by means of psychotherapy technique, delivered through a therapeutic relationship, an individual's serious disorder of thought, cognition, mood, emotional regulation, perception or memory that may seriously impair the individual's

judgement, insight, behaviour, communication or social functioning
■ Dispensing a drug (*Nursing Act,* 1991, s. 4)

Also, as discussed, NPs, may perform additional acts, provided they have met certain standards of education:

■ Communicating to a patient, or a patient's representative, a diagnosis made by the NP
■ Applying and ordering the application of a prescribed form of energy
■ Setting or casting a bone fracture or joint dislocation
■ Prescribing, dispensing, selling, or compounding a medication (*Nursing Act,* 1991, s. 5.1)

Moreover, NPs have the authority to order specified tests. Additional activities beyond their authorized scope (through legislation) are assumed through the use of medical directives or other authorizing mechanisms.

In Saskatchewan, the specific acts that nurses are authorized to perform are not detailed in the bylaws of the CRNS (*Saskatchewan Registered Nurses' Association Bylaws,* Bylaw VI, s. 2), made pursuant to *The Registered Nurses Act, 1988* of Saskatchewan. The Act includes a general authority to practice nursing s. 24. Rather than license nurses in areas of practice, Saskatchewan's system focuses on a broad authority to practice with competence requirements. Thus, an RN is not granted a blanket authorization to perform certain controlled procedures that the nurse may believe are part of the profession. The nurse may perform only those acts that they are specifically authorized to perform, given that nurse's specific qualifications and professional education.

Exemptions

In Ontario, an unregulated care provider may also perform certain controlled acts when providing ongoing care to a person. This would apply, for example, in the case of a personal support worker in a home or long-term care setting.

The *RHPA* does not apply to Indigenous healers or midwives when they are providing their services to members of an Indigenous community (*RHPA,* 1991, s. 35(1)). However, the Indigenous healer is subject to the jurisdiction, regulations, and bylaws if they are also a member of a college.

Delegation

Legislation allows nurses to delegate the performance of specific controlled acts to another regulated health care professional or an unregulated care provider (a worker who is not registered or licensed in a health care discipline) provided that the employer's policies support this and that the responsibilities of the organization, the nurse, and the unregulated care provider are clear. This allows for a greater degree of flexibility in the provision of health care services.

The act to be delegated would be one primarily performed by a nurse competent to do so and outside the role description of the other. The delegation is patient specific, based on that patient's particular needs and preferences. Generally, the nurse is responsible and accountable for the following:

■ Making the decision to delegate, based on patient factors (need, preference, risk), the task (complexity and risk), the care environment, and the ability of the provider (to whom the act is being delegated)
■ Ensuring the provider has the knowledge and skill, within defined limits, to perform the act in a safe manner
■ Ongoing supervision and support (BCCNM, 2023)

The fact that persons are permitted to perform certain acts (e.g., administering a drug, or putting an instrument or hand in natural or artificial body openings) facilitates the care of patients in the home. For example, to ensure the pain of a terminally ill patient is controlled, it may be appropriate for the RN coordinating care to teach a member of the family to administer morphine by injection. In this circumstance, this is not formal delegation because the family member is not accountable to the nurse, but the *RHPA* (1991) would allow this, provided that the provisions associated with the delegation process are followed. An important component of this plan is to assess the patient and the family member's openness to and comfort with assuming these responsibilities.

GOVERNANCE AND ORGANIZATIONAL STRUCTURE OF NURSING REGULATORY BODIES

Governance and Structure

In some provinces (i.e., Alberta, Nova Scotia, Ontario, Manitoba, Prince Edward Island, and British Columbia), the regulatory bodies are formally and legally called "Colleges." In some other provinces and territories (i.e., Yukon, Northwest Territories, Nunavut,

Saskatchewan, New Brunswick, and Newfoundland and Labrador), they are legally referred to as "Associations." Alberta's regulatory body was called the College and Association of Registered Nurses of Alberta, but in 2022, CARNA ceased operating as a professional association and continued solely as a regulator as the College of Registered Nurses of Alberta (CRNA). A new professional advocacy group was established as the Alberta Association of Nurses (AAN), representing all categories of nurses in the province. Despite the use of the word "College," CRNA is not involved in the post-secondary education of nurses.

As mentioned, in many provinces, the regulatory arm (the bureaucratic structure responsible for regulating entry to practice, licensing, continuing competence, and complaints and discipline) and the professional arm (the structure responsible for advocacy for members of the nursing profession) are combined. In Ontario, British Columbia and Alberta, these "arms" are completely separate: the regulatory aspect is entrusted solely to the CNO BCCNM and the CRNA (respectively), and the professional advocacy aspect, including the provision of professional malpractice insurance, the lobbying of governments in nurses' professional interests, and political action, is undertaken by the RNAO, NNPBC and AAN (respectively), which are separate entities.

In Ontario British Columbia and Alberta, because the professional nursing association is separate from the College, the duty to self-regulate in the interests of the public does not conflict with advocacy and lobbying on behalf of nurses in terms of work conditions, contracts, and benefits. However, because these arms are combined in most other provinces and territories, mechanisms must be available to resolve such potential conflicts. The foremost duty of all the regulatory bodies is to serve in the interests of the public. Because self-regulation is a privilege and not a right, a regulatory body that were to favour its professional self-interest over the public interest would risk losing the privilege of self-regulation. This knowledge helps ensure that such conflicts are kept in check.

Board or Council's Role

Colleges are governed by a voluntary board of directors or council, composed of registered members of the profession and, depending on the province or territory, may include members of the public usually appointed by the government. The boards are granted powers and responsibilities to fulfill the mandate provided in legislation and to govern the nursing profession in the interests of the public.

The board of directors provides oversight over the activities of the College and is ultimately held accountable for the protection of the public. The board monitors the operations of the organization and holds the executive team accountable for executing the responsibilities of the organization. Colleges are usually led by a chief executive officer (CEO), sometimes called an *executive director* or a *registrar*, who, with the leadership team and staff, is responsible for the ongoing operations and objectives of the organization. As the primary rule-making body, the board approves and enacts rules and bylaws regarding the development and enforcement of nursing practice standards; criteria for admission to nursing schools; the curricula and teaching standards of such schools (although the provinces also have a say in this); student membership; continuing education; reinstatement and renewal of membership; licensing, membership, setting of fees; rules governing types of duties; and so forth. In the acts of certain provinces and territories (e.g., British Columbia Act, s. 44(1); Yukon Act, s. 52(1); Saskatchewan Act, s. 34(1); Manitoba Act, s. 38(1); New Brunswick Act, s. 34(1); the regulatory body's board or council also hears **appeals** of decisions made by its disciplinary or professional conduct committee, discussed later in this chapter. (See Fig. 5.1.)

Statutory Committees

In addition to their board or council, colleges are required by legislation to establish statutory committees, also represented by members of the profession and the public. These committees report to the board and assist it in fulfilling its mandate to protect the interests and welfare of the public. The specific titles and structure of these committees vary across the colleges, but their functions include executive oversight, the complaints process, disciplinary procedures, finance, fitness to practise, quality assurance, and entry to practice (BCCNM, 2022b; CNO, 2016). Those committees related to complaints, discipline, fitness to practise, and quality are described later in the chapter.

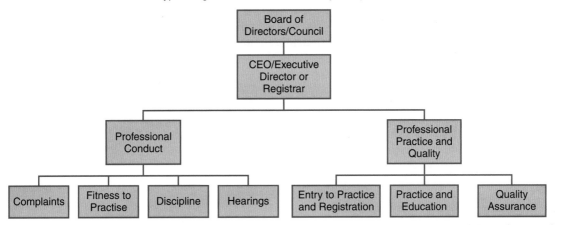

Typical organizational structure for regulatory bodies

Fig. 5.1 ■ This is an illustration of an organizational structure for regulatory bodies across the country, defining their mandate and responsibilities.

MANDATE OF REGULATORY BODIES

Legislation requires colleges to protect the public from incompetent, unqualified, or unethical health care professionals and provide the benchmarks against which professional practice is measured. Across the country, these bodies do this by managing entry to practice, establishing and communicating standards of practice and behaviour, ensuring ongoing competence, and enforcement.

Entry to Practice

A key component of a regulatory body's mandate is overseeing who enters the profession, ensuring they have the knowledge and competencies to provide safe and effective care. This is the first step in meeting their mandate to protect public interests.

Access to the Nursing Profession

To address public concerns regarding fair access to regulated health care professions, some provinces have put in place legal and supervisory mechanisms to ensure that all socioeconomic and cultural groups, particularly visible minorities, are given full opportunities to enter the health care professions, including nursing. Ontario, for example, passed amendments to its *Health Professions Procedural Code (HPPC, 1991)* that impose a duty on its college "to provide registration practices that are transparent, objective, impartial and fair" (*RHPA*, 1991, Schedule 2, s. 22.2). To ensure such

openness, a fairness commissioner is appointed by the government to assess and monitor these mandates and to provide advice as required (*Fair Access to Regulated Professions Act, 2006*; *RHPA*, 1991, s. 22.5).

Initiatives to attract Indigenous persons to the profession have been in place for a number of years. A report published in 2009 by the Aboriginal Nurses Association of Canada (ANAC), now the Canadian Indigenous Nurses Association, entitled "*Cultural Competence and Cultural Safety in Nursing Education*" was developed in recognition of the need to recruit more Indigenous nurses into the profession. This need identified by ANAC and the Canadian Association of Schools of Nursing led to a collaboration with the CNA and Schools of Nursing across the country, already engaged in active recruitment of Indigenous persons to the profession. The document was designed to "to assist educators to foster cultural competence and cultural safety among students," particularly those from Indigenous backgrounds (ANAC, 2009, p. 3).

The University of Saskatchewan Community of Aboriginal Nursing (UCAN), formerly known as the Native Access Program to Nursing (NAPN), began in 1984 with the goal of increasing the number of Indigenous people in healing careers, working toward balanced healthy communities. This program indicates that it has been a success in recruiting and retaining Indigenous students (https://nursing.usask.ca/indigenousinitiatives/ucan.php).

The Truth and Reconciliation Commission of Canada's (TRC) Calls to Action, released in 2015, addressed health and health care specifically. The TRC's 94 Calls to Action include number 23, which is related to access to health professions, including nurses:

> 23. *We call upon all levels of government to:*
> i. *Increase the number of Aboriginal professionals working in the health-care field.*
> ii. *Ensure the retention of Aboriginal health-care providers in Aboriginal communities.*
> iii. *Provide cultural competency training for all health-care professionals. (TRC, 2015, p. 3)*

In November 2021, several nursing organizations, including the Canadian Association of Schools of Nursing, Canadian Black Nurses Alliance, Canadian Federation of Nurses Unions, Canadian Nurses Association, Canadian Nursing Students' Association, among others, released the *Nursing Declaration Against Anti-Indigenous Racism in Nursing and Health Care*:

> *First Nations, Inuit, and Métis Peoples, as the original peoples of this country, and as*

> *self-determining peoples, have Treaty, constitutional, and human rights that must be recognized, respected, and protected. All Canadians, as Treaty peoples, share responsibility for establishing and maintaining mutually respectful relationships. . . .*

> *As nurses,*
> *1. We declare racism directed at Indigenous Peoples a national health crisis. We acknowledge that the current state of Indigenous health in Canada is a direct result of historical Canadian government policies and practices, including the residential school system (TRC Call to Action # 18). . . .*

> *7. We will call on all levels of government to . . .*
> ■ *Increase the number of Aboriginal Professionals working in the health and social work fields and ensure their retention in Aboriginal communities (TRC Call to Action #23 [i & ii]); and*
> ■ *Provide educational opportunities that support nurses and healthcare professionals in the provision of culturally competent and relevant care including incorporating Indigenous content into curricula for all (TRC Call to Action #23 [iii]). (pp. 1–3)*

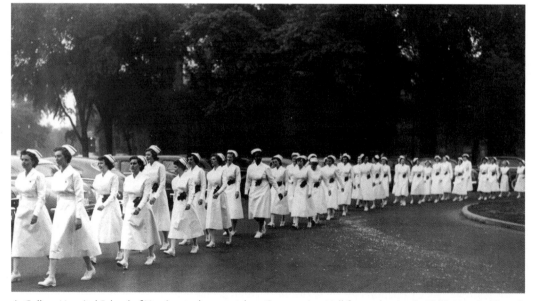

Women's College Hospital School of Nursing students march to Convocation Hall for graduation in 1951. Hospital-based nursing education provided hospitals with a reliable and inexpensive workforce. In 1973, responsibility for nursing education in Ontario was moved to the Ministry of Colleges and Universities. Women's College Hospital, the Wellesley Hospital, and the Hospital for Sick Children nursing schools were joined to form a nursing program at Ryerson Polytechnical Institute (now Toronto Metropolitan University). *Source: The Miss Margaret Robins Archives of Women's College Hospital, Photograph collection, L-00558.*

Educational Requirements

All provincial and territorial laws require those who apply for membership in their respective regulatory body to have graduated from an approved school of nursing. Regulatory bodies begin the process of protecting the public at the entry-to-practice level. This process starts with the establishment of competencies, designed to ensure that an entry level nurse is safe and competent to practice. These competencies inform the development of curriculum and the requirements of nursing education programs, which are approved and monitored by the regulatory body on an ongoing basis. Once a student successfully passes an approved program, they are then able to apply for registration with the college.

The Accreditation Program of the Canadian Association of Schools of Nursing (CASN) lists currently approved programs for RNs across Canada. Governing boards approve programs for LPNs and RNs based on key indicators, for example, demonstrating that the entry-to-practice competencies are evident. In some jurisdictions, the regulatory organization also fulfills a role in approving nursing education programs. For example, the College of Registered Nurses of Saskatchewan and the Ontario regulator approve nursing education programs and monitor the quality of existing programs. In a less formal role, some colleges like the Nurses Association of New Brunswick consult with educational institutions about programs and structure.

The Calls to Action of the TRC also addressed the education of health care providers, including nursing:

24. We call upon medical and nursing schools in Canada to require all students to take a course dealing with Aboriginal health issues, including the history and legacy of residential schools, the United Nations Declaration on the Rights of Indigenous Peoples, Treaties and Aboriginal rights, and Indigenous teachings and practices. This will require skills-based training in intercultural competency, conflict resolution, human rights, and anti-racism. (TRC, 2015, p. 3)

This TRC Call to Action mandates the teaching of various subject areas that must be covered by the program as a whole. Universities and colleges across the country are achieving this through dedicated courses or though the integration of the subject areas across the curriculum. Some programs, such as Thompson Rivers University, offer a comprehensive model that includes cultural safety, specific resources for Indigenous students, and Indigenous health career planning (https://www.tru.ca/nursing/indigenous-nursing.html). There are also schools, such as First Nations University of Canada, that were completely created and managed by Indigenous people, that offer degrees in Indigenous Health and that offer programs in social services and other areas (https://www.fnuniv.ca/academic/undergraduate-programs/indigenous-health/).

Eligibility for Registration/Licensing

When a student graduates from an approved program, they must apply to a college for registration in the profession in order to be authorized to practise as a nurse. As part of this process, the qualifications for an applicant are carefully reviewed to ensure that all of the requirements related to education and prelicensure hours of clinical practice are met. Once the applicant's educational requirements are successfully evaluated, additional approval processes are in place before they are deemed eligible (by the college) to write the Canadian entry-to-practice examination.

When assessing eligibility, the college may, depending on the province, require that the applicant (a newly graduated student, an internationally educated nurse, or individual who previously practised nursing but is no longer registered) meet criteria such as:

- Be a Canadian citizen or a permanent resident, or be authorized to practise through a work or study permit
- Have evidence of recent (within 3 years) experience in nursing (student placements qualify)
- Be fluent in English or French
- Have passed a jurisprudence examination that demonstrates knowledge of the laws, regulations, and regulatory processes related to nursing
- Disclose past offences or professional findings of misconduct (e.g., abusive conduct)
- Disclose health issues or disorders that could compromise safe practice (CNO, 2018).

For eligibility requirements in each province or territory, refer to the website of the respective college.

Once these eligibility criteria are met, applicants are required to pass a national examination to ensure that they meet the entry level standards of practice. Entry level competencies and the curriculum provided to students inform the development of these examinations.

Applicants for registration may obtain temporary permits if they have completed all elements of the application process other than the final licensing examination. Once nurses successfully pass the entry exam and meet all the criteria required by the college, they are granted a licence or issued a certificate of registration or permit to practise nursing in that province or territory. This is called the **licensing** process. Although the terms *registration* and *licensing* mean two different things, provincial and territorial regulatory bodies often use them interchangeably. **Registration** refers to the process of a nurse enrolling as a member of the regulatory body, essentially as a member of the profession. Through registration, the member is recognized as a person who is authorized to practise nursing in that jurisdiction. Registration allows the college to record the nurse's contact information, educational background, and qualifications. This information is accessible to the public.

This credentialing process is intended to assure the public and employers that nurses meet the appropriate standards of the profession and can safely practise nursing. Despite these measures, instances of impersonation have occurred, where a person has used the name of a member of the profession to work as a nurse when not licensed to do so.

In 2022, Brigitte Cleroux was convicted, in an Ottawa court, of impersonating a nurse and of assault (related to giving injections without the legitimate authority to do so) and was sentenced to 7 years in prison. Cleroux had a history of more than 60 criminal convictions and had a legacy of impersonating nurses in the United States and Canada (including a conviction for impersonating a nurse in Alberta). Previously an employee of BC Women's Hospital, she had numerous complaints against her for unprofessional behaviour. Her sentence demonstrates how the justice system takes the responsibilities given to nurses seriously. In speaking of Cleroux, Ontario Court Justice Robert Wadden noted that her actions "caused everyone to doubt the integrity" of that system "and the trust placed in the nursing profession, which is one of the most hard-working and highly regarded professions in this country" (*R. v. Cleroux*, 2022). Ms. Cleroux is awaiting trial as of May 2023 on additional criminal charges in BC.

This situation identified gaps in the screening of potential nursing employees, which requires the review of credentials as well as criminal background checks.

Criminal Background Checks

Many jurisdictions in Canada, the United States, and the United Kingdom have enacted laws to provide for mandatory criminal background checks for both nursing students and nurses seeking employment. The primary aim of any system of criminal background checks is, ideally, to exclude people with a history of inappropriate conduct, while not excluding people one would wish to employ (Devitt, 2004). The intent of such criminal check procedures is to exclude potential nursing candidates, both students and prospective employees, from the practice of nursing when there is a prior criminal record and if such persons would pose a threat to the safety of vulnerable persons.

In 1996, British Columbia passed the *Criminal Records Review Act* (*CRRA*), a law that provides a process for criminal record checks to help prevent (1) the physical and sexual abuse of children and (2) the physical, sexual, and financial abuse of vulnerable adults (*CRRA*, 1996, s. 2). It requires regulatory bodies to do criminal record checks on all members applying for registration (*CRRA*, 1996, s. 13). Those who wish to become nurses in British Columbia must authorize the regulatory body to initiate a criminal record search (*CRRA*, 1996, s. 15(1)). If such authorization is not provided, the member cannot be cleared to work with children. Furthermore, if a nurse (or other professional) refuses to authorize a criminal record check, the board of directors of the regulatory body must take that refusal into account in deciding whether to register the nurse or to set practice conditions (*Health Professions Act*, 1996, s. 20(3)). If persons who seek registration as a member of a professional regulatory body have a criminal record, including a "relevant offence," they will be subject to further examination by that professional body. The regulatory body must evaluate the nature of the offence; the time that has elapsed since the offence took place; the circumstances of the offence, including the age of the applicant at the time of the offence; and any other relevant factors, including any indications that the applicant might attempt a similar offence in the future and any attempts at rehabilitation. The main purpose of such an inquiry is to determine whether the conviction or outstanding charge indicates that the individual presents a risk of physical or sexual abuse to children. In this way, policymakers attempt to ensure the health and safety of children and to prevent cases involving the physical and sexual abuse of children by persons entrusted with their care and education.

The requirement of criminal background checks for nursing students and prospective nursing employees raises many ethical and legal issues. If a potential candidate for employment as a nurse denies having a criminal record but a subsequent check by a prospective employer (e.g., health care institution) reveals one, the employer may decide that the candidate's denial demonstrates untrustworthiness and deny employment on this basis (Devitt, 2004, p. 38). But what should such an employer do in cases in which the candidate has, in fact, disclosed a criminal record? Of course, the nature of the offence would be carefully considered since not all offences lead to the conclusion that the candidate may pose a threat to the safety of patients. One noteworthy pitfall of a criminal record check that should be considered is that it reveals a record of a criminal act committed at a past point in time. It would not reveal existing concerns, such as substance abuse or lack of trustworthiness. It might also identify a person who committed a criminal act a very long time ago which may not be relevant to their practice today (e.g., possession of a controlled substance, such as marijuana, or underage drinking). This is a difficult area for employers, and there are not always clear-cut answers (Canadian Civil Liberties Association, 2014).

A 1993 BC court decision involving an LPN illustrates how provincial human rights laws may protect an applicant's right to membership despite that person's prior criminal record (*Mans v. Council of Licensed Practical Nurses*, 1990). In this case, a person had applied for an LPN licence after having worked unlicensed as such for a number of years. The Council of Licensed Practical Nurses of British Columbia refused her application on the grounds that she had a prior criminal record consisting of a conviction for shoplifting in the early 1970s, nearly 20 years earlier.

The BC *Human Rights Act*, then in force (now called the *Human Rights Code*, 1996), prohibited discrimination in employment based on a person's past criminal record unless such a record was related to the person's intended occupation. The LPN took her complaint to the BC Human Rights Council, claiming that the Council of Licensed Practical Nurses' discrimination against her on this basis was contrary to the Human Rights Code. The Human Rights Council found in the nurse's favour and ordered the Council of Licensed Practical Nurses to grant the nurse a licence.

The Council of Licensed Practical Nurses appealed, and the case ultimately found its way to the BC Court of Appeal, which upheld the Human Rights Council's decision and confirmed that the *Human Rights Act* superseded the statute granting the Council of Licensed Practical Nurses authority to deny a licence to applicants deemed unfit to be licensed by it. The court further stated that the Human Rights Council was correct in asserting that the prior criminal record, in this case, was unrelated to the applicant's intended occupation as an LPN and that the discrimination was, therefore, illegal.

It is arguable that such a ruling as that by the BC Court of Appeal could apply to other provinces since most provincial human rights laws contain similar provisions with respect to discrimination on the basis of a criminal record. Of course, employers and regulatory bodies cannot deny employment or the awarding of a licence or registration on the basis of race, creed, ethnic origin, gender, religion, marital status, physical or mental disability, or sexual orientation.

Reciprocity

In the case of applicants who have received their education in a province other than the one in which they are applying, the curriculum must be either equivalent to that association's educational standards or from a board-approved institution. The requirements for Canadian and internationally educated nurses (IENs) are generally set out in each provincial or territorial act: see Alberta Act, s. 28(2)(b); Saskatchewan Act, s. 19(1) (i)(A)(II); Manitoba Act (for registration as a graduate nurse specifically), s. 9(2)(a)(ii), and *Registered Nurses Regulation*, Man. Reg. 128/2001, subparagraph 4(1)(a)(ii) and subsection 4(2); Nova Scotia Nursing Act c.8 (2019), PEI Regulated Health Professions Act, 2013, s. 12(4), Yukon,

Registered Nurses Profession Act and Regulation RSY 2002, c. 194 and OIC 2012/198 s. 4; and Newfoundland Act, s. 8. In British Columbia, the BCCNM's bylaws have set out the requirements for Canadian and IENs. In some provinces, applicants who are already registered and licensed to practise nursing in another province, who demonstrate that they are competent, and who are not currently the subject of disciplinary or competency proceedings in any other jurisdiction, will be entitled to registration in the province in which they are applying. The Yukon Territory requires nurses to register in another Canadian jurisdiction, as it is unable to register students for the national licencing exam.

Internationally Educated Nurses

Issues related to reciprocity, especially as it applies to Internationally Educated Nurses (IENs), are raised cyclically, especially when there are shortages of health care professionals. Consider the shortage of nurses that occurred across the country related to the COVID-19 pandemic and other system-associated factors, and the pressure placed on regulatory bodies to streamline and fast-track the regulatory process for IENs.

To ensure that international education programs meet Canadian standards, regulatory bodies have initiated methods of evaluating the credentials and experience of these applicants. Their websites include detailed information for new immigrants and those applying to come to Canada, which outlines the process and whether they are ready for registration and requirements for language proficiency in English or French. For example, in British Columbia, the BCCNM (http://bccnm.ca) provides a detailed step-by-step chart that outlines each requirement, including registration in the country where the applicant studied nursing, and in every other country where they practised. Applicants must also disclose information about any disciplinary or competency issues faced, their postsecondary nursing education, any criminal records or pardons, and so forth. Each application is examined on its own merits and, depending on the applicant's qualifications and challenges associated with obtaining the required documentation, this can take considerable time to process.

IENs have historically faced challenges in accessing entry into the nursing profession in Canada. The success rate after writing the national examination was low, as there were few supports in place to assist them. However, programs are now in place to educate and inform IENs about the Canadian health care system; the culture of the environment, including nursing-specific language and communication skills; and examination preparation. In some settings, clinical experience is offered through observation and shadowing opportunities. Also, pre-immigration supports and services are now in place to prepare them in advance and guide them through the application process. When they are successful in accessing employment, these programs also facilitate their transition to the workplace (CARE Centre for Internationally Educated Nurses, 2018). These services and supports appear to have improved access of IENs to the nursing profession. For example, in Ontario in 2022, there was a 132% increase in the number of IEN registrants as compared with the previous year (CNO, 2022). Interest in attracting IENs grows at times of nursing shortages in Canada.

Standards of Practice

Legislation requires that the nursing regulatory bodies establish standards of practice and professional behaviour. Professional standards serve as yardsticks to measure the actions and competence of nurses. Standards reflect the philosophy and values of the profession, the foundation of nursing practice, and its ethical and moral codes. Specifically, they focus on nurses' accountability to the public, knowledge requirements, the application of knowledge, ethics, ongoing competence, and professional behaviour. For each professional or clinical standard, there are indicators or descriptors that assist in clarifying the standard's application to practice, professional behaviour, and how they are measured or evaluated.

These standards make explicit nurses' accountability to the regulatory bodies, their employers, patients, and the public (see, as examples, the websites of the BCCNM, the CNO, and the CRNA). Clinical and professional standards are considered a component of the performance appraisal of nurses and serve as a guide for ongoing professional development, education, and quality assurance. Typically, the standards are defined as establishing the minimum requirements for safe and professional practice. These standards are used to evaluate the actions of any nurse who is the subject of a complaint or disciplinary process within the regulatory body or of a legal proceeding.

To hold nurses accountable to the public with respect to the delivery of safe, competent nursing care, in general, most standards of practice:

- Provide a guide for safe practice
- Describe the responsibilities and accountabilities of the nurse
- Provide performance criteria
- Ensure continuing competence
- Interpret nursing's scope of practice
- Provide direction for nursing education
- Facilitate peer review
- Provide a foundation for research-based practice
- Provide benchmarks for quality improvement (CNO, 2002)

Examples of standards include Guidelines for Professional Behaviour, the professional misconduct regulations; Nursing Documentation Standards; and the Professional Standards for Registered Nurses and Registered Practical Nurses in Ontario (CNO, 2018); Practice Standards: Medication Administration, Standards for Infection Prevention and Control, Standards for the Therapeutic Nurse–Client Relationship (Nurses Association of New Brunswick, 2018).

The BCCNM has identified four categories of professional standards that establish the level of performance nurses are required to meet:

- Professional responsibility and accountability
- Knowledge-based practice
- Client-focused provision of service
- Ethical practice.

Although legislation and regulatory bodies establish broad standards of professional practice, standards are developed more specifically in particular organizations or institutions to represent nursing practice in that setting. Nurses are required to meet these standards, and their actions are evaluated accordingly. Standards of practice also exist for specialty areas within nursing. For example, standards of practice for a nurse in critical care will differ from those for a nurse in a community or psychiatric setting.

Practice and professional standards are of great relevance in negligence and malpractice issues, as discussed in Chapter 7. They are a guide to the evaluation of the nurse and serve as a benchmark with respect to the extent that the standard is achieved. They are evidence against which a nurse's actual conduct relevant to expectations is judged in a professional negligence lawsuit or when disciplinary action is taken by the regulatory body. The practice standards are reviewed to understand the minimum quality of practice required of all nurses in the same category. Failure to meet professional standards is often enough for the court or the regulator to make a finding of negligence or professional misconduct. Meeting these standards is only one part of the assessment of the actions of the nurse and is often referred to as the "minimum" expectation of professional practice. Nevertheless, a failure to follow a clear written policy is often difficult evidence of negligence to overcome.

When there is a finding that a nurse has breached the standard and where that breach has resulted in harm or injury to a patient, a nurse may be found legally responsible in an action in negligence. Thus, standards are critical not only to ensure patient care is of the highest quality but also as a measure against which nursing practice is judged. A nurse can still be found guilty of professional misconduct or negligence based on other evidence, but the relevant standards are usually very persuasive.

Standards are updated on a regular basis to stay current with issues, trends, and emerging research. For example, when the Medical Assistance in Dying (MAiD) amendments to the *Criminal Code* were brought in, standards to guide the practice of nurses were introduced. Regulatory bodies also responded in a timely way during the COVID-19 pandemic by communicating expectations and professional standards for nurses. For example, the statement that appears in Box 5.1 was issued in Ontario by the CNO (2021).

Nursing regulators also respond to situations that reveal issues and challenges within the profession. The story of Joyce Echaquan, introduced in Chapter 2, regulated the existence of systemic discrimination within the health care system and reinforced the urgency of addressing racism within the nursing profession.

Joyce Echaquan was a 37-year-old Indigenous woman from the Atikamekw First Nation. Her story reveals exceptionally poor conduct by the team, including a nurse, caring for her. While a patient at the hospital, she recorded a video that documented the

BOX 5.1
NURSES SUPPORTING PUBLIC HEALTH MEASURES

Public health protection measures, such as handwashing, masking, social distancing, and vaccinations are effective strategies to prevent the spread of COVID-19. As the pandemic continues, College of Nurses of Ontario (CNO) is taking this opportunity to make its expectations about providing advice on evidence-based public health protection and prevention measures clear to nurses in Ontario.

CNO's Statement

Nurses are leaders in the community, and the public's trust in nurses may extend to their views on health matters communicated on social media and other forums. Statements made by nurses in public forums have the potential to impact the health and safety of the public.

Nurses have a professional accountability to:

- use accurate sources of information based in scientific theory and evidence, to inform their professional service and practice
- support patients and the public to make informed health care decisions, including decisions about public health prevention and protection measures
- role model and follow public health directives that keep patients and the public safe.

CNO's expectations are outlined in the Code of Conduct and Professional Standards.

CNO's practice standards do not apply to all aspects of a nurse's private life. However, when a nurse communicates with the public and identifies as a nurse, they invoke their professional position as a nurse and are accountable to CNO and the public it protects.

Nurses are expected to adhere to the standards of practice in carrying out their professional responsibilities. Nurses have a professional responsibility to not publicly communicate anti-vaccination, anti-masking, and anti-distancing statements that contradict the available scientific evidence. Doing so may result in an investigation by CNO, and disciplinary proceedings when warranted.

College of Nurses of Ontario. (2020, December). *Nurses supporting public health measures.* https://www.cno.org/en/news/2020/december-2020/nurses-supporting-public-health-measures/

---

indifference and mistreatment she received. She did not speak French well; therefore, she recorded her meetings with her caregivers so that a cousin could interpret for her.

Echaquan was admitted to the hospital with stomach pains, and the team discussed whether to give her morphine. When she objected, as she believed that she was allergic to morphine, she was spoken to in an abusive way and was administered the morphine in spite of her expressed concerns. In the video, at least two members of staff are heard insulting her in French. While Echaquan was moaning in pain, someone asked her if she was "done acting stupid." Another told her that she "made some bad choices" and questioned what her children would think if they saw her, where she quietly responded with: "That's why I came here." She was told that she was only "good for sex," that they were the ones "paying for this," and that she was "stupid as hell." Echaquan died later that day. Her cause of death was pulmonary edema. She had been treated for several years for cardiomyopathy.

Although the coroner determined that Echaquan's death was accidental, she also concluded that it was di-

rectly related to the care Echaquan received during her hospitalization and that her death was preventable. Due to their prejudice, the staff quickly labelled her as dependent on narcotics and trivialized her cries for help and claims of pain. Also, contrary to institutional policies, Echaquan was placed in physical restraints, sedated, and isolated without constant monitoring.

The nurse involved admitted to verbally abusing Echaquan and for failing to conduct the required assessments when Echaquan fell.

The Disciplinary Council of the Ordre des infirmières et infirmiers du Québec (OIIQ) sentenced the nurse to a 1-year suspension, as well as a 6-month suspension, to be served concurrently, for her role in this tragedy (*Infirmières et infirmiers (Ordre professionnel des) v. Rocray*, 2021). Echaquan's family have now sued the hospital, the local health authority, a nurse, and a doctor involved in her care for nearly $3 million.

The OIIQ acknowledged the existence of systemic racism in the health care system and the urgency of re-establishing trust between nurses and their First Nations and Inuit patients and communicated their intention to implement concrete actions to address these issues (OIIQ, 2022). Political leaders in Quebec have been less ready to concede the existence of systemic racism, with the premier in 2021 denying the existence of such discrimination (Bruemmer, 2021).

The Responsibility of Regulatory Bodies for the Ongoing Competence of Nurses

Colleges are responsible for introducing and maintaining mechanisms or processes to evaluate the continuing competence of nurses. Most of these processes involve a component of reflective practice and an alignment with established professional and clinical standards. Consult the websites of the provincial and territorial colleges for a more comprehensive review of their programs. In this section, the examples from various colleges serve as illustrations.

Continuing Competence Program Requirements

In Ontario, a quality improvement program called the *CNO Quality Assurance Program* is in place, and all nurses who are registered with the College are expected to participate in it. The program has three parts: reflective practice, competence assessment, and practice setting consultation. Each nurse must participate in one of these components each year. Full details and documentation concerning the program can be found on the CNO's website.

The reflective practice component of this quality improvement program is intended to identify strengths and improvement opportunities. The process involves a self-assessment based on the standards and guidelines for practice, feedback from peers, the development of a learning plan, implementation of the plan, and evaluation.

Other means of evaluation of a nurse's competence to practice include formal processes, such as examinations, and observation in the clinical setting. On a regular basis, the CNO randomly selects nurses from the registrant list to be assessed. Also, an individual nurse or a practice setting may choose to volunteer for an assessment, or the College may initiate an assessment based on a referral from a statutory committee (e.g., as part of a complaint or disciplinary process) (CNO, 2018).

In Nova Scotia, the College's Continuing Competence Program (CCP) is a mandatory requirement for licensing as a nurse. Continuing competence "is career-long enhancement of knowledge, skill, and judgment required to practice safely and ethically." Nova Scotia merged the different regulators into a single college (the Nova Scotia College of Nursing [NSCN]) and has integrated the requirements for the different categories of nurses into a single document, the *NSCN Continuing Competence Program Guide for Nurses* (2021) (https://www.nscn.ca/sites/default/files/documents/CCP/CCP_Guide_For_Nurses.pdf).

The College recognizes that nurses use a variety of approaches to maintaining competence, including formal education programs and consultation with colleagues. The CCP is a formal mechanism to further develop and record these processes and is based on the philosophy that nurses are competent and committed to lifelong learning. Tools are offered as a mechanism to engage nurses in reflective practice and learning.

The tools formalize processes most nurses already engage in: reflecting on the standards and code of ethics; identifying strengths and learning opportunities; developing learning plans; and implementing and evaluating learning plans (NSCN, 2021). Those applying for or renewing their licence must complete the tools or an equivalent to meet the requirements of the College.

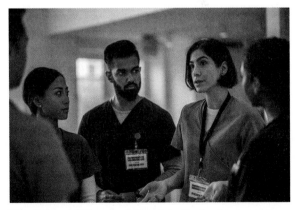

The College of Nurses of Ontario's Quality Assurance Program has three parts: reflective practice, competence assessment, and practice setting consultation. *Source: iStock.com/FatCamera.*

In Alberta, the CRNA's CCP is also based on a reflective practice model. Registrants assess their nursing practice, obtain peer feedback, and implement a learning plan to address their learning needs. The CRNA website provides online guidelines for nurses to meet the standards.

In British Columbia, nurses are required to meet continuing competence requirements annually. "The Annual QA [quality assurance] cycle involves three main components. During registration renewal, nurses complete a self-assessment of their practice. Once they have renewed their registration, they are required to seek peer feedback on their nursing practice, and create a professional development plan, that includes at least two learning goals, and activities to achieve those goals" (BCCNM, 2022a).

In addition to these quality assurance requirements, in many provinces, eligibility for continued licensing requires ongoing education. Each regulatory body has its own requirements. For example, in Quebec, each year nurses must have at least 7 hours of accredited ongoing education or professional development as well as 13 hours non-accredited education (such as being current in reading research, or attending seminars/conferences) (https://www.oiiq.org/formation/norme-de-formation-continue)

ENFORCEMENT: COMPLAINTS, DISCIPLINE AND APPEALS PROCESSES

Because regulatory bodies have the responsibility to protect the public, they are mandated to respond when these standards are not being met, and when there are allegations of incompetence, unacceptable conduct, or the incapacity of a member. Regulatory bodies have mechanisms in place to address complaints and engage disciplinary processes. They also have rules and mechanisms for mandatory reporting, for example, in circumstances where there are allegations of sexual misconduct. Through the complaint process and mandatory reporting mechanisms, concerns related to the practice or behaviour of a nurse come to the attention of the regulatory body. Reports or complaints are usually submitted to the CEO, registrar, or executive director of the college.

Whenever possible, concerns are resolved through education and remedial action. These interventions are intended to correct and improve the nurse's

practice and ensure that ethical and practice standards are met.

Mandatory Reporting

Employers are required by law to report when they terminate, discipline, or suspend a nurse for professional incompetence or misconduct. This is treated as a complaint and proceeds through a similar review process. The college expects that employers will manage professional competence and conduct issues through internal human resource processes. Ethical leadership practices, as discussed in Chapter 12, would ensure that nurses are supported through education, counselling, and health interventions to improve their practice. In the case of health, mental health, and addiction concerns, many programs are available for an employer to access for nurses. Most often, these approaches lead to improvement in the nurse's practice and conduct.

A formal complaint or report should be issued only after all avenues have been exhausted and the employer has no option but to terminate or discipline a nurse. In all circumstances where a nurse is terminated, the employer is mandated to report this to the regulatory body, which determines whether any action is required.

As stated, if an employer's internal disciplinary or performance review procedures are not able to resolve the issue, the employer would be required to file a formal complaint with the regulator. Ontario's *Regulated Health Professions Act* (1991) and Alberta's *Health Professions Act* (2000, s. 57) require that members' employers file a detailed report outlining the incidents or events that gave rise to termination or the intention to terminate, whether they involved misconduct, incapacity, or a failure to observe the standards of practice, the response of the member to these incidents, and the ultimate action taken by the employer against the nurse. Similar requirements are in place in Saskatchewan and Manitoba.

Ontario law specifically requires a member of the CNO to report a nursing colleague who the member has reasonable grounds to believe has committed an act of sexual abuse of a patient. In the case of nonsexual improper conduct, the nurse would first report the matter to the employer, who would invoke an internal practice review or disciplinary procedure before lodging a formal complaint with the regulator. British Columbia's *Health*

Professions Act (1996) and Alberta's statute contain similar requirements but also require mandatory reporting of all conduct or situations in which a health care professional's conduct, fitness to practise, competence to practice, or sexual misconduct poses a threat to the safety of the public. British Columbia's legislation additionally requires a medical practitioner in charge of a public hospital to report to the College a registrant (i.e., a member) who has been admitted to the practitioner's institution for psychiatric care or treatment.

Addressing Complaints

An extensive process is in place to address concerns brought forward about the practice of a nurse. This is part of a college's process for ensuring the ongoing competence of nurses. Colleges rely on input from health care professionals, employers, and the public to ensure that this legislative requirement is met. Concerns brought forward may relate to issues of neglect or abuse, safety, competence, breaches of privacy and confidentiality, theft or fraud, conflict of interest, rude and inappropriate behaviour, relationships with patients, and so on.

Submitting a Complaint

When a **complainant** (i.e., the person who makes a complaint) has concerns about a nurse's practice or conduct, a complaint can be submitted to the regulatory body. The complaint must be in writing or, in some settings, in audio format; signed and dated by the person making the complaint; and should name the nurse concerned. The submission must outline the facts and particulars of the alleged misconduct. Usually, concerns that are not in writing and made anonymously are not considered unless the college obtains further information that supports the need for investigation (CRNA, 2023; CNO, 2018; CRNM, 2018).

Complainants can be nursing colleagues, patients receiving care or members of their immediate family, other members of the health care team, or employers. It is the ethical and, in many cases, the legal obligation of nurses to report (to the employer or to the college) improper professional conduct or incidents that involve a nursing colleague's failure to meet the standards of professional practice, whether that colleague has acted in an unprofessional manner; has shown a lack of skill, knowledge, or judgement that poses a

threat to the safety of patients in the nurse's care; or is, by reason of addiction to alcohol or drugs or mental or physical illness, unable to discharge his or her nursing duties competently or safely. In Alberta, New Brunswick, and many other provinces, failure to report such conduct or situations constitutes professional misconduct on the part of the nurse whose duty it was to disclose it.

The duty to disclose unprofessional conduct or incompetence is an exception to the general prohibition on the communication of confidential information disclosed by the patient in the course of treatment and the provision of nursing care. If, in the course of providing treatment to a patient, a nurse gained knowledge from that patient that another nurse was acting in an unskilled manner, that nurse may disclose such information to the employer, the college, or both. Communication of a complaint to the college is confidential and does not violate the obligation to preserve confidentiality in the nurse–patient relationship. Communications to other authorities, such as the police, is improper unless the patient or their substitute decision maker consents or there is a legal duty to report. There are provisions in many provincial nursing and other health care professions' statutes that authorize disclosure of a patient's identity in a complaint only with the patient's consent or that of a substitute decision maker (in the case of a patient who is mentally incapable of consenting). It will usually be possible to disclose the information without divulging the identity of the patient or other details that would readily identify them. The patient who feels strongly about the professional's conduct may choose to waive privacy rights and authorize full disclosure.

The formal complaint is usually submitted to the CEO or registrar of the college. Once a complaint is registered with the college, it is subject to a preliminary review by the CEO, complaints committee, or investigator to ascertain whether it is well founded or merely frivolous or malicious (i.e., brought deliberately to injure a person's reputation) (Nova Scotia Act, s. 63 and 76, s. 31; Manitoba Act, s. 21; Yukon Act, s. 24; New Brunswick Act, s. 29 and Part IV.1).

The CEO or delegate, depending on the seriousness of the issue, encourages the complainant to discuss the matter with the nurse or employer because many complaints related to poor communication or misunderstandings may be resolved at that level. If this is not possible or successful, then the CEO has a number of options, including:

- Dismissal of the complaint if there is insufficient or no evidence of unprofessional conduct, or if satisfied that the complaint is trivial or intended to harass or damage a member's reputation
- Undertaking an expert assessment
- A referral for a fitness-to-practise assessment
- Recommending that both parties agree to an alternative resolution process
- Referring the complaint for further investigation CRNA, 2023.

Alternative Dispute Resolution

The nature of some concerns makes them amenable to a conflict- or dispute-resolution process. This option is available when both parties, the complainant and the nurse, agree. An expert facilitator is engaged to work with the parties to exchange ideas about how the matter can be resolved. This process allows nurses to reflect on their practice and to identify opportunities for professional growth. The resolution agreement is confidential, and the results are not published or available to the public (CRNA, 2023; CNO, 2018; CRNM, 2018).

Interim Investigation

By statute, members whose conduct or competence is the subject of an investigation must be notified immediately by the college upon receipt of a written complaint. The investigation process entails the gathering of information relevant to the complaint. An investigator has powers under statute to inspect nursing records, conduct interviews, enter the nurse's place of practice, inspect equipment, conduct tests, and so forth. The investigator also considers the past experience of the nurse regarding any issues involving the college. Nurses are under a legal duty to cooperate with an investigator and to allow examinations without interference.

It is also entirely appropriate, and sensible, that nurses immediately avail themselves of all legal and procedural rights during an investigation, including the engagement of a lawyer. Nurses' professional organizations, or provincial or territorial nursing regulatory bodies in those provinces where the regulatory and advocacy "arms" are combined, may provide for the services of a lawyer to

represent nurses in such proceedings. Insurance may also be purchased to fund the defence of disciplinary charges on top of standard practice insurance (professional liability protection [PLP]).

Nurses are expected to make submissions during this phase of the investigation (e.g., see Yukon Act, s. 24(4); Manitoba Act, ss. 29 (3) and 35(1)), including responding to the complaint that has been brought forward. Usually, they are provided with all of the documentation related to the investigation to facilitate their response.

At this stage, the complaint may be dismissed if it is unwarranted or unsupported by the results of the investigation. If the criteria are met, the matter is referred to a complaints or inquiry committee for further review and investigation (CRNA, 2023; CNO, 2018; CRNM, 2018).

Committee Review

If a complaint is well founded, the concern is reviewed by a panel of nurses and lay members who are appointed by the board or council. The committee is usually chaired by a member of the college's board or council. The inclusion of lay persons ensures the public input aspect of self-regulation.

The committee undertakes further reviews, and their deliberations are not usually open to the nurse, the complainant, or the public. If it becomes immediately clear to the panel that the allegations show that the nurse being investigated poses a threat to the safety or security of patients, the committee usually has the power to order that the nurse's right to practise be suspended or restricted pending the conclusion of the disciplinary proceedings.

The panel in their deliberations considers the evidence, the seriousness of the allegations before them, and whether the nurse had a past history of concerns with the college. In most circumstances, the panel attempts to resolve matters through remedial or rehabilitative activities but may take a number of other actions. The panel may:

- Take no action, if there is insufficient evidence to support the complaint that standards were breached
- Counsel the nurse about standards of practice and professional conduct related to the complaint

- Have the nurse appear for a caution or reprimand
- Require the nurse to complete a remediation program, as well as self-reflection, monitored by the college
- Accept the voluntary surrender of the nurse's certificate of practice
- Refer some or all of the issues in the complaint to the disciplinary committee (CRNA, 2023; CNO, 2018; CRNM, 2018)

Disciplinary Committee

The procedures for disciplinary hearings and the findings and penalties that can be assessed by the disciplinary committee are fairly similar in all provinces and territories. Professional disciplinary proceedings, although open to the public, are entirely an internal matter governed by the nursing regulatory body and are designed to ensure nurses' professional conduct conforms to practice standards, codes of ethics, and the regulations of the professional body. Any findings of misconduct would normally be punished by a range of measures, from a reprimand to outright revocation of a nurse's right to practise.

Before a hearing is scheduled to consider the matter, the disciplinary committee (in some provinces, the practice review committee) must first notify the nurse against whom the complaint was brought. The date and time of the hearing will usually be coordinated with the nurse's lawyer, if any. The notice usually specifies the nature of the conduct being reviewed, and the college must fully disclose the evidence it intends to rely on, as well as any other evidence in its possession that may be relevant to the hearing. Although the hearing is part of an administrative law process, the consequences for the nurse can be very serious, and nurses are, therefore, well advised to treat the process more like a criminal law matter than a civil law matter.

The hearing follows a formal process, similar to court proceedings. The nurse is entitled to be represented by a lawyer. The college will present its evidence first. The nurse will then have the right to cross-examine the college's witnesses and require the college to prove all elements of the case. The nurse has the opportunity to present evidence and witnesses. Both sides will be able to make closing arguments. The burden of proof lies with the college, and the nurse is not obliged to testify.

The committee, after hearing the evidence and the arguments from both sides, will make its decision. Among the possible findings it may make are that the nurse is:

- Innocent of any wrong-doing
- Incompetent, unskilled, or otherwise lacking in essential knowledge
- Guilty of professional misconduct
- Habitually impaired by the use of alcohol or drugs and unable to discharge nursing duties and obligations safely

Penalties

The penalties that may be levied against the guilty nurse include:

- A fine or award of costs of the investigation
- Censure or reprimand before the committee or in writing
- Conditions on the nurse's right to practise, including a requirement to take additional courses or education and pass further examinations
- Suspension from practice for a specified period of time (e.g., for the completion of such additional training or education)
- Revocation of the right to practise and expulsion from the regulatory body

Penalties vary across the country. In Ontario, for example, a nurse who has been found guilty of sexual misconduct can be ordered to reimburse the College for expenses incurred and for providing a program for therapy and counselling for patients who were sexually abused by that nurse (HPPC, 1991, s. 51(2), para. 5.1). Guilty nurses may have their licence revoked if the sexual abuse consisted of certain specified acts (s. 51(5)). In such a case, the patient is allowed to make, and the panel must consider, a statement describing the impact of the abuse.

If a nurse's practice demonstrates lack of knowledge, skill, or judgement, or if the nurse exhibits disregard for the welfare of patients, the nurse may be deemed incompetent. This finding of professional incompetence is different from a finding of professional misconduct.

Regardless of the nature of the finding, the panel must render its decision in writing and give it to all parties. The college is required to publish its decisions and the reasons for these, usually including the member's name, in its annual report and in any other of its publications. A member's name may be excluded from publication if the complaint was dismissed, if the name would reveal confidential patient information, or if the publication would be unfairly prejudicial to the member.

The processes for investigating and prosecuting complaints have developed to protect the public and to ensure the rights of the subject of the complaint to due process are maintained. Recall the case scenario of nurse P. W. in Chapter 4. They were alleged to have engaged in sexually abusive behaviour toward a child in their care. Their employment had been terminated, and their conduct was reported to the police and to their provincial regulatory body. P. W. has the right to due process and natural justice. The procedures above, which would likely be followed, provide for notice to P. W. and an opportunity to be heard and to defend themselves. These procedures are designed to respect and ensure that the requirements of natural justice are met. Failure to follow them opens any disciplinary proceedings brought against P. W. to attack on the grounds that P. W. has been denied due process. Of course, any criminal charges brought against them by the police would also entitle them to procedural and legal rights in a court of law. But in the case of disciplinary proceedings to determine their continued status as a nurse, P. W. would be entitled to due process.

A disciplinary decision from New Brunswick illustrates the type of matters considered and disciplinary action that may be taken against a nurse. In this particular case, the disciplinary committee of the Nurses Association of New Brunswick (NANB) considered the case of a nurse who had treated at least two patients in his care in a rough manner, had used verbal and nonverbal inappropriate behaviour against other nursing staff and patients, and had demonstrated a serious lack of judgement in the care of patients and lack of respect for their dignity. The association ordered that his registration be revoked and that he pay investigation and legal costs of $10,000 to the association before any application for readmission to the practice of nursing in New Brunswick. The committee further ruled that he could not reapply for admission for 3 years. David Lloyd Green (NANB 2007).

Appeals

The decision of a disciplinary/complaint committee as to the finding of guilt, the penalty handed down, or both may be appealed, usually to the board of directors or the council of the college by notice in writing within a specified time. If the decision on the appeal is still unfavourable, the nurse may appeal, in most provinces, to the provincial superior court (in Alberta, to the Court of Appeal, which may order a new hearing before the Court of King's Bench). Nova Scotia also allows appeals to the provincial appeal court directly. Yukon does not allow appeals to the courts. In the Northwest Territories and Newfoundland and Labrador, the decision of the Trial Division of the Supreme Court on an appeal from a disciplinary committee's decision is final and may not be appealed further to their respective Courts of Appeal. In Ontario, appeals are taken to the Health Professions Appeal and Review Board (see *Ministry of Health Appeal and Review Boards Act,* 1998). In Quebec, they are heard by the **Professions Tribunal** (see *Professional Code,* R.S.Q., c. C-26).

In Canada, the courts have a general power (judicial review) to review the actions of administrative tribunals, like a college's discipline committee. This is not a new hearing, but a review of the decision to ensure that the tribunal respected the procedural rights of the nurse, there was no fraud, and the committee correctly applied the law.

Fitness to Practise

Not all provincial and territorial regulatory bodies have a fitness-to-practise committee. In British Columbia, for example, the inquiry committee is charged with reviewing, among other issues, the ability or fitness of a nurse member to engage in the practice of nursing. In Manitoba, this task is the responsibility of the investigation committee.

Some colleges use a fitness-to-practise committee as a particular structure within the regulatory body responsible for reviewing a nurse's capacity. As noted, the process and particular regulatory sub-body responsible for carrying out such a function will vary by province or territory; however, many of the essential considerations and features described in this section will be similar among all provinces and territories.

The investigation of a nurse's fitness and capacity to practise does not necessarily raise questions of professional misconduct. The nurse's behaviour may be such that there is concern about that nurse's physical or mental abilities.

Inquiries as to a professional's capacity will usually be commenced by the CEO or the registrar, using the extensive investigatory powers granted under the relevant legislation. (See for example, *Health Professions Procedural Code,* 1991). If the registrar has reason to believe that the member in question may be incapacitated, the registrar must report the supporting findings to the executive committee for further action (*HPPC,* 1991, s. 57). If further action is warranted, and it has received the registrar's report or a referral from a panel of the complaints committee, the fitness-to-practise committee may appoint a board of inquiry to determine whether the professional is incapacitated. Some of that committee's members must be drawn from among the College's general membership. In this way, the professional's fitness to practise is evaluated by peers.

As part of its inquiry, the board may order the member to undergo physical or psychological examinations conducted or ordered by a health care professional (i.e., a physician or psychiatrist). Further, the member's licence may be suspended until further examination or until the inquiry is complete (*HPPC,* 1991, s. 59). Upon conclusion of the inquiry, the board is required to submit its report to the executive committee, which, in turn, may refer it to the fitness-practise committee if it decides that further proceedings are necessary.

If the executive committee refers the report to the fitness-to-practise committee, the latter then selects a panel of at least three of its members to hold a hearing into the fitness of the professional to practice nursing. Unless the professional requests otherwise, the hearing must be closed (i.e., not public). The professional's request for a public hearing may be refused if this would compromise public security or any person's safety or privacy (*HPPC,* 1991, s. 68(2)). The professional is entitled to be represented by legal counsel at the hearing, as are any witnesses who will testify, including any person who may have suffered harm or have been otherwise affected by the member's conduct. Evidence at the hearing may include testimony by medical or psychiatric experts. However, the professional who is the subject of the hearing must be given a copy of the expert's report or a summary of the evidence before it is presented at the hearing.

If the panel concludes that the professional is incapacitated, their certificate of registration may be revoked or suspended, or conditions, terms, or restrictions may be imposed on it. If a certificate is revoked, the professional may apply to the registrar to have a new certificate issued or the suspension removed no earlier than 1 year after the suspension or revocation (*HPPC,* 1991, s. 72(1)).

The Quality Assurance Committee

Several provinces' and territories' regulatory bodies have a quality assurance committee. In other provinces and territories, quality assurance is carried out by an investigations committee or the disciplinary committee itself. In Manitoba, this work is carried out by a continuing competence committee.

In Ontario, every college of health care professions is required under the *RHPA* (1991) to establish a quality assurance committee whose task is to review and examine individual members' practices to identify incompetence, incapacity, professional misconduct, and, in particular, the sexual abuse of patients by health care professionals. For example, if the executive committee, the complaints committee, or the Health Professions Appeal and Review Board receives from the registrar a report of sexual remarks or behaviour directed toward a patient following an investigation into a member's conduct, it may refer the matter to the quality assurance committee.

The *HPPC* defines sexual abuse of a patient as "sexual intercourse or other forms of sexual relations between the member and the patient, touching of a sexual nature of the patient by the member, or behaviour or remarks of a sexual nature by the member towards the patient" (*HPPC,* 1991, s. 1(3)), unless it is touching, behaviour, or remarks of a clinical nature that are appropriate in the context of the treatment being provided by the member.

The quality assurance committee will conduct its own investigation into the professional's practice, not only to identify incompetence or incapacity, but also to pinpoint inadequacies in their practice's operations and facilities. If the quality assurance committee concludes that on the basis of its assessment, the professional may have committed an act of misconduct or may be incompetent or incapacitated, it may disclose the professional's name and the allegations against the person to the executive committee. On receipt of such information, the committee would refer the matter to the discipline committee or to the fitness-to-practise committee, as required (*HPPC*, 1991, ss. 79.1, 80.2, 83). Similar procedures exist in all other jurisdictions, but the terminology may vary.

Other Offences

Nursing statutes of virtually all provinces and territories set out various offences that are designed to prevent unauthorized practice and contravention of the laws and regulations. In British Columbia, for example, these include a provision that forbids a person from providing a health service when that person is not registered with the regulatory body that regulates the service (e.g., nursing) unless the person provides the service under the supervision of a registered member (see *Health Professions Act*, 1996, s. 13).

An important distinction should be drawn at this point. The term *competent* is usually used to mean that a professional has the necessary skills, experience, and knowledge to carry out the duties of the particular position. But saying such a professional is "competent" is quite different from saying that the professional is "registered" or "authorized" to perform those duties. The latter expressions convey the notion that an official regulatory agency has assessed and passed judgement on that person's skills and knowledge and has found these to meet the requirements of registration. For example, an employment agency that found a position for a private nurse who was not a member or was not properly qualified in British Columbia, and that knew that that person was legally unable to perform any of the controlled acts that nurses are permitted to perform, even if trained to do so, has contravened the law.

To illustrate, offences in many jurisdictions, including Ontario, include:

- Obtaining a registration certificate from any one of the colleges by false pretenses or knowingly assisting a person to do this (*HPPC*, 1991, s. 92)
- Obstructing an investigator appointed by the registrar of the college in an investigation into professional misconduct, incompetency, or incapacity of a member (*HPPC*, 1991, s. 93(2))

- Disclosing any information revealed at a hearing or inquiry that is closed to the public (*HPPC*, 1991, s. 93(1))
- Failing to permit an assessor of the quality assurance committee of a college to inspect a member's records or premises (*HPPC*, 1991, s. 93(3))
- Failing to report a member (of the same or any other college) when there are reasonable grounds to believe that that member has sexually abused a patient (*HPPC*, 1991, s. 93(4))

Finally, no professional may treat a person if it is reasonably foreseeable that serious physical harm may result from the treatment or advice, or from an omission of such treatment or advice (*RHPA*, 1991, s. 30(1)). Counselling about emotional, social, educational, or spiritual matters, however, is not prohibited by the *RHPA*. Despite this, it would certainly be unethical to counsel someone if psychological harm might foreseeably result. Perhaps including psychological or mental harm in this prohibition would have placed too onerous a burden on health care professionals, as the human mind, its workings, and the genesis of mental disorders are still imperfectly understood.

Criminal Matters

It should be stressed from the outset that disciplinary proceedings against nursing professionals are a matter entirely separate and different from criminal proceedings. Criminal proceedings would be initiated against a nurse if there is an allegation of an offence under the *Criminal Code*. Serious criminal charges would normally be laid by the Crown attorney following a complaint filed either by a member of the public (e.g., a patient) and a police investigation, or by a police investigator who has found sufficient evidence to allege that a criminal offence of some kind has been committed. A finding of guilt following a criminal trial would lead to a fine or perhaps imprisonment. (In some provinces, a nurse convicted of an indictable offence under the *Criminal Code* or an offence under the *Controlled Drugs and Substances Act* (1996) or the *Food and Drugs Act* (1985) may be liable to suspension from nursing practice, in some cases, without any hearing.)

Generally, where there are criminal proceedings and professional misconduct hearings, the professional misconduct hearings will be delayed until after the conclusion of the criminal process. This is done so that the professional misconduct hearings will not prejudice the fairness of the criminal process. Also, if there is a criminal conviction, this may simplify the professional misconduct hearing as well, the conviction being proof of facts that support a finding of professional misconduct. This situation occurred with respect to the Ontario nurse who murdered several patients (*College of Nurses of Ontario v. Wettlaufer*, 2017). The hearing to revoke Elizabeth Wettlaufer's registration was held only after she had been sentenced to prison for multiple life terms. The professional misconduct of deliberately harming her patients was a separate matter and could only be fairly dealt with after her criminal procedures had been resolved.

SOME DISCIPLINARY DECISIONS

The following decisions illustrate some of the disciplinary matters heard by regulatory bodies across Canada and are provided as examples for further discussion.

Decision 1—Saskatchewan

The nurse was charged with professional misconduct for his activities in aggressive picketing of Planned Parenthood Regina. The nurse had carried placards and handed out brochures that used inflammatory and challenging language. Planned Parenthood had made complaints to the College about the nurse's conduct. The College found that the nurse's activities constituted professional misconduct. The Court of Appeal set aside the College's decision on the basis that the activities of the nurse represented protected free speech under the *Canadian Charter of Rights and Freedoms*. As such, the decision of the College could not be justified and was set aside (*Whatcott v. Saskatchewan Association of Licensed Practical Nurses*, 2008).

Decision 2—Ontario

An LPN, who was a member of the CNO, was found guilty of three counts of professional misconduct in that on three separate occasions, with respect to three separate patients, the nurse failed to take a blood sugar reading pursuant to a physician's order. In each of the three cases, the nurse subsequently documented that she had taken such readings when, in fact, she had not. She was found guilty not only of having failed to take the readings but also of having falsified records relating

to her practice by claiming to have taken the readings when she had not done so. The nurse pleaded guilty to all three counts. During the disciplinary hearings, she admitted that she was tired on the day that these acts were committed and that her judgement had been impaired as a result. She fully cooperated with the College, was forthright, and took full responsibility for her actions. The disciplinary committee, after finding her guilty on all counts, ordered that she appear before the committee at a later date to be reprimanded; that her registration be suspended for 60 days; that on return to practice, she inform the Director of Investigations and Hearings of her new place of employment; that she supply any prospective new employer with a copy of the committee's decision; and that her new employer confirm this disclosure and receipt of a copy of the proceeding to the committee (CNO v Julie Pouget, 2011).

Decision 3—Manitoba

An RN was found guilty of professional misconduct for several offences related to handling and providing medication to patients. She pleaded guilty to all the charges, and numerous conditions were imposed on her nursing practice entitlement, such as reporting to the college on her place of employment, providing her employer with a copy of the disciplinary orders made against her, undergoing a competence assessment, and writing a paper demonstrating learning and insight into the issues that had been raised during her disciplinary hearing.

Decision 4—Manitoba

An NP provided a private agency with letters regarding patients on the basis of verbal information and paper files, supporting the transition of the patients to 24-hour supportive care. However, the NP did not conduct any physical assessments of the patients, did not disclose the very limited nature of her review, was paid for this work, and signed 25 identical letters. This was found to be professional misconduct and the member was suspended for 1 month from practice and ordered to pay investigation costs of $5,000 (*Decision on Shahid Shams, CRNM #138111*).

Challenging Regulatory Body Decisions

The nursing regulatory bodies are granted authority by statute to administer the profession in relation to entry to practice, professional misconduct, quality assurance, and other matters as described earlier in this chapter. The decisions of the regulatory bodies are made by specific subcommittees, formulated for the purpose, such as a "fitness-to-practise" or a "disciplinary" committee. The decisions of these committees may be challenged by the affected parties. The way in which a decision can be challenged is a procedural issue and varies from province to province. Usually, an appeal will initially involve an internal process, and if that is unsuccessful, a request for a judicial review of the decision may be made to the Superior Court in the jurisdiction. (See, for example, ss. 89 and 90 of the *Health Professions Act, 2000* [Alberta]).

A judicial review is generally limited to ensuring that the process followed by the regulatory body was procedurally fair and did not involve any errors in the application of the law. These appeals are not a rehearing of the case. If a judicial review application is successful, generally, this will result in the matter being sent back for a new hearing.

The provinces of Ontario, British Columbia, and Quebec have an intermediate administrative tribunal between the regulatory body and the Superior Court. Those tribunals are called the Health Professions Appeal and Review Board (HPARB) in Ontario, the Health Professions Review Board (HPRB) in British Columbia, and the Office des professions du Québec (OPQ). The functions and duties of Ontario's HPARB and British Columbia's HPRB are confined to hearing appeals from complaints, registration, and accreditation committees of the lower-tier health care professions' colleges (i.e., those of nurses, physicians and surgeons, chiropractors, psychiatrists, dentists, etc.). In contrast, in Quebec, the OPQ regulates all professions, both health-related and non–health-related ones. In Quebec's system, however, the OPQ is not directly involved in appeals from disciplinary or registration matters. Its primary mandate is to ensure that the province's 45 self-regulated professions carry out their legal responsibilities in accordance with their governing legislation, that they self-regulate in the public interest, and that they adopt proper regulatory and professional standards for their respective professions. Disciplinary matters in Quebec are appealed to the Professional Tribunal, a government-appointed administrative tribunal that closely resembles Ontario's HPARB. Thus,

there are notable structural and functional differences among the two-tiered Ontario, British Columbia, and Quebec systems. Quebec appears to have the most unified system of professional regulation in Canada.

SUMMARY

This chapter has demonstrated how the interplay of ethics and the law is manifest in the legislation and regulations that govern the profession of nursing in Canada. Nurses throughout the country are held accountable for decisions and actions that influence safe, effective, and ethical practice. Professional regulatory or governing bodies, guided by legislation and regulation, have been established to develop and enforce standards of behaviour, practice, education, research, and leadership. The primary purpose of these regulatory bodies of nursing is the welfare of the public. The primary purpose of these regulatory bodies of nursing is the welfare of the public, accomplished through a legal framework that is intended to protect the public from incompetent, unqualified, or unethical health care professionals and provide the benchmarks against which professional practice is measured.

Nurses in Canada have been afforded the privilege of self-regulation that allows nursing the autonomy to govern its own members. Having the authority to self-regulate reflects the trust the public has put in the profession.

This chapter has reviewed the basic structures, roles, and workings of nursing regulators across Canada. An overview of common approaches was provided with some specific examples of the function of regulatory bodies in various provinces and territories. It is important for nurses to review these regulations because it is essential that nurses understand the expectations associated with being a member of a regulated profession and the responsibilities and obligations that come with that privilege. Regulatory bodies identify standards of professional and clinical practice, which provide clarity to the public with regard to what they can expect from nurses. Therefore, these standards are significant not only in the ongoing evaluation of nurses with respect to safe, competent, and ethical care but also in measuring the nurse's behaviour with respect to legal and professional expectations. The public interest to ensure that the integrity of nurses is validated through rigorous processes and mechanisms, as well as through evolving requirements that determine whether a person entering the nursing profession, and those who continue to practise, demonstrates the high standards to which nurses are held in Canadian society.

CRITICAL THINKING

Discussion Points

1. What are the structure and purpose of the professional nursing body in your province?
2. How does your provincial nursing governing or regulatory body manage complaints against nurses? Suggest ways in which the process might be improved or be made more accountable to nurses and to the public.
3. Are there any other approaches that regulatory bodies can take to better protect the public? What are your perspectives on whether regulatory and professional associations should be combined or separate bodies? Do you see any potential conflict of interest? If so, how can this be remedied?
4. What role should such bodies play in shaping legislation affecting nursing?
5. Critically evaluate the standards of practice of the regulatory body in your province against the standards within the organization where you are presently employed or receiving clinical experience. Evaluate the extent to which these standards assist you in understanding the expectations of you as a nurse.
6. How are the standards of practice in your setting measured? What mechanisms are in place to ensure these standards are maintained? Can you think of ways to improve this process? Do these standards help you reflect on your own performance as a student or as a nurse?

REFERENCES

Statutes

Controlled Drugs and Substances Act, S.C. 1996, c. 19.
Criminal Records Review Act, R.S.B.C. 1996, c. 86 (British Columbia).
Fair Access to Regulated Professions Act, 2006, S.O. 2006, c. 31 (Ontario).
Food and Drugs Act, R.S.C. 1985, c. F-27.
Health Professions Act, R.S.B.C. 1996, c. 183 (British Columbia).
Health Professions Act, R.S.A. 2000, c. H-7 (Alberta).

Health Professions Procedural Code, 1991, S.O. 1991, c. 18., Sch. 2 (Ontario).
Human Rights Code, R.S.B.C. 1996, c. 210 (British Columbia).
Ministry of Health Appeal and Review Boards Act, 1998. S.O. 1998, c. 18, Sch. H. (Ontario).
Nurses Act, R.S.Q. c. I-8 (Quebec).
Nurses Act, S.N.B. 1984, c. 71, as amended (New Brunswick).
Nursing Act, 1991, S.O. 1991, c. 32 (Ontario).
Professional Code, R.S.Q., c. C-26 (Quebec).
The Registered Nurses Act, 1988, S.S. 1988–89, c. R-12.2 (Saskatchewan).
Registered Nurses Act, S.N.S. 2006, c. 21 (Nova Scotia).
Registered Nurses Act, 2008, S.N.L., 2008, c. R-9.1 (Newfoundland).
Registered Nurses Profession Act, R.S.Y. 2002, c. 194 (Yukon).
The Regulated Health Professions Act, C.C.S.M., c. R117 (Manitoba).
Regulated Health Professions Act, R.S.P.E.I. 1988, c R-10.1 (Prince Edward Island).
Regulated Health Professions Act, 1991, S.O. 1991, c. 18 (Ontario).

Regulations

Nursing Act, 1991, O. Reg 275/94 (Ontario).
Nurses (Registered) and Nurse Practitioners Regulation, 284/2008 BC (British Columbia).
Registered Nurses Regulation, Man. Reg. 128/2001.

Regulatory Body Bylaws

Saskatchewan Registered Nurses' Association Bylaws, Bylaw VI (Saskatchewan).

Case Law

College of Nurses of Ontario v. Cecilioni [2008] CanLII 89793 (ON CNO). http://canlii.ca/t/g0k58
CNO v Julie Pouget, 2011.
College of Nurses of Ontario v. Wettlaufer [2017] CanLII 77173 (ON CNO).
Decision on Shahid Shams, CRNM #138111. https://crnm.mb.ca/wp-content/uploads/2022/02/CRNM-138111-Shahid-Shams_Decision.pdf
NANB and David Lloyd Green, *Info Nursing,* p. 25, Volume 38 Issue 3, Fall 2007.
Infirmières et infirmiers (Ordre professionnel des) v. Rocray [2021] QCCDINF 34.
Mans v. Council of Licensed Practical Nurses [1990], 14 C.H.R.R. D/221; aff'd. (1993), 77 B.C.L.R. (2d) 47 (C.A.).
R. v. Cleroux, [2022] ONCJ 188.
Whatcott v. Saskatchewan Association of Licensed Practical Nurses [2008] SKCA 6 (CanLII).
CRNM re Shahid Shams #138111 (2020) https://www.crnm.mb.ca/rns-nps/complaints/discipline-decisions/

Texts and Articles

Aboriginal Nurses Association of Canada. (2009). *Cultural competence and cultural safety in nursing education: A framework for First Nations, Inuit, and Métis nursing: Making it happen: Strengthening First Nations, Inuit and Métis health human resources.* https://www.indigenousnurses.ca/resources/publications/cultural-competence-and-cultural-safety-nursing-education-framework-first
British Columbia College of Nurses & Midwives. (2022a). *Annual requirements.* https://www.bccnm.ca/RN/QA/annual/Pages/Default.aspx

British Columbia College of Nurses & Midwives. (2022b). *Bylaws of the British Columbia College of Nurses and Midwives.* https://www.bccnm.ca/Public/regulation/Bylaws/Pages/Default.aspx

British Columbia College of Nurses & Midwives. (2022c). *How to apply: Applications for initial nurse practitioner registration in British Columbia.* https://www.bccnm.ca/NP/applications_registration/how_to_apply/Pages/Default.aspx

British Columbia College of Nurses & Midwives. (2023). *Delegating tasks to unregulated care providers; practice standard for registered nurses.* https://www.bccnm.ca/RN/PracticeStandards/Pages/delegating.aspx

Bruemmer, R. (2021, October 5). After Echaquan report, Legault repeats there is no systemic racism in Quebec. *Montreal Gazette.*

Canadian Civil Liberties Association. (2014). *False promises: Hidden costs. The case for reframing employment and volunteer police record check practices in Canada.* https://ccla.org/recordchecks/

Canadian Council of Practical Nurse Regulators. (2013). *Standards of practice for licensed practical nurses in Canada.* http://www.clpna.com

Canadian Council of Registered Nurse Regulators. (2018). *Nurse practitioners.* http://www.ccrnr.ca/nurse-practitioners.html

Canadian Council of Practical Nurse Regulators. (2019). *Entry-to-practice competencies for licensed practical nurses.* http://www.ccpnr.ca/resources/

Canadian Nurses Association. (2009). *Position statement: Clinical nurse specialist.*

Canadian Nurses Association. (2015). *Framework for the practice of registered nurses in Canada* (2nd ed). http://www.cna-aiic.ca/CNA/documents/pdf/publications/RN_Framework_Practice_2007_e.pdf

Canadian Nurses Association. (2016). *The nurse practitioner: CNA position.*

CARE Centre for Internationally Educated Nurses. (2018). *Home page.* https://care4nurses.org/

College of Registered Nurses of Alberta. (2023) Scope of Practice. Retrieved from https://www.nurses.ab.ca/protect-the-public/understanding-nursing-regulation/scope-of-practice/

The College of Registered Nurses of Alberta. (2023). Submit a Complaint. Retrieved from https://www.nurses.ab.ca/protect-the-public/complaints/

College of Nurses of Ontario. (2002). *Professional standards for registered nurses and registered practical nurses in Ontario.* http://www.cno.org/docs/prac/41006_ProfStds.pdf

College of Nurses of Ontario. (2014). *RN & RPN practice: The client, the nurse and the environment.*

College of Nurses of Ontario. (2016). *Committees.* https://www.cno.org

College of Nurses of Ontario. (2018). *Addressing complaints: Process guide.* https://www.cno.org

College of Nurses of Ontario. (2020, December). *Nurses supporting public health measures.* https://www.cno.org/en/news/2020/december-2020/nurses-supporting-public-health-measures/

College of Nurses of Ontario. (2022, June). *CNO sets new record for registering internationally educated nurses* [Press release]. https://www.cno.org/en/news/2022/june-2022/cno-new-record-registering-iens/

College of Registered Nurses of Nova Scotia, & College of Licensed Practical Nurses of Nova Scotia. (2013). *Guidelines: Effective utilization of RNs and LPNs in a collaborative practice environment.*

College of Registered Nurses of Manitoba. (2018). *Complaints, discipline and appeals process.* https://www.crnm.mb.ca

College of Registered Nurses of Saskatchewan. (2023). *About the CRNS.* https://www.crns.ca/about-us/

Devitt, P. (2004). Safeguarding children through police checks: A discussion. *Paediatric Nursing, 16*(9), 36–38.

DiCenso, A., Martin-Misener, R., Bryant-Lukosius, D., et al. (2010). Advanced practice nursing in Canada: Overview of a decision support synthesis. *Nursing Leadership, 23,* 15–34.

Guidelines On Advanced Practice Nursing 2020; https://www.icn.ch/resources/publications-andreports? category=_all&topics%5B0%5D=81&year=_all&page=1.

International Council of Nurses. (2018). https://www.icn.ch.

Narrative Research. (2021, February 9). *Canadians place the highest level of trust and confidence in healthcare professionals, including doctors and nurses, followed by a high degree of trust in school teachers and police services. Confidence and trust are significantly lower for provincial governments and federal politicians.* https://narrativeresearch.ca/wp-content/uploads/2021/02/feb9_pressrelease-1.pdf

Nova Scotia College of Nurses. (2021). *NSCN Continuing competence program guide for nurses.* https://cdn1.nscn.ca/sites/default/files/documents/CCP/CCP_Guide_For_Nurses.pdf

Nurses Association of New Brunswick. (2018). *Resources.* http://www.nanb.nb.ca/resources

Ordre des infirmières et infirmiers du Québec. (2022). *Dans la foulée de ses travaux, l'OIIQ reconnaît le racisme systémique envers les Premières Nations et Inuit [In the wake of its work, the OIIQ recognizes systemic racism against First Nations and Inuit]* [Press release]. https://www.oiiq.org/dans-la-foulee-de-ses-travaux-l-oiiq-reconnait-le-racisme-systemique-envers-les-premieres-nations-et-inuits

Registered Nurses, Association of Ontario. (2023). *About RNAO.* https://rnao.ca/about

Registered Psychiatric Nurse Regulators of Canada. (2018). *Registered psychiatric nursing in Canada.* http://www.rpnc.ca/registered-psychiatric-nursing-canada

Truth and Reconciliation Commission of Canada. (2015). *Calls to Action.* https://rcaanc-cirnac.gc.ca/eng/1450124405592/1529106060525

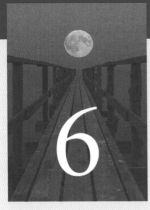

6

INFORMED CONSENT: RIGHTS AND OBLIGATIONS

LEARNING OBJECTIVES

The purpose of this chapter is to enable you to understand:

- The meaning of a valid and informed consent as an ethical/legal concept
- The relationship of ethical principles and individual rights to informed consent
- The various levels of, and approaches to, consent
- The concepts of competence and capacity
- The role of advance directives and substitute decision making
- The concept of proxy or substitute consent
- The advocacy role nurses play in ensuring that informed consent is obtained through an ethical and respectful process
- Challenges with respect to consent for the most vulnerable
- Professional responsibilities for consent in emergency situations
- Consent legislation across the country

INTRODUCTION

In health care, the strongest manifestation of human rights, autonomy and freedom, is evident in the processes associated with **consent**. Through consent, persons are able to exercise their rights to determine what happens to their bodies and what interventions they authorize, including nursing care. Through consent processes, they are able to be in control of their care and make decisions about what is most important for them—decisions based on what they value and what they believe.

In health care, consent happens when a person gives permission to a health care professional to follow through on a proposed plan of care. Over the past century, legal and ethical standards have evolved to ensure that consents are valid and informed. Standards and processes associated with informed consent are intended to ensure that persons are protected from exploitation and harm and are grounded in human rights and in principles of freedom and autonomy. Essentially, health professionals have a duty to inform, and patients have the right to accept, reject, or request alternatives to the options offered to them. Nurses play an advocacy role in ensuring that these rights are protected.

The term **informed consent** speaks to the fact that individuals need information to be able to make a decision and to select the right choice for themselves. The individual requires sufficient and clear information to be able to comprehend and evaluate the offered choices and alternatives. A valid informed consent involves distinct processes. First, the person must be capable of making the decision; second, the information required to make that decision must be provided; and third, the person must be assured that the choice is totally voluntary. The process must be free of deceit and coercion.

The right to self-determination is acknowledged through a valid informed consent process, founded on ethical standards, policies, guidelines, legislation, and rules. The historical evolution of informed consent, its ethical underpinnings, and the legal framework for consent will be described. Also, the ethical dimensions associated with the process of obtaining consent will be explored, especially as they relate to nursing.

The rights of patients extend to personal autonomy and the right to be informed of all risks material to a particular intervention, including the risks, both real and probable, in forgoing such a procedure. (A material risk is one that a reasonable person would wish to know in deciding whether to consent to or forgo a given procedure.) These rights include the rights of patients not to be subjected to any treatment to which they have not given free and informed consent, if mentally capable, and the moral right to be treated with respect, dignity, and courtesy throughout the process.

HISTORICAL PERSPECTIVES: THE EVOLUTION OF INFORMED CONSENT

In earlier chapters, the concept of paternalism, based on an interpretation of beneficence—that is, health care professionals thinking that they know what is best for their patients—was described. In the past, this way of thinking led to physicians and nurses influencing or directing patients toward what they thought was in the best interests of patients. This would have led, for example, to only one option being proposed to a patient—the one favoured by the health professional. Frequently, risks were minimized to protect patients from "needless" worry.

Less altruistic approaches were used in research, leading to serious abuse. In some settings, the focus on scientific inquiry superseded concerns about the rights and welfare of human subjects and led to serious offences, as occurred in Nazi Germany. In the evolution of informed consent in research and in the clinical environment, the recommendations resulting from the Nuremberg Trials, held after World War II, played an instrumental role. The discovery of Nazi atrocities related to research led to the development of the Nuremberg Code (1947), a guide for the ethical undertaking of research involving human subjects (Annas & Grodin, 2008). Prior to the Nuremberg Code, there was no generally accepted code of conduct governing the ethical aspects of human research. This code focused on informed consent, clarified the requirements related to capacity, information, voluntariness, and the person's right to withdraw from a study at any time.

Following the establishment of the Nuremberg Code, the Declaration of Helsinki, introduced in 1964,

was the first effort by the international medical research community to regulate research on human subjects (Ashcroft, 2008). To remain current, the Declaration has been revised several times.

History reveals that Canada has not been immune to abuses associated with consent. Sadly, a pattern and culture of coercion with respect to consent was prevalent in Indigenous communities throughout the nineteenth and twentieth centuries that contributes to their ongoing distrust of the health care system. Beyond the experience of paternalism in health care at the time, there appeared to be a system-wide approach to consent (or lack thereof) with Indigenous people that aligned with the overall strategy of control, regulation, and assimilation associated with colonization. In 1945, Percy Moore, acting director of the Indian Health Service at the time, explicitly noted, "we certainly do not feel that our program should be left to the whim of an Indian, as to whether he will accept treatment" (Lux, 2016, p. 95).

One example of this approach is evident with respect to the management of tuberculosis (TB) in Indigenous communities. In spite of emerging evidence that led to a more cautious approach to surveillance across Canada, mass annual X-rays and bacille Calmette-Guérin (BCG) vaccinations continued in Indigenous communities. It was "rationalized" that in spite of the risks of adverse reactions from BCG vaccinations and high radiation exposure, the risk of TB was greater. Therefore, an aggressive surveillance program was considered defensible to control TB in Indigenous communities and to protect the broader, non-Indigenous Canadian public.

When it came time for these annual assessments, teams of doctors accompanied by Indian agents and police would descend upon Indigenous communities. Though such assessments were generally voluntary in other Canadian communities, "reserve" communities were denied the same autonomy, and treaty annuity payments were withheld until every family member consented (Lux, 2016). This strategy was launched in the early 1940s and continued through to the late 1960s (Lux, 2016).

Further, there are numerous reports that research, medical experimentation, and pioneering treatments were conducted on patients in Indian hospitals and residential schools without adequate consent processes (Lux, 2016; Mosby, 2013). This continued to be a pattern even after the Nuremberg Code was introduced.

In Canada, a joint policy statement—the *Tri-Council Policy Statement: Ethical Conduct for Research Involving Humans* (TCPS2)—was written by Canada's three federal research agencies: the Canadian Institutes of Health Research (CIHR), the Natural Sciences and Engineering Research Council of Canada (NSERC), and the Social Sciences and Humanities Research Council of Canada (SSHRC) (CIHR et al., 2022). The ethical principles, standards, and values contained in that statement guide Health Canada's Research Ethics Board (REB) and are broadly accepted by the research community across the country and by research ethics boards (Health Canada–Public Health Agency of Canada & Research Ethics Board, 2023). The statement affirms, based on respect for the principle of autonomy, the capable person's right to make free, informed decisions through consent. (CIHR et al., 2022). This work was updated to reflect evolving issues related to research and clinical trials:

An important mechanism for respecting participants' autonomy in research is the requirement to seek their free, informed and ongoing consent. This requirement reflects the commitment that participation in research, including participation through the use of one's data or biological materials, should be a matter of choice and that, to be meaningful, the choice must be informed. An informed choice is one that is based on as complete an understanding as is reasonably possible of the purpose of the research, what it entails, and its foreseeable risks and potential benefits, both to the participant and to others. Respect for Persons also includes a commitment to accountability and transparency in the ethical conduct of research (CIHR at al., 2022, p. 6)

The clinical context, and common law approaches to informed consent, which are grounded in case law, evolved and were subsequently refined and codified in legislation. As part of this legislative process, administrative tribunals and procedures were developed to facilitate access to resolution of issues of consent for health care professionals and the capacity to give consent for patients.

Case Scenario 6.1 highlights the complex issues and challenges associated with consent.

CASE SCENARIO 6.1

WHOSE DECISION?

A 75-year-old widow lives alone in a suburban bungalow that she and her late husband owned for 30 years. Over the past few years, some of her close friends have died. She has two adult children who live in a distant city. For the past 6 or 7 months, her general health has been declining. She has lost weight, has been experiencing episodes of fatigue, and finds it difficult to leave home to go about her daily activities.

One day, the area's postal worker notices that her mail has been left uncollected for a few days, and when he knocks on the door, there is no response. Concerned, the postal worker, who knows this woman's daily routine and is always informed when she plans to go out of town, calls the police, who discover her lying semiconscious on the kitchen floor.

She is rushed to the emergency department, where the attending physician makes a preliminary diagnosis of gastrointestinal bleeding and, because it is an emergency and she is nonresponsive, orders some preliminary tests and blood transfusions. A few days later, she is alert and apparently competent, but the nurses caring for her have noticed that she occasionally seems confused by her surroundings.

The physician informs her that there is an urgent need for further tests and suggests an endoscopy and colonoscopy. She becomes agitated and upset, fearing that the doctors will discover cancer and that she will soon die. Consequently, she refuses to authorize the tests. The members of the team know that any number of easily treatable factors could be causing the bleeding, and they are concerned that this course of action is not in her best interests. Some nurses question whether, in her present state of mind, she is capable of making such a decision.

The team wants to involve her children, but she refuses to give any contact information. She does not want her family involved; she has always been able to take care of herself and does not wish to worry her children.

Continued on following page

CASE SCENARIO 6.1 *(Continued)*

Over the next few days, the team finds evidence that the bleeding is recurring. Something must be done soon, or she will die.

Issues

1. Does this person have the mental (and hence legal) capacity to make the decision to accept or refuse treatment? How would capacity be determined?
2. Has she been given an adequate amount of time to make an informed and meaningful decision?
3. Can the nurses or other team members legally and ethically attempt to contact and disclose information to her children?
4. What are the competing ethical interests in this situation, and how can they be resolved?
5. Would the team be able proceed with further investigation and intervention on the assumption that she is not capable of giving or withholding consent?

Discussion

If this woman is deemed capable, then the health care team cannot legally proceed without her consent.

Although the nurses and physicians are genuinely motivated by good intentions and have her best interests in mind, they are not free to exercise their own judgement and proceed on their own authority. If the team is concerned about her competence, the team would be authorized to proceed only if she was deemed incapable through a more thorough capacity assessment. The legal options available to the team are described later.

As a first step, the team should ensure that a clear, compassionate approach to informed consent is undertaken. This would include listening to her concerns, ensuring that she understands the risks and benefits of agreeing or refusing the procedure. A compassionate, caring approach would include giving her time to reflect on her situation and the options presented to her. The team needs to respond to her questions and clarify any misconceptions. Nurses play a role in exploring with patients the factors that might motivate their decisions (e.g., fear, past experiences, misconceptions).

Reflect on this story as the ethical and legal considerations are explored throughout this chapter.

ETHICAL FOUNDATIONS OF CONSENT

As discussed in Chapter 2, autonomy, a significant ethical principle, was highlighted by Beauchamp and Childress in their book *Principles of Biomedical Ethics.* They described personal autonomy as the notion of self-governance by the individual, promoting "personal rule of the self while remaining free from both controlling interferences by others and personal limitations such as inadequate understanding, that prevent meaningful choice" (Beauchamp & Childress, 1989, p. 68).

The principle of autonomy is based on respect for the person's individual liberty and the right to self-determination, all grounded in ethical theory, including Kantian ethics and utilitarianism.

However, autonomy is limited when one has limited capacity or when its exercise causes harm to oneself or others. When harm to others is sufficiently grave, the principle of autonomy is overridden. In some cases, the team may not be able to fully respect autonomous

choices if they are considered unreasonable, futile, or illegal, or if they conflict with the team's values and beliefs. For example, a patient with metastatic cancer requesting bone marrow transplantation after aggressive chemotherapy has failed could be considered to be making an unreasonable request. Carrying out such a request would cause moral distress in the team members because they know it would be futile and would cause needless pain and suffering for the patient.

Questions related to autonomy, coercion, and the consequences of refusing consent were brought to the forefront during the COVID-19 pandemic with the debate over vaccine mandates. Arguments against mandates focused on persons' rights to personal liberty, grounded in autonomy, to refuse vaccination. Others, including members of the Association of Bioethics Program Directors, with members across Canada and the United States, argued that "coercion" was morally justified in these unusual circumstances (Wynia et al., 2021). They noted that rights are limited when there is the risk of harm to others. They argued that early public health restrictions to freedom were justified and that the imposition of vaccine mandates was appropriate when other strategies to manage hesitancy (such as education and incentives) proved inadequate, except in cases of justified medical exemption.

Early in the pandemic, the World Health Organization (WHO) produced a policy brief on the ethical considerations associated with vaccine mandates (WHO, 2019). The WHO suggested that a vaccine mandate may be appropriate in certain contexts and offered six ethical considerations to help guide decision makers:

1. Is the mandate necessary and proportionate to the desired societal or organizational goals? Are there less extreme actions that could have the same effect? How long does the mandate need to be in place? Is the mandate less disruptive than the alternatives?
2. Has the vaccine been proven safe? A vaccine that has not been proven to be safer than not being vaccinated cannot ethically be mandated. Vaccinated persons who are harmed by the vaccine must be automatically compensated.
3. Will the vaccine achieve the desired goal? If the goal is to reduce the burden on the health care system, does the vaccine keep patients out of hospital? If the goal is to stop the spread of the illness, does it reduce infection and transmission?
4. Is the proposed distribution and supply of the vaccine just? Is there enough vaccine that it can be given to everyone, and does the proposed implementation address the circumstances of historically disadvantaged groups through outreach, transparency, and communication?
5. Will the mandate support the public trust in the scientific community and vaccination generally? Public trust can be damaged by a poorly implemented vaccine mandate or by a failure to impose a mandate when it is clearly required and within the power of the authority. Does the mandate take into account the need to work with marginalized and disaffected groups to ensure that the mandate is not seen as targeting these groups?
6. Has the ethical process of decision making behind the mandate been transparent? Will emerging evidence from the mandate be monitored to ensure that the mandate is revised or altered to reflect the evidence?

In summary, recommended in all contexts, these ethical considerations need to be evaluated, and mandates should only be used where they are ethically supportable. This approach makes clear that there are numerous ethical concerns beyond personal autonomy that influence these decisions.

In Canada, mandates were also used to encourage vaccination. As these mandates were introduced, persons had the option to refuse vaccinations, but with this refusal came consequences, including exclusion from certain public spaces and limited travel options, such as exclusion from planes or trains. For those employed in settings of higher risk, such as hospitals and police services, these consequences included suspension without pay and loss of employment. For health care professionals, a higher duty to promote the well-being of patients and minimize harm was also a factor in these deliberations (Olick et al., 2021). Issues associated with public health restrictions and vaccine mandates will be explored further in Chapters 10 and 11, where the rights of patients and nurses will be discussed.

Codes of Ethics

As discussed in Chapter 3, the importance of autonomy and informed consent has been made explicit in nursing codes of ethics. For example, the *Code of Ethics for Registered Nurses* of the Canadian Nurses Association (CNA, 2017) mandates nurses to respect and promote the autonomy of patients—the foundation of informed consent. This code clarifies nurses' responsibilities to safeguard the autonomy and the rights of persons to self-determination by supporting them in expressing their values and health needs and by ensuring that they have the right information, guidance, freedom, and support to make informed choices. Included in this code are specific nursing responsibilities associated with informed consent; these responsibilities include respecting the wishes of a capable person who does not want detailed information, who wants to engage family and community in decision making, and who adopts lifestyles or health treatment plans that the nurse and the team do not support. Furthermore, nurses are required to protect the rights of those who are not capable, ensuring that they are engaged in decision making as much as they are able. Nurses are also cautioned to be aware of the power differential between them and their patients and to ensure that this power is not abused.

Although informed consent is grounded in the principle of autonomy and is based on individual rights and freedoms, other ethical perspectives, such as narrative ethics and relationship and caring ethics, influence how consent is obtained, and this will be discussed later.

VARYING DIMENSIONS OF CONSENT

There are various levels of consent, depending on the nature and complexity of the decision to be made. Whitney et al. (2004) proposed a model that describes consent on a continuum from low risk to high risk and from high certainty to low certainty.

Consent is more straightforward, or simpler, when the interventions proposed are of low risk and have a high certainty of success. Frequently, in situations of a simple consent, a straightforward explanation is sufficient. In this context, consent is usually implied through action or expressed verbally. These circumstances occur frequently with respect to consent for many nursing actions, such as taking vital signs or changing a dressing. In these instances, the actions of persons allowing these interventions to occur implies consent, for example, when patients roll up their sleeve for a blood pressure reading. Examples of interventions of somewhat higher risk would include insertion of a catheter or establishment of an intravenous line. Usually, a written consent form is not obtained in such circumstances; however, these interventions require a more detailed explanation, including why they are necessary and the risks involved, such as the possibility of discomfort, infection, and so on. This discussion and the patient's agreement or refusal to have the procedure should be documented in the record. Other examples include the filling of prescriptions. Sometimes, a physician or nurse practitioner may simply alter the dosage of long-standing medications and explain this to the patient. Consent is implied when that person goes to the pharmacy to have the prescription filled. However, in the situation where a person is given the option of diet versus medication to manage cholesterol levels, a deeper discussion is required. This conversation would include the risks,

benefits, and current evidence for each option. The explicit authorization of one choice or the other would also be necessary, and this, again, should be documented in the health record (Whitney et al., 2004).

Complex nursing situations offer options that pose varying degrees of risk. Consider a patient with end-stage cancer, where the cancer has metastasized to the patient's bones, causing severe pain. The standard of care is to turn patients every 2 hours to prevent pressure sores and to minimize the likelihood of pneumonia and other complications. However, turning causes this patient so much pain that additional sedation is required, and this results in extended periods of drowsiness. Should the nurses give this patient the choice of being turned or not? Are other treatment alternatives available? For example, special mattresses can be used to protect skin integrity, gentle passive exercise and massage can improve blood flow, and frequent chest physiotherapy can minimize the risk of pneumonia. Taking on an advocacy role, the nurse should engage in a conversation with the patient to explore the options available and the risks and benefits associated with each. In this circumstance, the conversation might include how these risks can be mitigated. The nurse would support the patient in making the choice that aligns with this person's needs, values, and preferences, knowing that the care plan can be altered. Again, the discussion and the agreed-upon care should be documented in the patient's record.

Higher-risk areas of consent obviously include invasive procedures, such as surgery or image-guided procedures. These interventions require a more comprehensive consent process, with the person being provided the necessary information to authorize or decline the options presented. Many of these are straightforward because the only reasonable choice is to agree or not agree. For example, angioplasty and stent insertions have a high certainty of success. It makes more sense to take that approach first before moving to higher-risk cardiac surgery. Also, consider the patient with diabetes and vascular neuropathy who has developed gangrene in his toes. There is little option but to amputate the toes, and the risks and benefits are clear. It is not always inappropriate to guide the patient toward a decision, especially when only one option makes sense or if there is greater certainty of a positive outcome, while still respecting the person's rights to choose.

The consent process becomes more complex when there is less certainty about the outcome of an option, compared with the situation where the evidence overwhelmingly points to one option over others. Consider an 80-year-old person newly diagnosed with acute lymphocytic leukemia, for which three treatment options are available. The first option is aggressive chemotherapy requiring a 6-week hospitalization with many risks, including the possibility of death, but this option has a 50% chance of remission and a prognosis of about 3 to 5 years' survival. The second option is less invasive chemotherapy administered at home, with fewer complications and, perhaps, a better quality of life in the short term, but it has a limited prognosis of 1 to 2 years' survival. The third option is no chemotherapy, but management of symptoms with blood and plasma transfusions, delivered in an ambulatory setting and a prognosis of 3 to 6 months' survival. Clearly, each of these options comes with serious risks, side effects, and implications for quality of life. The consent process would take longer. This conversation would require a deeper exploration of the options and more time for the patient to reflect on them. The person would perhaps want to consult with friends and family. Many factors would be involved in making this decision, including the person's quality of life, values, and emotional and social needs.

Emergency situations pose other challenges with regard to consent, especially when there is no advance directive and when the next of kin or substitute decision maker is not readily available. When there is no other information available to the team members, they are morally and legally expected to act in the patient's best interests and do what a person would reasonably do in that circumstance.

A VALID CONSENT: AUTONOMOUS AUTHORIZATION

Consent may be given in writing, verbally, or simply implied (e.g., by holding out an arm to have blood drawn); however, for consent to be valid, it must be based on the relevant information required by the patient to make that choice. Consent must be free from coercion, and it must be made by someone capable of making that level of decision. The patient, to the extent that they are able, is an active participant in what

should be a shared decision-making process that leads to consent or refusal. Even if consent is given, it can be withdrawn at any time.

Capacity to Consent

As argued by Beauchamp and Childress (1989), to be truly autonomous and hence able to make a valid informed consent, the person must be capable of doing so. A person's capacity to consent depends on a number of factors, including the nature of the decision. For example, persons with dementia may not be capable of consenting to major surgery, but through their actions, they can consent to such interventions as physiotherapy exercises.

Because persons may have varying degrees of dementia, some may be able to agree to a particular intervention. For example, in some instances, dementia may cause a person to have severe short-term memory loss yet be able to comprehend and understand conversations in the moment. Thus, even though a substitute decision maker or family member may be required to consent on the patient's behalf to surgery, for example, the conversation with the person, who may or may not assent, should still occur. Although others would ultimately give the consent, the response by the person in the moment should be considered, especially if the person's comprehension can reasonably be determined. It is helpful to think of autonomy not as an intangible principle or as something that is entirely lost if a right to give informed consent cannot be upheld but, rather, as a matter of the degree to which it is respected and valued.

To be capable of giving valid consent, a person must be able to understand the information provided, retain it—that is, be able to repeat what was heard—and weigh the options presented. This is usually evident in the questions that are asked, the extent of deliberation, and the communication of concerns. Assessing for capacity may be a complex process, and it may take time. In many settings, there are resources available to assess for capacity if it is beyond the scope or expertise of the team members. Even health care settings in remote areas of the country have access via teleconferencing to guidance in challenging circumstances. In the context where someone is deemed incapable, the team needs to identify whether the person has an advance directive, a legal next of kin, or a substitute decision maker, or, in the case of children, parents or a court-appointed guardian. When none of the above is available, the team needs to consider whether there is time to pursue legal guardianship. Depending on the urgency of the situation, the team may be required to act on the basis of the person's best interests. The complexities related to children and emergency situations are discussed later. In circumstances where others are consenting on behalf of an incapable person, the team must be reassured that they are acting in the person's best interests, even when it is parents acting on behalf of their children. There are legal options available to the team if they have concerns about the welfare of an incapable person. These pathways are discussed in detail later in the chapter.

Even when there is no formal determination of incapacity, nurses and other team members should be conscious of the fact that the controlling, bureaucratic nature of the health care environment, as well as the nature of illness, has the potential to influence anyone's ability to think clearly and to make complex decisions. A person in pain or in an impaired physical or emotional state may not be able to make fully deliberative or meaningful decisions. Nurses must be aware of the multiple factors—social, cultural, or otherwise—that influence patients in these circumstances. Previous emotional trauma, fear, or anxiety can be a factor, as was the case in Case Scenario 2.9. Recall that the resident believed that they had followed the rules of informed consent; however, they had failed, from an ethical perspective, to engage in a meaningful conversation to understand M. M.'s fears and previous negative experience with the same procedure. Also, consider the 75-year-old widow in Case Scenario 6.1 and the fact that the absence of family and friends to support her and her apparent fear and anxiety may be influencing her decision. In such instances, care must be taken by the team to support patients, listen, and, when possible, give them the time to process the current circumstances. Even a health care professional who becomes a patient or has a family member who is ill may lose perspective when dealing with a highly emotionally charged situation.

Consider the person who presents at the emergency department with extreme abdominal pain and is told that they have colon cancer. The person would not be in a position to deliberate on the treatment options available to them in the first instance until they have understood and processed this news. Unless an emergency, this is a process that takes time. Informed consent should be viewed as an ongoing journey, rather than as a discrete or one-time choice that takes place in a given moment of time (Corrigan, 2003).

Information Sharing

For informed consent to be valid, an individual must have adequate and reasonable knowledge to explore and examine all available options relevant to the health care decision to be made. Often, this specialized knowledge is beyond the scope of most patients, so they must rely on health care professionals to present them with the information they need. Many patients, especially those with chronic conditions, are extremely knowledgeable about their illness and, in some circumstances, more so than even their health care provider. However, the higher the risk of the decision and the greater the complexity and uncertainty of the options, the more they rely on the opinion and expertise of health care professionals to provide them with the information and guidance they need to make these difficult decisions.

Informed consent is a shared process between the health care professional or team and the patient. Through the process of information sharing, the individual professional, or the team must ensure full disclosure and understanding on the part of the patient. This includes complete, comprehensive disclosure of all information about the nature of the proposed intervention or treatment and why it is necessary, the procedures involved, and other alternatives and options available (including doing nothing), as well as the consequences, risks, and benefits of each. Risks specific to that person must also be made clear. For example, consider the rare complication of radiation-induced brachial plexopathy resulting from radiation to the chest (Warade et al., 2019). This complication may manifest as weakness of or inability to use the muscles in the hand, arm, or shoulder. Although this is a rare complication, its consequences would have serious implications. Take, for example, a female artist who is exploring options for the treatment of her breast cancer. This complication is a risk that she might consider when making the decision whether or not to agree to radiation, especially if the evidence demonstrating its efficacy is uncertain.

In all circumstances, but more so when the decision to be made is of a higher risk and complexity, it is of importance how consent is obtained and how the conversation unfolds. Compassion and respect for the dignity of the person and concern for their well-being must always be at the forefront of the conversation, ensuring, as much as possible, that the patient has control of the process. It is important to appreciate that some people may need more time than others to consider the information they have received and to reflect on their choices. In some circumstances, the person is receiving difficult news for the first time and may need to assimilate this information. More than one session or conversation may be required.

Ideally, the setting of the conversation is suitable in that it allows for as much privacy, comfort, and equality for the person as is possible. For example, the perceived imbalance of power may be mitigated when both patient and provider are sitting and facing each other at eye level. This is especially important when interacting with children and persons requiring ability aids. It is the individual's call as to whether family or friends should be involved, but if the news is difficult, the team should encourage the patient to invite others to provide support, but, again, only if the person chooses to do so. Family members can also help interpret or clarify the information being presented and remind the patient of the details later.

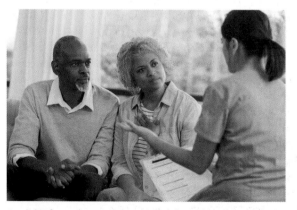

A valid informed consent is achieved through a shared process where the person is provided with the knowledge and support they need to decide on the best course of action. *Source: istockphoto.com/asiseeit.*

The team or the individual health care professional should clarify that this is a shared decision and ask about the person's preferences regarding the extent of their involvement and how best to share information. For example, some people may prefer to be given as little information as possible, whereas others may want to know every detail available. It is argued that it does not make sense to disclose every conceivable harm or risk that has not been proven. The team must also consider when it is not in a person's best interests to be burdened with every fact when it might not be material to their circumstance (Kocarnik, 2014).

The person might prefer a verbal discussion, written/printed information, use of pictures or diagrams, or access to online resources and videos endorsed by the team. The same approaches and materials may not apply to all patients. The materials should be consistent but suited to patients with different levels of sophistication and different learning styles. The team must also accept the rights of patients to defer the decision to others, such as family members. In some cultures, patients may prefer to defer to a community or spiritual leader. A member of an Indigenous community may prefer to have a community Elder or healer participate. Some persons may ultimately hand over the decision making to the physician or the team, seemingly against the principle of autonomy. However, this does respect this principle and the patient's right to self-determination because the person is making the choice to hand over the decision making to others. The team, however, must ensure that this is done freely and not through coercion or any imbalance of power.

The team must also be sensitive to cultural and language issues. Challenges with language may affect comprehension, and the person's values may influence their reactions and choices. Where there are language challenges, it is important to ensure that a qualified interpreter is engaged. In most settings, there is access to interpreters through teleconferencing, even in remote areas. A family member or friend should be used as a last resort as a translator because professional interpreters can better communicate the true meaning of the health care professional's message and ensure that the patient fully understands the circumstances and options for treatment. Interpreters have special skills related to the process and are comfortable with health care terminology. Without an interpreter, it is also challenging for the team to evaluate whether the family member is acting in the person's best interests.

The *Report of the Aboriginal Justice Inquiry of Manitoba* documented that qualified translators were frequently not available within the court system for Indigenous accused (Aboriginal Justice Implementation Commission, 1999). In Iqaluit, an investigation in 2012–2013 documented that similar language issues had been a source of concern for many years in the area's only regional hospital. Despite a need for services in Nunavut's official languages of English, Inuktitut, and French, most services were only available in English. The lack of professional interpreters was a major factor in problems with care and patient satisfaction. Language communication problems were cited as a persistent issue in Indigenous health delivery (Office of the Languages Commissioner of Nunavut, 2015).

The team must also be sensitive to patients with a hearing impairment. In this circumstance, a qualified hearing interpreter and/or a deaf interpreter would, with the patient's consent, facilitate the process of consent.

Conversations related to consent should be free of jargon, simple language should be used, and there should be ample opportunity for questions and clarification.

The team must confirm the person's understanding of the information and options presented and the choice made. The discussion may need to be repeated several times for some people to fully comprehend the choices available to them. It is also appropriate to communicate at the level of simplicity or sophistication the person is familiar with. The team may ask probing questions to ensure comprehension of what is being communicated. Questions from the person and their family, as appropriate, should also be encouraged.

At the conclusion of the discussion, there should be a summary of the discussion and the risks and benefits of the choice made. Although a written consent form is signed, the person should be reassured that it is not final and that they can withdraw consent at any time. Beyond this, the process should involve the use of appropriate moral reasoning, clear communication, comprehensive ongoing assessment of the process, respect, and empathy.

As mentioned previously, persons unable to give a valid consent also have the right to information. When an incapable person is alert and responsive, such as a person with dementia, the treatment or procedure can be explained with the use of visual aids, as appropriate. With young children, nurses and (in some settings) child life specialists engage in play to help a young child understand what is happening. For example, dolls can be used to illustrate the insertion of an intravenous injection or a surgical procedure. The approach would be appropriate to the age and stage of development of the child.

It is the obligation of the health care professional who is proposing treatment to share the relevant information needed to enable the patient to make an informed decision. Sometimes, if a patient makes a decision that does not seem reasonable or may cause moral distress within the team, it might be necessary to determine, through a more comprehensive capacity assessment, as in Case Scenario 6.1, whether there is a full appreciation of the implications of the decision. Consider the situation of an 11-year-old Indigenous girl, who was receiving chemotherapy for high-risk acute lymphoblastic leukemia (ALL) (discussed later in this chapter and in Chapter 10). Part of the treatment protocol had been completed when her mother withdrew her consent and indicated that she preferred to follow traditional health practices. The team did not believe that this choice was in the best interests of the child because the cure rate with this chemotherapy protocol was high, and without it, there was a high likelihood of death. In this case, the team sought assistance from the Children's Aid Society (CAS).

Voluntariness

As discussed, the culture of the health care environment and the person's illness and emotions can influence the consent process, including whether it can always be totally voluntary (Mueller, 1997). Many patients assume that physicians, nurses, and other members of the team are acting in their best interests and may be inclined to follow through on a proposed option without consideration of other choices. Some patients might be inclined to ask the team to do what the team thinks is best and may be influenced by a desire to please, especially when there is a perceived imbalance of power. It is important for the team to be aware that the dependent relationship the patient may have with the health care team may influence their decision.

It is also important to understand that the person may have had many contacts with health care, and these experiences may affect their response, especially if in previous encounters the team was more controlling of the plan. Lack of experience with health care may also be a factor because the process may be intimidating.

One strategy to ensure that consent is freely given includes how the conversation is undertaken. It is important to reinforce to the person that although this is a shared process, ultimately, the choice is theirs to make. The approach taken by the team can mitigate the risk of a perceived power imbalance. For example, the team member, as mentioned previously, should position themselves at the same level as the patient, display body language that communicates empathy and concern, maintain eye contact, and, most importantly, listen. The person should be reassured that they have time to reflect on their decision, be encouraged to discuss the issue with family and friends again, and be informed that consent can be withdrawn at any time.

In summary, competent people have the right to refuse consent to treatment, even if that treatment is in their best interests. In some situations, nurses may face a conflict between respect for the individual's wishes and their obligation to help their patients and protect them from harm. But it is the responsibility of nurses to support patients through such decisions and to respect their choices. It is also the nurse's responsibility to ensure that patients have the information required to make such choices as well as sufficient time to reflect on the alternatives available. Whether or not the nurse is part of an informed consent process, the nurse is obligated to advocate for the patient if the patient has not been duly informed or if the patient's wishes are not being respected.

NAVIGATING THE MORAL JOURNEY TO CONSENT

Clearly, respect for a person's autonomy and ensuring a valid informed consent involves more than a signature on a consent form. It is a process where a patient and the caregiver discuss a problem, exchange ideas, and choose an intervention together. At the core of informed consent is a conversation that respects the dignity of people at varying stages of health and illness and varying degrees of vulnerability. It is an ethical process that considers cultural perspectives and the values and beliefs of others.

Fairness and justice necessitate an equitable caregiver–patient relationship based on trust and mutual respect. As with the resident in Case Scenario 2.9, a caregiver cannot assume that once information relevant to treatment is made available and the patient is deemed capable of making treatment decisions, the health care professional has met their duty and moral obligations. It is problematic if the caregiver focuses only on the rules and legal parameters without ensuring that moral and ethical obligations to the person are met.

When models or approaches to informed consent assume that when presented with adequate information and given time to assess it, autonomous individuals will make mindful and sensible decisions, they ignore other considerations, such as the principles of beneficence and nonmaleficence, and other moral concepts, such as caring, therapeutic relationships, and the importance of the person's story. An emphasis on autonomy alone can reduce the significance of these important factors, especially when the cultural context, the process by which consent is obtained, and the role of relationships important to the patient, such as family, are discounted. It is important to gain a deeper and more meaningful understanding of the context, the relationships involved, and the social aspects of the consent process (Sugarman et al., 1999, p. 2).

A moral approach to informed consent empowers that person and is an important element of patient-centred care. Respect for persons demands that there be a meaningful and thoughtful process, not just a bureaucratic process or what has been called a *logical model of decision making,* intended only to ensure a person's autonomous authorization of the agreement regarding care (Corrigan, 2003).

The ethical theories discussed in Chapter 2 come into play here when it comes to the process that nurses and other health care professionals engage in with patients when seeking consent.

Principlism, with a focus on autonomy, has dominated the approach to informed consent, but other considerations that enrich an understanding of the moral nature of informed consent include narrative ethics, caring ethics, and relationship ethics. Consideration of these approaches, as well as the principles involved, can enhance the morally challenging decision-making process. Complementary approaches that accentuate the relational and communicative aspects of moral situations help explain ethical decisions and ultimately ensure satisfaction and comfort with the chosen option (McCarthy, 2003).

The narrative is not only an important form of communication and relationship building, but also a means of understanding the moral values and beliefs of a person and what matters most in the specific context of making an informed choice; it recognizes the uniqueness of that person's story, thus mitigating the temptation to generalize (McCarthy, 2003). Also, being present and listening to the individual's story builds empathy (Charon, 2001).

Caring ethics fosters active listening and encourages sensitivity and awareness of the person's emotional and physiological responses to the situation. A caring approach fosters empathy and compassion for the circumstance the person is facing (Halpern, 2014). For example, in Case Scenario 2.9, this approach would have given the nurse and the team insights into and clues regarding a traumatic reenactment of the patient's previous experience—essentially, what is at the heart of the person's reaction. This is also an important consideration with the woman described in Case Scenario 6.1. By engaging in a conversation with the patient, the team could uncover her story. What is at the core of her fear that she may have cancer? Perhaps if encouraged, she would share her personal experiences with friends that led her to believe that this likely would be the result of the proposed tests. By listening and demonstrating interest and concern, the nurse in the situation might ask her to share stories about her children. Perhaps in doing so, the patient might come to understand that she is not a burden on them as she thinks. It is also important for the team to consider and reflect on how emotions can influence a response or a decision.

Relationship ethics ensures a therapeutic connection built on trust. This approach recognizes that there is a correct time and a correct way to have a conversation. Effective communication conveys empathy, curiosity, and active listening; builds the relationship; and

establishes trust (Roter et al., 2006). The consent process has a profound influence on the development of trusting therapeutic relationships between the patient and the caregiver. It is a giving and receiving process that ensures reflection and a shared understanding of the person's perspectives and concerns.

Table 6.1 summarizes the responsibilities of nurses and provides guidance for an ethical approach to informed consent.

THE LEGAL FRAMEWORK FOR INFORMED CONSENT

A person has both legal rights regarding consent and moral rights to respect, dignity, courtesy, and so on. Some of these rights are enshrined in legislation and, if not respected, may be enforced through litigation. See for example, the *Health Care Consent Act, 1996*, as well as the *Personal Health Information Protection Act, 2004*. Moral rights may be implied in the law; for example, the medical clinic and the staff of that clinic enter a contract with the patient to treat the patient, and obligations of courtesy, respect, and privacy are implied in that relationship. In practice, health care professionals, including nurses, and, more particularly, the agencies that employ them, have comprehensive procedures in place to ensure that consent is properly obtained and documented. These procedures are often spelled out in the legislation, and health care agencies and professional colleges then interpret and apply the steps that need to be taken to ensure suitable documentation of consent.

As described, the ethical principle of autonomy supports the capable and competent person's right to determine and act independently. However, as discussed earlier, autonomy can be meaningful only when persons are given access to full and complete information as to their condition, the risks that the condition poses, and the benefits and drawbacks of any proposed treatment. From a legal perspective, the risks, material facts, and alternatives, including the consequences of nontreatment, must be explained to the competent patient using easily understood terminology.

If the patient is ill informed or is misled by the information provided, any consent given is, in law, no consent at all. Conceivably, the patient may have

TABLE 6.1

A Nurse's Guide to Informed Consent

- Confirm that the person is capable of giving consent.
- Ensure, when possible, that the environment is suitable to the discussion and enhances the nature of the conversation. Take every measure to promote comfort and safeguard privacy, confidentiality, and equality. For example, the perceived balance of power may be mitigated when both patient and provider are facing each other at eye level.
- Appreciate that some people may need more time than others to consider the information they have received and to reflect on their choices. In some circumstances, the person is receiving difficult news for the first time and may need to assimilate this information. More than one session or conversation may be required.
- Ensure that the person understands the information and options presented. The discussion may need to be repeated several times for some people to fully comprehend the choices available to them. It is also appropriate to communicate in simple terms but to also accommodate to the level of sophistication and experience of the person. This might include a person with a long-standing chronic illness or who works within the health care field. The team should ask probing questions to ensure comprehension of what is being communicated. They must also encourage questions from the person and family, as appropriate, and ask them to summarize what they have heard.
- Understand that the person may have had many experiences with health care, or this may be the first. Past experience, or lack thereof, may affect responses.
- Supplement verbal information with written material, web-based education, videos, pictures, and so on. This is especially important when the patient is a child; nurses must also consider the stages of child development.
- Give the person a choice as to whether to have a friend or family member present not only to provide support but also to help interpret or clarify the information being presented.
- Be sensitive to cultural and language issues and the influence these may have not only on comprehension but also on how the patient's values may influence their reactions and choices. Professional health care interpreters may be required. They can communicate the true meaning of the health care professional's message and ensure that the patient fully understands their condition and options for treatment.
- Be an active listener and be aware of the patient's emotional and physiological responses to their situation.
- Build a relationship of trust by engaging in the person's story and communicating empathy and compassion.
- Ensure the person understands that although this is a shared process, the decision is ultimately their own and that it can be changed at any time.

decided differently if informed fully and properly. The patient has the right not to be deprived of the opportunity to make a free and *informed* decision as to whether to undergo or forgo treatment. Depriving the patient of the opportunity to make a fully informed decision infringes on that patient's right to autonomy.

Respect for the patient's autonomy is likewise compromised when, in the absence of consent, the health care professional presumes to decide whether the treatment should proceed or decides what is or is not a material risk; all of this should be disclosed to the patient. (There are exceptions to the need for such consent in emergencies, as we will see later in this chapter.)

The final decision as to whether any nursing care, medical treatment, or plan of care should proceed rests with the patient. The nurse or other health care practitioner who proceeds without the patient's consent

runs the risk of professional sanctions, civil liability, and potentially criminal charges.

Lack of Consent (Battery)

As discussed in Chapter 7, battery, a category of intentional tort, is legally defined as battery is defined in common law as intentionally bringing about a harmful or offensive and nonconsensual contact upon another. Thus, it is an unwanted intrusion on the physical person. In the health care context, the administration of any medical treatment, surgical procedure, nursing action, diagnostic test, or other such intervention, no matter how necessary or beneficial to the patient's health and well-being in the health care professional's opinion, is forbidden unless the professional who is administering the treatment has obtained the patient's prior consent or the patient is unable to give consent having suffered a serious injury, and a lack of prompt medical attention would result in serious bodily harm or death.

Elements of Consent

Capacity to Consent

It is a fundamental principle of ethics and the law that people who are mentally competent have the right to their bodily integrity and personal autonomy about health care treatment. This right applies even to mentally incompetent people to the extent that their wishes, when they were competent, are known. If the patient is not competent, their prior wishes, as expressed to others or in an **advance directive** (discussed in Chapter 8), must be respected to the greatest extent possible. Also, a patient's capacity to consent may vary from time to time, depending on their condition, the proposed treatment, and the individual's capacity to make decisions. Consent to treatment should be considered a process, rather than a single event. Consent and capacity are discussed in detail later in the chapter.

Legal Conditions for Informed Consent

The components of a truly informed consent have been reviewed by courts many times. The courts have reinforced (through case law) the required conditions of a truly informed consent. These are summarized in Table 6.2.

TABLE 6.2	
Components of Truly Informed Consent	
Consent must:	**Explanation**
Be voluntary and genuine.	■ There must be no coercion or undue pressure from another person to obtain that consent. ■ Consent must be given without the influence of intoxicants, such as drugs or alcohol. For example, a patient who has received preoperative sedation may not have the capacity to give informed consent.
Be given with the knowledge that agreeing to treatment is not consent.	■ The patient must be told of all material risks inherent in a proposed procedure, together with its benefits and drawbacks, as well as the risks of forgoing the treatment and an explanation of possible alternatives. ■ The patient must understand the treatment options and benefits.
Be specific.	■ The consent must be specific to the proposed treatment or procedure. For example, a consent to an appendectomy does not authorize the removal of other infected or diseased tissues unrelated to that condition unless discussed during the consent process.
Specify the person providing treatment.	■ The consent process must specify who will perform the procedure or treatment. ■ If a patient has consented to its performance by a particular specialist, this would not authorize the substitution of another, less qualified, or different type of health care practitioner.
Be obtained by the person providing treatment.	■ The health care provider proposing the treatment is responsible for obtaining consent. ■ Where a patient will be treated by a physician, that physician should obtain the consent and not a nurse on the team.
Be given by a capable patient.	■ The patient must be legally capable of giving consent. ■ A minor under a certain age may not be legally qualified to consent, depending on the province. (Minor children have been able to consent to treatment or refuse treatment when they can demonstrate an appreciation for the nature and consequences of a particular treatment.)
Be given by a mentally competent patient.	■ Is the patient mentally capable of understanding the nature and consequences of the procedure, notwithstanding their mental condition? ■ The health care professional obtaining the consent is responsible for assessing the capacity of the patient to consent. ■ Capacity is usually presumed, and the health care provider does not have to explore the patient's ability to make treatment decisions, unless there is reason to believe that the patient does not understand the nature of the decision or its consequences. (See for example, s. 4(1) of the *Health Care Consent Act*, 1996.) ■ Where there is a concern about capacity, an experienced capacity assessor should be consulted, and the decision to refer to a substitute decision maker or to accept the consent of the patient should be carefully documented.

Types of Consent

There are two basic types of consent: expressed and implied. *Expressed consent* is a clear statement of consent from the patient. This may not be any specific wording; an expression, such as "Okay, nurse, go ahead" is sufficient. Many provinces require that a written consent also be obtained as evidence that the patient has consented to a procedure or treatment. Sound practice dictates that consent should always be obtained in writing so that it can be reviewed should any dispute occur later.

Implied consent is inferred from a patient's conduct. For example, a nurse advises a patient whose hand has just been punctured by a rusty nail that they will be administering a tetanus vaccine as a precaution to prevent "lockjaw." The patient then holds out their arm to receive the injection. Clearly, through this action, the patient has consented to the treatment without written or verbal means.

Documentation and Recording of Consent

Consent represents a type of agreement between the health care practitioner and the patient. Legally, the consent can be verbal or in writing and is binding and effective either way. However, because consent is such an important issue, when there is a higher degree of risk, it is best to document the consent in writing so that the precise consent can be reviewed later, if necessary. In the case of an unexpected outcome, a patient and their family will question if consent was given and what information regarding risks was provided. A written record can help prove what was said and what was agreed to by the patient. However, the written record is only part of the story, and its effectiveness can be diminished by other evidence.

Many nurses may be concerned when no expressed written consent is found in the patient's chart and the patient is ready for surgery and perhaps already sedated. Must a written consent be obtained in this instance? The written consent form itself cannot stand alone; it is documentary evidence of consent, but the mentally competent patient can withdraw consent at any time despite the existence of such a document. What matters is that an *informed* consent has been given. If the physician has documented somewhere in the patient's chart the fact of the patient's consent and the disclosure relating to the risks, consequences, and benefits of the procedure, this will usually be sufficient.

General consent forms are problematic as they are not specific to a particular procedure or treatment. Such forms may be so general that they cannot be safely relied on as proof that the patient gave informed consent to the treatment or procedure performed.

After obtaining consent, the health care professional should document the fact that the procedure was explained to the patient, along with its risks and consequences, and that the patient verbally consented. Moreover, the nurse in such a situation must be competent to provide the patient with information about the risks of the procedure; that is, the nurse cannot go beyond the scope of authorized nursing practice in explaining such procedures and risks. In some situations, it may be more appropriate for another professional in the health care team to provide such explanations. The best practice is always for the person who is to perform the treatment to explain the risks and benefits to the patient and obtain the consent.

In many cases, the gravity of the situation or the risks in delaying treatment may preclude obtaining signed consent; thus, documenting the fact of an informed consent is very important. Any such note should be signed and dated by the physician. It can also be signed by any other health care professional who is present at the time when such disclosure is made to the patient.

Withdrawal of Consent

Unlike a contract, the patient can withdraw or alter their consent at any time. If consent is altered or withdrawn, the treatment or procedure should stop as soon as it is safe to do so. A mentally competent patient has the right to withdraw consent or revoke (cancel) a previously given consent at any time, even verbally. Continuing with a treatment after consent has been withdrawn constitutes battery "unless terminating the treatment would be either life-threatening or pose immediate and serious problems to the health of the patient" (*Ciarlariello v. Schacter*, 1993, p. 619). If the patient is incompetent to withdraw consent, the health care practitioner can continue unless the patient's substitute decision maker also decides that the treatment should be withdrawn. Cases have turned on the interpretation of words spoken by the patient if they cried out during treatment. If the words were intended to be withdrawal of consent, then the health care practitioner should verify whether the patient still consents to the treatment (*Ciarlariello v. Schacter,* 1993, note 71, p. 618).

LEGISLATIVE AND REGULATORY CONSIDERATIONS FOR NURSING

Nurses have the responsibility to do all they can to facilitate a decision-making process that is thoughtful and reflective. They should also be aware that failure to obtain consent when there should be consent can be considered professional misconduct. For example, the regulations under the *Ontario Nursing Act, 1991* specifically define professional misconduct as "doing anything to a client for a therapeutic, preventative, palliative, diagnostic, cosmetic, or other health-related purpose in a situation in which consent is required by law, without such a consent" (*O. Reg. 799/93*, s. 9).

Case Law on Consent

Informed Consent

The most important case dealing with battery and the requirement of informed consent to medical treatment is the Supreme Court of Canada decision in *Reibl v. Hughes* (1980). In the *Reibl* decision, the plaintiff suffered from a blocked left carotid artery. Accordingly, he was scheduled for an elective internal carotid endarterectomy, which was performed by the defendant, a neurosurgeon. During the surgery, or immediately thereafter, the plaintiff suffered a stroke, which resulted in unilateral paralysis, impotence, and permanent disability. The plaintiff sued the neurosurgeon for negligent performance of the operation and for failure to inform him adequately of the risks of the surgery.

The case ultimately reached the Supreme Court of Canada, where the Court held that the surgeon was liable in that he had, indeed, failed to inform the plaintiff of all material risks related to the surgery. Although there was a real risk of stroke, paralysis, and possibly death, the surgeon had told the patient only that it would be better for him to have the surgery. Furthermore, as the plaintiff had difficulty with the English language, it was incumbent on the surgeon to ensure that the information conveyed was fully understood.

If such disclosure is not made, the health care practitioner risks being found liable. Consent was obtained,

but it was not a fully informed one and, thus, was considered defective because of the negligence of the doctor. The complete failure to obtain any consent at all or obtaining consent through fraud would leave the practitioner open to a civil suit for battery.

Refusal of Consent for Religious or Other Reasons

Along with the issue of informed consent is that of refusal of consent to certain procedures or treatment on moral or religious grounds. The Ontario Court of Appeal dealt with such a case in its decision in *Malette v. Shulman* (1990). In that case, the plaintiff had been seriously injured in a motor vehicle accident and rushed to a nearby hospital. She had sustained serious injuries to her head and face and was bleeding profusely. The physician on duty in the emergency department, who attended to her on her arrival, determined that she would need blood transfusions to maintain her blood volume and pressure lest she succumb to irreversible shock. The surgeon who examined her before radiographs were taken made the same determination. The patient was barely conscious at the time.

Meanwhile, shortly after the patient's arrival at the hospital, a nurse discovered in the patient's purse a card printed in French and signed by the patient, identifying her as a Jehovah's Witness follower and indicating that the patient refused treatment using blood or blood products (*Malette v. Shulman,* 1990, p. 419). The nurse brought the card to the attention of the physician who had first seen the patient.

Before radiographs could be obtained, the patient's blood pressure dropped markedly, her respiration became increasingly distressed, and her level of consciousness decreased. She continued to bleed profusely. At that moment, the physician determined that a blood transfusion was necessary to preserve her life. He decided to administer the transfusion to her personally and on his own responsibility, notwithstanding the card that had been brought to his attention.

Usually, nurses would administer blood transfusions pursuant to an order by a physician. The question then becomes: What are the legal obligations of nurses to follow a physician's order when they know that order to be contrary to the patient's wishes and that the patient has not consented to such treatment? In such a case, the law would apply equally to nurses as to physicians. Nurses and physicians must respect the patient's wishes and should not administer treatment for which consent has been withheld, no matter how necessary that treatment or how irrational the patient's decision may seem.

Returning to the *Malette* case, shortly after the physician administered the transfusion, the patient's daughter arrived at the hospital and became furious when told that a blood transfusion had been administered to her mother. She confirmed her mother's instructions that no blood be given to her and signed a document specifically prohibiting further blood transfusions to the patient, saying that her mother's faith forbade blood transfusions and that she would not want them administered to her.

Despite these objections, the physician refused to follow the daughter's instructions. In his professional opinion, transfusions were necessary to save the patient's life, and it was his professional duty to ensure that she received them. He did not believe that the card signed by the patient expressed her current wishes. He could not be sure that she had not changed her religious beliefs or that she had been fully informed of all the risks of forgoing a blood transfusion. (Again, if a nurse were carrying out an order for a blood transfusion under similar circumstances, despite having similar misgivings about the instructions, that nurse would be bound by the patient's limitations on consent to treatment.)

After making a full recovery from her injuries, the woman brought a lawsuit for battery, negligence, and religious discrimination against the physician and the hospital. Her action was allowed, and she was awarded damages on the grounds that blood transfusions had been administered against her specific wishes and that this constituted battery on her. The physician appealed this judgement in the Ontario Court of Appeal.

The Court of Appeal reviewed the law dealing with informed consent. It found that the common law recognized the right of a patient to refuse consent to medical treatment and that this right would override the health care practitioner's professional opinion about what might be best for that patient. Although it was true that informed consent was not required in an emergency when the patient was unable to give consent (and the physician had no reason to believe that the patient would refuse consent if conscious or able to do so), the physician was not free to disregard the patient's instructions in the presence of clear instructions,

such as those contained in the Jehovah's Witness card in this case. There is no corresponding doctrine of "informed refusal" requiring or authorizing a health care practitioner to proceed with emergency treatment when the practitioner has not been able to inform the patient of all the consequences and risks of refusing treatment (*Malette v. Shulman,* 1990, p. 432).

The Court of Appeal upheld the trial judge's finding that there was no rational basis or evidence on which the physician could base his belief that the card was not valid or that the patient's religious views had changed. Hence, there was no justification for the doctor's refusal to adhere to the patient's advance instructions. The treatment having thus been administered without the patient's consent, the Court of Appeal upheld the finding of liability for battery against the physician (*Malette v. Shulman,* 1990, p. 434).

The patient asked only that her spiritual beliefs be respected, and was willing to risk death for them. She consented to the use of alternatives other than blood transfusions. This case illustrates a limit on the doctrine of emergency treatment wherein the requirement for consent is waived. It further reinforces the principle that a patient's wishes are the final word on whether treatment shall be administered, no matter how necessary to life that treatment may be.

The case of an 11-year-old Indigenous child, mentioned earlier in the chapter, highlights the challenges associated with consent and children. In 2014, this young girl from the Six Nations of the Grand River, near Brantford, Ontario, was in treatment for ALL. The child had undergone part of a treatment protocol when her mother withdrew her consent and indicated that she preferred to follow traditional Haudenosaunee health practices. The oncologist did not believe that this choice was in the best interests of the child and reported the situation to the CAS. After an investigation, the CAS declined to act, and the hospital applied to the court to have the child apprehended as a child in need of protection. The court declined to act because it considered that the mother was entitled, because of her Indigenous rights, to follow traditional health practices. The court accepted that the mother believed that she was acting in the best interests of the child:

[3] . . . In constructing its reasons, it was this court's view that section 35 of the Constitution afforded the

mother the constitutionally protected right to pursue traditional medicine in the treatment of her daughter. [83b] In law as well as in practice, then, the Haudenosaunee have both an aboriginal right to use their own traditional medicines and health practices, and the same right as other people in Ontario to use the medicines and health practices available to those people. This provides Haudenosaunee culture and knowledge with protection, but it also gives the people unique access to the best we have to offer. (Hamilton Health Sciences Corp. v. D.H. et al., 2014)

A competent adult can refuse medical treatment, even if the consequences of that refusal will be death or injury. The refusal of treatment, even if irrational to most persons, is a fundamental right of a person. A patient dependent on a respirator for survival was permitted to withdraw her consent to the treatment, even though death would be the consequence. The court held that the death was "nature taking its course" and did not violate the provisions against assisted suicide in the *Criminal Code* at the time (*Nancy B. v. Hôtel-Dieu de Québec* (1992).

Withdrawal of Consent

The Supreme Court of Canada reviewed the law of informed consent in a situation in which the patient withdrew consent during a medical procedure to which she had previously consented. Although this case involved an action for battery and negligence against the attending physicians, the principles contained in this decision and developed by the Supreme Court are equally applicable to nursing professionals.

In *Ciarlariello v. Schacter* (1993), the Supreme Court was asked to consider whether a doctor still owed to a patient a duty of disclosure of all material risks inherent in a medical procedure if the patient withdraws a previously given informed consent during that procedure. The plaintiff was asked to be at a hospital for the first of two angiography procedures that were intended to determine the exact location of a suspected aneurysm. On the patient's arrival at the hospital, the physician who was to administer the test explained the risks inherent in the procedure, including possible blindness, paralysis, and death. Although the plaintiff's first language was Italian and her English was poor, she claimed at that time to have understood the doctor's explanation.

The plaintiff's daughter acted as interpreter during these explanations. The patient then signed her consent to the tests. Despite this, the doctor had misgivings as to the free and informed nature of the consent.

The doctor, therefore, destroyed the patient's consent and asked her to consult her family. This she did and returned with a consent signed by her daughter. The patient took the test; it failed to reveal the location of the aneurysm conclusively but indicated a possible site. The doctors in charge of her case decided that a second angiography was advisable.

In the meantime, the plaintiff suffered a second severe headache indicating a "rebleed" of the aneurysm, and this supported the need for a second angiography. The patient consented to this second test. Beforehand, a second radiologist (who had worked with the radiologist who administered the first test) carefully explained the test to her, including all possible material risks (skin rash; on rare occasions, blindness; stroke, paralysis, or both; or death). He stated that the patient appeared to understand, so he proceeded with the angiography.

During the procedure, the plaintiff began moaning and yelling. She started to hyperventilate and flex her legs. She calmed down sufficiently to tell the radiologist, "Enough, no more, stop the test." The test was stopped, and both radiologists proceeded to investigate her complaint that her right hand was numb. She was unable to move it or grasp with it. Her left hand was also slightly weak. Gradually, the strength returned to her right hand and both arms, although her left hand remained weak. Her sensory perception was normal. Both radiologists concluded that the residual weakness in her left hand was caused by her hyperventilating. Both expected the weakness to be temporary. The rest of her motor function appeared to return to normal.

At this point, the plaintiff became quiet and cooperative. The first radiologist took over the test and explained to her that one more area needed investigation and that this procedure would take 5 more minutes. She asked the plaintiff if she wished to continue the test, to which the plaintiff replied, "Please go ahead." The final injection of dye was administered, during which the plaintiff suffered an immediate reaction, which ultimately resulted in quadriplegia. The patient sued the doctors involved in treating her for negligence and battery. She died soon after her lawsuit came to trial, and her family and estate continued the suit.

This case is of relevance to nursing in that it illustrates that a patient has the right to withdraw consent to treatment at any time. Such withdrawal may occur in difficult circumstances, as in the *Ciarlariello* case, and it is important for the health care practitioner to ascertain whether the consent has been withdrawn. This may not always be clear. A professional who continues to administer treatment, regardless of a patient's instructions to stop, risks being found liable for battery. In the *Ciarlariello* case, at a point during the procedure, the patient clearly withdrew her consent, even though she had given an informed consent that met the requirements laid down in *Reibl v. Hughes* (1980).

A further crucial issue with respect to resumption of treatment after consent has been withdrawn was addressed in the case. The criteria laid down by the Supreme Court governing the health care professional's actions include a consideration of whether the risks have changed materially during the procedure and whether a reasonable patient would wish to know of such changes. In the *Ciarlariello* case, there was no evidence that the patient's condition had deteriorated to the point that she could not properly consent to the resumption of the treatment. Thus, her consent to resume the tests was valid.

As discussed in Chapter 7, one of the elements that must be proven in a negligence action is that the plaintiff's injury is a result of the defendant's breach of duty toward the plaintiff. In an action for negligence, such as that in *Reibl v. Hughes* or *Ciarlariello v. Schacter,* the question becomes whether a reasonable person in the plaintiff's position would still have consented to the procedure having known the information and risks that the health care practitioner failed to disclose.

In *Ciarlariello v. Schacter* (1993), the court found that the plaintiff's consent was an informed one and that there was no negligence on the doctors' part. It also found that as the risk of quadriplegia resulting from angiography was far less than the risks of not locating the aneurysm, a reasonable patient in the plaintiff's position would still have consented to the procedure.

COMPETENCY, CONSENT, AND SUBSTITUTE DECISION MAKERS

It is extremely stressful to be placed in a situation in which one must make very difficult choices—for example, whether to accept treatment that may be life-threatening or may have serious side effects, or when surrogates must make a decision that may influence the well-being of vulnerable populations, such as incapable persons, children, or persons with a mental illness.

Incompetent Adults

Returning to Case Scenario 6.1, before her children can be consulted, the patient's health care team must determine whether she is mentally competent to make an informed decision regarding the diagnostic tests. If it is determined that the patient is competent, her wishes that her children not be contacted must be respected, even if the team is concerned that this is not in her best interests. (As discussed earlier, this does not mean that the team should not listen to her story, further explore her reasons for this decision, and encourage her to engage with her family.)

In cases involving older persons, the initial and seemingly irrational refusal to consent may not necessarily be evidence of mental incompetence. The nurse or other practitioner must remain patient (if the situation is not urgent or life-threatening). Older patients may have fears of impending illness as they age. They may have friends or relatives, including their spouse, who have been ill or have recently succumbed to a serious illness. For example, a person whose brother has died of cancer may fear that he will be stricken with the disease himself. This fear may paralyze some people's thinking. They may be in a state of denial and may rationalize their refusal to consent on the basis that "if cancer is not detected, then that means I don't have it." We do not know what is going on in a patient's mind when they say, "No! I don't want to go through those tests. Leave me alone; I'm all right!"

The law allows any competent adult to refuse consent to treatment even when it may not be in their best interests. How, then, can the cognitive capacity of a patient be determined? Sharpe (1986) suggested the following test: "Can the patient appreciate the nature and consequences of the proposed treatment so as to be capable of rendering an informed judgment?" (p. 77). A method of testing for this appreciation is to explain to the patient, carefully and in detail, the risks and nature of the proposed procedure and then to ask the patient to repeat their understanding of the risks and treatment while carefully noting the responses and words used (Sharpe, 1986). On this basis, the health care practitioner is then able to form an opinion of the patient's ability to appreciate the nature, risks, and consequences of the proposed procedure. In many settings, health care providers with special training and expertise in capacity assessment may be available. For example, in Ontario, the local authorities responsible for providing home care for older persons have experienced capacity assessors, who can provide information to the health care team about which patients may require substitute decision makers and which patients are still capable.

Of course, patients may be capable of making decisions concerning some matters yet not others, and their mental capacity may fluctuate over time. Consider the example of a resident in a long-term care facility—the person has dementia and may not have the capacity to decide on a surgical procedure but is competent to refuse a shower or meals. However, if a person has stated an intention that a procedure can commence but has displayed an irrational or a confused understanding of that procedure or an incapacity to comprehend its nature or its risks, the nurse should be reluctant to proceed without the consent of an authorized substitute decision maker.

In some provinces, any health care professional faced with a question of administering treatment to a mentally incompetent patient must obtain the consent of the patient's spouse, parent, a person in lawful custody of that patient, or the patient's next of kin (*Health Care Consent Act*, 1996; *Substitute Decisions Act*, 1992). If no such persons are available, and the situation is not an emergency, a physician may have to obtain the consent of the patient's guardian, appointed under statute (e.g., Ontario's *Health Care Consent Act*, 1996), or a substitute decision maker designated by the patient pursuant to the *Substitute Decisions Act* (1992). Under such law, a court may be asked by any interested party, usually a spouse or relative, to appoint a person to act in the patient's best interests, including the giving or withholding of consent to medical treatment. This person then has the authority to consent to any medical treatment on behalf of the patient legally found incompetent by the court. In such a case, the physician may obtain the necessary consent from the guardian of the person.

For example, consider the person in the later stages of Alzheimer's disease who is rushed to the emergency department for sharp abdominal pain. His son, who has been appointed by the court to make medical decisions for his father, Committee of the Person accompanies him. The father exhibits classic symptoms of Alzheimer's disease: he is confused and incoherent and at times does not recognize his son. The emergency team will have to obtain the son's consent to tests and treatment for the father. In such a consultation, health care professionals should encourage the son to consider his father's expressed views on treatment (if any) when he was competent and take those views into account in making decisions on his behalf.

The *Civil Code of Québec* (1991) provides that if a person is incapable of giving consent, such consent may be given by a person (or a group) authorized by the court. This person is appointed by the court to act in the incapable person's best interests and to ensure proper care for that person. In the absence of a court-appointed person or persons, the person's spouse or, if there is no spouse or the spouse cannot consent because of incapacity, a close relative or adult showing a special interest in the patient may give consent (*Civil Code of Québec*, art. 15). If neither the patient nor the court-appointed person can consent, or if the patient or court-appointed person refuses consent, a health care professional in Quebec cannot proceed with treatment until and without obtaining an order from the court authorizing the procedure (*Civil Code of Québec*, art. 16, para. 1).

Children

There are likewise unique challenges when determining competency with respect to children. In some provinces, a child who is old enough and mature enough to understand the nature and risks associated with care is given the right to consent to treatment of their own accord. This approach is formally set out in the relevant Ontario legislation, which provides that the wishes with respect to medical treatment of any mentally capable person 16 years of age or older must be adhered to (*Health Care Consent Act*, 1996). Even in the case of a child under the age of 16 years, the child's wishes with respect to the granting or withholding of consent to treatment must be respected where the child is "able to understand the information that is relevant to making a decision about the treatment, admission or personal assistance service, as the case may be, and able to appreciate the reasonably foreseeable consequences of a decision or lack of decision" (*Health Care Consent Act,* 1996, s. 4(1)). A person (including a child) is presumed to be capable, and a health care practitioner is entitled to rely on such a presumption unless the practitioner has reasonable grounds to believe that the person is not, in fact, capable (*Health Care Consent Act,* 1996, ss. 4(2), (3)). The capacity of the child will depend on each child's age, intelligence, maturity, experience, and other such factors. The information that the child must understand in giving or refusing consent will be provided by the health care practitioner and includes information about the following:

- The nature of the treatment
- The expected benefits of the treatment
- The material risks of the treatment
- The material side effects of the treatment
- Alternative courses of action
- The likely consequences of not having the treatment (*Health Care Consent Act,* 1996, s. 11(3))

This is the same information that must be provided to any patient, regardless of age, when obtaining the person's informed consent.

In Quebec, any child over age 14 years may give consent freely without need for recourse to their parent or guardian (*Civil Code of Québec,* 1991 art. 14, para. 2). However, if such a child refuses consent, a court order is necessary before treatment may proceed, even if the health care professional has obtained the consent of that child's parent or guardian (*Civil Code of Québec,* 1991, art. 16, para. 2).

The Children's Aid Society (CAS) may apply to the courts to have a child in need of protection made its ward so that it can make treatment decisions on that child's behalf. This usually occurs in situations in which the health care professional and the CAS workers have reasonable grounds to believe that a child is not capable of giving informed consent because of the child's lack of maturity, young age, and so forth. This procedure has been followed in numerous cases involving parents who had refused medical treatment for their children on religious grounds. If their refusal places the child's life at risk by denying life-saving treatment, the court can deem the child a "child in need of protection" and can authorize the CAS or other such body (in some

provinces, the Director of Child Welfare) to give the required consent if it is in the child's best interests. In *Alberta (Director of Child Welfare) v. B.H.* (2002), a 16-year-old girl had been diagnosed with acute myeloid leukemia (AML). With the full support of her parents, she advised her medical team at the hospital that she would not consent to the prescribed treatment (blood transfusion or administration of blood products) because she, like her parents, was a devout member of the Jehovah's Witnesses faith. The health care professionals refused to proceed with treatment in the face of her refusal of consent, accepting that she was sufficiently mature to make such a decision. A few days later, a judge attended a hearing at the hospital on the application of the Alberta Director of Child Welfare for an apprehension order and a medical treatment order directing that the treatment be administered to the girl. The court subsequently granted the order that she be removed from the custody of her parents and that the medical treatment be administered to her.

It was clear from the evidence of the medical experts consulted by the treating physician that blood transfusion was the best treatment option under the circumstances, that the survival rates the physician had relied on were accurate, that the treatment could not be administered without use of blood products, and that the physician had not overlooked any other reasonable treatment options. The child's lawyer argued that the court had no right to make the order because she was a mature minor who had decided to refuse treatment. She was, therefore, not a child in need of protection and could not be subject to Alberta's child welfare laws. The court ruled that despite the opinion of the hospital's bioethics committee that she was sufficiently mature to refuse treatment, the father's opinion that she was not was most compelling. The girl had, in effect, decided not only to refuse medical treatment that would likely prolong her life but also to die. Moreover, an expert physician involved in the child's treatment was of the view that although the child was intelligent and had a sophisticated understanding of what she was facing, she was in no way concerned or fearful of the very likely consequences of her refusal, had no real understanding of the imminent physical death, and was childlike in many ways. She lacked the maturity to truly appreciate the nature and finality of death. Accordingly, the court granted the order requiring that the treatment be administered to her. Moreover, the court ruled that although the *Canadian Charter of Rights and Freedoms* rights to life, liberty, and security of her person had been infringed by the granting of the order, such an infringement was justified under section 1 of the Charter and that a reasonable limit was demonstrably justified in a free and democratic society. The state had a valid interest in intervening to save the life of a child who had refused treatment. The court's decision was upheld on appeal to the Alberta Court of Queen's Bench (*Alberta (Director of Child Welfare) v. B.H.,* 2002).

Other challenges arise when parents who are separated or divorced have differing views on their child's treatment. For example, during the COVID-19 pandemic, sometimes separated parents disagreed with each other over the administration of vaccines to their children. In the context of vaccines, the courts were prepared to allow for the administration of vaccines on the ground that vaccination was in the best interests of the children.

For example, in a case where the custodial parent, the mother, objected to vaccination, the father with access rights was able to obtain an order that he could have the child vaccinated. The mother argued that vaccination was only required where a child was attending school in person. The court held that as vaccination was recognized as a safe and effective treatment, the father could arrange for vaccination of his daughter even though medical decisions related to the daughter were part of the mother's custodial rights. (A.C. v. L.L., 2021 see also A.V. v. C.V., 2023 ONSC 1634 (Div. Ct.))

The decision indicated that:

The responsible government authorities have all concluded that the COVID-19 vaccination is safe and effective for children ages 12–17 to prevent severe illness from COVID-19 and have encouraged eligible children to get vaccinated. These government and public health authorities are in a better position than the courts to consider the health benefits and risks to children of receiving the COVID-19 vaccination. Absent compelling evidence to the contrary, it is in the best interests of an eligible child to be vaccinated (A.C. v. L.L., 2021).
This analysis and conclusion are consistent with the approach taken by other courts addressing vaccinations prior to COVID-19.

The issue is not, as argued by the respondent mother, whether obtaining the vaccination is "crucial" to in-person attendance. [This was often the issue in disputes about standard childhood vaccines in the past.] That is not the legal test. The question is whether it is in the best interests of the child. Given the government statements above, there can be no dispute that, as a general presumption, it is in the best interests of eligible children to get vaccinated before they attend school in person (*A.C. v. L.L.,* 2021).

Emergency Treatment

The law in Canada allows physicians and other health care professionals to administer treatment in an emergency, even if the patient's consent cannot be obtained. Such a situation might arise because of the nature of an injury or illness or because no time can be spared in administering treatment. Health care professionals acting in extreme emergencies will be absolved of any liability for administering treatment, provided there is no gross negligence on their part (Canadian Nurses Protective Society, 2004).

Proxy Consent

Traditionally, common law did not allow **proxy consent** to treatment—that is, consent granted by a third party designated by the incapable person (when capable) to make decisions on their behalf. The only situations in which third-party consent was recognized were in cases of parents consenting on behalf of minors and court-appointed guardians over mentally incompetent persons. However, in some situations, the patient may be unable to consent, not because of some current or progressive mental infirmity but because of a physical condition, for example, coma. A proxy decision maker is clearly desirable in such situations.

In Case Scenario 6.1, the medical team would have to resort to a proxy decision maker if the patient were not competent to give or withhold consent and if they were not able to contact her family.

The following discussion of recent legislative reform of common law in this area focuses on Ontario's legislation because it is presently the most detailed such legislation in Canada.

LEGISLATIVE REFORM OF COMMON LAW RESPECTING CONSENT TO TREATMENT

The main components of the Ontario legislation affecting consent to treatment are contained in the

Health Care Consent Act (1996) and the *Substitute Decisions Act* (1992).

The *Health Care Consent Act* (1996) enshrines into statute law the existing common law requirements for an informed consent to treatment, as discussed earlier. It preserves the right and duty of caregivers to restrain or confine persons when necessary to prevent serious bodily harm either to themselves or to others (s. 7). The Act requires all health care professionals (including nurses) to ensure, first, that the patient to be treated is capable of consenting and, second, that the patient, in fact, consents. If the patient is not capable, the health care professional must obtain the consent from another person authorized to give consent under the Act (s. 10(1)). The Act also provides for other consents by patients to admission to a care facility, such as a long-term care facility, or to personal assistance services, such as assistance with dressing, hygiene, eating, grooming, and so forth (ss. 2(1), "personal assistance service," 4(1)).

Ontario's statute defines informed consent in much the same way as discussed earlier in this chapter: that is, it allows the consent to be expressed or implied, provided that (1) an informed consent has been given, (2) it relates to the treatment proposed, (3) it is voluntary, and (4) it has not been obtained through fraud or misrepresentation (*Health Care Consent Act*, 1996, s. 11). Consent is informed if, before giving it, a patient received information about the nature of the treatment, its expected benefits, material risks, material side effects, alternative courses of action, and the consequences of not having the treatment (s. 11(3)). A health care professional (including nurses, under this Act) is entitled to presume that consent to a treatment includes consent to variations or adjustments in the treatment or the continuation of the treatment in a different setting, provided the benefits, risks, and material side effects of such alterations do not differ significantly from those of the original treatment.

This provision has a practical purpose. It would be quite impractical to demand that the health care professional obtain renewed consent, along with having to restate all the information required every time a course of treatment was altered in even the slightest way. This legislative provision also addresses the issue that arose in the *Ciarlariello v. Schacter* case (discussed earlier), in which there were few or no significant changes to the risks and side effects from one angiography procedure to the next.

A person is always presumed to be capable unless a health care professional has reasonable grounds to believe otherwise (*Health Care Consent Act*, 1996, s. 4). For example, a health care professional cannot assume that a patient is capable if the patient demonstrates erratic or confused behaviour or lack of lucidity or rationality. Although such an observation does not necessarily mean that the patient is incapable of consenting to treatment, a health care professional must investigate capacity further.

Capacity can vary over time and the Act allows for this (*Health Care Consent Act*, 1996, s. 15). This provision addresses concerns that arise when a capable person has not yet given consent and then later may no longer be capable, for example, while under heavy sedation. It also addresses such situations as patients with Alzheimer's disease having periods of lucidity but relapsing into a confused state only moments later.

The health care professional in charge of the patient's care is responsible for determining whether the patient is capable or incapable of consenting to a proposed treatment. If the patient's capacity to consent returns after another person has made a decision with respect to the patient's treatment, the patient's own decision to give or refuse consent will be respected and implemented (*Health Care Consent Act*, 1996, s. 16). If the physician determines that the patient is not capable of consenting to treatment, the patient must be informed of that fact and of the consequences of such a finding in accordance with the guidelines laid out by the governing body of the health care practitioner's profession. For nurses in Ontario, these would be the guidelines set out by the College of Nurses of Ontario (CNO) (s. 17). Once the health care professional has determined that the patient is incapable (or, if before the treatment is begun, the professional is informed that the person intends to apply to the Consent and Capacity Board for review of the finding of incapacity or has applied for appointment of a representative to give consent to treatment), the professional must not begin treatment or must take steps to prevent such treatment being given until the matter is decided by the board (s. 18).

The Consent and Capacity Board is an administrative tribunal. Its role is to hear appeals from findings of incapacity by health care professionals. It also hears applications brought on behalf of incapable persons for the appointment of representatives who can give consent to treatment in specific situations. In the event that the health care professional has found a patient incapable of giving consent, the patient may disagree with this finding, and, if so, has recourse to this tribunal. This mechanism protects patients' autonomy and prevents abuses of patients' rights—for example, in a case in which a nonconsenting patient might be subjected to treatment that is not in that patient's best interests or is unnecessary. Without such review, a person, refusing to consent to a treatment, might be incorrectly deemed incapable of giving consent and then be subjected to treatment simply because a health care professional was of the opinion that the patient lacked capacity.

If an incapable person has appointed a person who is acting under a **power of attorney for personal care** or the court has appointed guardian of the person (see next two sections), such an agent can give the required consent, but only in accordance with the instructions, limitations, and authority contained in the power of attorney or court order (*Health Care Consent Act*, 1996, s. 20).

If a substitute decision maker has been chosen, the known wishes of the patient must be considered and govern the substitute's decision to give or refuse consent to treatment. The wishes may be contained in the power of attorney itself or any other document or may have been communicated orally by the patient to the substitute decision maker. When such documents provide detailed directions on behalf of the maker that take effect after that person has lost the ability to make those decisions on their own behalf, they may be known as **living wills**. If there are no known wishes regarding the giving or refusal of consent to a given treatment, the substitute decision maker must make the decision in the patient's best interests and in accordance with the incapable person's values and beliefs. In particular, the substitute decision maker must consider whether:

- The proposed treatment will likely improve the patient's condition or well-being
- The proposed treatment would prevent the patient's condition or well-being from deteriorating

- The proposed treatment would reduce the extent to which (or the rate at which) the patient's condition or well-being is likely to deteriorate
- The patient's well-being or condition would likely improve, remain the same, or deteriorate without the treatment
- The benefits of treatment outweigh the risks
- If a less intrusive or restrictive treatment would be as beneficial as the one proposed (*Health Care Consent Act*, 1996, s. 21(2))

The *Health Care Consent Act* (1996) establishes a hierarchy of alternative substitute decision makers (ss. 20(1), (3)). The persons set out in this list may give or refuse consent if no person described in the next higher ranking is available and meets the requirements of the Act:

1. A guardian appointed by the court under the *Substitute Decisions Act*, 1992
2. An attorney for personal care acting under a power of attorney for personal care that confers that authority
3. The incapable person's representative, appointed by the board, if the representative has authority to give or refuse consent
4. The incapable person's spouse or partner (a "partner" is defined in section 20(9) of the Act as one with whom the incapable person has lived for at least 1 year and share a close personal relationship of primary importance to both their lives; this would apply to same-sex couples.)
5. The incapable person's child, or parent, or the CAS or other person lawfully entitled to give or refuse consent in place of the parent (this does not include parents having only a right of access over the child and does not include the child's parents if the CAS is lawfully entitled to give or refuse treatment in the parents' place)
6. The person's parent with only a right of access
7. The person's brother or sister
8. Any other relative of the incapable person

CASE SCENARIO 6.2

RECURRING CHALLENGE FOR NURSES

Nurses working in an acute care facility approach their manager regarding concerns they have with the end-of-life care for one of their patients.

The patient, a woman in her late seventies, has end-stage liver disease. The medical team has determined that they have exhausted all treatment options and that the family should be consulted

CASE SCENARIO 6.2 *(Continued)*

regarding next steps. The patient does not have an advance directive, nor has she designated a power of attorney (POA) for personal care.

During the family meeting with the patient's five children, it becomes clear that there are a range of divergent opinions, from those who want everything possibly done for the patient to those who believe palliative care is the best option. The patient's children also have different opinions on who should make the decision. The youngest daughter, who lives with the patient, believes that their mother would not want any more aggressive treatment. Two siblings (a sister and brother who live nearby) agree,

but the oldest brother and sister (who live in another province) disagree.

The nurses are asking the manager for advice on next steps:

- When there is no formal arrangement made by the patient, where do you look for substitute decision-making authority?
- When there is more than one person in the same relationship to a person who is not competent to make personal care decisions, how can the team try and help them resolve their differences? If they cannot, then an application can be made to the court or the Consent and Capacity Board for guidance.

Other requirements are that the substitute decision maker be:

- At least 16 years of age
- Capable of deciding with respect to the treatment
- Not prohibited by court order or separation agreement from having access to the incapable person or giving or refusing consent
- Available, and willing to assume the responsibility of giving or refusing consent (*Health Care Consent Act*, 1996, s. 20(2))

In the event of a conflict between two or more people claiming to have authority to give consent, the person who ranks highest in the categories listed earlier prevails. If two persons of equal ranking disagree about whether to give or refuse consent, the public guardian and trustee (see "Attorneys for Personal Care" section) may give or refuse it (*Health Care Consent Act*, 1996, s. 20(6)).

As mentioned earlier, the *Health Care Consent Act*, (1996) provides that the wishes of a minor aged 16 years or older in giving or refusing consent to treatment must be respected. The Act does not explicitly set out a minimum age for consent. Rather, the guidelines that would likely govern would be the person's capacity to understand the proposed treatment, its risks, benefits, and consequences. As discussed previously, a child less than 16 years of age might be capable of giving informed consent if of sufficient intelligence and maturity to appreciate the consequences of their decision and all the relevant information surrounding the proposed treatment.

Emergency treatment poses a special challenge for the health care professional, and the Act provides special rules for such situations. If a patient is found incapable, in the health care professional's opinion, of understanding a proposed treatment to alleviate severe suffering or if the patient is at risk of serious bodily harm if the treatment is not administered promptly and it is not possible to find a substitute decision maker without delaying such treatment, then the practitioner may administer the treatment. The practitioner may do so even when an application has been made to the Consent and Capacity Board for the appointment of a representative to give such consent on the patient's behalf.

The authority to proceed extends to any examination of the patient or diagnostic procedures (if these are reasonably necessary) to determine whether the patient is at risk for serious bodily harm or is experiencing severe suffering. The emergency treatment can continue for as long as is reasonably required to find someone who can give the necessary consent from among the list of persons authorized to do so. The Act obliges the health care professional to ensure that a continuing search is made for any substitute decision makers willing to assume responsibility to give or refuse consent. If the patient becomes capable once again, his or her wishes govern.

The health care professional is also required to note in the patient's chart the opinions required by the Act to permit treatment without consent in an emergency (*Health Care Consent Act*, 1996, s. 25(5)).

If the health care professional has reasonable grounds to believe that the incapable patient, while capable and after the person reached the age of 16, expressed a wish to refuse treatment in such circumstances, the treatment may not be administered. Thus, for example, if the patient is unconscious and an attorney for personal care advises the health care professional that this patient once expressed the desire that no blood transfusions be administered during an emergency, the professional may not administer such treatment (*Health Care Consent Act*, 1996, s. 26).

Despite a refusal of consent by someone on the list provided earlier, the health care professional may proceed if the treatment is believed to be necessary to alleviate suffering or to avoid serious bodily harm and that the person refusing the consent has done so against the patient's previous wishes or has not acted in the patient's best interests in accordance with the guidelines and considerations enumerated in the Act. The authority to proceed, as discussed earlier, extends to having the person admitted to a hospital or psychiatric facility for treatment. However, a health care professional must respect the wishes of a patient who objects to such admission primarily for treatment of a mental illness. This provision was included to cover situations in which a person might be forced to undergo psychiatric treatment against his or her will. There are separate procedures for admission of patients with mental diseases to psychiatric facilities set out in the *Mental Health Act* (1990). These include legal safeguards to ensure that otherwise mentally healthy persons are not detained against their will in psychiatric institutions.

Attorneys for Personal Care

With respect to substitute decision makers or attorneys for personal care, Ontario's *Substitute Decisions Act* (1992) provides that a person aged greater than 16 years may exercise the power of decision making on behalf of an incapacitated person who is also at least 16 years of age (ss. 43 and 44). In most cases, the parents of an incapacitated adolescent would presumably continue to make treatment decisions and give the necessary consent. The determining factor under this statute for incapacity (thus the need for a substitute decision maker) is similar to that under the *Health Care Consent Act* (1996), but in this case, patients must be unable to understand information regarding their health care, nutrition, shelter, clothing, hygiene, or safety,

or be unable to appreciate the reasonably foreseeable consequences of a decision (or lack of decision) respecting these matters (*Substitute Decisions Act*, 1992, s. 45).

Under the *Substitute Decisions Act* (1992), there are two methods of providing a substitute decision maker for an incapable person. The first is an appointment of a person or persons in a written document (called a *power of attorney for personal care*) in advance of the person (usually referred to as the **grantor**) becoming incapable. Those named in the power of attorney are authorized by the grantor to make decisions concerning personal care on his or her behalf (s. 46(1)). The person named in the power of attorney (the attorney is seldom a lawyer) for personal care may be the grantor's spouse, partner, a relative, or close friend. It cannot be anyone who provides health care to the grantor for compensation or who provides residential, social training, or support services to the grantor for compensation (s. 46(3)). This provision is important because in some situations, the grantor may be tempted to name a physician or a respected and trusted nurse as an attorney. The legislation prevents any such conflict of interest. However, critics point out that a nurse may be one of the people more knowledgeable about care and treatment issues, particularly in the case of an incapable patient, and thus is a practical and beneficial choice to be the attorney. This provision may, therefore, be viewed as a questionable limitation on the incapable patient's right to choose and appoint an attorney.

The attorney may act only in accordance with this statute and the limitations stipulated by the grantor in the power of attorney. A person who does not have a trusted friend, partner, spouse, or relative to name as attorney can name the public guardian and trustee of Ontario (with the public guardian's permission, obtained before signing the power of attorney) (*Substitute Decisions Act*, 1992, s. 46(2)). This person is a government official charged with ensuring that mentally incompetent persons, orphaned children having no legal guardians, and their property are cared for and that their legal rights are protected when there is no one else available to act in their interests.

In Ontario, the power of attorney for personal care is a fully and legally valid document from the moment the grantor becomes incapable of making treatment decisions and giving consent to treatment within the requirements of the *Health Care Consent Act* (1996) and the *Substitute Decisions Act* (1992).

Of course, the grantor making the power of attorney must be mentally capable of doing so. The test for determining this capacity is: Does the grantor understand whether the proposed attorney has a genuine concern for their welfare, and appreciate that the grantor may need to rely on the attorney to make decisions (*Substitute Decisions* Act, 1992, s. 47(1))? The power of attorney for personal care can be revoked at any time, provided the grantor is mentally capable when doing so. The grantor must also have had the capacity to make decisions with respect to any instructions contained in the power of attorney for personal care.

The formalities for making a legally valid power of attorney for personal care in Ontario are not complicated but should be carefully observed. Otherwise, there is a risk of the power of attorney being declared invalid by a court. The power of attorney for personal care must be signed by the grantor in the presence of two witnesses, who cannot be:

- The proposed attorney or that person's spouse or partner
- The grantor's spouse or partner
- A child of the grantor or a person that the grantor has treated as if that person were his or her child
- Someone whose own property is under a guardianship (this prevents a potentially incompetent person from being a witness)
- A person under 18 years of age (*Substitute Decisions Act,* 1992, ss. 10(1), (2), 48(2)).

The power of attorney for personal care authorizes the attorney to make decisions regarding the grantor's personal care if the *Health Care Consent Act* (1996) authorizes the attorney to make the decision or if the attorney has reasonable grounds to believe that the grantor is incapable of making the decision. This power may be subject to any precondition in the power of attorney document (*Substitute Decisions Act,* 1992, s. 49(1)(b)). For such a condition to be legally effective, the grantor must establish that they have the capacity to grant or revoke the power of attorney document.

The legislation protects grantors against having decisions made without their consent. For example, a grantor has the right to request the attorney's assistance in arranging an assessment by an assessor, who may be a physician, a psychologist, or a psychiatrist, as designated by government regulation to make such an assessment. A grantor may place conditions on the authority of the substitute decision maker and can specify the way their capacity is to be assessed (*Substitute Decisions Act,* 1992, s. 49(2)). The assessor is responsible for determining whether the grantor is in fact incapable of making some, if not all, treatment decisions. The attorney is not required to make such arrangements, however, if the person was assessed within 6 months before the request for an assessment (s. 55(1)).

In addition, the *Substitute Decisions Act* (1992) provides the attorney with the authority to use such reasonable force as is necessary to determine the grantor's capacity, to confirm whether the grantor is incapable of personal care, to take the grantor to any place of treatment, or to admit the grantor to such place for detention and restraint if treatment is required (s. 59(3)).

Court-Appointed Guardians of the Person

The second method of providing a substitute decision maker under the *Substitute Decisions Act* (1992) in Ontario is through an application to the court for the appointment of a guardian of the person (s. 55(1)). This is more difficult. The court must consider whether there is an alternative course of action (e.g., one that is less restrictive of the patient's decision-making rights) for making decisions that does not require it to declare the applicant incapable of his or her own personal care (s. 55(2)). Thus, the legislation is aimed at encouraging alternatives to court proceedings in these matters.

Any person (i.e., a physician, close friend, relative, spouse, partner, or any person who has an interest in the applicant's care) may apply for the appointment of a guardian. In any event, the appointed guardian cannot be someone who provides health care for compensation (*Substitute Decisions Act,* 1992, s. 57(1)) but may be the applicant's attorney for personal care. An exception may be made if there is no other suitable person who can act as guardian (s. 57(2.1)). The appointment of an attorney could expand their decision-making power over and above the authorization contained in the power of attorney for personal care. If it is made in a court order for full guardianship, it might include the power to:

- Determine the person's living arrangements, shelter, and safety

- Take charge of any lawsuits by or against the applicant
- Gain access to personal information about the applicant
- Make decisions about the applicant's health care, nutrition, and hygiene
- Give or refuse consent to medical treatment on the person's behalf pursuant to the *Health Care Consent Act* (1996)
- Make decisions about the applicant's employment, education, training, clothing, and recreation, and any other duties and powers specified in the order

In short, full guardianship may (depending on the exact provisions of the court order) grant power to the guardian over all facets of the incapable person's life.

Before appointing a guardian, the court must find that the patient is, in fact, incapable according to the definition outlined earlier. The appointment of the guardian may be for a limited time or may have other conditions attached to it as the court considers appropriate. In deciding the application, the court must consider (1) whether the proposed guardian is the attorney under a power of attorney; (2) the incapable person's wishes, to the extent that these can be ascertained; and (3) the closeness of the relationship between the person applying for the guardianship and the incapable person.

A partial guardianship order may be made when the court considers the patient incapable with respect to some, but not all, aspects of personal care and health. In such a case, the guardianship order will specify those matters in which the guardian has the power to make decisions, leaving other matters to the patient's own discretion. In this way, any court order can be tailored to be as unobtrusive as possible to the incapable patient's life while still affording the protection of a competent guardian to make crucial decisions on his or her behalf.

DUTIES OF GUARDIANS AND ATTORNEYS FOR PERSONAL CARE

The philosophy behind the law is to involve the incapable person in the process of consent to the greatest extent possible under the circumstances. This accords

with the basic principle of autonomy, as discussed in Chapter 2. Thus, both guardians and attorneys are required to exercise their powers diligently and in good faith and to explain their powers and duties to the incapable person. As mentioned, the wishes of the person, made while capable, must guide the guardian or attorney when faced with decisions relevant to these wishes; the guardian or attorney must make diligent efforts to ascertain the existence and substance of prior wishes; and the most recent wish made while the person was capable must prevail over an earlier related wish. To determine these prior wishes, the guardian or attorney must take the incapable person's values and beliefs into account. In addition, the guardian must consider whether the decision is likely to improve the quality of the incapable person's life, prevent that quality of life from deteriorating, or reduce the extent to which (or rate at which) the person's quality of life is likely to deteriorate. Further, the guardian must weigh the relative risks and benefits the person may derive from the decision against those that may arise from an alternative decision.

If it is not possible to decide in accordance with an incapable person's wish, or if such wishes or instructions cannot be determined, the guardian or attorney must make the decision in the person's best interests. The least restrictive and least intrusive course of action under the circumstances must be chosen, and in making any decision, the guardian should foster the incapable person's independence as much as possible. The guardian should consult with the person's family, friends, and health care professionals. Here, nurses caring for such patients have an opportunity to make their perspectives and views known and to contribute to the quality of care. Unlike attorneys for personal care, however, court-appointed guardians of the person must have written guardianship plans (usually written by lawyers, with the assistance of the health care professionals involved) to which they must adhere. Guardians and attorneys are also required to maintain records of all decisions affecting the incapable person.

Manitoba and British Columbia

Manitoba's substitute decision maker legislation, *The Health Care Directives Act* (C.C.S.M. c. H27), is similar to that of Ontario. In Manitoba, the document signed by the grantor is called a **directive**, and the grantor is referred to as the *maker of the directive*. The person who is appointed to be the substitute decision maker is the **proxy**.

The Manitoba Act is silent on court-appointed guardians; however, this area is covered through other legislation. The directive need not be witnessed so long as the maker has signed it. However, the Manitoba Act does permit another person to sign for the maker in the maker's presence and in the presence of a witness. Neither the person who signs for the maker nor the witness may be nominated as the proxy in the directive. This is intended to cover directives made by blind persons or others who, although mentally competent, are physically unable to sign the document.

British Columbia has enacted the *Representation Agreement Act* (1996), which establishes procedures respecting agreements with substitute decision makers, like Ontario's and Manitoba's Acts. Under the *Representation Agreement Act*, a competent adult also has the right to appoint a substitute decision maker (called a *representative*) to make treatment and care decisions on his or her behalf. The document making the appointment is called a *representation agreement,* which must be signed by the patient's representative (unlike Ontario's or Manitoba's legislation). The signatures of each party to the agreement must be witnessed by two people. The representative of the incapable person is also supervised by a monitor whose duty it is to ensure that the representative carries out all their obligations under the agreement and in accordance with the wishes of the incapable person (as expressed when capable). British Columbia also has the *Health Care (Consent) and Care Facility (Admission) Act* (1996), which codifies much of the law on informed consent and is broadly like Ontario's *Health Care Consent Act* (1996).

Other Provinces and Territories

Several other Canadian jurisdictions, notably Newfoundland and Labrador, Prince Edward Island, Nova Scotia, Saskatchewan, and Yukon, also have legislation respecting the power of persons to make advance directives or allowing for substitute decision makers. See the following:

- Newfoundland and Labrador: *Advanced Health Care Directives Act* (1995)

- Prince Edward Island (PEI): *Consent to Treatment and Health Care Directives Act* (1988)
- Nova Scotia: *Medical Consent Act* (1989)
- Saskatchewan: *Health Care Directives and Substitute Health Care Decision Makers Act* (1997)
- Yukon: *Enduring Power of Attorney Act* (2002)

Of these other jurisdictions, only PEI's legislation codifies the law requiring a patient to give consent to treatment as does Ontario's *Health Care Consent Act* (1996). The statutes of the other four jurisdictions address the powers of substitute decision makers and advance directives to make treatment decisions for incapable persons. The PEI statute, interestingly, makes legal any advance directive made before the law was passed (*Consent to Treatment and Health Care Directives Act,* 1988, s. 1(e), "directive"), acknowledging that the practice of making so-called living wills arose before the law had a chance to respond to this societal change. The directive in PEI may set out the maker's wishes with respect to treatment, may be limited simply to appointing a proxy, or may both set out wishes and appoint a proxy.

The PEI statute, like Ontario's, sets out what does and does not constitute treatment. Included in this list are:

- An examination or assessment conducted under PEI's *Adult Protection Act, Mental Health Act, Public Health Act, Public Trustee Act,* or any other statute respecting capacity or guardianship of the person
- The assessment or examination of a person to determine his or her general health and condition
- The taking of a person's health history
- The communication of an assessment or diagnosis
- The admission of a person to a hospital or other facility
- A personal assistance service
- A treatment posing little or no risk of harm
- Counselling that is primarily in the nature of advice, education, or motivation
- Any other act prescribed by regulation

The provisions in this statute are subject to any contrary provisions in the *Mental Health Act* and the *Public Health Act* of PEI.

PEI's statute sets out specific "consent rights," including the right of the patient to give or refuse treatment on any grounds, including moral and religious grounds, even if death results consequently (*Consent to Treatment and Health Care Directives Act*, 1988, s. 4). A patient is also permitted to have a trusted advisor, referred to as an "associate," for assistance and has the right to select the health care professional and form of treatment on any grounds. The provisions respecting the giving of consent and prohibitions on administering treatment without consent are like Ontario's provisions. The requirements for determining capacity and whether consent is informed are also similar; however, a person may waive the right in writing to receive information as to the nature of the proposed treatment (*Consent to Treatment and Health Care Directives Act*, 1988, s. 6). In determining capacity, a health care professional must inform the patient of his or her right to the assistance of an associate but must also consider the associate's assistance.

As in Ontario, PEI provides for specific people to act as substitute decision makers in decreasing order of priority (*Consent to Treatment and Health Care Directives Act*, 1988, s. 11(1)). The order is quite like that outlined in Ontario's legislation. A substitute decision maker is not authorized by the Act to give consent to electric shock therapy, the removal of nonregenerative tissue, an abortion (except in cases in which there is likely immediate danger to the life or health of the patient), sterilization not medically necessary for the protection of the patient's health, or a procedure whose primary purpose is research, except where the research is for the patient's own benefit. This is somewhat different from Ontario's legislation, which does allow consent to electric shock therapy if consent is given in accordance with the *Health Care Consent Act* (1996).

Unlike Ontario's legislation, PEI's legislation does not provide for a consent and capacity board. In both Ontario and PEI, health care professionals acting because of an apparently valid consent are shielded from legal liability for their actions. Neither is a substitute decision maker, or a proxy in PEI, liable for a decision made while acting in good faith and in accordance with the law. "Good faith" means that the substitute decision maker must have an honestly held belief that the patient is either capable of giving an informed consent or incapable of doing so and acts appropriately.

In Ontario, two persons must witness the making of a power of attorney for personal care, whereas only one witness is required in PEI. In PEI, any interested person may file a complaint about a proxy with a public official designated by the Minister of Health and Social Services (*Consent to Treatment and Health Care Directives Act*, 1988, s. 27). A proxy cannot delegate the authority to make decisions to anyone else. Further, a decision by a proxy under an advance directive takes precedence over a decision made by a court or any other person, including a guardian, unless the directive provides otherwise. A directive made outside PEI is valid in that province if it meets the requirements of the PEI legislation or accords with the laws of the province (or country) where it was made and if the maker was habitually resident in that other province or country.

Saskatchewan's *Health Care Directives and Substitute Health Care Decision Makers Act* (1997) is fairly similar to the acts described earlier but does not codify completely the common law relating to informed consent. It provides for the making of health care directives in a similar manner.

In Saskatchewan, the proxy must be an adult—that is, a person aged greater than 18 years. However, the maker of a health care directive may be anyone who is capable and aged greater than 16 years. As in PEI, only one witness is required to the making of a health care directive.

Yukon's legislation (*Enduring Power of Attorney Act*, 2002) is like that of the other provinces. It provides that a regular power of attorney becomes an "enduring power of attorney" if it is in writing, is signed by its "donor," is dated, and contains a provision that it is to continue to be in force after the donor's incapacity or is to take effect at such time (*Enduring Power of Attorney Act*, 2002, s. 3). The Yukon statute also requires that certain notes on the enduring power of attorney be included in it. These notes relate to the donor's appreciation of the nature of the document, the powers it grants to the attorney, when it takes effect, and when (and under what circumstances) it can be cancelled. A lawyer must attest in writing that the donor understands the document, was competent when it was signed, and was an adult, and that the power was given freely and voluntarily. The legislation does not explicitly set out what powers or restrictions may be contained in the enduring power of attorney. Without the permission of the court, the attorney is prohibited from renouncing an appointment once it has taken effect. Consent to treatment in Yukon is dealt with under that territory's health act, insofar as the attorney as substitute decision maker is concerned.

Best Practices in Situations of Substitute Decision Making

The health team can ensure the best outcome where a substitute decision maker is or may become involved by:

- Determining who has the legal consent to treatment and clearly documenting this in the patient's chart.
- Devising a plan of care based on the patient's current and potential status. The plan can consider the withholding or withdrawal of consent and the necessary time and opportunity to obtain informed consent.
- Documenting the actions and decision-making process of the health team, especially if there is an emergency or urgent situation.
- Reviewing the facility's policies and procedures in relation to consent and substitute decision maker consent on a regular basis to ensure that they reflect current best practices.

SUMMARY

This chapter focused on the ethical and legal foundations of consent and provided examples to clarify their application in practice. Nurses face many challenges while seeking to protect their patients' autonomy: advances in technology, the complexities within the health care system, increasing emphasis on individual choice, questions regarding whether a person has the capacity to provide consent, and concerns regarding potential litigation, to name but a few. Furthermore, legislation pertaining to consent is constantly being revised to achieve a balance between respecting the patient's choice and protecting individuals from harm.

Issues of consent are more complex where the most vulnerable are concerned. These include children, persons with cognitive impairment, and persons with a mental illness. Even when considered incapable of providing consent, they must be engaged in the process, and where possible, their consent should be considered. With adults, their wishes, if known in advance, should be respected, and reflected in the deliberations.

Nurses are in the best position to ensure that the process is compassionate, and that the person's story is shared and understood.

Consent policies, rules, and legislation are very much based on the principle of autonomy, which recognizes that a capable and competent individual is free to determine and act in accordance with a self-chosen plan. Other equally important ethical principles that nurses must consider, such as beneficence and nonmaleficence, at times may conflict with this principle.

Each clinical environment or setting in which nurses practice needs to establish nursing guidelines relative to consent. Ethics committees to assist nurses and other members of the team to deal with challenging situations should be in place. Ongoing education, peer review, and continuous quality improvement are necessary to ensure that standards are kept consistently high.

There are many complex dynamics involved in dealing with ill people, whose capacity to make informed choices in the context of a confusing bureaucratic setting may be challenged. Nurses must give serious consideration to their role in caring for and supporting these patients and making sure that patients have the time and resources to make the decision best for them. In doing so, nurses ensure patients' rights are respected and that they are protected from harm.

CRITICAL THINKING

The following case scenario is for further reflection, discussion, and analysis.

Discussion Points

1. Identify 10 nursing interventions in which the patient's consent is implied.
2. In what circumstances should nursing interventions require a more explicit consent?
3. Provide some examples of when the principle of beneficence is in conflict with the person's right to choose. How might this dilemma be resolved? What action would you consider to address the challenges for the patient in Case Scenario 6.1?
4. Your patient is about to go for an exploratory laparotomy, has received preoperative education, and was seen by the surgeon the evening before. The patient's family has travelled a long distance to be present on the morning of surgery.

It is only after you give the patient the preoperative sedation that you notice that the consent form has not been signed. What would you do? What would be the practice in your facility if this were to occur?

5. Should parents be permitted to give or refuse consent for their young children regardless of the circumstances? Why, or why not? Should the child's best interests govern? Are there any legal avenues open to ensuring that the child's best interests are considered?

6. It is a busy evening, and one of your confused older patients is restless and keeps trying to climb over the bed rails. You believe your only option to protect this patient is to restrain her.

As you prepare to do this, the patient—appearing lucid for the moment—asks simply to sit up in the chair and does not want to be tied down. What do you do?

7. You are a nurse in the obstetrical wing of a busy teaching hospital. A woman comes in for a pelvic examination under general anaesthesia a few days before her due date. A young nursing student asks you whether he can observe the examination. What do you tell the patient? Can you assume that the patient knows that students will observe procedures as part of their training? What are the risks of proceeding without properly informing the patient and obtaining her consent?

CASE SCENARIO 6.3

OLD ENOUGH TO CHOOSE?

L. L. who 3-year-old with acute lymphocytic leukemia is presently undergoing treatment in the pediatric unit of a large tertiary cancer centre. The leukemia was diagnosed when L. L. was 8 years old, and at that at time had undergone several rounds of chemotherapy. The cancer went into remission, but because this was a severe form of leukemia, the team asked the parents to consider bone marrow transplantation. A sibling , who 2 years older, was a perfect match. The bone marrow retrieval was scary for the sibling as it required general anaesthesia, and there was much pain afterward. However, this pain and suffering did not compare to that experienced by L. L. In preparation for the transplantation, L. L. received high doses of chemotherapy and underwent total body

radiation. A short time after the transplantation, L. L.'s body started to reject the new marrow (graft versus host disease).

However, L. L. recovered, but now 5 years later the cancer has returned, and the team is proposing more chemotherapy and possibly another bone marrow transplant.

L. L. reveals to the primary nurse, who has cared for L. L. since the beginning, that although L. L.'s parents favour more treatment, they is tired and has "had enough." Furthermore, two friends and fellow patients at the hospital had undergone similar treatments and died. Although wanting only to go home and spend time with family and friends, L. L. plans to go ahead with the treatment not wanting to upset them.

REFERENCES

Statutes

Advanced Health Care Directives Act, S.N.L. 1995, c. A-4.1 (Newfoundland and Labrador).

Civil Code of Québec, CQLR c. CCQ-1991 (Quebec).

Consent to Treatment and Health Care Directives Act, R.S.P.E.I. 1988, c. C-17.2 (Prince Edward Island).

Enduring Power of Attorney Act, R.S.Y. 2002, c. 73 (Yukon).

Health Care Consent Act, 1996, S.O. 1996, c. 2, Sch. A (Ontario).

Health Care (Consent) and Care Facility (Admission) Act, R.S.B.C. 1996, c. 181 (British Columbia).

The Health Care Directives Act, C.C.S.M., c. H27 (Manitoba).

Health Care Directives and Substitute Health Care Decision Makers Act, S.S. 1997, c. H-0.002 (Saskatchewan).

Medical Consent Act, R.S.N.S. 1989, c. 279 (Nova Scotia).

Mental Health Act, R.S.O. 1990, c. M.7 (Ontario).

Nursing Act, 1991, S.O. 1991, c. 32 (Ontario).

Personal Health Information Protection Act, 2004, S.O. 2004, c. 3, Sch. A, s. 13 (Ontario).

Representation Agreement Act, R.S.B.C. 1996, c. 405 (British Columbia).

Substitute Decisions Act, 1992, S.O. 1992, c. 30 (Ontario).

Regulations

Professional Misconduct, O. Reg. 799/93 (under the *Nursing Act*, 1991, Ontario).

Case Law

A.C. v. L.L. [2021] ONSC 6530 (CanLII). A.V. v. C.V., 2023 ONSC 1634

Alberta (Director of Child Welfare) v. B.H. [2002] ABPC 39 (CanLii), affirmed B.H. v. Alberta (Director of Child Welfare), 2002 ABQB 371.

Ciarlariello v. Schacter [1993] 2 SCR 119.

Hamilton Health Sciences Corp. v. D.H., P.L.J., Six Nations of the Grand River Child and Family Services Department and Brant Family and Children's Services [2014] ONCJ 229 and 2014 ONCJ 608.

Malette v. Shulman [1990], 72 OR (2d) 417 (CA).

Nancy B. v. Hôtel-Dieu de Québec, [1992], (CanLII) 8511 (QC CS).

Reibl v. Hughes [1980] 2 SCR 880; (1980) 14 CCLT 1; 114 DLR (3d) 1; 33 NR 361.

Texts and Articles

Aboriginal Justice Implementation Commission. (1999). *Report of the Aboriginal Justice Inquiry of Manitoba.* http://www.ajic.mb.ca/reports/final_toc.html

Annas, G. J., & Grodin, M. A. (2008). The Nuremberg Code. In E. J. Emanuel, C. C. Grady, R. A. Crouch, et al. (Eds.), *The Oxford textbook of clinical research ethics* (pp. 136–140). Oxford University Press.

Ashcroft, R. E. (2008). The Declaration of Helsinki. In E. J. Emanuel, C. C. Grady, R. A. Crouch, et al. (Eds.), *The Oxford textbook of clinical research ethics* (pp. 136–140). Oxford University Press.

Beauchamp, T. L., & Childress, J. F. (1989). *Principles of biomedical ethics.* Wadsworth Publishing Company.

Canadian Institutes of Health Research, Natural Science and Engineering Research Council, & Social Sciences and Humanities Research Council of Canada. (2022). *Tri-council policy statement: Ethical conduct for research involving humans.* https://ethics.gc.ca/eng/policy-politique_tcps2-eptc2_2022.html

Canadian Nurses Association. (2017). *Code of ethics for registered nurses.*

Canadian Nurses Protective Society. (2004). Consent of the incapable adult. *InfoLaw, 13*(3), 1–2.

Charon, R. (2001). Narrative medicine: A model for empathy, reflection, profession, and trust. *Journal of the American Medical Association, 286*(15), 1897–1902.

CIHR/NSERC/SSHRCC, (2018) *Tri-Council Policy Statement: Ethical Conduct for Research Involving Humans – TCPS 2 (2018).* https://ethics.gc.ca/eng/policy-politique_tcps2-eptc2_2018.html

Corrigan, O. (2003). Empty ethics: The problem with informed consent. *Sociology of Health & Illness, 25*(7), 768–792.

Halpern, J. (2014). From idealized clinical empathy to empathic communication in medical care. *Medicine, Health Care and Philosophy, 17*(2), 301–311.

Health Canada – Public Health Agency of Canada, & Research Ethics Board. (2023). *Research Ethics Board: Policies, guidelines and resources.* https://www.canada.ca/en/health-canada/services/science-research/science-advice-decision-making/research-ethics-board/policy-guidelines-resources.html

Kocarnik, J. M. (2014). Disclosing controversial risk in informed consent: How serious is serious? *The American Journal of Bioethics, 14*(4), 13–14.

Lux, M. K. (2016). *Separate beds: A history of Indian hospitals in Canada, 1920s–1980s.* University of Toronto Press.

McCarthy, J. (2003). Principlism or narrative ethics: Must we choose between them? *Medical Humanities, 29*(2), 65–71.

Mosby, I. (2013). Administering colonial science: nutrition research and human biomedical experimentation in Aboriginal communities and residential schools, 1942–1952. *Social History, 46*(91), 145–172.

Mueller, M. (1997). Science versus care: Physicians, nurses and the dilemma of clinical research. In M. A. Elston (Ed.), *The sociology of medical science and technology.* Blackwell.

Office of the Languages Commissioner of Nunavut. (2015). *If you cannot communicate with your patient, your patient is not safe: Systemic investigation report: Investigation into the Qikiqtani General Hospital's compliance with the Official Languages Act, R.S.N.W.T. 1988: Final Report.* https://langcom.nu.ca/sites/langcom.nu.ca/files/QGH%20-%20Final%20Report%20EN.pdf

Olick, R., Shaw, J., & Yang, T. (2021). Ethical issues in mandating COVID-19 vaccinations for health care personnel. *Mayo Clinic Proceedings, 96*(12), 2958–2962.

Roter, D. L., Frankel, R. M., Hall, J. A., et al. (2006). The expression of emotion through nonverbal behavior in medical visits: Mechanisms and outcomes. *Journal of General Internal Medicine, 21,* 28–34.

Sharpe, G. (1986). *The law and medicine in Canada* (2nd ed.). Butterworths.

Sugarman, J., McCrory, D. C., & Powell, D. (1999). *Empirical research on informed consent: An annotated bibliography.* A Hastings Center Report, Special Supplement.

Warade, A. C., Jha, A. K., Pattankar, S., et al. (2019). Radiation-induced brachial plexus neuropathy: A review. *Neurology India, 67*(Suppl S1), 47–52.

Whitney, S. N., McGuire, A. L., & McCullough, L. B. (2004). A typology of shared decision making, informed consent, and simple consent. *Annals of Internal Medicine, 140*(1), 54–59.

World Health Organization. (2019). *COVID-19 and mandatory vaccination: Ethical considerations Policy brief.* https://www.who.int/publications/i/item/WHO-2019-nCoV-Policy-brief-Mandatory-vaccination-2022.1

Wynia, M. K., Harter, T. D., & Eberl, J. T. (2021, November 3). Why a universal COVID-19 vaccine mandate is ethical today. *Health Affairs Blog.* https://www.healthaffairs.org/do/10.1377/forefront.20211029.682797/

7

THE NURSE'S LEGAL ACCOUNTABILITIES: PROFESSIONAL COMPETENCE, MISCONDUCT, MALPRACTICE, AND NURSING DOCUMENTATION

LEARNING OBJECTIVES

The purpose of this chapter is to enable you to understand:

- The professional responsibilities and accountabilities of the nurse
- Nurses' ethical and legal responsibilities to the patient, other health care professionals, and the public, including professional competence, torts, misconduct, and malpractice
- The legal concepts of negligence, duty of care, vicarious liability, standard of care, and causation
- Criminal law with respect to standard of care and negligence
- The importance of meeting standards for timely, accurate, and complete documentation in ensuring safe and effective nursing care
- The role of the coroner's office and the implications of a coroner's inquest
- The legal requirements of nursing documentation, its significance, and how it is used in legal proceedings

INTRODUCTION

Nurses, as professionals, have an obligation to serve the public interest and to operate within a set of professional standards and ethical rules. They are accountable to the public through a legal framework aimed at ensuring competent and safe care while preserving respect for individual rights. This framework includes nursing-specific statutes and **regulations**, the nursing regulator's practice standards, the *Criminal Code*, provincial and federal legislation, and the principles of civil liability embodied in common law and the *Civil Code of Québec*.

The *Code of Ethics for Registered Nurses* (Canadian Nurses Association [CNA], 2017) makes clear the nurse's responsibility not only to practise ethically but also to be accountable to both professional and legal standards and rules:

> . . . nurses, as members of a self-regulating profession, practise according to the values and responsibilities in the Code of Ethics for Registered Nurses and in keeping with the professional standards, laws and regulations supporting ethical practice (p. 16)

As discussed in Chapter 5, Canadian society places its trust in nurses and allows the nursing profession to regulate its members through self-governing bodies. As noted in Chapter 4, the legal system measures the performance and behaviour of nurses against professional and ethical standards and imposes significant consequences when nurses fail to meet them. Ignorance of the law is not a defence; therefore, nurses must have a deep understanding of the expectations and the consequences when standards and rules are not met.

While describing the legal consequences that nurses face when failure to meet professional standards results in harm, this chapter focuses on the civil and criminal legal systems in Canada. The competence and conduct of nurses are gauged through the disciplinary powers of nursing regulatory bodies, criminal law, and civil liability. Through these mechanisms, nurses are made accountable to their patients, their colleagues, employers, the community, and society. Criminal law can impose significant consequences for nurses who act carelessly and recklessly or, who in their nursing role, engage in deliberate criminal activity. Nurses have been convicted of crimes, such as fraud, theft, and child pornography (Zhong et al., 2016).

The structure and processes of investigation and reviews of unexplained deaths, and the implications for nursing, are described. The coroner system or the similar medical examiner system, in every province, investigates unexplained deaths to determine cause and to make recommendations to prevent such occurrences in the future. Frequently, nurses are involved in such investigations and may be called to testify at inquests.

In all of these contexts, documentation provides key evidence against which the actions of nurses are evaluated. Nurses must understand the relevance of the duty of care, practice standards, and documentation when issues are brought before the legal system. These will be described and illustrated with case law.

STANDARDS OF CARE AND PUBLIC EXPECTATIONS: IMPLICATIONS WHEN THEY ARE NOT MET

Legal concepts, such as a professional's duty of care, competent practice, professional misconduct, malpractice, and negligence, should be understood by nurses. The ethical and legal aspects of these expectations are interrelated and relevant to both the legal system and regulatory processes. Nurses have responsibilities to many different people. These responsibilities are separate but related. Nurses' primary legal responsibilities are the (1) maintenance of professional competence; (2) legal obligation to compensate others injured by their conduct; and (3) criminal liability for conduct that violates the provisions of the *Criminal Code*. A nurse's conduct does not always violate all of these responsibilities in the same circumstance. Conduct that is unprofessional may not have civil liability consequences where no one is harmed by the unprofessional conduct. Negligence, which creates legal liability, does not always rise to the level of professional misconduct. Criminal liability is rare for a nurse acting in good faith and within the scope of their employment. Where criminal conduct does occur, usually all aspects of the nurse's legal responsibilities will be affected. For example, sexual interference with a cognitively compromised patient would result in

criminal and civil liabilities and a review of the nurse's professional conduct. (Zhong et al. [2016] found that only about 10% of crimes committed by nurses involve their patients.).

A tragic example of the alignment of these legal accountabilities occurred in June 2017, when former Ontario nurse Elizabeth Wettlaufer pled guilty to the first-degree murder of eight senior citizens, the attempted murder of four others, and the aggravated assault of two. While a nurse working in long-term care facilities between 2007 and 2016, she administered insulin overdoses to these people. In criminal court, she received a life sentence with no chance of parole until 2041. Subsequently, the College of Nurses of Ontario (CNO) deemed her actions "most egregious" and found her guilty of 14 counts of professional misconduct (*College of Nurses of Ontario v. Wettlaufer,* 2017). In addition, civil lawsuits were filed against her and her employers by families of the victims. The Government of Ontario launched a public inquiry to answer questions about the factors that led to these deaths and to ensure that a similar tragedy would not happen again (The Long-Term Care Homes Public Inquiry [2019], https://longtermcareinquiry.ca/en/).

The following sections describe those concepts that ground the framework for legal nursing practice.

Professional Duty of Care

Common law imposes on persons a duty of care to those people who are close to, or closely connected with, one's conduct or activities.

The classic definition of the duty of care can be found in *Donoghue v. Stevenson* (1932). Lord Atkin, one of the Lord Justices of the House of Lords, spoke of the duty thus:

The rule that you are to love your neighbour becomes, in law, you must not injure your neighbour; and the lawyer's question, Who is my neighbour? receives a restricted reply. You must take reasonable care to avoid acts or omissions which you can reasonably foresee would be likely to injure your neighbour. Who, then, in law, is my neighbour? The answer seems to be, persons who are so closely and directly affected by my act that I ought reasonably to have them in contemplation as being so affected when I am directing my mind to the acts or omissions which are called in question (Donoghue v. Stevenson, 1932, p. 580; 101 LJPC 119, at p. 127; 147 LT 281 (HL); see also Linden, 2018)

Professionals, such as nurses, owe a duty of care to those who require their services or are placed in their care to act in a competent and diligent manner according to reasonable standards and expectations. This includes the responsibility of a nurse, as with any other professional, to keep abreast of current developments and practices within the profession and to undertake ongoing education and professional development.

Competence

Professional competence is the broad professional knowledge, attitude, and skills one must have to work in a specialized area or profession. Disciplinary knowledge and the application of concepts, processes, and skills are required to test professional competence in any particular field. Regulatory bodies establish the standards and competence required of professional nurses. Each jurisdiction (province or territory) has a government-authorized regulatory body for nursing that defines the standards of the profession (CNA Regulated Nursing in Canada, Regulatory Bodies https://www.cna-aiic.ca/en/nursing/regulated-nursing-in-canada/regulatory-bodies).

When the regulatory body is told that a member's conduct falls below the standard, the member will be investigated and remedial action such as education may be imposed. If warranted, disciplinary action may be taken or the member may be subjected to charges, a hearing, and further sanctions, including removal from the profession. The internal process of the regulator can be reviewed by the courts (judicial review) to ensure that the relevant laws and legal principles were appropriately applied. This is not a rehearing but merely a review of the evidence and process to ensure that the result is consistent with the power of the tribunal.

The standards of the profession are often reviewed to assess whether the conduct of a nurse is negligent or criminal. Where a nurse's conduct appears to fall below the standard of competent practice, this fact may be evidence that the nurse has acted in a negligent or wrongful manner. To avoid legal complications, nurses should always ensure that they are in strict compliance with the standards, rules, and regulations of their profession.

Professional Misconduct

Professional misconduct occurs when a professional's behaviour fails to meet the ethical and legal rules and standards of the profession. Many provincial and territorial statutes regulating nursing and other health care professions provide a legal definition of *professional misconduct*. The CNO (2018) describes professional misconduct as "an act or omission that is in breach of these accepted ethical and professional standards of conduct (p. 3).

In Nova Scotia, section 2 of the *Nurses Act*, c. 8, 2019 defines professional misconduct as including:

includes such conduct or acts relevant to the practice of the profession that, having regard to all the circumstances, would reasonably be regarded as disgraceful, dishonourable or unprofessional, including

(a) *failing to maintain the standards of practice;*
(b) *failing to adhere to any codes of ethics adopted by the College;*
(c) *abusing a person verbally, physically, emotionally or sexually;*
(d) *misappropriating personal property, drugs or other property belonging to a client or an employer;*
(e) *inappropriately influencing a client to make or change a legal document;*
(f) *abandoning a client;*
(g) *neglecting to provide care to a client;*
(h) *failing to exercise appropriate discretion with respect to the disclosure of confidential information;*
(j) *falsifying records;*
(k) *inappropriately using licensing status for personal gain;*
(l) *promoting for personal gain any drug, device, treatment, procedure, product or service that is unnecessary, ineffective or unsafe;*
(m) *publishing, or causing to be published, any advertisement that is false, fraudulent, deceptive or misleading;*
(n) *engaging or assisting in fraud, misrepresentation, deception or concealment of a material fact when applying for or securing registration or a licence to practise or taking any examination provided for in this Act, including using fraudulently procured credentials; and*

(o) *taking or using a designation or a derivation or abbreviation thereof, or describing the person's activities as "nursing" in any advertisement or publication, including business cards, websites or signage, unless the referenced activity falls within the practice of nursing;*

Similar principles apply to all regulatory bodies across the country.

Malpractice

Malpractice does not necessarily include professional misconduct but, rather, involves the negligent performance of acts in a manner that does not conform to a generally recognized practice, such as standards of care in the nursing profession. Nurses can perform lawful acts in a way that does not involve any professional misconduct, but might perform such an act or function in a way that is careless or lacking in skill and that could lead to harm or injury to a patient or otherwise compromise a patient's course of treatment or health. For example, consider the nurse who fails to document and flag that a person is allergic to an antibiotic. A urinary tract infection develops, and the patient requires antibiotics. However, the patient is no longer alert, and the team cannot confirm allergies, so assuming the patient has none, they go ahead and administer the drug, which causes anaphylaxis. Also consider a nurse working in the neonatal intensive care unit (NICU) of a busy teaching hospital, educated in the latest therapies and medications in this specialty. A court might find that such a person would be held to a higher standard of care with respect to the care provided in this setting than a nurse working in a general setting.

CIVIL LIABILITY: IMPLICATIONS FOR NURSING

In Chapter 4, *civil law* is described as the body of rules and legal principles that govern relations, respective rights, and obligations among individuals, corporations, or other institutions. It includes the law related to tort and negligence, as well as rights and obligations between individuals, and it regulates how these rules are preserved and enforced in the courts. Through the disciplinary process, regulatory bodies determine the extent to which nurses fail to meet standards of practice and impose appropriate penalties, which, in the extreme, may take away a person's ability to practise nursing. Civil law also ensures that a person who is wronged can seek redress or compensation.

A **tort** is a civil wrong committed by one person against another causing that other some injury or damage, either to person or property. Torts may be *intentional* or *nonintentional.* "Intentional" refers to a deliberate action even where unanticipated consequences occur. An assault is an example of an intentional tort, in that the person who commits it intends the action that causes harm to the victim. Nonintentional torts generally constitute negligence.

In Quebec, torts are called **delicts** and come within the Civil Code provisions dealing with obligations. Specific provisions of the Civil Code define and govern the concept of delicts and the elements that must be proven in court for a party who has been injured to recover damages. Under the Civil Code, anyone under a duty not to cause harm to another fails in that duty by not acting according to the expected standard of care.

Intentional Torts

Battery

Of particular importance to the nursing profession is the concept of battery. Much of a nurse's work involves the physical touching of patients—for example, administering injections, suturing wounds, establishing intravenous lines, physically moving patients, and other invasive measures—procedures that may be done only with the consent of the patient. Treatment performed without consent is battery. Blood transfusions, injections, examinations, and diagnostic imaging are examples of interventions that would be considered battery if performed without consent and would entitle the patient to compensation.

Battery is defined in common law as intentionally bringing about a harmful or offensive and nonconsensual contact upon another (Fleming, 1983, p. 23; see also Linden, 2018). An obvious example of battery would be one person striking another. The harmful or offensive contact may be either direct, such as a slap in the face, or indirect, such as pulling on a person's chair, causing a fall. (Linden, 2018). In either case, there has been an *intentional* interference with the bodily integrity and security of another.

Moreover, these acts are seen as potentially leading to further violence because the victim may be provoked into retaliation. An aim of tort law is to prevent violence by making perpetrators of such acts civilly liable to their victims for damages. The law is also concerned with the need to restore the victim of the wrong to the situation prior to the battery, as much as is possible, through the award of monetary damages.

The offensive or intrusive conduct need not be violent, as even seemingly insignificant unwanted touching may amount to battery. The perpetrator need not intend any harmful result. Thus, even a pat on the back may amount to battery if it is not consented to by the recipient.

However, certain common, everyday acts will not usually amount to battery. For instance, the custom of shaking hands is not considered battery. One need not ask another's permission before shaking hands; consent would be implied by the holding out of one's hand. It must be noted, however, that in a diverse society, such as Canada's, nurses must be respectful of cultures that might not welcome such conduct. Further, the COVID-19 pandemic elevated concerns regarding infection control, so this may also influence a person's response. There is also the special consideration of nurses who care for children. Appropriate cuddling and holding, depending on the child's developmental age, is often essential to their care and well-being.

As mentioned treatment without consent is batter. Claims arising from battery are easier to prove than claims of negligence because the issue is not whether the treatment involved reasonable care but only that the touching occurred without consent. The health care professional must provide evidence that consent was obtained, and if not, is liable for all the direct consequences of the battery. The absence of consent creates a much larger risk for health care practitioners than negligence. Even if the patient suffers no harm and may even have benefited from the treatment, damages may be granted for mental distress and upset suffered by patients when they learn that they were treated without consent. Consider, for example, *Mohsina v. Ornstein* (2013). In this case, the patient had consented to surgery to treat ovarian cysts and during the operation, the surgeon had clipped the patient's left fallopian tube believing that any chance of pregnancy was already compromised. The patient claimed that the

procedure, as carried out, went beyond the scope of the consent given (consent was for biopsy or cutting adhesions). The court agreed that when the doctor knew that this patient was unwilling to consent to a procedure, the doctor should not ignore this knowledge and act without concern for the patient's instructions. The court found that the actions of the doctor constituted battery and entitled the patient to damages.

Consent

Consent to treatment is discussed fully in Chapter 6, but since its relevance to the discussion of torts is significant, it is summarized here.

Generally, if the aggrieved person has consented to a specific action or conduct, the perpetrator may escape liability for such conduct if they use generally accepted practices and procedures and do not go beyond the limits of the consent given. In *Mohsina*, the patient wanted to become pregnant again and wanted to ensure the surgery would not prevent this. The surgeon's action in clipping the fallopian tube and making pregnancy impossible was beyond the limits of the consent. If the action had been required by an emergency, the consent would have been sufficient.

Consent, which can be defined as permission given by persons for someone else to perform an act upon them, may be *explicit* (expressed) or *implied* by the circumstances or by the conduct of the aggrieved person. Expressed consent may be given orally or in writing. The written consent is not consent in and of itself but, rather, is evidence that the party giving it has consented to an act.

Implied consent is agreement to an act inferred from the actions of the recipient. An example of implied consent in a health care setting is a patient's holding out an arm to a nurse to have their blood pressure checked. A reasonable person would infer from the patient's conduct that consent had been given. This illustrates another aspect of implied consent—that is, the existence of consent is measured against an **objective standard**.

Where a dispute occurs over implied consent, usually the issue will turn on the quality of the evidence available to the health care practitioner. Because these disputes will be assessed years after the events in issue occurred, it is critical that consent be documented in writing, either by getting signed consent or by recording, at the time, the words and actions that implied consent and the names of any witnesses present.

For consent to be valid in law, the person giving it must be capable of doing so. In the case of a cognitively impaired patient, consent to treatment may or may not be valid, depending on whether that patient is able to appreciate the nature, quality, and consequences of the proposed treatment. Children under the age of majority (or under 16 years of age, in some provinces) usually cannot consent to treatment, in which case their parents or legal guardians would be called upon to give consent. However, if the child is mature enough to understand the nature and risks of the proposed treatment, the caregiver or the institution may rely upon that consent or assent (agreement by the child that treatment may proceed on the basis of informed consent from parents).

Consent will be invalidated if it was obtained by force or fraud. Coercion or the use of force invalidates any consent as recipients are obviously not deciding of their own free will. Only a freely given and voluntary consent is valid in law.

In the context of health care, it is important to remember that no treatment, no matter how crucial to the health or survival of the patient, may be ad-

ministered without that patient's consent, unless the situation is life-threatening and the patient is unconscious or mentally incompetent (e.g., see Saskatchewan's *Emergency Medical Aid Act,* 1978). Statutes, such as the *Emergency Medical Aid Act,* permit a registered nurse (RN) to administer emergency medical treatment to an unconscious person involved in an accident without incurring liability for negligence as a result of an act or omission on their part. It does not, however, excuse the nurse from *gross negligence*—that is, conduct that drastically departs from the standard of the reasonably competent nurse.

In a clinical setting, only that specific treatment that is consented to may be administered, and in most cases, only those health care professionals specified in the patient's consent may administer the consented-to treatment. The patient's consent must also be informed. This means that the nature of the treatment to be administered, its benefits and attendant risks, and any and all material information must be given to the patient for the consent to be valid.

Nonintentional Torts

Consider Case Scenario 7.1 as concepts related to negligence are explored.

CASE SCENARIO 7.1

ACCOUNTABILITY?

Several nurses in a nursing team rotate through the same schedule in a busy critical care unit (CCU) of a major hospital. One of the nurses, K. L., has recently been under extreme personal stress because of the breakup of a relationship and the death of a close family member.

Over the past 4 to 5 weeks, colleagues have noticed that occasionally K. L. arrived for the night shift smelling of alcohol. When the other nurses raised their concerns, K. L. admitted to having a glass or two of wine over dinner with some friends. As the weeks go by, these incidents increase in frequency. At times, K. L.'s speech seems slurred. The other nurses on the team hesitate to report these incidents to the nurse manager because they do not wish to add to K. L.'s stress. They hope that when these personal

challenges are addressed this issue will resolve itself. To protect K. L. and to minimize the risks to patients, the nurses in charge give K. L. easy assignments and send them on a break whenever the night supervisor visits the unit.

In this CCU, nurses are expected to have and to use specialized skills and to perform certain delegated medical acts. As well, under the hospital's nursing standards policy, each nurse is subject to an annual review of knowledge and skills. K. L. is 3 months overdue for this review. The unit educator has scheduled it three times, but on each occasion, K. L. has cancelled, citing illness or heavy workload. It is unclear when this review can be rescheduled because, as a result of budget cuts, the number of educators has been reduced.

One night, when K. L. again arrives smelling of alcohol, K. L. is assigned a patient who is relatively

Continued on following page

CASE SCENARIO 7.1 *(Continued)*

stable. Shortly after the shift begins, K. L. notices on the monitor that this patient is having episodes of a cardiac arrhythmia, which she identifies as ventricular tachycardia. Nurses in the CCU have been delegated the act of administering lidocaine, a drug that treats such an arrhythmia, so K. L. prepares and administers a bolus intravenously. A few minutes later, the patient has a respiratory and cardiac arrest. Fortunately, resuscitation is successful.

Upon further review, it is noted that the patient had, in fact, experienced supraventricular tachycardia, for which lidocaine is not indicated. Furthermore, another nurse noticed that the label on the ampoule indicated that it contained pancuronium, not lidocaine. These drugs are contained in similar-sized ampoules, and the lettering is the same colour. Pancuronium causes temporary paralysis and is used during general anaesthesia or, sometimes, for patients who are being mechanically ventilated in the CCU. Clearly, the drug led to the patient's cardiac arrest. Subsequently, it was discovered that the pancuronium ampoules had been placed in the wrong container, which was labelled *lidocaine*.

Issues

1. Do the nurses in the unit have an obligation to "blow the whistle" and report K. L. on the suspicion of alcohol use? Are they able to evaluate the risk K. L. poses to patients?
2. What are K.L.'s responsibilities for reviewing their knowledge and skills? What are the hospital's responsibilities?
3. Does the educator have any responsibility for ensuring that K. L.'s review takes place?
4. What responsibility, if any, does the second nurse have to report that the incorrect drug was given?
5. Does the charge nurse have any specific accountability or duty that is distinct from that of the other nurses?
6. Does the hospital have any obligation to disclose the occurrence to the family of the patient (and to the patient)?
7. Is K. L., the hospital, and the nursing team at risk of any legal, civil, or criminal actions against them?
8. Should any disciplinary action be taken with K. L. and her colleagues?

9. Is the fact that the pancuronium ampoules were placed in the wrong container a contributing factor?
10. How accountable are hospitals for making resource allocation decisions that ensure the provision of safe patient care?

Discussion

This scenario highlights a number of significant ethical and legal challenges. What is a nurse's ethical and legal responsibility when a colleague demonstrates incapacity or incompetence? What is the individual professional's responsibility to maintain competence, and what is the organization's responsibility to ensure the overall competence of staff? Further, what are nurses' responsibilities with regard to colleagues who are in need of help?

As noted in the CNA *Code of Ethics for Registered Nurses,* nurses have a responsibility to safeguard the quality of nursing care that patients receive. The code states:

> *Nurses question and intervene to address unsafe, non-compassionate, unethical or incompetent practice or conditions that interfere with their ability to provide safe, compassionate, competent and ethical care to those to whom they are providing care, and they support those who do the same. (CNA, 2017, p. 8)*

Therefore, nurses must take preventive and corrective action to protect patients from unsafe, incompetent, or unethical care. They must ensure that they have the skills and knowledge to remain competent. When they suspect unethical, incompetent, or unsafe care, or doubt the safety of conditions in the care setting, they must take the appropriate steps to resolve the problem.

It is clear, then, that when a nurse becomes aware of incompetence on the part of another nurse or other health care professional, that nurse is obligated to take action to ensure the safety of patients. When a nurse fails to take such action, then that nurse is also accountable for any subsequent consequences of that incompetence.

Delegation of added responsibilities to nurses should be appropriate, and processes must be in place to ensure ongoing competence with respect

CASE SCENARIO 7.1 *(Continued)*

to these responsibilities. In this scenario, K. L., and colleagues, and the educator also had a professional responsibility to ensure that patients continually received competent care.

Nurses have a responsibility to maintain their professional competence by meeting at least the minimum standards required by their regulatory body. When the health care facilities that employ them, such as hospitals or community agencies, impose a higher standard, then these higher standards must be met. In this case, both K. L. and the hospital bear the responsibility for ensuring her competence. The leadership within any organization must take steps to ensure the competence of its employees. If the employee does not respond to a requirement for reassessment or **recertification**, then reminders, counselling, and (if required) disciplinary action must take place.

Nurses are required to collaborate with one another to ensure the care environment is consistent with safe and ethical practice and to provide mentoring and guidance to ensure the continued competency and professional development of not only students but also practising nurses. This is of particular importance in highly technical critical care environments, where patients are most vulnerable and at risk of serious harm if not cared for by highly competent professionals.

What might have caused or contributed to K. L.'s behaviour? Did her colleagues understand the professional and legal consequences of her behaviour? Were they aware of the warning signs that K. L. was in crisis and needed help? K. L.'s colleagues, aware of these personal challenges, thought they were protecting her. They seemed to be hoping that this crisis would resolve itself and made efforts to shield K. L.

from further harm. Although one might sympathize with their concern, their strategy was counterproductive to K. L.'s needs, placed the lives of patients in jeopardy, and compromised their own professional integrity.

Nurses function within a highly stressful work environment. (In Chapter 11, the importance of a healthy work environment is discussed in detail.) When personal problems add to this stress, some nurses, like others in society, may become susceptible to substance abuse, such as alcohol or drugs, when seeking short-term relief from their problems. In fact, nurses may be more at risk for abuse given their easy access to controlled substances, such as narcotics. There are programs and support available for nurses facing addiction and emotional challenges (Dunn, 2005). K. L.'s colleagues, have a responsibility both to K. L. and to the patients to take their concerns to their leaders. An engaged and astute manager should also recognize K. L.'s need for help.

Early intervention in such situations can avoid risks to safe patient care, and to putting the nurse's career in jeopardy.

This scenario raises additional questions regarding the organization's accountability. The institution is responsible for assessing the competence of staff and also for ongoing staff development and learning. Furthermore, although it appears that K. L. failed to read the label accurately, the hospital should address the systems and processes that contributed to error. For example, when high-risk medications have a similar "look," additional precautions such as storing such medications in different locations, or posting signs to alert nurses to potential risks, should be considered.

Negligence

Negligence is a category of nonintentional tort. A nurse may still have liability to another even where no harm or injury was intended. For a defendant to be liable for negligence, three elements must be present (Linden, 2018). These are summarized in Table 7.1. If these three elements can be proven by the plaintiff on

a balance of probabilities, then the plaintiff is entitled to compensation.

To use a nursing example, a nurse owes a duty of care to a patient when administering a medication. Suppose the nurse misreads the label on a bottle containing a certain medication. What if the medication administered is, in fact, one that the patient is highly

TABLE 7.1

The Elements of Negligence

1. Duty of care owed to the plaintiff (e.g., a patient).
2. Breach of duty of care by the defendant (e.g., a nurse or physician) by failure to administer treatment or provide health care in accordance with a particular standard of care.
3. Patient suffers damage as a direct result of the breach of the duty of care.

allergic to? In reading the medication label incorrectly and failing to note that the patient is allergic to the medication, legally, the nurse has breached the duty owed to that patient. As a result of that breach, the patient receives a harmful substance and suffers a severe allergic reaction, which, in turn, causes brain damage. The patient's brain damage is a direct and foreseeable result of that breach.

Factors that help determine whether a defendant (the nurse) will be held liable (responsible) in a case of negligence include duty of care, standard of care, proximate cause, and contributory negligence. A case from Ontario serves to illustrate the application of these concepts in a health care setting. In *Latin v. Hospital for Sick Children et al.* (2007), a 14-month-old girl presented to a pediatric hospital in late January 1998 with a very high fever. It appeared that the infant had been suffering from croup for a month before her admission. On the day before her admission, the mother had called her family pediatrician about her daughter's high fever and was given an appointment for the following day. In the evening, the child was restless with fever, was not eating or drinking well, and wanted only to be held. The following day, the child's body jerked violently while she was sitting on her grandmother's lap. The mother eventually reached the family physician, who told her he thought the child was experiencing febrile seizures, that she might be dehydrated, and that it was better for her to be assessed at the hospital. She was taken to the hospital's emergency department, where, according to the hospital's triage classification system ("emergent," "urgent," and "nonurgent"), she was assessed as urgent and sent back to the waiting area. Her mother was advised to bring her child back to the triage nurse if her condition changed.

Ninety minutes after arriving at the emergency department, while still in the waiting area, and before a medical assessment had been done, the child began to have a generalized **tonic-clonic seizure**. She was immediately taken into a treatment room, where the team attempted to bring her seizure under control. Despite these efforts, seizure activity continued for more than 90 minutes. After about 5 hours, the child was transferred to the pediatric intensive care unit (PICU) of the hospital. An electroencephalograph (EEG) was performed the following day and showed a result consistent with diffuse encephalopathy.

Three days later, the infant was more alert, able to move all four limbs normally, and had no further seizure activity. She was transferred from the PICU to a general unit, but approximately 2 hours later, she began to have more seizures. Over a period of 8 hours, at least seven seizures were noted, and she was transferred back to the PICU, where she was unresponsive and demonstrated decreased power on her right side and abnormal movements.

A computed tomography (CT) scan showed diffuse cerebral edema, primarily in the frontal regions of her brain. She was discharged some weeks later to a rehabilitation facility, without confirmation of the cause of her brain injury that had resulted in profound brain damage and extreme and permanent disabilities.

The child in this case was a healthy, normally developing infant when she was brought to the emergency department of the hospital, and at the time of the lawsuit, she was 9 years of age and very disabled (*Latin v. Hospital for Sick Children et al.,* 2007, paras. 19–21). (Note: Litigation of complex medical malpractice cases will often take many years to complete.)

The infant's mother and grandparents brought the lawsuit against the hospital, the triage nurse, the charge nurse on duty that day, several other nurses involved in the child's treatment in the emergency department, the child's family physician, and the physicians at the hospital who had been involved in her care. The lawsuit against the doctors was discontinued before the trial (likely because the claim against the doctors was settled or withdrawn by the plaintiffs). A diagnosis as to what caused the child's brain damage was never made, but the parties in the lawsuit advanced numerous theories to explain the injury.

It must be noted that when a claim is made against a health care practitioner in negligence, the action is brought by the injured person and often their family.

These are the plaintiffs. The plaintiffs make a claim against all of the persons potentially responsible for their injuries. This ensures that as facts emerge, the plaintiffs can be sure that the responsible parties will appear before the court. Typically, in a claim arising out of a hospital visit, the defendants will include the hospital, the physicians, the nurses, other professional staff involved in the care of the patient, and, in some cases, the manufacturers of medications, medical equipment, and training materials.

The lawsuit brought by the child's family against the hospital, the triage nurse, and the charge nurse proceeded to trial. Their claim was that when they first presented at the emergency department, the girl was in a state of "early/compensated distributive shock due to sepsis as a result of bacterial pneumonia" (*Latin v. Hospital for Sick Children et al.,* 2007, para. 23). They alleged that this infection was not noticed by the team because the triage nurse had taken an inadequate history of the child. Furthermore, they alleged that the infant later progressed to a state of shock and that the medical team then tried to control the seizures, rather than managing the shock and ensuring that her brain was receiving an adequate supply of oxygen. They alleged that as a result of this, she suffered a hypoxic–ischemic brain injury. They had a number of experts testify on their behalf at the trial with respect to the level of nursing (among other medical) care the child received during treatment. Their experts alleged that the girl had been incorrectly classified as an "urgent" rather than an "emergent" case. As an emergent case, they claimed, she would have been seen sooner by a physician, who would have recognized that she was in shock and taken measures before decompensation occurred (*Latin v. Hospital for Sick Children et al.,* 2007, para. 24).

The hospital, on its own behalf and on behalf of the nurses involved in the infant's care, alleged that her brain damage was caused by an infectious process in her brain (in all likelihood, influenza A virus), which was not considered an explanation for her brain damage at the time of her hospitalization. With subsequent increased knowledge of influenza A in the years since the events in question, it is now known that this was the viral agent that caused the infection, but this would not have been detected with the knowledge available at the time. No treatment available then could have reversed this process. The plaintiff's shock theory was not supported by the evidence available, and even if the child had been classified as an emergent case and seen immediately by a doctor, no useful treatment could have been administered before the seizures began (*Latin v. Hospital for Sick Children et al.,* 2007, para. 26).

The court first had to determine the appropriate standard of care owed to the child by the nurses and the hospital. The girl's family alleged that the nursing care had fallen below the required standard and that this had resulted in her brain damage. The court determined the appropriate standard of care in this situation from several sources, including the testimony of nursing experts, the hospital's own written policies, information given to members of the public on procedures in the emergency department, nursing manuals and academic literature, and the testimony of physicians who were knowledgeable in emergency medicine (*Latin v. Hospital for Sick Children et al.,* 2007, para. 31).

The court found that the triage nurse (who was one of the nurses being sued) had met the standard of care expected of her in assessing the case as urgent rather than emergent. She had conducted an assessment of suitable length (5 minutes), and there was no evidence that the length of the assessment had any bearing on the standard of care. She had not taken the child's blood pressure or respiration rate on triage; however, the child was crying at the time, and the nurse had noted this on the triage form. The child's crying, the court noted from expert evidence, would have naturally prevented the nurse from being able to obtain a meaningful respiration rate or blood pressure (*Latin v. Hospital for Sick Children et al.,* 2007, para. 67).

In terms of the alleged failure of the triage nurse to record the child's respiration rate, the court concluded, on the basis of the evidence available and a review of the child's medical and emergency department nursing records, that there was nothing at the time to alert that nurse to any breathing difficulty in the child. Even the child's mother testified that she did not note any breathing difficulty in the child (*Latin v. Hospital for Sick Children et al.,* 2007, para. 80). The court finally concluded that with respect to the triage nurse's conduct, she had correctly exercised her clinical judgement in assessing the girl as an urgent case. Determining this classification was a function that fell within a nurse's clinical judgement, and in this case, it was in accordance with the hospital's own triage classification policy and was, on the available evidence, a reasonable and appropriate decision (*Latin v. Hospital for Sick Children et al.,* 2007, paras. 100–109). Even if the triage nurse's conclusion was wrong, she had appropriately exercised her judgement about the seriousness of the girl's condition. The court concluded that she had met the standard of care of a reasonable and prudent nurse in acting as she did then and in her subsequent reassessment of the child. The court noted, in passing, that the nurse should have documented the reassessment results but that her failure to do so did not amount to negligence (*Latin v. Hospital for Sick Children et al.,* 2007, para. 109).

The court also considered the conduct of the charge nurse. The child's family alleged that she had failed to meet the standard of care because examination rooms were available at the time the child arrived in the emergency department and yet the child was not sent to one of them; she allowed a more stable patient in the urgent category and a nonurgent patient to be seen ahead of this child (*Latin v. Hospital for Sick Children et al.,* 2007, para. 110). The evidence of the physicians and nursing experts indicated that the charge nurse's evaluation of when it would be appropriate to send patients to an examination room from the waiting room was a complex process. Availability of rooms was only one of the factors; other factors included availability of physicians; support staff, including discharge planners to assist patients about to be discharged; and cleaning staff to prepare rooms for new patients (*Latin v. Hospital for Sick Children et al.,* 2007, para. 112). On this point, the court found that although it would be inexcusable to keep patients waiting if a treatment room was available, there was nothing in the evidence to suggest that the child could have been seen any earlier. The presented evidence fell short of establishing that appropriate resources were available before then such as to indicate that the charge nurse had failed to assign the child to a treatment room at an earlier time (*Latin v. Hospital for Sick Children et al.,* 2007, para. 118). There was also no evidence that the child was critically ill before 1400 hours or that her condition was precarious. The charge nurse reprioritized patients in the emergency department as situations changed to ensure that available resources were assigned to the most serious cases. The court held that deference had

to be shown to the judgement of those who manage work in an emergency department—in this case, the charge nurse. The court concluded that the charge nurse had met the standard of care of a reasonable and prudent charge nurse that day (*Latin v. Hospital for Sick Children et al.,* 2007, para. 126).

Duty of Care

To be liable in tort, a defendant must owe a **duty of care** to the plaintiff, either personally or as a member of a class of persons, such as patients seeking health care or perhaps school children being transported to school on school buses (where the driver, the school, the school board, and the bus manufacturer, among others, would owe a duty of care to the children). The law imposes a duty of care in many, but not all, situations. If there is no duty of care in law, the defendant will not be liable to the plaintiff, even if the defendant's conduct was the immediate cause of the plaintiff's injuries. See, for example, *Hubley v. Hubley Estate* (2011), where the Prince Edward Island Court of Appeal held that a husband who died as a result of his own negligent driving owed no duty of care to his wife to not drive negligently. The wife had suffered considerable financial hardship as a result of the death of the husband but could not sue him (and his motor vehicle insurer) for negligence.

As we saw in the *Latin v. Hospital for Sick Children et al.* (2007), nurses have a special relationship with those whom they serve, and it is thus desirable to impose on them a duty of care (Linden, 2018). They have special education and expertise and are required to exercise a very high degree of care when practising as a nurse.

STATUTORY DUTIES. Most provincial nursing statutes explicitly or implicitly impose certain duties on nurses. Among these is the duty to report a fellow nurse whose conduct displays a lack of proper skill, judgement, knowledge, or training. (See, for example, Saskatchewan's *Registered Nurses Act,* 1988, s. 26(2)k; and Manitoba's The *Regulated Health Professions Act,* C.C.S.M., c. R117, s. 138(1)) This also includes, in many provinces, a duty to report a nurse who is under the influence of alcohol or drugs.

Thus, in Case Scenario 7.1, K. L.'s colleagues clearly have demonstrated professional misconduct by failing to report incidents of intoxication (which would be deemed unprofessional conduct under the Nova Scotia statute, for example). In covering up a potentially harmful situation, they are ethically, and probably legally, liable for any harm to patients that may arise.

Because K. L. is presenting as a qualified health care practitioner, she owes a duty of care to all of their patients. This duty has been described in law as "the duty to exercise a reasonable degree of skill, knowledge and care in the treatment of a patient" (*Thompson Estate v. Byrne et al.*, 1993, p. 423). K. L. has breached her duty not to practise when her ability to do so was impaired by alcohol.

DUTY OF CARE IN EMERGENCIES. There is no general duty to aid someone in peril except in Quebec (Linden et al., 2018, pp. 113, 121). This absence is one illustration of the potential divergence between the law and ethics. What may clearly be a moral or ethical imperative may not necessarily be a legal requirement.

For example, in common law provinces, a passerby may observe a person in cardiac arrest and not render assistance. Where there is a positive duty to act, a failure to act or a failure to act in good faith may constitute a crime *Criminal Code* (1985), section 215 (Duty of persons to provide necessaries); section 218 (Abandoning child); section 216 ("Duty of persons undertaking acts dangerous to life" [to use reasonable skill and care in so doing]), and section 217, which reads: "Every one who undertakes to do an act is under a legal duty to do it if an omission to do the act is or may be dangerous to life."

Absent a positive duty, many people acting morally, would likely intervene to save a person in obvious danger. If someone does act, the law imposes a duty of care to not conduct such a rescue negligently. A person who fails in a rescue bid may be civilly liable for any injury or death resulting to the person being rescued (Linden, 2018). Usually, however, for the rescuer to be found liable, their conduct must amount to gross negligence—that is, a substantial and marked departure from the standard of the reasonably competent and skilled rescuer.

Breach of the Standard of Care

How do courts determine whether or not a defendant's conduct has been negligent? Common law has developed the concept of the **standard of care** as an objective measure of such conduct. If a defendant's conduct is seen as having fallen below the standard of what a competent person, acting reasonably and responsibly in similar circumstances, would have followed, a court may find that defendant's conduct to be negligent. In *Latin v. Hospital for Sick Children et al.* (2007), the standard was determined by means of the expert testimony of nurses about the standards of the regulatory body, as well as by the standards and policies within the organization, emergency physicians, and literature and documentation illustrating hospital policies and procedures. The particular standard against which any given conduct is judged will vary, depending on the circumstances and people involved. For example, a doctor will be judged by the standard of the reasonably competent physician. Similarly, a nurse's conduct in the treatment of a patient who has suffered harm as a result of their acts or omissions will be judged by the standard of the reasonably competent nurse.

In any negligence lawsuit involving a nurse or other health care professional, the trial will essentially amount to an evaluation of the nurse's conduct and the degree to which an objective standard of care has been met. The nurse is legally required to operate and act at a level that meets or exceeds the standard of care of a reasonably prudent caregiver or health care professional. This, of course, implies that the nurse has a duty to maintain a level of expertise through continuing education to ensure a practice in accordance with current standards. For example, it would be inappropriate for a nurse educated in the 1990s to continue to practise according to the standards of that decade. Furthermore, the nurse must meet or exceed the standards established by the regulatory body regarding continuing education and quality assurance. Any failure to comply with the standards of the profession or the policies and procedures of an employer may constitute evidence that a nurse is not operating in a reasonable and prudent manner.

In Case Scenario 7.1, apart from the fact that K. L. was practising while under the influence of alcohol, of concern is the issue of mistakenly identifying the arrhythmia as ventricular tachycardia when, in fact, the patient was experiencing supraventricular tachycardia. If a reasonable and prudent nurse in similar circumstances would not have made this mistake, then legally K. L. has breached the standard of care.

The nurses in the *Latin* case were judged according to the average standards of triage and charge nurses—that is, having reasonable knowledge, skill, and ability related to these roles. These would also include the standards of competence and knowledge set by the governing body for nurses in the province and any applicable standards prescribed by the health care facility where that nurse is employed. Such standards also include the requirement to have current knowledge of the latest professional and technological developments. Additional education should be taken, as required, to maintain expertise to the appropriate standard. A professional who fails to be up to date with regard to new knowledge and standards runs the risk of employing methods that have been discredited or proven harmful by the latest research and thinking in that field. If that professional's conduct were ever called into question, such failure would be evidence of negligence.

THE STANDARD OF CARE AND CAUSATION. As seen in *Latin v. Hospital for Sick Children et al.* (2007), in legal proceedings, the nurse's practice is examined and compared with normal, competent, and reasonable standards of nursing practice to determine whether the conduct in question conformed with that expected of a reasonably competent and skilled nurse. Of course, standards change over time as new knowledge and technology are introduced and become widely available. Standards also differ from one institution to another and from one treatment setting to another. For example, the standards and expectations of a nurse in a critical care unit will differ from those of a nurse in a rehabilitation setting. Patients have the right to expect that a nurse employed in the critical care unit will have the specialized knowledge and skills required to provide the necessary care. In Case Scenario 7.1, the fact that K. L. administered the wrong drug (and, even if it had been the drug intended, one that was not indicated for this patient's condition) shows that K. L. did not meet the basic standard of care with respect to the administration of medication (i.e., checking the label carefully before administering the drug) and thus breached the common law duty to provide reasonably competent, knowledgeable, and skilled nursing care to the patient. K. L. was, therefore, negligent.

Many hospitals and other health care facilities that employ nurses have policies and procedures in place for an annual review of the nurses' skills and competencies. This practice would be recognized as evidence of the appropriate standard of care in any negligence

suit brought against such an institution. The institution is responsible for ensuring that these reviews take place, and nurses who fail to participate in them are opening themselves up to liability. In *Latin v. Hospital for Sick Children et al.* (2007), for example, the defendant hospital had written policies in place that were admitted into evidence and carefully considered by the trial judge in determining the appropriate standard of care with respect to the triage classification of a patient presenting in the emergency department as "emergent," "urgent," or "nonurgent" (*Latin v. Hospital for Sick Children et al.,* 2007, paras. 33–35).

In Case Scenario 7.1, nurses in the CCU were expected to perform certain specialized medical acts, including the interpretation of arrhythmias and, when required, the administration of lidocaine. K. L.'s competence and knowledge regarding the interpretation of arrhythmias should have been assessed on a regular basis. The failure to do this may have led K. L. to conclude that lidocaine was indicated when it was not.

Employers also have the common law duty to take active steps to ensure that nurses who fail to meet a standard receive the appropriate improvement plan. Such steps may include counselling, additional education, and, in some cases, disciplinary measures. This duty includes ensuring that the nurse's skills are reviewed on a regular basis (although the nurse also has such a duty). In K. L.'s case, counselling or substance abuse treatment would be in order, but the hospital may have to resort to disciplinary measures if K. L. persistently fails to meet the expected standards of practice. Such ongoing assessment of nurses' competence is a priority, and cuts based on financial constraints would not be a defensible excuse for failing to have systematic reviews.

In some institutions, the review of skills is completely the responsibility of the nurse, and appropriate action must be taken against the nurse if such expectations are not met. If this is the case, this stipulation should be made explicit at the outset of the nurse's employment.

Finally, K. L. breached the professional obligation not to work while impaired. All provincial and territorial nursing statutes prohibit a nurse from working while impaired. In fact, in Ontario and Saskatchewan, practising nursing while one's ability to do so is impaired by any substance constitutes professional misconduct (*Professional Misconduct, O. Reg. 799/93* [Ontario]; *The Registered Nurses Act*, 1988, s. 26(2)(k) [Saskatchewan]). It would also likely constitute misconduct under the legislation of the remaining provinces and territories (even though these statutes do not expressly refer to impairment of the nurse while on duty) because it would adversely influence the nurse's ability to practise safely and properly. It may also constitute a threat to the safety of patients.

Furthermore, K. L.'s fellow nurses may also be considered negligent. Because they were aware of the possible impairment they may, in permitting K. L. to continue to provide care, be contributing to the risk of injury to patients. It is clearly their professional and ethical duty to alert the manager of the issue. In some cases, failure to report improper, negligent, or unethical conduct could, in and of itself, constitute professional misconduct. The matter, in most cases, will then be taken up according to the disciplinary procedures and mechanisms of the provincial regulatory body (as discussed in Chapter 5).

Standards of care provide a baseline for assessment, planning, decision making, and action. They help ensure the provision of safe and efficient nursing care within the health care facility. Case Scenario 7.1 illustrates two crucial duties that the nurse must discharge properly: (1) the correct assessment of a patient's condition, and (2) the administration of the correct medication, if required. Also, it is a critical duty of the institution to ensure nurses are competent to practise and that their competence is reviewed on a regular basis.

CAUSATION AND HARM. A defendant will be liable for harm to a plaintiff if that harm was caused by the defendant's negligent conduct. This seems straightforward and logical. However, can a plaintiff be compensated for all possible harm that may occur as a result of the defendant's negligent act? Some results that follow negligent conduct can be so unlikely (i.e., removed from the foreseeable chain of events and consequences) that they should not be within the scope of what is compensable damage. To qualify as damage for which a plaintiff can recover compensation, damage must be something that a reasonable person could foresee as resulting from the negligent conduct—that is, the cause should be reasonably close (proximate) to,

or the reasonably foreseeable cause of, the ensuing damage.

In the *Latin* decision, the court applied the principle that if a defendant's negligence has caused or contributed to the plaintiff's injury and if that injury would not have occurred but for such negligence, the plaintiff has proved **causation**. The child's family in *Latin* alleged that it was a delay in diagnosing and treating the child that essentially caused her brain damage and that the delay was the result of the negligence of the triage nurse, the charge nurse, and other members of the health care team involved with the care in the emergency department. The court had three alternative theories about the causes of the child's brain injury: (1) idiopathic status epilepticus, (2) shock, and (3) viral encephalitis (*Latin v. Hospital for Sick Children et al.*, 2007, para. 148).

The court eventually found that the child's very high fever was caused by an underlying infection, but was unclear as to whether its source was bacterial or viral. The court, in the end, could not conclude whether, on a balance of probabilities (the civil standard of proof), the child's brain injury was caused by shock, a fever, or infection. Thus, the court could safely conclude that if the child was in a state of shock at triage, it was highly improbable that an emergent classification by the triage nurse would have resulted in any different treatment at that time. The nurses were, therefore, found not liable for the girl's injuries because nothing they did could have contributed to or caused those injuries.

Contributory Negligence

In earlier times, under common law, if plaintiffs were found to be partly at fault for the harm suffered (**contributorily negligent**), the law would deny them the right to recover **any** damages from the defendant. The consequences of this principle could be catastrophic for plaintiffs. The principle was changed by legislation to correct this unfairness. In Canada today, a plaintiff may recover damages even if partly at fault, but the damages awarded will be reduced by the percentage to which the plaintiff was to blame or contributed to the loss. (See, for example, Alberta's *Contributory Negligence Act*, 2000; and British Columbia's *Negligence Act*, 1996). Of course, if the evidence shows that the plaintiff was completely to blame for the harm, the plaintiff will have no claim. The court will apportion the liability among the parties—that is, it will determine, to the best of its ability, the percentage or proportion to which each party is to blame for the loss.

In this respect, the law is similar across Canada, including Quebec, where it is known as the *principle of common fault* (*Civil Code of Québec*, 1991; see also Linden, 2018).

CASE SCENARIO 7.1A

APPLICATION TO K. L.'S CASE SCENARIO

The analytical process that was applied in the *Latin v. Hospital for Sick Children et al.* (2007) decision will also apply in assessing K. L.'s conduct. K. L.s actions would be re-examined with the aid of expert testimony to determine whether and, if so, how the duty of care had been breached. As the hospital is under a duty to provide proper and competent medical and nursing staff to patients in its care (*Kolesar v. Jeffries,* 1976, p. 376), it also would likely be named as a defendant in any subsequent lawsuit if the patient had suffered harm.

K. L. and the hospital would be sued by the patient, their family, or their estate, if the patient subsequently died. The plaintiff might allege that K. L. had failed to meet the duty to the plaintiff and that the hospital had breached its duty to the patient to provide proper care by ensuring competent nursing and other health care staff were used to provide care. Thus, they could be held personally liable for any damage or injury caused by this negligence.

For example, the hospital may be considered negligent for failing to ensure adequate and safe emergency procedures and, in this case scenario, in failing to ensure that drugs were safely and properly stored (e.g., vials of pancuronium may have been placed in the container labelled "lidocaine"). The finding of liability is possible also because the hospital, through K. L.'s

supervisor, failed to ensure K. L. was competent and able to carry out these duties properly and effectively. K. L. was an employee of the hospital, and these actions were under its control. This is known as the *doctrine of vicarious liability,* where a person or entity is responsible for the negligence of persons under their care and control. This type of liability applies to employees, volunteers, and guardians of children, among others.

K. L. is under a duty to arrive at work in a fit and proper condition. K. L. clearly breached this duty in arriving at the hospital in an impaired state, and may have placed the patient in jeopardy and contributed to the risks of harm.

Another aspect of vicarious liability as it relates to hospitals is that physicians, who provide instructions to nursing staff in the care of their patients, are entitled to rely on the assumption that the hospital employs duly qualified and competent nurses. The doctors are not responsible for ensuring that nurses carry out their instructions properly unless they have actual knowledge that the nurses are not competent to carry out those instructions. Thus, in cases in which a claim of negligence is brought against physicians and their instructions were not properly followed, they may argue as a defence that the nurse was negligent. However, the instructions provided by the physician must not be negligent in and of themselves.

In summary, civil liability, the obligation to compensate another person, arises from three elements: the existence of a duty, a failure to meet that duty and a loss that is caused by that failure. In the complex world of health care, there are several duties owed to every patient, by the health care professionals in direct contact with the patient, by the agencies employing the health care professionals, by the manufacturers of equipment and medications, and by city planners and engineers who design the roads, just to name a few.

Logically, the best approach would be to just choose the persons most directly responsible and sue them. Two concerns result in many potential defendants being included in lawsuits. First, the actual causes of the plaintiff's loss and damages may be unknown or uncertain when the lawsuit is initiated. This is especially true in medical cases because health problems or issues can evolve over time. For example, consider a person who falls and sustains a knee fracture. The initial harm might involve pain, surgery, mobility challenges, and rehabilitation. Over time, arthritis may develop because of the injury, and the person may require knee replacement. The second factor is the existence of insurance. Each defendant may have available to them a pool of insurance, purchased individually or through their employer. The plaintiff's legal advisors would want to make sure that the defendants' insurance reserves are substantial enough to pay a claim. To ensure that the insurers for the hospitals are involved, plaintiffs frequently name any and all potentially responsible hospital staff, including nurses, as defendants. The concept of vicarious liability means that a breach of a duty by a nurse (in most cases) will result in the nurse's employer being liable.

Professional Liability Insurance

Many health care professionals who practise independently carry professional liability insurance to shield them from what may be financially catastrophic negligence claims. Physicians, for instance, carry insurance from the Canadian Medical Protective Association, a professional group insurer that offers liability insurance tailored to each physician's type and scope of practice.

Most nurses in Canada are employed by publicly funded health facilities, which carry negligence insurance. As mentioned above, health care facilities, as employers, are responsible ("vicariously liable") for the negligent acts of their employees. The employer institution's liability is not unlimited and extends only as far as the scope of the expressed or apparent authority of its employees. A nurse who performs acts outside the normal scope of nursing would not make the employer liable; the nurse would remain fully liable for negligence. Nurses should consider whether their employer has the appropriate liability insurance to meet possible claims. Most public institutions are backed by the governments and have sufficient resources, but small organizations not part of the public sector, such as volunteer clinics, charity-operated agencies, may not have the resources to respond to serious claims. Nurses may need insurance coverage to ensure adequate financial protection. The often-devastating consequences of liability claims to nurses without personal insurance can include bankruptcy, loss of professional status, and personal upheaval. Some provincial regulatory bodies now require nurses to obtain liability insurance to be able to cover potential claims. Coverage is available through

professional associations, private insurers, and the Canadian Nurses Protective Society. In addition to liability insurance, some issuers also offer insurance against disciplinary or professional misconduct claims.

Insurance coverage usually includes an obligation by the insurance company (usually referred to as the *insurer*) to defend the health care professional in any litigation involving allegations of negligence or malpractice. This means the insurer will retain and pay for the services of a lawyer to represent and defend the professional accused of negligent conduct. In some cases, the insurer will leave the choice of lawyer to the professional involved. Some policies, however, provide that the choice of lawyer and the source of the lawyer's instructions remain with the insurer. The professional is required to cooperate fully with the insurer in investigating and defending the claim, which may require attendance at meetings with insurance adjusters, claims representatives, and lawyers, as well as court appearances and examinations for discovery. Any insured professional who has knowledge of an actual or potential negligence claim is required to inform the insurer of the claim immediately and to cooperate fully with the insurer. Failure to follow the notice requirements of the insurance may lead to a refusal to provide indemnity.

Some insurance policies do not contain an obligation to defend and pay only for any negligence judgement ultimately pronounced against the professional. Therefore, in the meantime, the professional must hire and pay for their own lawyer to defend the negligence action, although these costs can be partially recovered from the plaintiff if the suit is unsuccessful.

CRIMINAL LAW SOURCES OF LIABILITY

Criminal law imposes significant consequences for nurses and other health care practitioners, who, in their professional roles, act carelessly or recklessly. The *Criminal Code* provisions concerning the legal duty of health care professionals to meet knowledge and competency standards are mentioned in Chapter 4. Section 216 of the *Criminal Code* (1985) states:

> *Everyone who undertakes to administer surgical or medical treatment to another person or to do any other lawful act that may endanger the life of*

another person is, except in cases of necessity, under a legal duty to have and to use reasonable knowledge, skill, and care in so doing.

This places an obligation on those who represent themselves as qualified and competent nurses to ensure that their qualifications are adequate to perform properly the treatment that they are called upon to administer. The section excludes "cases of necessity," which imply emergency or life-threatening situations. However, a nurse would not normally administer such treatment if a more qualified practitioner, such as a physician, were available to perform, for example, an emergency treatment. In the absence of a more qualified practitioner, a nurse, acting in good faith, and according to ability, could proceed. The legal policy here is to encourage people to render treatment to those in urgent need of it. In some extreme cases, such treatment could include a minor surgical procedure such as a tracheostomy.

Criminal Law Standard of Care

A person who represents herself or himself as a duly qualified health care practitioner will be held to the standard of the reasonably qualified practitioner if death, serious injury, or bodily harm ensues. In *R. v. Flynn* (2017), Justice Quinlan reviewed the standard of care in criminal negligence. The accused, Joanna Flynn, had been charged with manslaughter and criminal negligence causing death in relation to her termination of a patient's life support. After receiving information from other health care professionals and speaking with the patient's husband, Ms. Flynn discontinued the patient's life support without a doctor's order. Ms. Flynn admitted that by removing the patient from life support, she hastened the patient's death.

To prove criminal negligence causing bodily harm, the Crown must prove that:

> [13] a. *what Ms. Flynn did or failed to do showed a wanton or reckless disregard for the life or safety of Ms. Leblanc, and*
> b. *what Ms. Flynn did or failed to do was a marked and substantial departure from what a reasonably prudent nurse would do in the same circumstance. . . .*
> [15] *It is against the standard of a "reasonable person" that the jury will have to assess the dangerousness*

of any unlawful act. It is against the standard of a "reasonably prudent person" that the jury will have to assess whether Ms. Flynn's conduct was a marked and substantial departure from the norm. The "reasonable" or "reasonably prudent" person may be particularized to the circumstances of the accused and the nature of the conduct at issue. In this case, that may be the reasonable or reasonably prudent member of an ICU team, whether a nurse or health practitioner. (R. v. Flynn, 2017)

Ms. Flynn terminated the life support for Ms. Leblanc without a doctor's order. Her evidence was that she believed that Ms. Leblanc was brain dead, and that Mr. Leblanc was instructing her to cease life support. Although other physicians had concluded Ms. Leblanc was brain dead, the physician in charge on the night Ms. Leblanc died had not come to that conclusion himself. He had not met with the family, was not told by Ms. Flynn that life support was being terminated, and was surprised when advised that she had died. An expert testified that a patient like Ms. Leblanc should be kept on life support for at least 24 hours, as in rare cases some level of recovery occurred. Ms. Flynn took her action after about 16 hours. Ms. Flynn met with the family before life support was terminated. She discussed the process with them, answered their questions, shut down life support with the husband in the room, and stayed with the family in the room until Ms. Leblanc died. She reported the responsible physician for failing to deal with the family's desire to remove life support. She was terminated and a year later charged with manslaughter and criminal negligence causing death. The jury found Flynn not guilty on the criminal charges. Following her acquittal, she had a CNO disciplinary hearing and was suspended from practice for 5 months for turning off life support without the required medical authorization and failing to note that the responsible physician had not authorized the withdrawal of life support.

Criminal Negligence

Section 219 of the *Criminal Code* (1985) defines *criminal negligence* in this way:

Everyone is criminally negligent who (a) in doing anything, or (b) in omitting to do anything that it is his duty to do, shows wanton or reckless disregard for the lives or safety of other persons.

The "duty" of which this section speaks is a duty imposed by law, either by statute or common law (*R. v. Coyne*, 1958). This section must be understood in conjunction with section 217 of the Code, which states:

Everyone who undertakes to do an act is under a legal duty to do it if an omission to do the act is or may be dangerous to life.

Thus, if a nurse fails to perform an act that is part of expected nursing standards and duties, and, as a result, someone dies or suffers serious bodily harm, the nurse's omission may constitute a criminal offence of either criminal negligence causing death or criminal negligence causing bodily harm. Before this breach could be characterized as negligent, however, it would have to demonstrate a marked or substantial departure from the expectations required of a reasonable and competent nurse. There would have to be extreme carelessness or recklessness (i.e., a complete disregard for the consequences of one's actions); or such a grave or serious omission as to show that the nurse failed to recognize obvious risks; or, if aware of those risks, chose to take them anyway, "reckless" and oblivious to the consequences. Such a formulation in the law shows how extreme and outrageous carelessness must be to be judged criminally negligent.

In *R. v. J.F.* (2008), the Supreme Court discussed the essential elements of the offence of criminal negligence by omission. At paragraph 68, the Court wrote:

Turning to the offence of criminal negligence, the [criminal conduct] will be established if it is proved

(1) that the accused was under a legal duty to do something; (2) that, from an objective standpoint, he or she failed to perform the duty; and (3) that in failing to perform the duty, he or she showed, again from an objective standpoint, wanton or reckless disregard for the lives or safety of other persons. Proof of the [criminal intent] will flow from a finding that the conduct of the accused was wanton or reckless. Wanton or reckless behaviour has been equated with a marked and substantial departure from the norm, (H. Parent, Traité de droit criminel (2nd ed. 2007), vol. 2, at p. 299) which necessarily includes behaviour that constitutes a marked departure.

In the case scenario, K. L.'s intoxication and failure to realize the wrong drug was being administered might arguably be classified as reckless behaviour.

Necessity for Causation

By definition, criminal negligence must cause death (*Criminal Code*, 1985, s. 220) or bodily harm (s. 221) to another. That is, there must be a connection between the voluntary act of the accused and the outcome. So, for example, where an accused has consumed alcohol or drugs and becomes impaired, the accused may be found criminally negligent if someone is either hurt or killed in a motor vehicle accident. In such cases, the fact that the accused freely became intoxicated is evidence that may lead a court to decide that the driver acted with wanton or reckless disregard for the lives or safety of others (*R. v. Anderson*, 1985, p. 133). Intoxication is, therefore, a relevant factor in determining whether a person acted wantonly or recklessly.

CASE SCENARIO 7.1B

APPLICATION TO K. L.'S CASE SCENARIO

In this case, if the patient had died, the fact that the nurse was impaired would be relevant in a charge of criminal negligence causing death. The fact that being intoxicated rendered K. L. incapable of appreciating the probable consequences of these actions would not be a defence. Whether a conviction could

be successfully obtained, however, would depend on whether the mistake of administering the wrong drug demonstrated a wanton or reckless disregard for the life or safety of the patient. Even if this conduct was found to be grossly negligent in a civil law context, that conduct may not be sufficient to show the degree of wanton or reckless disregard required for a

Continued on following page

CASE SCENARIO 7.1B *(Continued)*

criminal negligence conviction. The patient would have to have suffered some harm or have died.

There is a substantial difference between being negligent in a civil lawsuit and being criminally negligent. The latter type of negligence requires conduct that does not meet what one would normally expect of a reasonable person (in this case, a reasonable nurse). The intent of the accused is irrelevant. It is sufficient that the accused acted in such a manner as to demonstrate either recognition of the obvious risk of danger to another and took that risk anyway or ought to reasonably to have foreseen such a risk yet failed to do so (*R. v. Sharpe*, 1984). In other words, the accused was completely indifferent to the risks and the consequences of the actions taken, to the life or safety of others who might reasonably be expected to be so affected.

THE PROVINCIAL CORONERS' AND MEDICAL EXAMINERS' SYSTEMS

The coroners' and medical examiners' systems are integral to both the criminal justice system and the provincial responsibility under the Constitution for administering justice within the province. In every province, an unexplained death must be investigated with a view to determining its causes and identifying ways to prevent similar occurrences in the future. Thus, if there is any evidence of negligence on the part of nursing or medical staff contributing to the death of a person, an inquest may be ordered by a coroner or a court to determine the circumstances and all possible causes of the death. It is important for nurses to have a basic understanding of the coroners' and medical examiners' systems in use across Canada because nurses may be called upon to testify at such proceedings.

The **coroner's inquest** is primarily a fact-finding and investigatory endeavour. In earlier times, a coroner's court could also find criminal or civil responsibility; however, the modern coroner's inquest is not a criminal trial. There is no accused person. In some provinces, the coroner has the authority, upon conclusion of an inquest, to order the arrest of anyone who has been found to be responsible for the death investigated. However, none of the evidence and testimony given at an inquest may be used in a criminal trial. Coroners have reported nurses to their regulatory body where their care was in question (Canadian Nurses Protective Society [CNPS], 2003).

The inquest process is often part of the public exploration of societal issues and the need for change. A coroner's inquest into the death of Joyce Echaquan, an Indigenous woman who died while a patient in a Quebec hospital (Bureau du Coroner Quebec, 2021), found that her death was due, in part, to discriminatory and the racist behaviour of nursing staff. These facts led to the discipline of nursing staff by the regulatory body and initiated a discussion about systemic discrimination in Quebec health care.

Ontario, Quebec, New Brunswick, Prince Edward Island, Saskatchewan, British Columbia, Yukon, the Northwest Territories, and Nunavut use the coroner's system adopted from English common law. The remaining provinces have moved to a medical examiner's system. Both systems, however, operate similarly to investigate suspicious deaths. In the medical examiner's system, the function of holding an inquiry is usually left to a judge, or, in the case of Alberta, the Fatality Review Board (*Fatality Inquiries Act*, 2000). In the traditional coroner's system, the inquiry is led by the appropriate coroner.

A detailed review of each province's system is beyond the scope of this book. However, Ontario's system will serve as an example. Under Ontario's *Coroners Act* (1990), a chief coroner for Ontario is appointed to supervise coroners appointed to represent regions in the province. The coroner must be a resident of that region and be a legally qualified medical physician.

Under the Act, a death under any of the following circumstances must be reported either to a coroner or to the police (*Coroners Act*, 1990, s. 10(1)):

- As a result of violence, misadventure (e.g., an accident), negligence, misconduct, or malpractice
- By unfair means
- During pregnancy or following pregnancy in such circumstances to which the death could be attributed to the pregnancy

- Suddenly and unexpectedly
- From disease or sickness for which the person was not treated by a legally qualified medical practitioner
- From any cause other than disease
- Under circumstances that require investigation

Similarly, if a person dies while in a retirement home, a long-term care facility, a children's residence, a home for developmentally delayed persons, or a mental health facility, the coroner should be informed. In addition, if a person is transferred to a public or private hospital from one of these facilities, and dies, the coroner must also be informed. Pending an order from the coroner, no person may in any way alter the condition or interfere with the body of the deceased.

Once notified, the local coroner can give permission to proceed with signing a death certificate and release the body for burial or review the documentation around care and then release for burial or issue a warrant to take possession of the body as part of the investigation. The investigation and fact-finding into the circumstances of the death begin at this point. The coroner has the power to enter any place where the death occurred, inspect and extract information from any records or documentation relating to the deceased, and seize anything that the coroner believes is material to the purposes of the investigation. In Ontario, some coroners will review a death electronically by examining video or still images of the decedent and issue a death certificate based on this and the person's medical history.

In cases in which someone has died under care of a health care facility, and there is a concern regarding the circumstances of the death, it is likely that the coroner would seize the deceased's health records immediately upon being notified of the death. This is a precaution to preserve the character of the evidence and to avoid the possibility of additions being made to such records that might obscure the circumstances and condition of the deceased at the time of death.

This emphasizes again the importance of ensuring that records are made as contemporaneously as possible. The nurse involved in the care of the deceased is, at the very least, a potential witness to the circumstances surrounding the treatment, care, and condition of that person immediately prior to death. Although in most cases of death there is no inquest, the coroner has the right to

investigate the death and may call for evidence about the care of the deceased. The nurse may be called upon to testify at the coroner's inquest, if indeed there is one, and will have to rely on the records to recall the events leading up to the death. Questions asked of witnesses in such cases may be quite specific and require precise and detailed interpretation of the nursing progress notes and other records. Therefore, as discussed in this chapter, the necessity of making clear and accurate records as close as possible to the time when the nursing act was performed cannot be overstressed for both civil and criminal liability issues as well as quality assurance in health care.

A coroner can order that an inquest be held into the circumstances of the deceased's death if it is deemed advisable. Otherwise, the matter will proceed no further.

If an inquest is held, the coroner will convene a hearing, in some provinces, with the aid of a jury (usually smaller than a criminal trial jury of 12; in Ontario, for example, the jury consists of five persons). The jury's function is to determine the cause of death based on the evidence heard at the inquest and to aid in making recommendations as to any improvements to procedures, policies, and standards that may help to prevent similar occurrences in the future.

Specifically in provinces with coroner's juries, the jury is charged with answering five questions when investigating a death:

- Who was the deceased?
- Where did the death occur?
- When did the death occur?
- How did the death occur (i.e., the medical cause)?
- By what means did the death occur? (i.e., classification or manner of death—natural, suicide, accident, homicide, or undetermined)

The jury may also make nonbinding recommendations related to the issues in the matter. The jury may not offer a verdict that attributes guilt for the death.

In Quebec, the formulation is very similar. Sections 2 and 3 of the *Coroners Act*, (Chapter C-68.01) states:

2. The coroner's function is to determine by means of an investigation or, as the case may be, an inquest,
(1) the identity of the deceased person;
(2) the date and place of death;

(3) *the probable causes of death, that is, the disease, pathological condition, trauma or intoxications having caused, led to or contributed to the death;*
(4) *the circumstances of death.*
3. If pertinent, the coroner may also, at an investigation or an inquest, make any recommendation directed towards better protection of human life.

The inquest will usually proceed along similar lines to a trial. However, as mentioned earlier, the inquest is not a criminal trial; there is no prosecution and no accused. Depending on the province, the coroner, a judge, a retired judge, or a lawyer may conduct the inquest. The coroner may conduct the hearing themselves, calling and examining witnesses under oath. More often, a lawyer appointed by the coroner, the coroner's counsel, will handle the calling of witnesses and obtain their evidence in open court. The coroner may question the witnesses at any time. Members of the jury are also permitted to ask questions.

The Crown attorney may assist the coroner in obtaining evidence by acting as coroner's counsel, by providing evidence about the outcome of criminal proceedings, or by providing advice about the legal position being taken by the Crown. Any other parties who are material witnesses or participants in the events leading up to the person's death may be called to testify at the inquest.

In some cases where a group has a particular interest in an inquest, its members may request a report on status at the inquest. This right is called *standing* and entitles the party to question witnesses and make arguments to the jury about conclusions in the inquest. In some cases, they may also be given the right to call witnesses. The coroner may grant or refuse standing to group members based on the reason for their interest in the proceeding. A person charged with a criminal offence related to the death cannot be compelled to testify at an inquest. Any person called to testify will have the right to the aid of a lawyer. However, the lawyer's involvement may be limited to advising on answers to questions and the rights of the witness. In most provinces, witnesses have the right not to have any evidence that they give at an inquest used against them in any ensuing criminal proceedings. This is to ensure that the witness's rights, under the *Canadian Charter of Rights and Freedoms* (1982), against self-incrimination are maintained (s. 13).

This does not mean, however, that the witness has the right to refuse to answer any proper questions. A refusal to answer may place that witness in danger of being found in contempt of court, a judgement that carries with it fines and a possible jail term.

The inquest is more flexible in terms of the strict rules of evidence normally applied in a court. However, coroners tend to follow such rules, especially in recent years.

In provinces with a medical examiner's system, the medical examiner takes the place of the coroner. Appointed by the provincial government, a medical examiner must be a physician given the medical complexities and technicalities that tend to be the focus of such inquests. Coroners historically were laypersons, but this has evolved so that now coroners in most provinces must be duly qualified and licensed physicians. The procedures across the country are fairly similar, except that in some provinces (i.e., Nova Scotia, Manitoba, and Alberta), the inquest may be held by a provincial court judge. The investigative and inquiry functions are, thus, kept separate.

Once the inquest is concluded, the coroner or judicial officer conducting the hearing may give a decision (taking into consideration any recommendations made by the jury) on the cause of death and anything that could have been done to prevent it. For example, the jury might recommend changes to certain policies, procedures, or systems that it feels may have contributed to the death. Although these recommendations are not binding, they often lead to policy changes and influence standards established by other agencies, such as Accreditation Canada and the Institute for Safe Medication Practices Canada (ISMP Canada). Further, if the coroner's decision suggests criminal responsibility, it is possible that criminal charges may be laid in the wake of the decision. The criminal justice process would then take over to determine the guilt or innocence of any accused person.

Interaction Between Coroner's Inquests and Criminal Law

A coroner's inquest that took place in Ontario in 2000 illustrates the interface between the criminal law system and the coroner's inquest system. Both systems are distinct and separate from one another, and a finding of liability in a coroner's inquest does not necessarily lead to a criminal conviction. In one case, a 10-year-old girl attended a pediatric hospital for treatment of (unusual) pain associated with an earlier fracture of her tibia (*Shore v. Law Society of Upper Canada*, 2009). The girl was experiencing considerable leg pain and a burning sensation because of a rare condition known as *reflex sympathetic dystrophy syndrome* and, at the direction of the treating physicians, was started on a morphine infusion for pain control. The girl died a few hours after the infusion was initiated. The coroner's jury concluded that the girl had died from respiratory and heart failure caused by a severe reaction to the morphine and its interaction with another drug she was receiving. The jury ruled that the death was a "homicide."

Homicide, for the purposes of a coroner's inquest, is the death of a person caused by the actions of another person or persons. It is the pure physical act that causes the death of a human being. The verdict in a coroner's jury only determines how the death occurred. There is no assignment of blame or criminal responsibility as in a criminal trial. As stated earlier, coroners' juries do not have the power to assign legal liability—that is, to determine civil (as in a lawsuit) or criminal responsibility on the part of any person involved in the death. The inquest's chief purpose is to determine how a person died when the death was unexpected or was the result of an accident or unexplained circumstances.

If criminal charges are later laid by the police against an individual, the ensuing criminal trial will determine whether the act of killing was the result of an intentional act or criminal negligence (discussed earlier). In the case of the 10-year-old girl, criminal charges were initially laid by the police against the two nurses directly involved in the girl's treatment (*Shore v. Law Society of Upper Canada*, 2009). Shortly into the preliminary hearing (a pretrial process in which the Crown must set out sufficient evidence to support the matter proceeding to trial), the charges were stayed (halted) by the Crown (the prosecution) because Crown counsel believed that there was insufficient evidence for a conviction. Ironically, the mother of the 10-year-old girl had withheld a medical record in the criminal case until the preliminary inquiry and her loss of credibility was a factor in the charges being stayed. The mother had become a law student by the

time of the criminal trial and faced a complaint by the nurses to the Law Society of Upper Canada over her conduct (*Shore v. Law Society of Upper Canada*, 2009). She was found to have made a serious error but since she had disclosed her misconduct and was previously of good character she could be admitted to the practice of law.

NURSING DOCUMENTATION

Background

Careful and accurate documentation is an important component of professional nursing practice. The nurse's assessment and progress notes monitor, on a continuing basis, the course of treatment and the effect of interventions. Comprehensive and complete documentation ensures that a clear picture emerges of the patient's progress toward the stated goals and outcomes and that complications or risks can be identified before they become problematic. Further good documentation is essential to ensuring:

- Continuity of care
- Effective communication and team collaboration
- Patient safety
- Compliance with regulatory requirements
- Quality improvement
- The retrieval of data for research, evaluation, and funding purposes
- Adherence to legal standards

The patient's health record, whether it is paper or electronic, is an important tool in planning, implementing, and evaluating the plan of care; it ensures accurate tracking of the patient's status, which, in turn, promotes quality care and the achievement of optimal outcomes. Proper documentation includes a plan of care that reflects the nurse's critical thinking and judgement, including identification of problems and recommendations on the action to be taken and how they will be evaluated. A documented plan enables others to follow through on the recommendations and to follow up on the efficacy of actions taken. Effective and accurate communication through documentation is absolutely critical to achieving effective team function. This record is vital during the course of treatment in that it facilitates communication between nurses and other health care professionals actively involved in the patient's care. Without it, effective, safe, quality care would be impossible (Fischbach, 1996; Lapum et al., n.d.). For example, what if a nurse encountered a patient who was extremely agitated? Should previous documentation not assist the nurse in understanding the source of the agitation and what was effective in managing this in the past?

Key aspects of the initial assessment that should be recorded in the patient's chart include things such as emergency contacts, substitute decision makers, and advance directives, including cardiopulmonary resuscitation (CPR) status.

Documentation is highly relevant in legal proceedings. The health record is used to validate the actions and to evaluate the standards of practice of nurses in these circumstances. Consider a situation where the assessment of a patient's pain is only documented as "severe." How adequate is such a description? For example, it does not indicate whether the pain was of sudden onset or a recurring pattern, or whether there were actions implemented to manage the pain and their effectiveness.

The health record provides evidence of the adequacy of any treatment that is administered, the appropriateness of care, and the quality of care received. This is especially important for the evaluation of standards of care; as discussed, in any disciplinary proceedings for alleged improper or unprofessional conduct; and in any negligence actions, criminal proceedings, or coroner's inquests in the event of the patient's death under circumstances requiring investigation. Failure to document specific acts or treatment accurately and contemporaneously can have serious consequences for the health care professional in a negligence action (CNPS, 2022).

The frequency of documentation and repeat assessments is based on patient need, complexity of care, and employer protocols. For example, in most settings, the initial assessment includes a person's risk of falling. To prevent harm, if a person is assessed as being at risk, then frequent reassessment would be necessary. If this component of the assessment were omitted and the patient subsequently fell, this would increase the risk of a finding of negligence. The court would question why the assessment was incomplete and would likely conclude that hospital staff was negligent in (a) failing to foresee that the plaintiff was prone to falling and (b) failing to take appropriate precautions to prevent this.

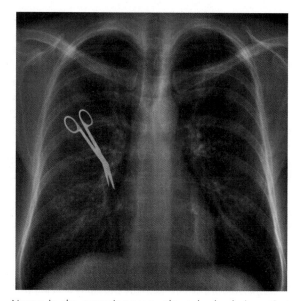

Nurses in the operating room play a lead role in patient safety by ensuring and documenting that items such as instruments, sponges, sutures etc. are not retained in the person's body during surgery. *Source: istockphoto.com/Lukasz-Panek.*

In most cases, the patient's record constitutes the only documented evidence of what care a patient has received. Nursing documentation is used by the courts as evidence of what was done or not done. Documentation standards imposed by the regulatory authority and the employer are used to assess the conduct of nurses. Failure to meet these standards can contribute to findings of professional misconduct and can be used to discredit evidence in a lawsuit.

Accurate and Complete Documentation

Documentation must be an accurate record of the patient's journey. This would include initial and ongoing assessments of the person, a clear plan of care and ongoing evaluation of that plan, the ongoing documentation of the patient's progress, and the notation of any interventions and their effect. As discussed in earlier chapters, it should also include the person's story, especially as it influences the course of their care.

CASE SCENARIO 7.2

DOCUMENTING: IS IT ENOUGH?

An 8-month-old boy is brought into a hospital emergency department late one evening with vomiting and diarrhea and a history of toxoplasmosis. Upon arrival, his pulse rate is 120 beats per minute; his respiration rate is 24 breaths per minute. He is seen by the physician on duty in the emergency department and then by the hospital pediatrician, who admits the child and writes treatment orders for an intravenous (IV) line, as well as tests for hemoglobin and blood urea nitrogen (BUN) electrolytes.

That night, the child's condition deteriorates. Over a period of 4 to 5 hours, his heart rate increases to 164 beats per minute and his respiration is 64 breaths per minute. Nurse H., who is looking after the boy, is concerned. She speaks to the charge nurse, who echoes her concerns. Nurse H. phones the child's physician at his home, even though it is the middle of the night.

She informs the physician of the child's condition, vital signs, and of abnormal values for hemoglobin, BUN, and electrolytes. In particular, the carbon dioxide (CO_2) level is at 10.9, well below the normal range of 22 to 32. The physician replies: "That's fine. Just continue doing what you've been doing."

Not satisfied with the doctor's response, Nurse H. again speaks to the charge nurse, who says, "Well, you're not the doctor; he is. Whatever he says is what we do; don't worry about it."

All the abnormal results and readings, including fluid balances, are duly recorded by Nurse H. in the boy's chart. Also noted are the conversations with the charge nurse and the boy's physician, and the times at which these took place. The boy dies that morning at 0600 hours.

Issues

1. What should the charge nurse have done when Nurse H. reported her discussion with the boy's physician?
2. Should Nurse H. have taken her concerns about the boy's abnormal test results to a higher authority when the physician and the charge nurse took no further action?

3. Should Nurse H. have called the physician back to confirm his instructions? In speaking with the doctor, should she have placed greater emphasis on the boy's abnormal vital signs and test results?

Discussion

Nurse H. should have contacted the physician a second time to impress upon him the urgency of the situation, especially because he had likely been roused from a deep sleep and that might have clouded his judgement.

A critical issue in this situation is the charge nurse's responsibility in assisting Nurse H. to obtain the help of the physician. Through her assessment, Nurse H. obviously realized the seriousness of the boy's condition. The standard of care would require that Nurse H. bypass the charge nurse and find a higher authority for instructions. Lack of support from a supervisor, even if accurately documented in the patient's chart, would not protect a nurse from liability. (However, this scenario raises serious concerns regarding safe nursing practice and the team culture in this unit. Patient safety, leadership, and collaborative team models are discussed in Chapters 11 and 12.)

Having determined the high risks of inaction, a nurse must act. A nurse cannot avoid liability by using the excuse that "the doctor said . . ." or by simply documenting the doctor's instructions. The nurse has a duty to protect the patient from harm. In this situation, the appropriate standard of care requires that the nurses appreciate the severe consequences of inaction. The conduct of both nurses clearly fell below the required professional and legal standards of care.

This scenario is based on an actual occurrence that led to a coroner's inquest. One of the issues that arose at the inquest was the documentation of fluid balance, particularly in the emergency department. It had not been totalled accurately, and it was difficult to determine how much fluid the patient had been given, in both the emergency department and the pediatric unit. (Sozonchuk v. Polych, 2013 ONCA 253; Ares v Venner [1970] SCR 608)

Continued on following page

CASE SCENARIO 7.2 *(Continued)*

The physician denied that the nurse had reported the patient's vital signs to him. He further denied that he had been given the electrolyte results, specifically, the CO_2 level. No other nurses on duty that evening witnessed the telephone conversation; thus, no one was able to corroborate the nurse's testimony. The doctor claimed to have been roused from a deep sleep and was very tired as he had been up all night the previous day and that if the nurse had really had such a pressing concern, she should have phoned him back to confirm his instructions and make sure he realized the severity of the situation. In such a case, he said, he certainly would have taken the appropriate action. It was obvious that regardless of which version of events was the correct one, the child died because of a serious breakdown in communication.

The coroner's jury found, first, that the nurse should have documented her concerns in greater detail. Second, she should have called the doctor back to repeat her concerns and had another nurse present to attest to the fact that she did so. Third, the hospital should have had procedures in place for the nurse to bypass the physician's instructions and to seek another doctor in the hospital to ensure that proper instructions were provided in the treatment of this child.

The cause of death, as determined by autopsy, was dehydration. The IV fluid that had been administered to the child was wholly inadequate. The inquest determined that the boy's intake and output should have been checked more frequently and recorded systematically. In particular, the levels might have been checked and recorded by nursing staff just prior to the child's leaving the emergency department and then again by the nurses in pediatrics immediately upon his transfer to that unit.

The jury did not accept the physician's excuse in this case, and he was found negligent for having given improper instructions. He was subsequently reported to the College of Physicians and Surgeons of Ontario and severely disciplined.

An important case for the establishment of legal precedent for documentation was that of *Meyer v. Gordon* (1981). The parents of a newborn who suffered severe brain damage during delivery and ensuing cerebral palsy brought an action of negligence against two nurses, the hospital, and the attending physician. In all, three nurses were involved in the delivery. The plaintiff had previously had a very short labour, her first child having been born within 4 hours of the onset of labour. The plaintiff's doctor knew this but had not advised the nursing or hospital staff when he had his patient admitted to the hospital at approximately 1130 hours on the morning her labour began.

Ascertaining the patient's birth history is a routine and standard part of any labour assessment performed by a nurse. However, the first nurse who examined the plaintiff, Nurse W., did not ascertain whether this was the woman's first or second birth and, in fact, failed to obtain any obstetrical history. It was made clear at the trial that had she done so, the history would have indicated that this patient should have been closely watched. Nurse W.'s failure to determine the obstetrical history of the mother in this case shows a marked departure from acceptable standards of practice in Canada.

Also, there was evidence that the charting done by the two nurses who were named in the suit was inaccurate and incomplete. As a result, their progress notes were rejected by the trial judge as unreliable. Upon the plaintiff's admission to the hospital, Nurse W. performed the initial examination and established that the patient was in the early stages of labour. She did not record this, however, and was imprecise as to the position of the fetus at that time, noting the position only as "mid." Neither did the nurse record the duration of the contractions during the first, and only, vaginal examination. At this point, she did ascertain and record that dilation was 3 cm, but the character of the cervix (an important indication of the progress of labour) was not recorded accurately.

A second nurse, Nurse M., assisted Nurse W. in these examinations. Neither nurse appeared to have recognized the danger of leaving the mother lying on her back, the position she remained in until delivery. The court found, among other things, that permitting the plaintiff to remain in this position contributed greatly to the fetal distress and constituted a marked departure from the standard of care at that hospital, which was known for excellence in obstetrics. The mother should clearly have been positioned on her side.

The fetal heart rate was checked at 1150 hours and again at 1200. However, this information did not appear to have been recorded until much later. At noon, the patient's doctor prescribed an injection of Demerol and Gravol to ease the patient's pain and nausea. Although this was not explicitly stated by the court or in the evidence as reported, the administration of Demerol would, no doubt, have had a sedative effect not only on the mother but also on the fetus and could have contributed to the onset of fetal distress. The physician did not instruct Nurse M. to conduct a vaginal examination before administering the Demerol, and, in fact, no examination was conducted before the drug was given at 1205 hours. This was also against generally accepted practice.

From the time the Demerol was administered until the child was born at 1232 hours, the plaintiff was left lying on her back, alone and completely unattended despite her excruciating and rapid labour pains and despite Nurse W.'s opinion that the fetal heart rate ought to have been checked every 15 minutes at that point. The court noted that the obstetrical unit appeared to have been extremely busy that day and that the plaintiff did not appear to have been assigned a specific nurse from that point on.

At 1215 hours, the plaintiff's husband, distressed by his wife's extreme pain, sought out Nurse W. He told her that he believed his wife was about to give birth and needed assistance. The evidence at trial indicated that Nurse W. may have brushed off his concern, dismissing him as a nervous husband. The court found it deplorable that there was no nursing care made available to the plaintiff when her husband sought it (*Meyer v. Gordon*, 1981, p. 15).

At approximately 1230 hours, the plaintiff's husband again sought out a nurse, saying that his wife was giving birth. A third nurse (Nurse T.) responded and went to the plaintiff. She found the baby's head already out with a very large amount of meconium around it. She completed the delivery; however, as Nurse M. (who assisted her) had failed to include a suction bulb

in the emergency bundle, Nurse T. was unable to suction the meconium from the baby's nose and mouth. The expert physicians who testified at trial deemed this a serious oversight.

The baby was not breathing when she was born. Nurse T. described the baby as "very flaccid and limp." The baby was brought to the case room for resuscitation, where another doctor was involved in her resuscitation with the use of initial suctioning, positive pressure ventilation, and oxygen with endotracheal suctioning. The resuscitation efforts continued for some time with the assistance of two other physicians and were ultimately successful. The child was moved to the hospital's intensive care nursery. It was soon discovered, however, that she had suffered brain damage because of asphyxia in conjunction with meconium aspiration (*Meyer v. Gordon*, 1981, p. 9).

The parents sued the mother's doctor, the doctors involved in the resuscitation efforts, the nurses, and the hospital. The court dismissed the suit against the doctors (except the plaintiffs' own doctor, who was found 25% liable on the basis that he had failed to instruct Nurse M. to conduct a vaginal examination of the plaintiff before administering the Demerol). The hospital was found 75% responsible for the baby's brain damage resulting from its negligence in failing to provide adequate and proper nursing care.

The court noted that both nurses had gone back and altered the chart some hours after the delivery to make the record appear more complete than it was, which meant that the court was unable to rely upon the nurses' progress notes as an accurate account of what had happened. Much was made of the fact that the nurses' notes were inaccurate and inadequate. For example, the time of the mother's arrival at the hospital was not recorded (*Meyer v. Gordon*, 1981, p. 7); upon initial examination of the patient, Nurse W. noted that the fetal heart rate was "normal," that the plaintiff's labour was "good," that the cervix had dilated 3 cm, and that "strong" contractions were occurring every 2 minutes (*Meyer v. Gordon*, 1981, p. 7). However, the duration of the contractions was not recorded, as it should have been.

The court found that the description of the labour as "good" did not indicate the fact (later brought out in Nurse W.'s testimony) that the plaintiff was in active labour, which would require a fetal heart rate check every 15 minutes (*Meyer v. Gordon,* 1981, p. 12). The court was equally critical of the inexact description of the fetus's position as "mid" and of the lack of record as to the character or effacement of the cervix. Such inaccuracies and inadequacies contributed to a poor appreciation of the advanced stage of mum's labour.

In most court cases, failure to document a particular act during treatment may mean that the court will assume the act was not done. Such failure seriously undermines how probative the evidence is—that is, how much the testimony proves or how convincing it is that the action was performed. Records that are sketchy and incomplete may not be accorded much weight by the court.

In assessing the quality and accuracy of Nurse W.'s recorded observations, the court relied on the expert evidence of two nurses (presumably, with obstetrical experience) who stated that an obstetrical nurse, when assessing fetal position, looks for the height of the presenting part of the fetus in relation to the ischial spines of the mother's pelvis. When asked about Nurse W.'s assessment of the fetal position as "mid," one of the experts commented that such a notation was not specific enough to aid in the evaluation of the labour. The other expert stated that the expression "mid" used in the record had no meaning (*Meyer v. Gordon,* 1981, p. 12). This case, thus, illustrates the importance of accurate and precise observations when documenting details of patient care and treatment.

Guidelines for Proper Documentation

Over time, as a result of the outcome of civil and regulatory hearings, the significance of effective documentation has been made abundantly clear. Nurses should be aware of the professional and legal standards associated with documentation. Table 7.2 summarizes these standards and guidelines.

TABLE 7.2
Legal Guidelines for Proper Documentation

Record contemporaneously.	Timely documentation makes a record more accurate and reliable, ensures safer care, and affords the record greater weight in any legal proceedings. Therefore, the record should be made at the time of occurrence of the event or action that is recorded. It is not always possible to record items, events, or actions at the time they occur, especially during emergencies. The longer the delay in documenting a fact, however, the more likely it is that the accuracy of the observation or detail will be questioned later, especially in a trial. For example, in *Meyer v. Gordon* (1981, p. 9), the nurses who treated the plaintiff had recorded some of their observations a considerable time after the fact and, further, had altered the record to make it appear that the observations had been recorded contemporaneously. Thus, the nurses' progress notes were deemed unreliable as an evidentiary source. Another reason for contemporaneous documentation is that memory fades with time. A fact is more likely to be recorded accurately and completely soonest after the occurrence. As a considerable length of time may pass before a trial or hearing is convened, a well-constructed and well-maintained record serves to refresh the memory of the person who made it. If it was not possible to record the act or event when it occurred (e.g., the nurse had other pressing obligations or simply forgot), the late entry should still be recorded, to the nurse's best recollection, and noted as a late entry, thus: *1230 h, patient regurgitated reddish coffee-ground fluid; recorded at 1330 h because called away on emergency to assist in another patient's resuscitation. [Signed, etc.]* A late entry is clearly better than no entry at all. The nurses in the *Meyer* case attempted to cover up the fact that some of their entries had been made late rather than contemporaneously. This destroyed the value of their evidence.
Record only your own actions.	The nurse should record only their own actions. In criminal or civil proceedings, the nurse will be permitted to testify only as to these actions. When documenting electronically, nurses should use only their own password or access card. This ensures that the system reflects the name of the particular nurse making the entry.
Record in chronological order.	All entries should be made in chronological order. Otherwise, a confused record would result, which could have serious consequences for the course of treatment, especially with respect to the administration of medication. It would also make the record of limited use in any litigation and undermine the nurse's testimony.

TABLE 7.2

Legal Guidelines for Proper Documentation *(Continued)*

Record clearly and concisely.	Entries should be clear, concise, factual, and as objective as possible. Any evidence that leads the nurse to draw a particular conclusion should be carefully documented. A subjective entry potentially creates problems in patient care and, in a court proceeding, might leave the nurse's testimony open to challenge.
Make regular entries.	The nurse should make sure that the record contains regular entries throughout. If there are significant gaps in the record, the benefits and evidence of continuous monitoring of the patient are lost. Further, a lengthy gap in the record (e.g., a gap of a number of hours prior to a patient's cardiac or respiratory arrest, pulmonary edema, or, in a psychiatric setting, a psychotic event or suicide attempt) would be questioned in court.
Record corrections clearly.	Any alterations, corrections, or deletions to the record should be carefully documented, dated (including the hour), and initialled by the nurse who makes the change. Otherwise, the nurse's credibility could be undermined. No attempt should be made to cover up one's mistakes by surreptitiously altering the record to make it look complete. In cases in which a coroner's investigation is underway, the coroner often seizes nursing notes and other patient records immediately in order to ascertain the circumstances of the patient's treatment or condition in the moments prior to death. An online entry is dated with the digital signature of the person making it. Because in most systems this can never be altered, the recorded act is "etched in time." Yet, there have been situations in which nurses have attempted to alter the record upon learning of a coroner's inquest, only to learn later that the coroner had already seized the record and made copies of it. The coroner thus had an accurate version of the record at the moment of the patient's death, as well as evidence that the nurses attempted to alter the record afterward. It is best to avoid such situations by making it clear that one is documenting a fact some time after its occurrence or that one is correcting a previous inaccuracy.
Record accurately.	Vague terms should be avoided. Nursing assessments are essential to care planning. The initial assessment of a patient entering the care process is crucial and should, therefore, be thorough and comprehensive. Most agencies and hospitals require that initial assessments be made within a specified period from the time of admission. Inaccurate or incomplete assessments can affect the outcomes of care and raise serious questions in any ensuing legal proceedings. The frequency of repeat assessments is based on patient need, complexity of care, and agency protocols. For example, in some settings, the initial assessment includes determining a person's risk of falling. If a patient is assessed as being at risk, then reassessment on a regular basis would be necessary. If this component of the assessment were omitted and the patient subsequently fell, a negligence suit against the nurse(s) and hospital could result. The court would question why the assessment was incomplete and would likely conclude that hospital staff was negligent in (a) failing to foresee that the plaintiff was prone to falling and (b) failing to take appropriate precautions to prevent this. Key aspects of the initial assessment that should be recorded in the patient's chart are: ■ The name of an emergency contact ■ The name of the patient's proxy (if any) ■ Any decision made by the patient or proxy regarding cardiopulmonary resuscitation (CPR) (see Chapter 8) ■ Whether the patient has made an advance directive ■ Any reassessment should likewise be documented to ensure a complete record. A notation in the patient's record such as "Slept well, had a good day" is of limited use. In a trial, the nurse who made the note could well be asked detailed questions about what was meant by "a good day" (e.g., any pain felt by the patient, symptoms, vital signs) in an attempt to pinpoint the patient's condition at the time when the notation was made. The nurse would probably be unable to answer such questions meaningfully, as the original meaning of "had a good day" would have been forgotten. It is far better to document, for example: "Patient reported sharp pains in chest radiating down the left arm of 10-min duration, relieved with rest," rather than: "Patient reported chest pain." The latter notation would not bear scrutiny in a legal proceeding. More important, it would be of limited use in an attempt to diagnose the patient's ailment accurately.
Record legibly.	The records, and any corrections, should be legible. Given the speed with which nurses sometimes are required to perform their duties, illegibility is a very real issue; however, nurses must be aware that illegible entries may result in misreading, which can have disastrous results.

Incident Reports

When critical incidents or mistakes occur, such as a patient fall or a medication error in addition to documentation in the patient record, the nurse should prepare an incident or occurrence report that describes the incident, all relevant facts, resulting harm, and any remedial action. The implications of error, disclosure, and patient safety from the perspective of quality improvement and the importance of a just culture are discussed in Chapters 5 and 10.

Incidents reports do not form part of the health record but are used, first, to document occurrences out of the ordinary for investigative or quality-assurance purposes. For example, an insurance company might investigate a claim made against a hospital's general liability insurance policy, or a hospital may monitor or audit the rate of occurrence of certain types of incidents over a specified period. Thus, such reports can contribute to the hospital's risk management processes by identifying opportunities for improvement or possible problem areas in systems or procedures.

Second, the information gained can be used to inform staff education and to address system issues that would prevent similar occurrences in the future. Furthermore, with the current emphasis on quality improvement and patient safety, the data and information gathered from these reports are key to these processes because they demonstrate trends and patterns over time. Such information can also influence and inform policy and procedures and further ensures that professionals and health care settings are held accountable for the delivery of high standards of care.

Finally, in the event that a negligence action is brought against the health care facility arising out of an incident, the incident report can form part of the evidentiary record at trial and assist the court in understanding the cause of the incident. Such a report is usually introduced along with the testimony of the health care professional(s) who made it.

Legal Requirement to Keep Records

In all provinces and territories, hospitals and other health care facilities are required to keep and maintain records on all patients. For example, in Ontario, the names of all attending physicians, dentists, midwives, and registered nurses in the extended class (RN-EC), a record of admission, diagnosis, consent forms, examinations, treatment, care plan, nursing notes, and so forth must be kept on each patient (see, for example, *Hospital Management Regulation, R.R.O. 1990, Reg. 965*, s. 19(3), made under the *Public Hospitals Act, 1990*). Physicians' orders must be in writing and signed or authenticated by the physician who made the order. All entries in the patient record must be initialled or signed and dated, with the exact time of the entry noted (*T.C. v R.J.A.*, 2016). Late entries must also be indicated.

Also, records must be kept for a specified time—for example, in Ontario, for 10 years (*Hospital Management Regulation, R.R.O. 1990, Reg. 965*, s. 19(f)).

USE OF DOCUMENTATION IN LEGAL PROCEEDINGS

Evidentiary Use

In many cases of malpractice, the trial of the actions of health care professionals will occur several years after the events leading up to and including the negligent acts. Memories fade with time, and the evidence given by witnesses will often be hazy or incomplete. Therefore, the notes and records prepared by the health care team assume added value and significance because these are often the only source of information regarding what occurred.

The goal of the courts is to obtain the truth. Meticulous, clear, legible, and well-organized records not only help the court (i.e., the judge and, in some cases, the jury) to determine the exact sequence of events and the circumstances of treatment; they also improve the credibility of the witnesses who made them. Thus, with a well-constructed health care record, those who made the notes will be able to impart their testimony with authority, and that testimony will be accorded greater weight than would be the case with an inadequate record.

The court will be interested in all aspects of the record, including nursing progress notes, care plans, checklists, flow charts, hospital policies in force at the time, and so forth. These will provide a more complete picture of events. In many cases, the record will also document the thought processes and frame of mind of the health care professional at the time. For example, the patient's chart may reveal that a certain treatment or intervention was or was not warranted under the circumstances and given that patient's condition. This no is a further reason for ensuring that records are made and kept according to the highest possible standards.

In Scenario 7.2 and in the *Latin v. Hospital for Sick Children et al.* (2007) decision discussed earlier in this chapter, the medical charts, nursing records, and notes surrounding the treatment given to the patient were essential. They provided evidence to show the type of care received and served as a means of communication between the various members of the health care teams. In the *Latin* case, for example, the triage nurse's contemporaneous notes of her observations of the child were carefully considered and her notations studied. Her notes taken in the emergency department that day showed that she noted the vital signs of each patient she examined, including a respiratory rate. In the child's case, she had written the word "cry" in the space where the rate was to be recorded. The court took this, along with evidence from the girl's mother, to mean that the child's crying made it difficult for the nurse to obtain the respiration rate. The following section discusses the uses and importance of proper documentation in nursing practice.

Nurses as Witnesses in Legal Proceedings

Assessing the conduct of nurses in a particular situation in relation to the appropriate standard of care often requires drawing upon expert testimony. The court calls upon experts because the judges trying a case rarely possess the necessary expertise to make valid conclusions and draw inferences from technical data. A nursing expert, however, can interpret the health care record and assist the court in reconstructing the events and drawing inferences. Experts can also be used by the parties to a lawsuit either to support the plaintiff's position and interpretation of the evidence or to refute these for the defence and perhaps suggest another cause for the injury. Although such inferences from the evidence are properly the function of the judge or jury, the expert, with unique knowledge and experience, is permitted to formulate and express an opinion. This is an exception to the general evidentiary rule that a witness's opinion on a matter at issue is inadmissible. More important, the nurse expert is able to describe the appropriate standard of care in a particular case and, upon review of the health care record and,

in particular, the nursing progress notes, give an opinion on whether proper documentation and nursing procedures were followed.

Prior to the nurse's testimony, the lawyer for the party wishing to rely on the nurse's evidence must first ask questions in court about his or her education, experience, nursing background, and continuing education. The purpose here is to establish in the trial record that the witness has the necessary qualifications to give such testimony or opinion.

In some cases, expert testimony may also be elicited as part of the nurse's own involvement in the care of the plaintiff. The nurse may be asked questions about notations in the patient's record. It is important that the nurse answers such questions truthfully and as accurately as possible. Again, this reinforces the importance of ensuring accuracy, clarity, and objectivity when first documenting.

As a rule of evidence, the person who recorded the note or observation will be allowed to use those notes to facilitate recall when testifying in court. However, the court must first be satisfied of the following:

1. The notes were, indeed, made by that person.
2. It was part of that nurse's duty to make such notes.
3. The notes were made contemporaneously (or reasonably so) with the event or act that they record.
4. There have been no alterations, additions, or deletions to those notes since they were made.

Usually, items 1 and 2 pose no problem, as the nurse witness will have been involved in the patient's care and will have been the one who made the notes in the first place as part of his or her normal duty.

Item 3 can pose a problem. For example, in the case of *Kolesar v. Jeffries* (1976), the court commented on the documentation practices in the surgical unit where the plaintiff was placed postoperatively. After surgery on his spinal column, the plaintiff was returned to the recovery room shortly after 1200 hours, sedated and unconscious, secured in the supine position to a Stryker frame. Although the standard of care in such a case would include rousing the patient at frequent and regular intervals for deep breathing and coughing, the plaintiff was permitted to sleep undisturbed by an overworked nurse, who according to the documentation, made one round at midnight. At 0500 hours, one of the nurses discovered that the patient had died.

He had suffered pulmonary edema and hemorrhage secondary to the aspiration of gastric juices.

The court heard evidence that no nursing notes were made for a period of 7 hours. Indeed, it was the practice in that nursing unit to record vital signs and any other observations as to the patients' condition on scraps of paper during the shift. Afterward, the nurses would get together and, with the aid of these scraps of paper, would reconstruct the record for each patient. The nurses would assist "each other to recall and record the events of the evening" (*Kolesar v. Jeffries*, 1976, para. 13). This practice does not fulfill the requirements of contemporaneous recording or standards of care.

Upon discovering that no entries had been made on the plaintiff between 2200 hours and 0500 hours the next day, the assistant director of nursing asked one of the nurses on duty that night to write up a report of the events. Here, the court noted:

One is always suspicious of records made after the event, and if any credence is to be attached to [the nurse's report], it shows that at all times the patient was quite pale, very pale, and was allowed to sleep soundly to his death. (Kolesar v. Jeffries, 1976, p. 48)

Thus, the absence of adequate nursing records served only to reinforce the court's opinion that the standard of nursing practised in this patient's care had been wholly inadequate. If efforts had been made to rouse the patient regularly to check and record his condition and vital signs, his death could have been avoided. The absence of documentation resulted in the court assuming "nothing was charted because nothing was done" (*Kolesar v. Jeffries*, 1976, at 48).

In *T.C. v. R.J.A.* (2016), an appeal to the Health Professions Appeal and Review Board of a decision by the College of Nurses of Ontario considered the record of actions taken by a nurse who was the subject of a complaint by a patient and his family. The family believed the nurse had not provided appropriate care and had not monitored the patient.

With respect to the Applicant's concern that the Respondent did not monitor or assess the patient properly and did not perform appropriate tracheostomy care, the Committee noted that the parties had conflicting accounts of what occurred. . . . The Committee noted that it cannot prefer one version to

another; rather, it looks to other information to assess what occurred. The Committee identified witness information and the contemporaneous documentation to be of assistance. . . . The Committee looked at the contemporaneous charting record which, it concluded, supported the accounts provided by the nursing staff. The Committee concluded that the Respondent did provide appropriate monitoring, assessment, and care during the period in question. (T.C. v R.J.A., 2016, para. 15)

Item 4 poses potential problems with respect to alterations, deletions, or additions made to the nursing notes after the original entries were made. In *Meyer v. Gordon* (1981), (the case involving the nursing negligence surrounding the birth of a child) discussed in the following quote, the alteration of the records prompted Justice Legg to remark:

The hospital chart contains alterations and additions which compel me to view with suspicion the accuracy of many of the observations which are recorded. The chart also contains at least one entry which was discovered during this trial [in May 1980] to have been made after the fact. That also casts suspicion on the reliability of those who made the entries and undermines the accuracy of medical opinions based upon these entries and observations. (Meyer v. Gordon, 1981, p. 15)

Thus, any attempt to conceal an alteration of the health care record can effectively cast doubt on the witness's evidence, as well as on any other evidence based on the entries and observations contained in the altered record.

CLINICAL INFORMATION SYSTEMS

Today, many organizations use clinical information systems for documentation. The same legal and ethical standards apply to electronic documentation. The benefits of online systems include:

- Improved clarity of documentation
- Structured and forced data entry
- Improved and timely communication across the team
- Continuity of care and more efficient access to providers

- Built-in templates, protocols, and alerts based on best practices
- One-time data capture (e.g., if one enters a laboratory value, it would automatically appear in all components of the system where that value should be documented)
- Timely and efficient retrieval of data or information
- Ability to aggregate data, providing greater opportunities for monitoring and improving quality of care

Further, integrated systems allow for shared databases and interfaces among departments, and access and exchange of patient information across health care systems, settings and geographical areas (CNA, 2022; Fischbach, 1996, pp. 28–29; Gagnon et al., 2012; Lapum et al., n.d.). All of these benefits contribute to patient safety and enhance a person-centred approach to care.

Concerns that arise with automated systems relate to security, confidentiality, and the legality of the electronic signature. Health care systems usually identify who is doing the documenting through access cards and passwords or a double-password system, which becomes the caregiver's electronic signature. When nurses share their access information with another caregiver, they are effectively allowing that person to use their signature; this could present legal liability at a future date.

To address the issue of confidentiality, most health care computer systems are designed to restrict access points (e.g., a technician in the laboratory may be able to access only information relevant to the test being conducted), limit access through the use of security codes and passwords, and monitor access of information. For example, programs are in place to monitor the extent to which patients' charts are accessed by those not involved in their care (Fischbach, 1996, pp. 535–536). In many facilities, access is monitored on a regular basis. Breaches of confidentiality are taken very seriously. It is up to each facility to ensure that safeguards (e.g., standards, guidelines, quality reviews) are in place to protect patients' privacy. These issues will be explored further in Chapter 10 in relation to a person's right to confidentiality.

Clinical documentation systems have the further advantage of ensuring greater accountability for documentation in terms of timeliness and accuracy

(Fischbach, 1996, pp. 251–254). For example, in online systems, it is difficult to tamper with or erase previous documentation. Properly used, it is also impossible to document later and attribute the documentation to an earlier time.

Patient Access to Health Information: Patient Portals

Technology now supports patient access to their own health information. Once registered to a secure portal (a website or app), patients can receive appointment reminders and view their appointments, consultation reports, laboratory results, and diagnostic reports at their convenience. If they choose, they can share this information with others, for example, a family physician or nurse practitioner in the community. These portals may also provide links to approved websites that offer health information and educational resources (University Health Network, 2022).

Access to a person's health information in a timely way respects their personal autonomy and right to have this knowledge. It gives the person more control over the information they seek, and that access, in many circumstances, can help diminish the anxiety of not knowing and of having to wait. Access to this resource also facilitates continuity of care, minimizes gaps in the system, and ensures that concerns or complications do not fall between the cracks. Furthermore, this resource holds the health care team accountable for accurate and timely documentation. However, at the same time, health information can be confusing and difficult to understand for some. There are potential challenges as well; for example, people reading a diagnostic report may interpret it as bad news, causing further anxiety until it is clarified by their provider. If processes are in place to provide support in these circumstances, then these systems can be helpful. Also, because it is voluntary, not all patients will choose to access this resource and may prefer to receive information directly from the health care team. In practice, some systems strictly limit communication from the patient to the physician. The flow is from the doctor to the patient, and the ability to respond is limited. Additionally, patients may inadvertently disclose their medical records, if they are not careful with passwords, providing access to other people or handling and storage of copies of their records.

SUMMARY

This chapter has demonstrated the complexity of the interrelationship among nursing practice, ethics, and nurses' accountabilities within the legal system. The significance of the societal expectations of nurses is evident in the serious consequences nurses may face when expectations are not met. The magnitude of the consequences is highlighted in the many cases summarized in this chapter.

It is critical for nurses to appreciate the gravity of these responsibilities and the extent to which their performance is measured according to professional, ethical, and legal standards. The professional responsibilities and accountabilities of nurses are made explicit by society to safeguard and protect the interests and well-being of vulnerable persons entrusted to their care.

Furthermore, this chapter has established why comprehensive and accurate documentation, whether electronically or in writing, is a key component of nursing practise. Nursing notes provide a continuous record of the patient's assessment and treatment, and the effect of interventions. From this record, the patient's progress toward stated goals and outcomes may be evaluated, and any impending complications can be identified before they become problematic.

With the introduction of electronic documentation, there is greater need for accurate, timely documentation. Once information is documented online, it is usually difficult to alter or erase. Also with patients now having greater access to their health record, documentation serves as an additional means of communication with patients therefore enhancing the quality and safety of care.

Nurses are held accountable for the care they provide and must meet multiple ethical and legal standards. In doing so they are able to provide safe and competent care to patients and avoid regulatory and legal consequences.

CRITICAL THINKING

The following case scenarios are for further reflection, discussion, and analysis.

Discussion Points

1. Discuss how concepts of negligence might apply in a nursing practice setting. Where do you see the biggest areas of risk?
2. What systems and guidelines are in place in your facility to guard against negligence?
3. How would you ensure that you do not put yourself at risk?
4. What actions would you take if you realized you had made a mistake? How would your leaders respond?
5. Identify the most important reasons for good documentation. Beyond meeting standards, how does good documentation ensure high-quality care? How would you evaluate the documentation standards in your setting?
6. How are documentation standards evaluated in your facility? What ideas do you have for improving them?
7. Would the quality of your documentation meet the standard during a legal proceeding? Why, or why not?
8. What are the risks inherent in using imprecise language when describing and documenting a patient's condition over time? How can you improve the precision of the language you use in your documentation?

CASE SCENARIO 7.3

NO HARM DONE?

There is only one registered nurse (RN) on the night shift at a long-term care facility. The nurse is working with a personal support worker (PSW). They have worked together on many occasions; and the nurse respects the PSW's judgement and caring approach to patients. One night, the nurse asks the PSW to clean an 80-year-old resident with Alzheimer's disease, who had just been incontinent. After helping the resident, the PSW leaves the room to dispose of the soiled linen and forgets to put up the bed rail, and, during her absence, the resident falls from the bed to the floor.

The nurse assesses the resident, who does not appear to have sustained any injury, and returns the resident to bed. The PSW is very worried and pleads with the nurse not to report it to their manager. The manager had recently chastised the PSW over a simi-lar incident when another resident fell after climbing over the bed rails, and the PSW did not believe this was fair. Also, the resident's daughter worries a great deal about the resident's care, and the PSW is afraid of being in serious trouble.

The nurse doesn't know what to do. The manager can be very harsh; the nurse does not want to get the PSW into trouble or worry the daughter unnecessarily.

Questions

1. What ethical or legal standards should guide the nurse in this scenario?
2. Is there risk of any civil or criminal liability?
3. What do you think the nurse should do?
4. Would this nurse also be accountable for this accident because the PSW is an unregulated care provider?

CASE SCENARIO 7.4

WHO IS RESPONSIBLE?

A public health nurse (PHN) has been asked to monitor a high-risk single mother who has been just discharged from the hospital only 24 hours after delivery. The mother is on welfare and also has a 2-year-old child, and although she has had parenting experience, the hospital nurse observes that she seems somewhat uncomfortable when bathing and feeding the baby. This nurse has suggested that she remain in the hospital another day or two to ensure that she is able to provide appropriate care for the baby. As well, in the hospital, she will be able to get some rest because her 2-year-old is staying with neighbours.

The unit manager thinks that the nurse was overreacting, and the unit is tight for beds. The nurse, therefore, requests an early visit from the PHN who manages a quick visit. Everything seems fine, although the mother is tired and reveals she is having difficulty feeding the baby.

The PHN promises to return the next day; however, the next morning, the PHN calls in sick. The unit is unable to send another nurse until the following day, who finds everything in chaos. The 2-year-old is screaming and seems to have a cold. The mother is very stressed. The new baby has been vomiting and is obviously dehydrated. The nurse calls for an ambulance; the baby is taken to the closest emergency department, and is stabilized.

Questions

1. What ethical or legal standards can guide the nurses in this scenario?
2. Is there risk of any civil or criminal liability?
3. Who is ethically and legally accountable for any potential harm to the baby—the hospital, the hospital nurse, the PHN, the public health unit, the system, or the mother?
4. How could this situation have been prevented?

CASE SCENARIO 7.5

SHOULD YOU STOP?

A nurse driving home after a very busy 12-hour shift in the cardiovascular critical care unit comes across a multivehicle accident. The nurse is only 5 minutes from home and is looking forward to spending the evening with friends. The nurse observes a number of people rushing to help, so assured that appropriate assistance will be provided, the nurse continues home.

The next day, the nurse arrives at work and is assigned to care for one of the accident victims, a 20-year-old who sustained serious chest trauma resulting in a tear to the aorta. Delays in the arrival of paramedics resulted in problems with early management of the patient's airway. Now, although

surgery has corrected the tear, it is unclear whether inadequate oxygenation to the patient's brain will result in permanent brain damage. The nurse feels responsible for not stopping to help.

Questions

1. Has the nurse in this scenario violated any ethical or legal standards?
2. Is there risk of any civil or criminal liability?
3. Did this nurse have any ethical or legal responsibility to provide assistance to the victims of this accident? Is there a difference between a nurse's legal and moral responsibilities?
4. What choice would you have made?

CASE SCENARIO 7.6

KNOWING THE PATIENT'S STORY?

A patient admitted to hospital with anemia and high fever was found to have a hydronephrosis of the left kidney caused by a stricture of the ureter. This was a result of chronic infection related to an ileal conduit she has had for about 30 years.

Because the patient's creatinine was also very high, it was decided that her left ureter must be dilated immediately. This procedure was extremely painful. Afterward, sepsis developed, and she was seriously ill for about 2 weeks. The episode was appropriately documented on the medical record. A few weeks later, just as she was improving, a nurse accidentally removed the stent (in place to ensure the ureter remained dilated), and the dilation had to be repeated.

The patient's daughter was present during the procedure and heard the physician state that it was important to monitor her mother's vital signs, in particular her temperature, blood pressure, and urine output, because sepsis was a risk. The daughter was concerned when after 2 hours the nurse had still not come to assess her mother.

The daughter approached the nurse, who told her that because this procedure was unusual on this unit (a medical unit), the nurse did not know the protocol. The daughter was further concerned that the nurse had not reviewed her mother's record; otherwise, the nurse would have appreciated the risks associated with this procedure.

Questions

1. Did the nurse in this case violate any ethical or legal standards?
2. Is there a potential risk of any civil or criminal liability?
3. Did the nurse involved after the second dilation meet the standards of practice with respect to documentation? What, if any, professional standards were not fulfilled in this case?
4. Would the facts that this procedure was rarely practised on this unit and that this nurse had never cared for a patient who has had this procedure excuse the nurse's behaviour?

CASE SCENARIO 7.7

A MODERN DILEMMA?

A nurse works in a busy emergency department at a hospital that has a fully integrated clinical information system.

One of the residents arrives to assess a patient presenting with severe abdominal pain. This resident has forgotten to bring along the access card that allows them to review patients' health care information online.

The nurse, aware of the urgency of this review (the patient's condition is rapidly deteriorating), lets the resident use their access badge. The nurse knows this is against the confidentiality policy they signed upon receipt of the access card. Nonetheless, while reviewing the data online, the resident notes abnormal findings that require immediate action and, via the system, orders further tests.

Questions

1. Has the nurse in this case violated any ethical or legal standards?
2. Is there risk of any civil or criminal liability?
3. What dilemma was the nurse facing in this scenario?
4. Can this nurse's actions be justified, given the circumstances?
5. What action should the nurse take now?

REFERENCES

Statutes

Canadian Charter of Rights and Freedoms, Part I of the *Constitution Act, 1982*, being Schedule B to the *Canada Act 1982* (UK), 1982, c. 11.

Civil Code of Québec, CQLR c. CCQ-1991 (Quebec).

Contributory Negligence Act, R.S.A. 2000, c. C-27 (Alberta).

Coroners Act, chapter C-68.01 (Quebec).

Coroners Act, R.S.O. 1990, c. C.37 (Ontario).

Criminal Code, R.S.C. 1985, c. C-46 (Canada).

Emergency Medical Aid Act, R.S.S. 1978, c. E-8, ss. 2(b), 3 (Saskatchewan).

Fatality Inquiries Act, R.S.A. 2000, c. F-9 (Alberta).

Negligence Act, R.S.B.C. 1996, c. 333 (British Columbia).

Public Hospitals Act, R.S.O. 1990, c. P.40. (Ontario).

Registered Nurses Act, R.S.P.E.I., 1988, c. R-8.1, s.1(s) (Prince Edward Island).

The Registered Nurses Act, 1988, S.S. 1988 -89, c. R-12.2 (Saskatchewan).

Registered Nurses Act, S.N.S. 2006, c. 21 (Nova Scotia).

The Regulated Health Professions Act, C.C.S.M., c. R117 (Manitoba).

Regulations

Hospital Management Regulation, R.R.O. 1990, Reg. 965. (Ontario).

Professional Misconduct, O. Reg. 799/93 (under the *Nursing Act, 1991*, Ontario).

Case Law

College of Nurses of Ontario v. Wettlaufer [2017] CanLII 77173 (ON CNO).

Donoghue v. Stevenson [1932] AC 562, at p. 580; 101 LJPC 119, at p. 127; 147 LT 281 (HL).

Hubley v. Hubley Estate [2011] PECA 19 (CanLII); 344 DLR (4th) 460.

Kolesar v. Jeffries [1976] 9 O.R. (2d) 41 at 48 (H.C.J.), varied (1976) 12 O.R. (2d) 142 (C.A.), aff'd (sub nom. Joseph Brant Memorial Hospital v. Koziol [1978] 1 S.C.R. 491).

Latin v. Hospital for Sick Children et al. (unreported, January 3, 2007, doc. No. 99-CV-174519) 2007 CanLII 34 (ON. S.C.) 2007. Carswell.

Meyer v. Gordon [1981] 17 C.C.L.T. 1 (B.C.S.C.).

Mohsina v. Ornstein [2013] ONSC 200 (CanLII).

R. v. Anderson [1985] 35 MVR 128, at p. 133 (Man. CA).

R. v. Coyne [1958] 124 C.C.C. 176; 31 C.R. 335 (N.B.C.A.).

R. v. Flynn [2017] ONSC 2290 (CanLII) http://canlii.ca/t/hn9nt

R. v. J.F. [2008] SCC 60 (CanLII), [2008] 3 S.C.R. 215.

R. v. Sharpe [1984] 12 C.C.C. (3d) 428; 39 C.R. (3d) 367; 26 MVR 279 (Ont. CA).

Shore v. Law Society of Upper Canada [2009] 250 O.A.C. 331 (DC).

T.C. v R.J.A. [2016] CanLII 9066 (ON HPARB).

Thompson Estate v. Byrne et al. [1993] 114 NSR (2d) 395 (SCTD).

Texts and Articles

Bureau du Coroner Quebec. (2021, October 1). *Death of Mrs. Joyce Echaquan. Coroner Géhane Kamel submits her investigation report.* https://www-coroner-gouv-qc-ca.translate.goog/medias/communiques/detail-dun-communique/466.html?_x_tr_sl=fr&_x_tr_tl=en&_x_tr_hl=en&_x_tr_pto=sc

Canadian Nurses Association. (2017). *Code of ethics for registered nurses.*

Canadian Nurses Association. (2022). *Nursing informatics.* https://www.cna-aiic.ca/en/nursing/nursing-tools-and-resources/nursing-informatics

Canadian Nurses Protective Society. (2003). *InfoLAW: Inquests and fatality inquiries* (under review). https://cnps.ca/article/inquests-and-fatality-inquiries/

Canadian Nurses Protective Society. (2022). *InfoLAW: Quality documentation: Your best defence.* https://cnps.ca/article/infolaw-qualitydocumentation/

College and Association of Registered Nurses of Alberta. (2018). *What does CARNA do?* http://www.nurses.ab.ca/content/carna/home/about/what-is-carna/what-we-do.html

College of Nurses of Ontario. (2018). *Professional misconduct.* Pub. No. 42007. https://www.cno.org/globalassets/docs/ih/42007_misconduct.pdf

Dunn, D. (2005). Home study program: Substance abuse among nurses—Intercession and intervention. *AORN Journal, 82*(5), 775–799.

Fischbach, F. T. (1996). *Documenting care: Communication, the nursing process and documentation standards.* F.A. Davis.

Fleming, J. (1983). *The law of torts* (6th ed.). The Law Book Co.

Gagnon, M. P., Desmartis, M., Labrecque, M., et al. (2012). Systematic review of factors influencing the adoption of information and communication technologies by healthcare professionals. *Journal of Medical Systems, 36*(1), 241–277.

Lapum, J., St-Amant, O., Ronquillo, C., et al. (n.d.). *Documentation in nursing* (1st Cdn. ed.). https://pressbooks.library.torontomu.ca/documentation/

Linden, A. M., Feldthusen, B. P., Hall, M. I., et al. (2018). *Canadian tort law* (11th ed., Student ed.). LexisNexis Canada.

The Long-Term Care Homes Public Inquiry. (2019). Inquiry report. https://longtermcareinquiry.ca/en/

University Health Network. (2022). *About myUHN patient portal.* https://www.uhn.ca/PatientsFamilies/myUHN

Zhong, E. H., McCarthy, C., & Alexander, M. (2016). A review of criminal convictions among nurses 2012–2013. *Journal of Nursing Regulation, 7*(1), 27–33.

8 COMPLEXITY AT THE END OF LIFE: ETHICAL AND LEGAL CHALLENGES

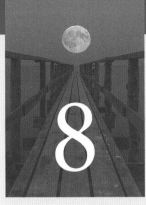

LEARNING OBJECTIVES

The purpose of this chapter is to enable you to understand:

- Important legal and ethical issues surrounding death and the process of dying
- Ethical and moral approaches to palliative care
- The values and challenges associated with advance directives
- The moral imperative of respecting the values, beliefs, and preferences of various cultures with respect to death and dying
- Special considerations of children and older persons at the end of life
- The legal and ethical implications of withdrawal of treatment
- The difference between euthanasia and assisted suicide
- The legal framework for Medical Assistance in Dying (MAiD)
- The legal and ethical challenges surrounding organ donation and transplantation

INTRODUCTION

Many of the most complex ethical and legal issues in health care today are associated with transitions at the end of a person's life. Notwithstanding the various cultural and religious views of death and any after-life, many people remain fearful of death and of the dying process.

Nurses play a vital role during this significant journey by providing compassionate care and comfort to the patient and family, and by ensuring that the process of dying is dignified for and respectful of all involved. Nurses have a significant role in minimizing suffering and in making it possible for the choices of the dying to be respected, such as ensuring those most important to them are present.

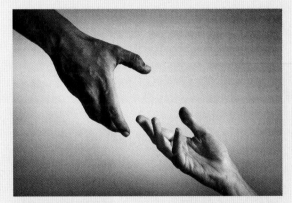

Nurses play a significant role at the end of a person's life. They minimize suffering and provide compassionate care and comfort to the patient and family. *Source: istockphoto.com/kieferpix*

Society and science have found many ways to extend life, leading to numerous options to improve life expectancy. Diets, exercise regimes, supplements, and meditation, to name a few, are espoused to be almost magical solutions to achieving health, treating illness, and avoiding an early death. Yet, extending life may diminish the quality and dignity that gives life meaning. Ethically, nurses are central to preserving dignity, and through the caring relationship they support the patient and those closest to them. While caring for the dying patient, nurses afford that person as much comfort, respect, and freedom from anxiety and pain as possible.

The financial and emotional costs of extending a person's life, even with a diagnosis of a terminal illness, can be high, posing challenges when resources are scarce. Science constantly finds new ways to extend life through research and advanced technology. Nursing care in such situations promotes the expression of dignity that ethically and morally respects the patient's values and wishes. When nurses provide gentle respect and comfort during these vulnerable moments, they allow persons to be their own navigators in achieving for them what constitutes a good death. Nurses also try to ensure consideration is given to the needs of the family or significant others when coping with their impending and subsequent loss (Canadian Nurses Association [CNA], 2017, pp. 13–14).

What constitutes a good death is person-specific and may include preferences for a specific dying process, acceptance that their life's journey is complete, having family present, being pain- and symptom-free, spiritual and emotional well-being, or receiving dignified and compassionate care (Meier et al., 2016).

DEATH AND DYING

The process of dying has become more complex and, in some circumstances, less humane. In previous decades, persons at the end of life frequently died in their own homes. Though able to have those most important to them present, the resources were not always in place to minimize pain and suffering. Now if a person dies in hospital—for example, in a critical care unit—the very technology that extends their life may create a barrier between caregivers, family members, and the person. Infection control protocols, as witnessed during the COVID-19 pandemic, may also serve to exclude family and friends when patients need them most. With advances in palliative care, persons are now afforded the opportunity to die at home, when the community supports are available, or in a hospice setting. In community settings, nurses play a significant role in assisting the family's engagement in care and in ensuring that the patient's wish to die peacefully in the setting of their choice is fulfilled.

In highly technological environments, patients may be denied the presence of family and friends, especially when death occurs during resuscitation efforts. In person- and family-centred settings, families are given the opportunity to be present during resuscitation efforts, even during the management of trauma in emergency departments.

In a hospital or long-term care facility, if a patient or resident's death is sudden or unexpected, and family members are not able to arrive in time, nurses can be present to provide comfort to the dying person. This reassures the family that their loved one had comfort and support, and may thus facilitate their grieving process. Although it may not always be possible, ensuring that someone is present in the final phase of a patient's dying should be considered a nursing priority for resource allocation and when organizing patient assignments.

A new era in end-of-life care began with the passing of Medical Assistance in Dying (MAiD) legislation, which gives some Canadians the choice to have medical assistance in dying. Since June 2016, physicians and nurse practitioners (NPs), at the request of an eligible person, can (1) administer a substance, or (2) prescribe or provide a substance for self-administration, either of which would result in that person's death. The ethical challenges and the legal implications for nurses and NPs are discussed in this chapter.

Advances in technology have achieved major successes in organ donation and transplantation. This became possible when "brain death" became the legal definition of death, and when life-support technology enabled perfusion of tissues and organs until retrieval and transplantation. Consequently, health care professionals have been obliged to explore and consider the distinction between life and death in such circumstances.

Canada is a multicultural society, and patients come from many religious and cultural backgrounds that view death and dying from varying perspectives. While being sensitive to these differences and respectful of the values and beliefs of others, in all settings and in all circumstances the goal of nursing is to play a central role in creating a humanistic environment while accompanying the patient through an end-of-life journey that is compassionate and caring.

This chapter will examine the complex ethical and legal issues that relate to the end-of-life continuum: death and dying.

CHALLENGES AT THE END OF LIFE

Communication

Patients and families can be overwhelmed when dealing with unfamiliar information at a time of incredible stress. They are expected to make complex and emotionally charged decisions as they struggle to comprehend and retain the information shared with them and be confident in the choices they make. A key role for nurses is to ensure effective communication and information sharing while creating an environment conducive to respectful conversations, and encouraging questions and listening to concerns. Patients and families struggle when facing end-of-life choices, so, when possible, it is best when these issues are discussed and options are explored in advance (Adams et al., 2011; Andershed, 2006; Heyland et al., 2009; Jezewski & Finnell, 1998; Lang & Quill, 2004). Various resources are in place to support advance decision making. Provincial and territorial governments offer tools and guidelines for advance directives that can be accessed on their respective websites.

Planning Forward: Advance Directives (Living Wills)

An *advance directive* allows persons to provide instructions regarding decisions about care if they become incompetent. When persons are not able to participate in decision making, advance directives ensure they retain some control of the care they receive. These directives can take the form of a verbal discussion with someone whom a person has identified as a substitute decision maker (SDM) or be made explicit in writing (Browne & Sullivan, 2006; Molloy et al., 2000; Singer et al., 1996).

A written advance directive may be created in the form of a *living will,* a document that enables persons to specify their informed choices well in advance of requiring such care. This takes effect only when a patient is incapable of making decisions. People who have living wills should update and revise them on a regular basis. Regardless of whether they are sanctioned by law, living wills are a useful resource for families and health care professionals when making end-of-life decisions on behalf of that person, as such wills are evidence of the wishes the person expressed when capable and able to reflect on various scenarios and options.

There are usually two components to living wills. An instruction directive allows persons to specify which life-sustaining treatments they would not wish in various situations. The proxy directive allows the individuals to identify a substitute decision maker should they ever be rendered incompetent.

For most people, it is difficult to envisage all possible scenarios in advance, especially when they have a limited understanding of the complexities of future health care decisions relating to the end of life. Ideally, individuals who complete a living will consult with physicians, nurses, and perhaps lawyers or other people so that they can anticipate the situations that might arise and comprehend the treatments available to them. This helps them make sound choices and ensures that these choices are clearly expressed and provide meaningful direction to health care professionals.

A living will can be revoked or altered at any time if the maker is competent. Advance directives may not be as helpful as initially intended as it is not possible for individuals to anticipate every possibility in advance or their future state of mind and circumstances (Porteri, 2018).

It is helpful to construct a life-values advance directive, thereby integrating the complexity of acceptable treatment with an expected level of independence, function, and quality of life (Kolarik et al., 2002; Murray et al., 2005). For example, persons can express in advance what they value most. Some may most value independence, being free from pain, or not wanting excessive use of technology when death is imminent or when the outcome might result in lifelong morbidity. Connection to family may also be an important value that might influence one's decision. For example, would a person want treatment withdrawn immediately if family members have to travel from out of town to say goodbye?

Individuals who complete a living will are advised to ensure that several appropriate people know that the will exists and that copies are shared, particularly with their doctor, lawyer, family members, and close friends. The will should be reviewed and updated regularly to ensure that it continues to reflect a person's current wishes.

All provinces and territories permit some forms of advance directives. The precise requirements vary from jurisdiction to jurisdiction (See for example: Ontario's *Substitute Decisions Act, 1992*; Manitoba's, *The Health*

Care Directives Act, C.C.S.M., c. H27; Nova Scotia's, *Personal Directives Act*, 2008; Alberta's, *Personal Directives Act*, 2000; and British Columbia's *Representation Agreement Act*, 1996). Most provinces and territories offer guides to completing advance directives on their websites.

END-OF-LIFE CHOICES

Resuscitation

Over the past few decades, advancements in pharmaceuticals and medical devices, such as defibrillators, have made cardiopulmonary resuscitation (CPR) a routine intervention unless the patient or the family has refused this in advance and a "no CPR" order is documented or included in some form of an advance directive. "No CPR" is frequently used interchangeably with "do not resuscitate" (DNR). However, DNR is a broader concept that may preclude other interventions, such as ventilation, antibiotic therapy, and so on. A person may agree to aggressive treatment but may choose not to receive CPR in the case of a cardiac arrest.

CPR has proven to be effective in specific cardiac events not related to another terminal condition (Booth, 2006). Such cardiac events may include sudden arrhythmias, such as ventricular fibrillation, or sudden asystole, related to cardiac disease. The positive results of defibrillation have led to public access to automated external defibrillators (AEDs) that are simple to use and available in many public settings. CPR is usually not as effective in circumstances in which a patient's condition is unrelated to a cardiac problem and when the patient's illness is in its final stage (e.g., emphysema or severe stroke) (Bigham et al., 2011; Booth, 2006). CPR in these circumstances, however, may negatively influence the quality and dignity of that person's death and the experience of that person's family and friends.

There has been some reflection on the burden placed on families when they have to make a "no CPR" or other end-of-life decisions on behalf of an incapable family member (Adams et al., 2011; Andershed, 2006; Cantor et al., 2003; Heyland et al., 2009; Lang & Quill, 2004; Venneman et al., 2008). Research suggests that the conflict and emotional distress the family faces may arise from the terminology used when they are asked to make this decision. From their perspective, they are being asked to make a decision not to do something. Some families feel they are making a deci-

sion not to prevent death, that they are signing a "death warrant" or "playing God," or that they are making a decision to terminate a loved one's life. The emotions associated with these thoughts would potentially have implications for the family's future bereavement process and if they worry that they played a role in causing the death, which was, in fact, inevitable (Jezewski & Finnell, 1998).

Framing the discussion around whether to "allow a natural death" enables a more positive experience in which one is contributing to a dignified and respectful death without the use of inappropriate interventions (Venneman et al., 2008). Knowing that the death was dignified and compassionate may also influence the family's experience and memories of the dying process (Cohen, 2004).

There are other considerations with respect to CPR that include whether this choice or intervention should be offered at all. For example, although one has the right to refuse any treatment offered, does a person have the right to demand a particular therapy when it is futile and has no likelihood of success (Bremer & Sandman, 2011)? Should the family or patient even be offered the option of CPR or other technologies when the patient is dying of a terminal illness, such as end-stage cancer, extreme cardiac failure, or severe traumatic brain damage? These questions are not straightforward when taking into consideration various cultural views or the family's or patient's reluctance to give up hope (Cantor et al., 2003). Such challenges are best met not through policy but via a fair process based on the shared relationship that the nurse and the team have with patients and their family. As these situations arise, they should be explored through a common understanding of the values and perspectives of all team members, including those of the patient and family. For example, what are the goals behind the family's or patient's wishes? A patient who is near death may want some minimal resuscitation if a close friend or family member is soon to arrive from out of town and the patient wants to say goodbye. At the same time, there are challenges within a complex system with limited resources that consistently attempts to meet the needs of all patients (e.g., a critically ill patient may be waiting in the emergency department until a bed is available on the unit).

These tensions occur in complex sociological, cultural, technological, legal, and political contexts. Making decisions in these circumstances are not easy and are made based on probabilities since there are few absolutes in health care. Each situation is unique and must be decided contextually, with the focus on what is best for the person. Ethical principles, similar cases, professional codes, positions, statements, policies, and procedures can serve as guides, but each circumstance requires a collaborative effort while deciding on the most ethical course of action (Hayes, 2004).

Palliative Care: Ensuring Relief of Suffering

Palliative care is an option for, but not restricted to, end-of life care. The focus of palliative care, derived from the Latin *palliare*, meaning to "cloak", is on symptom management, the relief of suffering and quality of life (Webster, 2022). Palliative care can be provided in the home, hospice, or other settings, such as hospitals, retirement homes, and LTC facilities. The goal of palliative care is to provide a holistic approach across the continuum of care, to ensure the relief of pain and suffering (physical, spiritual, emotional and psychological), as depicted in Fig. 8.1. Specific aspects, or elements of care, focus on the patient and family and those relationships important to them. Those relationships include the interprofessional team providing care. Though palliative care is provided across the continuum of the illness when the end of a person's life is reached this approach ensures a peaceful and dignified death.

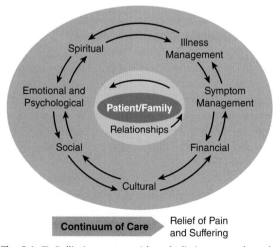

Fig. 8.1 ■ Palliative care provides a holistic approach to the relief of pain and suffering. *Source: https://www.pallium.ca/professionals/ Health Professionals: Pallium Canada.*

Regardless of the setting, nurses can provide superior supportive care to their patients. Nurses experience a sense of reward and satisfaction when guiding patients and families through this complex journey, more so when quality at the end of a person's life and a peaceful death are realized. At the end of life persons may express the need for closure, reconciliation and continuity. A dying person may want to recall important life events and ensure an ongoing connection with family by documenting their story in a journal or through video, and nurses can facilitate this. Nurses are in an important and significant position to give family and friends the opportunity to be involved in care and to aid in this significant transition, if they, and the patient, so choose. Nurses may enable opportunities for the dying person, friends, and family to engage in meaningful conversation and perhaps reach closure on past issues that have remained unresolved. For as long as possible, the nurse should ensure that the patient retains control over the process. Patients should lead the direction of their care, for example, decide on the right balance of pain management if they are alert and able to do so (Hayes, 2004).

Palliative Sedation

Palliation sedation is the administration of sedation to reduce a dying person's consciousness to relieve intolerable suffering from refractory symptoms. Continuous deep sedation is controversial as it ends a person's ability to interact meaningfully with others and has the double effect of shortening life.

The debate focuses on the ethical intention to use sedation for the relief of intolerable symptoms versus the intention of hastening death, a form of euthanasia. Further there are questions about what constitutes intolerable suffering (Bruce & Boston, 2011). Some raise concerns about the risks of this becoming a substitute for other palliative care options while others argue that suffering can only be defined by the person, and that all suffering cannot be relieved in spite of advances in palliative care.

Nurses play a significant role during this process, including supporting the patient and family in the decision-making process, the administration and monitoring of sedation, and providing compassionate care (Heino et al., 2022). Making this decision is a difficult one for patients and families who must appreciate the consequences once the process begins.

UNIQUE DEATH AND DYING EXPERIENCES: DYING YOUNG

Most expect that the death of a child does not precede that of parents and grandparents. For nurses caring for terminally ill and dying infants and children, the need for compassionate care seems magnified and extends to the entire family.

Neonates

Advances in technology have led to complex ethical dilemmas with respect to the care of newborns with uncertain prognoses. Interventions to support and treat high-risk newborns have become more effective, to the extent that it is now possible, in some circumstances, for the child to achieve a normal life. However, these interventions may alternatively result in a life with disability or developmental delays. In some cases, these interventions compromise the quality of the infant's life and prolong the dying process (Committee on Fetus and Newborn [American Academy of Pediatrics], 2007).

The limits of viability have changed, and an infant born at 22 weeks is now considered viable. This, in part, is the result of specialized neonatal transport units, where teams go to the delivery setting to facilitate the birth, support resuscitation efforts, and, when necessary, transport the infant to sophisticated neonatal units (Dr. H. Whyte, personal communication, March 27, 2018). When a child is born at 22 to 32 weeks' gestation, parents are forced to make very difficult decisions that balance quality versus extension of life (Paris et al., 2006). Parents must choose between aggressive interventions or palliation when long-term outcomes for the baby are difficult to predict. Those looking forward to parenthood and the birth of a child are now suddenly faced with making decisions for their baby, whose future values and wishes are not known, and whose future life is yet undetermined (McAllister & Dionne, 2006). Decisions are particularly challenging when an infant presents with a disease or injury for which outcomes are totally unpredictable. For example, infant hypoxic ischemic encephalopathy (HIE), a brain dysfunction caused by a reduction of oxygen in the brain, is a primary source of severe impairment and death. The effects can be mild, moderate, or severe and may result in neurodevelopmental and motor skill delays, epilepsy, and cognitive challenges. Often, the extent of damage is

difficult to predict. The challenging choices may include allowing a natural death, short-term interventions to assess the extent of damage, or sustaining life with a permanent tracheostomy and chronic ventilation. The ethical issues that are balanced in the decision-making process include sanctity of life, the quality of life for the child and parents, and futility (given the unpredictability of outcomes and the potential for survival). Also, the principle of justice, is relevant given the resources that would be required to support the child for many years to come. It is a challenging balancing act, as well as an ethical grey zone (Dr. H. Whyte, personal communication, March 27, 2018).

Further ethical debate centres on the notion of futility and, in some circumstances, whether options other than allowing for a natural death should be offered at all. Challenges in making these decisions are amplified as technology evolves and conditions that would have resulted in certain death a few years ago now entail the possibility of survival, although with an uncertain quality of life for both the child and the family. Take, for example, an infant born with central hypoventilation syndrome ("Ondine's curse"), a congenital respiratory disorder that results in respiratory arrest during sleep. These children are normal in every other way, cognitively and physically. In the past, because the condition was considered permanent and the prognosis for a good quality of life was poor, frequently the approach was to provide palliation rather than aggressive intervention. Now, emerging evidence shows that with more aggressive use of technology, this condition may improve as the child develops. Experience is showing that by providing respiratory support with a tracheostomy and chronic ventilation in the home, they may improve after a few years to the point of needing only minimal support, such as continuous positive airway pressure (CPAP). The options have evolved from thinking that allowing a peaceful death would be in the best interests of the child to offering the option of respiratory support with the hope of improvement. With more resources to support in-home ventilation, this has become a more viable option. Still, for parents, making this decision continues to be challenging. The future prognosis and quality of life for the infant may still be uncertain, but there is no doubt that the child's care needs would be extremely high and taxing on the parents, potentially stressful for the family dynamic, and resource intensive. There are ethical questions related to whether, in these circumstances, the parents should have a choice. For example, what would be the ethical and legal implications if the parents refuse to provide such support while a health care team considers that doing so would be in the best interests of the child (Dr. H. Whyte, personal communication, March 27, 2018)?

Babies born prematurely may simply have arrived early or may have medical challenges, such as cardiac, gastrointestinal, or congenital anomalies. In some cases, multiple challenges are anticipated; in others, they are not, and may not be discovered until birth. These various scenarios influence the timing and extent to which the health care team can collaborate with the parents to decide on the best course of action. Regardless, parents of premature babies need the special support of nurses and the health care team. Communication and how the message is delivered are extremely important.

In these extremely challenging and emotional moments, the health care team and the parents must weigh the benefits and burdens of aggressive intervention in circumstances such as the following:

- Early death is very likely, and survival would be accompanied by a high risk of severe morbidity.
- Intervention would only prolong dying.
- The prognosis is uncertain, and survival may be associated with diminished quality of life.
- Significant neurodevelopmental disability is possible.
- The infant would suffer significant discomfort (e.g., pain).
- Survival is likely, and the risk of morbidity is low (Janvier & Barrington, 2005).

In situations where the infant's future is highly uncertain, the parents' decisions are even more difficult (Meadow, 2006). It is important that the decisions be made collaboratively and that the team respects the wishes of the family and ensures that the best interests of the infant are met. Because these decisions are made in very stressful situations, a collaborative team approach (with the parents as members of the team) to decision making is essential (Baumann-Hölzle et al., 2005).

For the parents and the family, continuity of care is extremely important; therefore, whenever possible,

one nurse should be designated to provide ongoing support for the family, and a core team of nurses should be consistently assigned to caring for the infant. In these difficult circumstances, the parents need to see strong interprofessional collaboration that can enable effective and meaningful communication (Kowalski et al., 2005). Parents may view nurses as their primary source of information, so nurses are in a leadership position to promote parents as active participants in the infant's care.

When the decision is to provide palliative care, nurses must support the parents and the family through this very difficult transition. They do this by respecting the special needs of these parents whose child's life is about to end just as it has begun. Nurses may support the family through this emotional transition by:

- Facilitating the opportunity for the parents to provide direct care to their infant
- Creating memories by taking pictures or videos or making sculptures of the infants hands or feet
- Facilitating breastfeeding, if possible, or supporting pumping to ensure the infant receives the mother's milk
- Creating the opportunity for the infant to go home
- Ensuring sibling participation
- Influencing organizations to make available family-centred, home-like environments that offer privacy and dignity (Epstein, 2007; Ives-Baine, 2007)

Nurses have a responsibility to ensure the comfort of the dying neonate and to provide the parents (and siblings) the opportunity to create memories that can sustain them through their loss. It is important for families to have memories of the infant in settings other than the hospital. In many settings, rooms are set up to provide a more home-like and peaceful environment where parents can hold and comfort their child and each other.

The Special Circumstances of the Dying Child

The world of the dying child is highly charged emotionally and involves highly complex moral and ethical issues. Parents and the team must make difficult choices on behalf of the child who may not be competent or of an age to make these decisions on their own. Competent youth may refuse to consent or assent to treatment that may have the potential to extend life. These dilemmas are more challenging when the outcomes of specific therapies may not be clear and when the quality of life of a child may be compromised (Carlet et al., 2004). Nurses have expressed crises of conscience when caring for a critically ill or dying child when they believe the treatments to be overly burdensome or when they believe that use of technology is inappropriate (Solomon et al., 1993). Rarely do nurses cite examples of the health care team giving up too soon (Solomon et al., 2005), which is not surprising because our frame of reference assumes that children should have a long life ahead of them. Society is programmed to care for and protect children, and therefore, it is to be expected that every attempt is made to prevent their premature death. That being said, health care teams need to address these moral and emotional challenges to ensure that children die with dignity, free of pain, and receive the compassionate care that ought to be afforded to persons of all ages (Jordan et al., 2018).

There are challenges when there is conflict between the team and family about continuing care or withdrawing treatment (Canadian Paediatric Society, 2004). Consider a child with a serious brain injury that might evolve to brain death or might leave the child in a persistent vegetative state. The family may not be ready to accept this outcome and may need some time to adjust. Yet, the team may think that continuing life support is a burden on a strained system and is disrespectful of the child.

When not managed effectively, the experience of moral distress (for the team and the family) in these circumstances is not uncommon. These situations are more complex when there is limited ability to predict outcomes adding to the ethical challenges faced by the team and family. The team is challenged to balance the complexities of autonomy (the parents as substitute decision makers) against harm and suffering, and the conflict in personal values. This is especially so when there is conflict with the personal values of the team and family relative to their respective views of quality as opposed to sanctity of life (Mills & Cortezzo, 2020).

These conflicts and their consequences, for the patient, the family, and the team can be mitigated with collaborative conversations regarding the plan of care and the advantages and disadvantages of the options available. What is key is that the family is supported, and their values and beliefs are respected. For the team, this is an opportunity for value clarification so that all positions can be understood. At times, if conflicts cannot be resolved, there are opportunities for outside mediation (Meller & Barclay, 2011) and consultation with ethics committees where possible, prior to any legal intervention.

Nurses often develop long-term relationships and emotional bonds with patients and their families when caring for children who require continuing care, for example, those with cancer, cystic fibrosis, or transplant recipients. When the child they have grown to know so well and cared for over time is nearing death, it can cause great emotional trauma. In these circumstances, nurses may not find it helpful to draw on traditional reasoning processes. Instead, an ethic of care that focuses on the relationship with the child and the family can enable nurses to understand and accept what is right from all perspectives and continue engaging with and supporting the child and the family. Nurses are rewarded when they know they have contributed to a dignified journey for that child.

Issues of consent are challenging for parents who must decide on behalf of their child, even more so when their child is dying or is diagnosed with a terminal illness. These challenges associated with consent are discussed in Chapter 6.

Some of the most difficult circumstances involve making decisions about whether to provide life support or not. A decision may be made to forgo life-support when a child is terminally ill or permanently unconscious, in instances of medical futility, or when the burdens of treatment outweigh any benefits. However, there may be some families with religious and cultural views that might not accept this and may insist on continuing care beyond accepted medical standards. These situations are never easy. They become increasingly challenging when they relate to the withdrawal of treatment already begun versus making the choice to allow a natural death. Although the family may decide against highly complex technological support for their child, decisions related to the withdrawal of nutrition, particularly given the symbolic nature of nurturing a child through the provision of food and water, are even more difficult (Canadian Paediatric Society, 2004; Kirsch et al., 2018).

Nurses are empathetic to the needs of the family by encouraging their involvement in care, in pain and symptom management, and in making the situation as normal as possible for the child, which may be achieved by enabling the child to die at home. If this is not possible, even a hospital room can be arranged to create a home-like environment. In all circumstances, it is important that nurses support parents in enacting their parental role with their child. The importance of patient- and family-centred care is discussed in Chapter 12.

As discussed, many children are not able to make difficult end-of-life decisions for themselves. They may be too young, too ill, or cognitively impaired. There are unique consent challenges regarding treatment decisions when one is dealing with an adolescent. A 13-year-old who is newly diagnosed with cancer may want to refuse treatment due to fear of pain and of feeling sick. However, a 13-year-old with a long history of leukemia who has relapsed on several occasions, having been through that experience, would be in a

more informed position when making a decision not to accept further treatment.

Of particular importance in pediatric cases is a child's need to develop emotionally and socially even when they are ill or dying. Consider the story of the teen who was diagnosed with osteosarcoma of the tibia at age 10 years, discussed in Case Scenario 8.1.

MEANINGFUL LIVES: THE FINAL JOURNEY

Persons who die late in life may no longer be able to care for themselves. It is distressing when those who, throughout their lives, contributed a great deal to society, their profession, their families, and others become unable to care for themselves because of physical inability, frailty, end-stage chronic disease, and dementia. They may experience the loss of dignity and yearn for the same degree of respect they received earlier in their lives. Some may be abandoned by their families; others may worry that they are a burden on them. People who have been independent their whole life find it difficult to rely on others to accomplish even

---

CASE SCENARIO 8.1

I MAY BE DYING, BUT I AM STILL GROWING UP

A 13-year-old teen, L. H., was actively engaged in conversation with the nurses about all the things teens want to talk about. When she was going through chemotherapy, she enjoyed displaying all the stylish wigs she was able to wear and enjoyed her sense of fashion. L. H. had been cared for by the same nursing team for almost 3 years before the cancer returned and spread to her lungs.

L. H. deteriorated quickly during this relapse and suffered major respiratory distress. She was very upset that she would not be able to attend her Grade 8 graduation ceremony. L. H.'s primary nurse mobilized the team, organized an ambulance, and, along with one of the physicians, escorted her to the graduation ceremony. L. H. was able to maintain her stamina and was wheeled into the graduation hall where she received a standing ovation from her teachers and fellow classmates as she

received her diploma. L. H. died after returning to the hospital that evening.

At this important milestone in L. H.'s life, her primary nurse understood what mattered to L. H. and her family. To the end, L. H. continued to grow and develop as any 13-year-old girl would. She was still a child graduating from Grade 8 and in need of this important rite of passage. In fact, she was not ready to die until she reached this milestone. This act of caring ensured that her family, despite their grief, would retain the happy memory of their child's achieving her goal—receiving her Grade 8 diploma along with her friends.

This story illustrates one aspect of the developmental stage of a young adolescent. How might nurses consider the phases of development in others? What about the infant? The young mother? A person who has just lost their spouse? The older person who has had so many life experiences? How should these factors be considered in nursing practice?

basic bodily functions. Nurses who engage in conversation with older persons about their lives, listen to them, and learn from them are richer for the experience. Older persons need stimulation and socialization and frequently want to share their stories with others.

When older persons transition to a long-term care facility, they understand that they are entering the final phase of their life's journey. Nurses play a critical role in helping these residents achieve a high quality of life until their death and ensure that they retain as much control over their lives as possible. A palliative care approach to care guides the journey with a focus on quality of life, relationships, spiritual care, and pain and symptom management.

An integrated evidence-informed and equity-based online resource is available for nurses to guide their practice and strengthen their relationships with residents and families as they prepare for death: *Resources for Strengthening a Palliative Approach in Long-Term Care* (SPA-LTC; https://spaltc.ca/resources-2/). SPA-LTC was developed by a Canadian team of health researchers who integrate and evaluate best practices in palliative care, nationally and across the globe.

The COVID-19 pandemic led to catastrophic consequences for older persons in long-term care settings across the country, particularly in Ontario and Quebec (Canadian Institute for Health Information [CIHI], 2021). Most devastating was that the lockdowns, intended to protect residents, isolated them from their families and close friends. Sad and lonely, many residents died alone, and many staff experienced moral distress because they were unable to provide the compassionate care needed. The extent of the suffering is detailed in a report issued by Nursing members of the Canadian Armed Forces who provided support at five long-term care homes in Ontario during the height of the pandemic Canadian Armed Forces, 4th Canadian Division Joint Task Force [Central], 2020).

CULTURAL CONSIDERATIONS AT THE END OF LIFE

A respectful understanding of another's culture leads to trust, openness, and more productive ongoing relationships. It is important not to judge other cultures in relation to one's own values and customs. It is also important not to make assumptions that just because a person present as a member of a specific

culture or religion that they follow all of their traditions or beliefs

While engaging with a patient, it is important to keep in mind that culture is layered and multidimensional and that each person or family is unique in how cultural behavioural patterns may be practised (Solomon & Schell, 2009). (For a better understanding of this theory, see https://www.palomar.edu/anthro/tutorials/cultural.htm) Although it is helpful to understand the generalities of specific cultures, this is just the starting point in learning about others and developing a global mindset. Such understanding provides general guidelines to support conversations with others while refraining from stereotyping or making assumptions.

Value clarification can facilitate the understanding of other cultures. As discussed in Chapter 2, this process helps individuals come to understand their respective values and their relative importance. To facilitate understanding across multiple groups, open dialogue, active listening, and a commitment to mutual respect are necessary.

An ethical approach to care requires the nurse to understand the views, religious, and cultural traditions of the patient and family. It is important to build these considerations into the overall initial assessment to understand people's values and traditions. The nurse's attention to such needs can improve the quality of the dying process and constructively influence the bereavement that follows. A general familiarity with the fundamental concepts of various cultural, spiritual, and religious traditions allows nurses to provide competent, compassionate, and respectful care as patients from differing backgrounds approach the end of life (Ross, 2001). By undertaking cultural assessments of patients and their families, nurses gain a basic understanding of the values and practices important to them and can, thus, play a crucial role in supporting the patient and the family at the end of life. Understanding these factors further influences relationships, communication, and decision making in the practice setting. Understanding a person's culture also helps the team interpret observations and facilitates a shared understanding of that which has meaning. When nurses do their best to facilitate traditional practices, the family experiences the true meaning of care and respect, and nurses feel valued when the best possible outcomes are achieved.

To understand the importance of these assessments, three examples of various cultural perspectives on the end of life are presented. Note that, as mentioned, even within these perspectives, individuals may have a range of views, and this reinforces the importance of asking. It is not possible to know in advance the beliefs and rituals of all cultures; therefore, it is important to ask the patient and the family what is most significant to them to understand and accommodate their beliefs.

Indigenous Views on End of Life

There is no single Indigenous culture, so one cannot assume that all views and practices within a community are uniform. As with many other cultures, varying beliefs and values exist within Indigenous communities. Some individuals may value quality of life rather than the exclusive pursuit of a cure, whereas others may want aggressive intervention complemented by traditional medicine. Some believe medical intervention should be minimal and that the Creator determines the time of death. Diversity of beliefs exists between and within Indigenous communities as a result of differences in traditional, acculturated, or religious perspectives.

The concept of health in Indigenous communities is probably best understood as a set of assumptions about the holistic nature of a person. Both physical health and emotional health are considered to result in the balance of mind, body, and spirit and in the strength of interpersonal relationships. This holistic view means that modern healing practices that focus purely on physical problems may not always be accepted. They might prefer to be treated by traditional healers who use healing circles, spiritual approaches, and traditional medicines. Not all Indigenous peoples want traditional healing; others may see it as being complementary to conventional medicine (Anderson, 2002). The *Report of the Aboriginal Justice Inquiry of Manitoba* indicated that some Indigenous Elders and healers believe that Indigenous people who are ill must have their body, mind, and soul heal fully in the Indigenous way (Aboriginal Justice Implementation Commission [AJIC], 1999). They believe that involvement with non-Indigenous medicine means that a person cannot be healed properly in the traditional way. Other Elders and Healers believe that traditional approaches can be complementary to non-Indigenous medicine. (AJIC, 1999). Again as with all cultures, it is important that nurses not make assumptions but

explore the values, beliefs, and wishes of the patients and families they are caring for. Indigenous patients might wish to involve Elders in their care and treatment decisions. Elders, valued for their wisdom and experience, might be invited participants in decision making because they are highly respected and valued for their life experiences.

Generally, Indigenous people view life in four stages. The "Circle of Life" includes birth, life, death, and the after-life, with ceremonies and rituals associated with each. In death, mother earth reclaims the physical form, the Creator takes the spirit to the place of origin, and the cycle of life is complete. When a person is dying, ceremonies may include traditional medicines and prayers intended to guide the spirit back to the spirit world. These rituals are often performed by a spiritual leader or another respected Elder, with family and often community members present (Anderson, 2002; Johnston et al., 2013).

The nature and practice of such rituals and ceremonies vary across communities and may include pipe ceremonies, as pipes and tobacco are considered sacred items. Other sacred medicines, such as sage, sweetgrass, or cedar may be burned to help purify the person who is encouraged to be at peace within themselves and the Creator. All who are present pray for the safe passage of the spirit and hold vigils to bring comfort and to ease pain. Stories are shared and ancestors are invited to guide the spirit in its travels. It is important not to interrupt these ceremonies; understanding the importance of these rituals demonstrates compassion and respect (Anderson, 2002).

Nurses play a key role in facilitating these ceremonies and rituals, especially in the hospital setting. Nurses must recognize that the Indigenous culture embraces the community beyond the immediate family and respects the role of Elders, even in decision making. Indigenous patients often prefer to have immediate and extended family members involved in decisions about their care, demonstrating the centrality of family and community (Kelly & Minty, 2007). Therefore, the care team can expect many visitors. Where possible, private rooms are preferable not only to facilitate the process but also to respect the needs of other patients and families. In communities where there is a high population of Indigenous peoples, specific rooms can be designated for these processes (Anderson, 2002; Kelly & Minty, 2007).

Islamic Views on End of Life

In Islam, death is not viewed as final but, rather, as a transition from this world to eternity. Just as the fetus develops in the womb, Muslims believe that the soul undergoes growth and change in the grave in preparation for the Day of Resurrection (Chittick, 1992; Kramer, 1988). As Muslims approach death, they must be placed in the supine position, facing Mecca (the spiritual centre of the Muslim faith, located in Saudi Arabia). The room must be perfumed, and anyone "unclean" must leave it. Excerpts from the Quran are read by the dying person or a close friend or family member, and the basic tenet of Islam—"There is no God but Allah, and Muhammad is his prophet"—is recited (Chittick, 1992; Kramer, 1988), thus making the connection from birth to death, as this is the first statement read to the newborn. Traditionally, families prepare the body for burial almost immediately, and, when possible, the dead are buried on the day they die. Ideally, family members are present at the time of death, both to mourn and to prepare the body (Ross, 2001).

Buddhist Views on End of Life

In Buddhism, death is not viewed as the end of life but merely the end of the body. The spirit remains and seeks attachment to a new body and new life which is influenced by the person's past actions. Accumulated actions, or *karma,* influence future lives, and in this sense, death is not feared as it leads to rebirth (Keown, 2005; Tang, 2002).

If a person has brought happiness to people, that person will be happy in this life and in a future life. If a person has led a responsible and compassionate life and has no regrets when death approaches, that person is at peace and in a state of grace at the time of death.

A dying Buddhist person is likely to request the service of a monk or nun in their tradition to assist in this process further, making the transitional experience of death peaceful and free of fear (Keown, 2005; Tang, 2002).

Before and at the time of death, and for a period after death, the monk, nun, or spiritual friends may read prayers and chant. Death bed chanting is regarded as very important and is ideally the last thing the Buddhist hears. Buddhists believe that one can actively assist and bring relief to the dying person through these processes (Keown, 2005; Tang, 2002).

The final moment of consciousness is considered paramount, the most important moment of all. If the ill person is in hospital and is unlikely to survive, the family may call in a Buddhist priest to pray so that at the final moment, their loved one can find their way into a higher state of rebirth (Keown, 2005; Tang, 2002).

Persons are not supposed to touch the body for several hours after death because of the belief that the spirit of a person will linger on for some time and can be affected by what happens to the body. It is important that the body is treated gently and with respect; and it is believed that the priest can help the spirit continue its journey calmly to higher states, not causing the spirit to become angry and confused (Keown, 2005; Tang, 2002).

Undertaking these rituals might be challenging in the institutional setting; however, Case Scenario 8.2 is a compelling illustration of the incredible role nurses can play in supporting a family through the death of a loved one. In this situation, a newborn child with a serious congenital condition was dying, and the child's nurses supported the parents and grandparent through this emotional time.

CASE SCENARIO 8.2

HONOURING BELIEFS

When 26 days old, an infant was diagnosed with a fatal congenital condition. The parents were devastated because earlier, they had given birth to a child with the same condition, and that child had died shortly after birth. Why did they have the misfortune to give birth to two children with the same condition?

Why them? What had they done in their previous lives to warrant such a tragedy? The notion of *karma* in the Buddhist tradition is the belief that one's actions in past lives have consequences in future lives. The parents understood their child would die soon and, in discussions with the health care team, agreed that palliative care was in their infant's best interests.

CASE SCENARIO 8.2 *(Continued)*

The parents were not religious, however, the infant's grandparent, who had just arrived from northern China and did not speak a word of English, had strong Buddhist beliefs. The grandparent had been informed prior to leaving China that things did not look good for their grandchild; however, this gentle elder came to assist their grandchild through this very significant transition. When the grandparent entered the hospital room, they began to chant and continued to chant in spite of their fatigue after such a long journey. The nurses discovered that Buddhists believe that chanting helps connect the living with the higher being. They were chanting to encourage the higher being to lead their grandchild's spirit to a happier place. Although the grandparent had not slept for more than 2 days, they continued chanting, sometimes falling asleep while doing so. They also wrote messages in Chinese on small cards, which were placed on their grandchild's chest. These were also intended to help the child get to the next place. The nurses were careful to put the cards back in place whenever they provided care that required moving them.

The nurses soon discovered that the grandparent's belief was that more voices chanting would strengthen the request for calling the coming of the higher being, so they began to chant with the family. They further discovered that after death, it was important for the chanting to continue for an additional 16 hours because it would take this long for the spirit to leave the body and ensure the connection with the higher being. Although clearly not the norm that the deceased remain in the acute care setting that long, the nurses made this possible and transferred the infant and family to a private, more peaceful setting in the hospital. In doing so, they made a significant difference.

The nurses learned a great deal. They gained insight into the importance of faith to some families and how faith and tradition give people strength and the ability to survive adversity, such as the death of a child. The experience reinforced that language barriers can be overcome by being present and by sharing in rituals, whether understood or not. It also validated that by asking and listening, "nurses begin to understand the values and beliefs of that person rather than make assumptions based on what is generally known about that culture." (Ives-Baine, 2007).

Questions

1. What are your learnings from this story?
2. How do you gain insight into the cultural values and beliefs of your patients and their families?
3. The nurses were able to make a difference in this situation. What are the barriers that must be overcome to ensure all families in these circumstances have a meaningful experience?

With the increasing diversity of society, a single policy for the care of the dying and of the person after death is not possible. A meaningful death goes a long way in supporting the family's grieving process and in providing comfort. By facilitating and engaging in traditional practices, nurses can help achieve the right outcomes for the dying (Ross, 2001).

Organizational processes and resources can facilitate the provision of culturally sensitive care. Supports to the team include but are not limited to:

- A directory of spiritual and Indigenous healers, as a resource to the teams or a support to the patient and family
- Educational material for patients and families that communicates to them that various cultural, religious, and traditional ceremonies are welcomed and can be accommodated
- Staff education and online resources regarding respect for diversity and best practices associated with cultural sensitivity
- Formation of cultural/spiritual care committees to create staff awareness, to foster relationships of mutual respect, to provide education, and to facilitate the adoption of best practices

CHOOSING DEATH

As science and technology advanced over the past number of decades, ethical debates regarding the choices associated with prolonging versus ending life intensified. Specifically, attention focused on various approaches to end of life, such as the withdrawal of treatment, assisted suicide, and Medical Assistance in Dying (MAiD). Considering these ethical debates and in response to individual legal challenges, the law regarding end of life in Canada has evolved. High profile cases guided the transition to Canadian legislation on MAiD, enacted in 2016.

Euthanasia

Euthanasia, derived from the Greek words *eu* meaning "good," and *thanatos*, meaning "death," is a means for ending the life of a person with the goal of eliminating pain and suffering and ensuring a peaceful dignified death. The Supreme Court of Canada endorsed the view that the distinctive quality of euthanasia is that a third party is taking an intentional action that will result in the death of the patient (*Rodriguez v. British Columbia (Attorney General)*, 1993). Euthanasia can be indirect or direct.

Direct euthanasia:

■ It involves active steps (such as the administration of a drug or drugs intended to cause death) to end the life of a person. This action might be as a result of a request from the patient, from a substitute decision maker or a decision by the person taking the action. Such a request might arise in cases of irreversible injury or terminal illness, when persons deem their quality of life no longer acceptable, and they want to choose the time and means of their death. When the decision is not made by the patient themselves, the action is criminal except in very limited circumstances.

Indirect euthanasia:

■ Involves actions that allow persons to die of their disease or condition. Actions may include the withholding or withdrawing of treatment necessary for the continuation of life, or the administration of increasingly higher doses of analgesia and sedation with the intent of relieving pain, understanding that the medication has the potential to hasten death.

A heightened awareness of euthanasia arose partly from advances in health care technology and partly from the growing number of persons with chronic or terminal conditions whose quality and dignity of life were diminished. Circumstances where the death of a person is intended have been extremely problematic, and there are severe restrictions on the circumstances where it might be permitted. Where the patient was a participant in the decision, courts were sometimes prepared to consider the option. Where the decision maker was acting without the consent of the patient, criminal sanctions were imposed. Examples of both situations will be discussed below.

For those who support euthanasia, it is viewed as an act of compassion as the intention is to do good by relieving pain and suffering. Some who argue against euthanasia base their reasoning on the principle of sanctity of life and the traditional rules and laws prohibiting the taking of life except in situations of self-defence or war. (Strong advocates of this principle would argue that it is unacceptable to kill even in these circumstances.) Others are concerned about the potential for abuse. They argue that it would be difficult to limit the act to situations in which patients are terminally ill and actively dying; conceivably, it might extend to the chronically ill, the infirm, the aged, and those with dementia. This is the **"slippery slope"** argument.

Those who agree with euthanasia believe that not all life is worth living. They believe that when someone is dying and it is no longer possible to eliminate their physical, emotional, and psychological pain, then euthanasia should be permitted at the request, and with the consent, of the competent patient. Supporters believe that sanctity of life is not an absolute principle and can be overridden out of respect both for patient autonomy and for the dignity of human life. They believe that when death is inevitable or suffering unbearable, euthanasia only makes a person's end of life more compassionate and dignified. If rules were in place to control the process of euthanasia, they argue, then the potential for abuse would be lessened.

Case Scenario 8.3 highlights some of the legal and ethical challenges associated with these issues.

CASE SCENARIO 8.3

A CRY FOR HELP?

A 40-year-old mother of two teenage children had been diagnosed 2 years earlier with ovarian cancer. She has always been independent and active, a devoted mother who ran a corporate law practice and participated in many volunteer organizations.

Early in her illness, she was treated with chemotherapy, radiotherapy, and surgery. For a time, the cancer seemed to be in remission. However, after a year, it metastasized to her liver and lower intestines. Since then, she has been in and out of hospital, receiving various treatments. Over the past 2 months, her health has deteriorated to the point that she has constant intense pain, especially in her bones. During her last admission to hospital, the team decided that nothing they could do would slow the disease process. After discussions with the team and her family, she decided to enter a home palliative care program that would provide her with home care services, a pain control protocol, and nursing care. As well, her spouse has taken a leave of absence from work to remain at home with her.

For the past few weeks, her condition has remained unchanged, although the pain is becoming difficult to control, and she suffers frequent bouts of nausea and constipation (side effects of the medication). She has become despondent and distressed by her loss of dignity and the effect her illness is having on her family.

One day, she exclaims to the nurse: "I've had enough! I cannot stand the pain; I've become a burden on my husband and children. Please help me end it!" The next day, the nurse finds her confused and disoriented.

Questions

1. What actions can the nurse take, (a) legally and (b) ethically?
2. What options are available for this patient?

Discussion

Even with the best palliative care, not all pain and suffering can be relieved. When death is preferred, the means toward achieving it may place caregivers and family under great moral distress—for example,

in the case of withholding food and fluids at a patient's request. These situations are more difficult when the patient is no longer competent, has left no advance directive, and a substitute decision maker is left to make the decision. Hence, it is not surprising that questions around advance directives, withdrawal of treatment, euthanasia, and assisted suicide have intensified in recent years.

Nurses may experience extreme emotional and moral distress when dealing with challenges related to death and dying. In most settings, they have sustained and close contact with patients and their families. Consequently, they are able to empathize with their physical, emotional, and spiritual experiences. Conflict arises when the patient's wishes, the nurse's loyalty to the patient, and the principle of beneficence (i.e., concern over providing good and avoiding harm when pain control and symptom relief fails) clash with the principle of sanctity of life and the law. These situations represent true dilemmas that nurses face in their practice and provide a poignant reminder that what is legal may not, for some, be what is right.

This scenario offers an illustration of one that challenges the ethical and professional integrity of the nurse and the nature of the nurse–patient relationship. Nurses are encouraged to empathize—that is, to enter the patient's way of seeing and being—so that they can attempt to appreciate the patient's experience and understand the situation from the patient's perspective. A nurse working closely with a patient, as in this scenario, might understand this request and notwithstanding their ethical values and beliefs, would experience frustration due to their limited ability to reduce all physical and emotional pain and suffering.

Nurses have a duty to care for the physical, emotional, and psychological needs of those entrusted to them. The CNA *Code of Ethics for Registered Nurses* (2017) includes the following responsibilities:

"In all practice settings, nurses work to relieve pain and suffering, including appropriate and effective symptom to allow persons receiving care to live and die with dignity" (p. 13). dignity....When a person

Continued on following page

CASE SCENARIO 8.3 *(Continued)*

receiving care is terminally ill or dying, nurses foster comfort, alleviate suffering, advocate for adequate relief of discomfort and pain and support a dignified and peaceful death. This includes support for the family during and following the death, and care of the person's body after death." (CNA, 2017)

Within the context of the caring relationship, the nurse in this scenario cannot assume that this patient has thought through all the issues and choices available to her and has made a reasoned decision to end her life. The nurse has a responsibility to explore the reasons behind this request. Has it arisen out of fear and uncertainty about the future and how death will occur? Has her pain become unbearable? Does she believe she is a burden to her husband and family? Is she living her own grieving process, is she angry or resigned to the journey ahead? Finally, is she frustrated with the growing lack of control and dignity in her life?

By understanding the reasons behind the patient's statement, the nurse may be able to develop a creative plan with the patient, family, and health care team to enhance the quality of her living and her dying.

Those living with cancer can tolerate extremely high levels of pain medication. The ethical and caring nurse ensures that such patients receive appropriate pain management while attempting to minimize the related complications of drowsiness, confusion, constipation, and diarrhea. Patients should be given choices

regarding the level of pain control they receive; some may elect to experience some pain in order to remain lucid, for other patients, the pain may be so severe that they want it controlled even if it means falling into a semi- or unconscious state. Nurses may be concerned that high levels of pain medication may bring about or hasten the patient's death. The ethical concept of **double effect** attempts to resolve this dilemma. The notion of double effect justifies the provision of appropriate pain relief in that the good intention is to eliminate pain, and a subsequent effect of that good intention may or may not result in hastening the person's death. Ethically, the nurse's primary obligation is to respect the patient's wishes and to provide a good by minimizing the pain, which may or may not hasten death. The obligation to provide palliative care and adequate pain control is also supported in law (Law Reform Commission of Canada, 1980).

In this scenario, the nurse may assist her in taking control over her remaining time. There are ways that her family and caregivers can give her back some control. Perhaps she needs more opportunity to talk about her feelings and the meaning this experience has for her. Her husband and family may have similar needs; the nurse could facilitate such conversations.

At times there is nothing nurses can do to relieve a patient's physical and emotional suffering. It is in such situations that nurses face the most challenging ethical and legal dilemmas in health care today.

Withdrawal of Treatment

With withdrawal of treatment, nothing active is done to end a person's life; rather, all life-sustaining treatment is withdrawn, and death is allowed to occur through natural processes. The issue of withdrawal of treatment began to gain prominence in the mid-1970s with the case of Karen Ann Quinlan in the United States (*Re Quinlan*, 1975, 1976), followed by Nancy B. in Quebec (*Nancy B. v. Hôtel-Dieu de Québec*, 1992), and Sue Rodriguez in British Columbia (*Rodriguez v. British Columbia (Attorney General)*, 1993).

The following two Canadian cases highlight the issues related to the withdrawal of treatment and the ethical conflicts that arise.

In Manitoba, in 2008, an 84-year-old man who had a portion of his brain removed years earlier, injured after a fall, was placed on life support when he became unable to speak, breathe, or eat on his own (*Golubchuk v. Salvation Army Grace General Hospital et al.*, 2008). The treating physicians determined that his chances of recovery were extremely remote, and recommended to his family that life support be withdrawn. The man was an Orthodox Jew, and his family argued against the decision to end life support, as they believed doing so would be a sin because their religious beliefs required that all life must be preserved to a natural conclusion. Ending life support, they argued, would hasten his death and would, in fact, constitute an assault. Accordingly, his family sought a court order (an injunction) requiring the hospital to continue to provide life support (a ventilator and feeding tube). The court granted a temporary injunction preventing termination of life support and ordered the matter to proceed to a trial. Typically, unless there is urgency, courts will grant an interim injunction to preserve the status quo until there can be a full examination of the merits of the case.

In this case, the physicians relied on the College of Physicians and Surgeons of Manitoba guidelines for such situations, which stipulated that if the patient was unable to communicate, physicians would consult with the patient's family to determine what course of action should be taken, but that the ultimate decision on withdrawing treatment would rest with physicians. They and the hospital maintained the view that given the man's terminal condition and the extremely poor prognosis, keeping him on life support would needlessly prolong his suffering and would be wasting limited medical resources while other patients were in serious need of those same resources.

The man ultimately died, but not before several physicians at the hospital withdrew their services rather than continue to perform what they deemed unethical continued treatment (CTV, 2008; *Golubchuk v. Salvation Army Grace General Hospital et al.,* 2008).

An Ontario case (*Cuthbertson v. Rasouli,* 2013) went to the Supreme Court of Canada in 2013 based on similar issues. Mr. Rasouli, a 62-year-old man who had recently come to Canada from Iran, had developed meningitis following surgery for a benign brain tumour. He was left in a minimally conscious state and reliant on mechanical ventilation, tube feeding, and hydration. The physicians at Sunnybrook Medical Sciences Centre in Toronto advised Mr. Rasouli's family that there was no realistic hope of recovery and recommended that he be removed from life support and given palliative care. According to the family's religious belief, removing life support was not acceptable. Furthermore, they saw signs (hand movements, responses to stimuli) that led them to believe recovery was possible.

Mr. Rasouli's wife and substitute decision maker sought an injunction to prevent the removal of life support. Ultimately, the injunction was granted, and Mr. Rasouli remained in Sunnybrook until a bed in a long-term care setting with the ability to provide the advanced support became available. He died shortly after being transferred to this facility.

In this case, the decision was based on a narrow interpretation of the term "treatment" as defined in the *Health Care Consent Act, 1996.* Consent is required under the *Health Care Consent Act* for "treatment." The question for the court was whether the withdrawal of life support by the medical team was "treatment" and required consent from Mr. Rasouli's family or if it was not "treatment" and could be done without consent. In other words, having started active treatment to keep the patient alive, was the medical team required to continue to provide life-sustaining care until the patient's family consented to a change in care, or could the medical team withdraw care that they believed had become futile?

The court concluded that the withdrawal of life support in Mr. Rasouli's case did constitute treatment and required consent, which his wife was not prepared to give. As part of the decision, the Supreme Court reviewed the practice of the Ontario Consent and Capacity Board. The Consent and Capacity Board consider conflicts over consent. The Board has permitted the withdrawal of life support in some cases without consent and in others has required consent. The specific facts of each case are considered to determine the "best interests of the patient."

Assisted Suicide

Suicide, defined as the act of taking one's own life, was a crime in Canada until 1972, when the provision of the *Criminal Code* (1985), making it an offence to commit suicide, was repealed by the *Criminal Law Amendment Act* (1972, s. 216).

In **assisted suicide**, persons are mentally capable of making a decision to end their life, yet are too debilitated by illness to act on this decision and require the assistance of another (e.g., a physician, nurse, family member, or friend). Such assistance might involve someone providing the person with a lethal dose of medication and or assisting with its ingestion.

The demand for legal assisted suicide arose in cases where persons with a chronic disease wished to live as long as possible, and determine for themselves when the quality of their life was no longer acceptable. An example might be patients with amyotrophic lateral sclerosis (ALS) who, when they transition to a state of total paralysis, no longer have the means to end their own life. Without the option of assisted suicide, they might choose suicide earlier to avoid living in a state they consider intolerable.

The arguments for and against assisted suicide are like those of euthanasia. However, those who support assisted suicide also argue that by not aiding, we set limits on disabled people's autonomy by denying them the opportunity to perform an act of which able-bodied persons are capable. The attention given to patients' rights and respect for patient autonomy has provoked questions regarding the right to die and the right of patients to choose the time and means of their death. (Physician-Assisted Suicide, 1992).

Assistance in Dying: Shifting Options

As mentioned earlier, advances in health care technology and a growing number of terminally ill patients living longer with a compromised quality of life have played a large part in bringing euthanasia to the fore. Pivotal cases dealing with "mercy killing" have been before the courts over the past few decades.

The Robert Latimer Case

Passionate public debate regarding the case of Robert Latimer in Saskatchewan (*R. v. Latimer*, 1997, 1 SCR 217; 2001 SCC 1) renewed and reenergized controversy over the ethical and legal justifications for and against euthanasia. Latimer, a farmer, had a daughter Tracey, who, at the time of her death, was 12 years old. She had cerebral palsy and was immobile and nonverbal. She was assessed as having the mental capacity of an infant. Since birth, she suffered from seizures, experiencing five to six a day. Although she was not dying, she had several health challenges and experienced severe ongoing pain. She had already had several surgeries and was scheduled for more. Her father decided that his daughter's life was "not worth living" and that as a father, he had an obligation to protect her from ongoing torture. In 1993, he ended Tracey's life by poisoning her with carbon monoxide (Historica Canada, 2018).

In 1994, Latimer was convicted of the second-degree murder of Tracey. He was sentenced to a mandatory minimum of life imprisonment with no parole for 10 years, a conviction and sentence upheld by the Saskatchewan Court of Appeal.

In 1997, the Supreme Court of Canada ordered a new trial. At the second trial, although Latimer had a sympathetic judge and jury, there was no provision for leniency in Canadian law, so he was again found guilty of second-degree murder. This judge found that the original sentence was "grossly disproportionate" to the offence and granted Latimer a "constitutional exemption" from the mandatory minimum sentence.

Latimer was sentenced to time served plus 2 years in jail, notwithstanding the fact that the minimum sentence for second-degree murder is imprisonment for life without possibility of parole for at least 10 years. The judge held that to sentence Latimer to the minimum term specified in the *Criminal Code* would have constituted cruel and unusual punishment under the circumstances and violated his constitutional rights. In granting the extremely rare (and equally controversial) constitutional dispensation from the legally mandated sentence for this offence, the judge recognized the agonizing choices and decisions that Latimer had to make in the face of his daughter's suffering. Some argue that the Latimer decision signalled a turning point in the law's attitude toward euthanasia. Latimer's sentence, however, was subsequently overturned on appeal by the Crown to the Saskatchewan Court of Appeal, which substituted the minimum 10-year sentence mandated by the *Criminal Code*. Latimer's subsequent appeal to the Supreme Court of Canada in 2001 was dismissed (*R. v. Latimer*, 2001). The Supreme Court of Canada ruled that the harm had inflicted was out of all proportion to the harm he sought to avoid. Latimer was granted full parole in 2010.

A number of special interest groups participated in the Latimer proceedings, including groups advocating for the disabled. These groups were particularly concerned that Latimer might succeed on the defence of necessity or the jury deciding that he should be judged based on what he thought was "right" according to his own conscience rather than following "the letter of the law," among other concerns. They were essentially concerned that the human rights and constitutional rights of disabled persons would be gravely and adversely affected were Latimer to succeed (*R. v. Latimer*, 1995). These groups were permitted to participate as intervenors in Mr. Latimer's appeal.

On the subsequent appeal to the Supreme Court of Canada in 2001, other interest groups also intervened, including the Canadian Civil Liberties Association, the Canadian AIDS Society, and the Disabled Women's Network of Canada, as well as a number of religious groups representing various Christian denominations. The religious groups sought to argue that allowing the defence of necessity in this case would legalize euthanasia, a concept to which they were opposed on religious grounds. Women's groups argued that the decision might undermine the autonomy of disabled women.

The Dr. Nancy Morrison Story

Similarly, the situation involving Dr. Nancy Morrison in Nova Scotia in 1996 highlighted the divergent views of the legal system and the public at large on the issue of euthanasia. Dr. Morrison enjoyed a groundswell of public support for her cause after she was charged with the murder of a patient with terminal cancer. It was alleged that she had injected a patient at the Queen Elizabeth II Health Sciences Centre with potassium chloride (Robb, 1997, 1998).

The charges against Dr. Morrison were dropped at a preliminary hearing because of insufficient evidence that she had done anything to hasten the patient's death. Subsequently, Dr. Morrison accepted a reprimand from her provincial College of Physicians and Surgeons.

THE EVOLUTION OF THE LAW TO MEDICAL ASSISTANCE IN DYING

The legal journey toward legislation supporting MAiD began in 1993 with the tragic case of Sue Rodriguez. Mrs. Rodriguez brought a court application in British Columbia for an order declaring section 241(b) of the *Criminal Code* (1985) unconstitutional.

This section of the *Criminal Code* stated that anyone who "aids or abets a person to commit suicide, whether suicide ensues or not, is guilty of an indictable offence and liable to imprisonment for a term not exceeding fourteen years." This case, *Rodriguez v. British Columbia (Attorney General)* (1993, 3 SCR 519), received much public attention and debate.

The Sue Rodriguez Story

In 1991, Sue Rodriguez was diagnosed with ALS, a motor neuron disease, also known as *Lou Gehrig's disease*, and was given 2 to 5 years to live. A progressive disease of the nervous system, ALS eventually results in complete paralysis and the loss of one's ability to speak, swallow, or breathe without a ventilator. Those afflicted by ALS gradually lose control of all bodily functions. Finally, even the heart succumbs to paralysis, and the person dies. Throughout the course of the disease, the person's mind remains clear, and the ability to reason is unaffected by the deterioration of the nervous system. ALS is accompanied by painful muscle spasms, although these can be controlled to some degree with medication. Clearly, the rigours of this disease can take a heavy emotional toll on the person, family, and friends.

Mrs. Rodriguez was married and the mother of a young son. Her concern throughout was that although she wished to live as long as possible, she did not wish to live through the last and most debilitating stages of ALS and die as a result of asphyxiation. Fearing complete loss of control over her bodily functions, and hence the ability to end her own life when she wished to do so, she sought a legal exemption, in her home province of British Columbia, permitting her to obtain a physician-assisted suicide, when necessary.

Mrs. Rodriguez sought this declaration on the grounds that the effect of section 241(b) of the *Criminal Code* prohibiting anyone from counselling, aiding, or abetting another to commit suicide was to deprive her of several of her rights under the *Canadian Charter of Rights and Freedoms*, namely, life, liberty, security of person (*Canadian Charter of Rights and Freedoms*, 1982, s. 7), equality before the law (s. 15(1)), and freedom from cruel or unusual treatment (s. 12). She argued that the effect of the law was to deprive her of control over her body and her life. Further, she argued that this prevented her from obtaining the assistance of another person in ending her life when she could no longer do so on her own and that this subjected her to cruel and inequitable treatment at the hands of the state. Finally, she argued that since suicide was no longer a criminal offence in Canada (the provision in the *Criminal Code* making it an offence to commit or attempt to commit suicide was repealed in 1972, she was being discriminated against and treated unequally by the law solely by reason of her physical disability because she was effectively being prevented from doing that which able-bodied people could do legally.

Mrs. Rodriguez's application was dismissed by the British Columbia courts. An appeal to the Supreme Court of Canada was heard on May 20, 1993, and the Court rendered its decision in September of that year. The Supreme Court of Canada delivered a five-to-four decision against Mrs. Rodriguez's application. This narrow margin illustrates the complexity of the ethical issues and the lack of consensus in the court. Most of the judges felt that while the effect of section 241(b) was to impinge on Mrs. Rodriguez's right to life, liberty, and security of the person, such intrusion was not contrary to the principles of fundamental justice. The majority also felt that her right to equal treatment was violated but that this was permitted as being a "reasonable limit which [was] demonstrably justified in a free and democratic society" (*Canadian Charter of Rights and Freedoms*, 1982, s. 1). The minority judges wrote that both her right to life, liberty, and security of the person, and her right to equality before the law had been infringed and that the infringement by the state through section 241(b) could not be justified in any way under the Charter. Thus, they felt that the section could not stand as valid under the Constitution and that, therefore, Mrs. Rodriguez should be free to seek assistance in committing suicide when she wished it.

Chief Justice Sopinka, writing the decision for the majority, undertook a historical review of the ethical and legal principles behind the legislative prohibitions against both suicide and assisted suicide. The chief ethical principle that he identified was the state and society's concern for the sanctity and value of human life and human dignity (*Rodriguez v. British Columbia (Attorney General)*, 1993, p. 592), as well as society's role in protecting those who are vulnerable and who could be coerced or encouraged, in a moment of weakness, to commit suicide. The purpose of section 241(b) in the *Criminal Code* was to protect such members of society. In recent times, the concept of protecting human life at all costs has become tempered with limitations premised on personal independence and dignity and with quality-of-life considerations (*Rodriguez v. British Columbia (Attorney General)*, 1993, pp. 595–596). Furthermore, common law has recognized the right of

an individual to withdraw or withhold consent to medical treatment, even if the absence of such treatment would likely result in death.

The majority judgement suggests that the law recognizes a form of *passive euthanasia*—that could be legal. For example, inadvertently hastening a terminally ill patient's death by administering larger and larger doses of pain medication with the intent to control pain and the withdrawing (with the patient's consent) of all treatment and artificial means to prolong life once such treatment has become therapeutically futile. Palliative sedation, discussed earlier, would be an example of such an approach.

Although the law has always had great aversion to the participation of one person in the death of another, passive euthanasia could be considered acceptable because artificial means to prolong life are withdrawn on the patient's request and death ensues as a natural consequence. In the case of passive euthanasia, the exact time of death cannot be known, and death does not result directly from the actions of another.

Another argument used to justify the blanket prohibition on assisted suicide was the risk of abuse, together with the difficulties in formulating guidelines and conditions under which assisted suicide would be legally permissible. In relation to abuse, as reasons justifying the continued prohibition, Justice Sopinka cited a working paper of the Law Reform Commission of Canada (1983) that points out examples of mass suicides or of persons who for financial gain, takes advantage of the depressed state of another to encourage their suicide. Furthermore, noting the challenges in developing guidelines, he reviewed the record in the Netherlands, which at the time had the most liberal guidelines on euthanasia and physician-assisted suicide and noted evidence (without stating his source) of a disturbing rise in cases of voluntary active euthanasia, not permitted by their guidelines (*Rodriguez v. British Columbia (Attorney General)*, 1993, p. 603). Thus, this "slippery slope" argument, in the opinion of the majority, justified a complete prohibition on physician-assisted suicide. To hold otherwise would "send a signal that there are circumstances in which the state approves of suicide" (*Rodriguez v. British Columbia (Attorney General)*, 1993, p. 608).

The minority opinion was that section 241(b) of the *Criminal Code* infringed on the rights of disabled persons, such as Sue Rodriguez, because it effectively deprives them of choosing suicide, an option available to able-bodied persons (*Rodriguez v. British Columbia (Attorney General)*, 1993, p. 544). Thus, disabled persons were not being treated equally before the law as guaranteed under the Charter. Further, it is a fundamental aspect of personal autonomy in common law that citizens have the right to make free and informed decisions about their bodies and to consent (or withhold consent) to specific medical treatment, even when to do so would likely result in death.

With respect to the "slippery slope" argument, the minority noted that despite the concern that decriminalizing assisted suicide would leave the physically disabled vulnerable and open to manipulation by others, this still would not justify depriving a disadvantaged group (i.e., the disabled) of equality before the law, specifically, the right to determine the circumstances in which they end their life. In Mrs. Rodriguez's case, there was no evidence of such vulnerability and plenty of evidence of her free consent (*Rodriguez v. British Columbia (Attorney General)*, 1993, pp. 566–567). The minority opinion was that Mrs. Rodriguez could have an exemption to compliance with section 241(b), provided that:

1. She had applied to a superior court for authorization.
2. She had been certified by her attending physician and a psychiatrist to be competent, had made her decision freely and voluntarily, and at least one physician would be with her when she committed assisted suicide.
3. The physicians certify that (a) she is or will become physically incapable of committing suicide unaided, and (b) they have informed her of her continuing right to change her mind about terminating her life.
4. Notice and access be given to the regional coroner at the time.
5. She be examined daily by the physicians.
6. The act actually causing her death be her act alone, unaided by anyone else (*Rodriguez v. British Columbia (Attorney General)*, 1993, p. 579).

The exemption was to expire 31 days after the date of the physicians' certificate. The conditions were described as having been designed with Mrs. Rodriguez's circumstances in mind. With the assistance of an unknown doctor, Sue Rodriguez committed suicide in February 1994, in the presence of Svend Robinson, a New Democratic Party Member of Parliament and a champion of her cause.

The Supreme Court of Canada: The *Carter v. Canada* Decision

Over the years following the *Rodriguez* decision, public opinion polls demonstrated growing support for persons having greater control over their life and death. In June 2014, just over 20 years after the *Rodriguez* decision, the province of Quebec took the lead in passing legislation, *An Act respecting end-of-life care,* legalizing physician-assisted suicide for consenting adult patients who suffer from a "serious and incurable illness," are in "an advanced state of irreversible decline in capability," and "experience constant and unbearable physical or psychological suffering which cannot be relieved in a manner the patient deems tolerable." However, Quebec has no power to change the *Criminal Code,* as this is the jurisdiction of the federal government, hence this change was more symbolic than real.

In 2015, the Supreme Court of Canada was asked to reconsider the issues raised in the *Rodriguez* case in another case. (*Carter v. Canada (Attorney General)* 2015). The British Columbia Civil Liberties Association (BCCLA) had challenged the law against assisted suicide on behalf of the families of Kay Carter and Gloria Taylor, both of whom suffered from debilitating medical conditions. Kay Carter, who had degenerative spinal stenosis, died in 2010. Gloria Taylor died in 2012 as a result of ALS. In June 2013, the Supreme Court of British Columbia ruled in favour of the BCCLA, agreeing that the law that prohibits aiding a person to commit suicide violates sections 7 (the right to "life, liberty, and security of the person) and 15(1) of the *Canadian Charter of Rights and Freedoms* (equality). Appeals resulted in a 2015 decision of the Supreme Court of Canada that the *Criminal Code* prohibitions on voluntary euthanasia (s. 14) and assisted suicide (s. 241(b)) violated the Charter.

Most *Canadian Charter of Rights and Freedoms* cases involve an assessment of whether the complained of legislation violates the rights enshrined in the Charter. If the rights are violated, then the courts will consider whether the violation of Charter rights is permissible under section 1 of the Charter. Section 1 has established the following: "The *Canadian Charter of Rights and Freedoms* guarantees the rights and freedoms set out in it subject only to such reasonable limits prescribed by law as can be demonstrably justified in a free and democratic society." As discussed earlier, the majority opinion in *Rodriguez* had relied on section 1 to save the challenged provisions of the *Criminal Code.*

In *Carter v. Canada (Attorney General)* (2015), the court revisited the issue of the prohibition of physician-assisted death and held that section 7 of the Charter ("Everyone has the right to life, liberty and security of the person and the right not to be deprived thereof except in accordance with the principles of fundamental justice") was violated by sections 241(b) and 14 of the *Criminal Code* because the prohibition:

deprives some individuals of life, as it has the effect of forcing some individuals to take their own lives prematurely (para. 57)

denies people in this situation the right to make decisions concerning their bodily integrity and medical care and thus trenches on their liberty (para. 66)

by leaving people like Ms. Taylor to endure intolerable suffering, . . . impinges on their security of the person. (para. 66)

The Court found that the prohibition was too broad in its application and that the objective of the prohibition, protecting "vulnerable persons from being induced to commit suicide at a time of weakness" (para. 74) could be achieved within a less restrictive structure. The conclusion, therefore, was that section 1 of the Charter did not save the challenged sections of the *Criminal Code.*

Madam Justice Smith, at trial, held that a system for physician-assisted suicide operating within reasonable limits could alleviate concerns and ensure protection for the disabled and other disadvantaged groups. Justice Smith wrote that "it was feasible for properly qualified and experienced physicians to reliably assess patient competence and voluntariness, that coercion, undue influence, and ambivalence could all be reliably assessed as part of that process" (para. 106).

Furthermore, with respect to the potential abuse of the vulnerable and the "slippery slope" concerns, she concluded that there was "no evidence from permissive jurisdictions that people with disabilities

are at heightened risk of accessing physician-assisted dying"; "no evidence of inordinate impact on socially vulnerable populations in the permissive jurisdictions"; and "no compelling evidence that a permissive regime in Canada would result in a 'practical slippery slope'" (*Carter v. Canada (Attorney General)*, 2015, para. 107).

Sections 14 and 241(b) of the *Criminal Code* were declared invalid in relation to the prohibition of:

physician-assisted death for a competent adult person who (1) clearly consents to the termination of life; and (2) has a grievous and irremediable medical condition (including an illness, disease, or disability) that causes enduring suffering that is intolerable to the individual in the circumstances of his or her condition. (Carter v. Canada (Attorney General), 2015, para. 147)

The Court suspended the effect of its ruling for 12 months to permit Parliament to formulate appropriate legislation. Subsequently, a 4-month extension was granted to June 6, 2016, to permit the legislation to be completed. During the extension, persons who wanted a physician-assisted death could apply for court approval based on the grounds laid out in *Carter.* Many successful applications were made before the new legislation came into effect. Courts routinely granted the exemption to criminal liability to the health care team, including nurses involved in providing an assisted death (Canadian Nurses Protective Society [CNPS], 2021).

Carter did not specifically refer to the role of nurses in medically assisted dying. Therefore, until the new legislation became law, nurses were advised that they should not participate in MAiD unless they received a specific exemption in a court order (CNPS, 2021).

Without the exemption order, persons involved MAiD faced liability for criminal conduct and the potential of a professional conduct complaint.

LEGISLATION: MEDICAL ASSISTANCE IN DYING (BILL C-14)

The first countries to legalize euthanasia were the Netherlands and Belgium in 2002. Subsequently, it has been legalized in Canada, Colombia, Luxembourg, South Korea, New Zealand, Spain, several Australian states, and India. Assisted suicide is legal in the same countries and Switzerland, Germany, Austria, Japan, and in some states in the United States. Bill C-14, a legal framework for assisted dying in Canada, was passed on June 17, 2016, over a year after the *Carter* decision.

Given the diverse opinions on this significant social policy issue, the government undertook extensive consultation in the development of the legislation. Although the majority of Canadians supported formulating an approach to assisted dying, the issue was ethically challenging for many. Even the views of those supporting the legislation ranged from very liberal to more conservative perspectives on the parameters of the legislation.

Amendments to the *Criminal Code*

The legislation required changes to the *Criminal Code* (1985). Section 241 of the *Criminal Code* provides that it is a crime for anyone to counsel "a person to die by suicide or abet a person in dying by suicide or aid a person to die by suicide." In response to the legislation, this section in the *Criminal Code* was amended. Section 241(2) excludes medical practitioners and NPs from criminal sanctions if they provide a person with Medical Assistance in Dying (MAiD), and ensures they and other team members are protected "if they do anything for the purpose of aiding a medical practitioner or nurse practitioner to provide a person with medical assistance in dying in accordance with Section 241(2)" (*Criminal Code* s. 241(3)) and "if they do anything, at another person's explicit request, for the purpose of aiding that other person to self-administer a substance that has been prescribed for that other person as part of the provision of medical assistance in dying in accordance with Section 241.2" (*Criminal Code,* s. 241(5)). If a person has a reasonable, but mistaken, belief that the exemption conditions under section 241.2 have been met, they are able to rely on the exemptions in section 241(2)–(5) and will not have committed an offence. Furthermore, the legislation explicitly makes clear that providing information about lawful MAiD is not an offence.

Two forms of MAiD are exempt from criminal sanctions: (1) the administration of a substance to persons, at their request, to cause death; and (2) the prescription of a substance to persons, at their request, so that they may self-administer the substance.

Role of Health Care Professionals

The *Carter* decision referred only to physicians as providing assistance in dying; the federal legislation extended the exception (in the *Criminal Code*) to the prohibition on MAiD to NPs. Clinicians (physicians and NPs) are required to have "reasonable knowledge, care, and skill" and comply with any applicable provincial laws, rules or standards if they are providing MAiD (*Criminal Code,* s. 241.2(7)). Canada is the only jurisdiction where legislation permits NPs to provide MAiD; however, because credentialling of health care professionals is in the jurisdiction of provinces and territories, NPs were not licensed in all provinces immediately. By 2023 all Canadian jurisdictions except Quebec indicate that NPs may provide MAID.

Recognizing an interprofessional approach to health care, the legislation also provided for the involvement of pharmacists. Clinicians are required to advise the pharmacist dispensing the required drugs about their intended use to bring about the death of a person who has requested MAiD. A new offence of providing MAiD while knowingly failing to comply with the safeguards in the *Criminal Code* (s. 241.2(3)) or the requirement to inform the pharmacist of the purpose of the substances prescribed was created with a penalty of up to 5 years' imprisonment.

Nurses—those not in the extended class—participate in the process by providing nursing care to the patient, supporting the family and assisting a NP or a physician in the provision of MAiD (CNPS, 2021). Although they can provide technical support, such as the insertion of intravenous lines, nurses may not administer the substance or obtain consent for MAiD. Nurses play a vital role during this significant transition by providing education, care, and comfort to the patient; providing support to the family; and ultimately ensuring that the process is dignified and respectful for all involved. The CNPS recommends that RNs should verify that a medical practitioner or NP has documented their conclusion that the conditions in section 241.2 of the *Criminal Code* have been met (College of Registered Nurses of Manitoba, 2021). This can be done by reviewing the chart to ensure that the presence of all requirements has been noted or by asking the MD or NP providing MAiD. The nurse should document in the chart the steps they took to confirm that eligibility criteria and safeguards have been met (CNPS, 2021).

Counselling (i.e., encouraging, soliciting, or inciting) suicide is still considered a criminal activity (*Criminal*

Code, s. 241(a)). Nurses may inform patients and respond to their questions about MAiD but should take care that their communication does not verge on encouraging or inciting a patient to seek MAiD. Requests for information can be referred to the treating physician, NP, or a specific MAiD team.

Nurses who are providing health care services or personal care services to the person making the request are permitted to witness the written MAiD request, but best practice is that the request and any witnessing should be done by persons independent of the health care team who has been providing care to that person. Furthermore, all persons with an interest in the estate of the person requesting MAiD are excluded from being independent witnesses or clinicians.

Access and Eligibility

Section 241.2 of the *Criminal Code* outlines the eligibility criteria that must be met before physicians and NPs are able to provide MAiD:

241.2 (1)   A person may receive medical assistance in dying only if they meet all of the following criteria:

(a)   they are eligible for health services;

(b)   they are at least 18 years of age and capable of making decisions with respect to their health;

(c)   they have a grievous and irremediable medical condition;

(d)   they have made a voluntary request for medical assistance in dying that, in particular, was not made as a result of external pressure; and

(e)   they give informed consent to receive medical assistance in dying after having been informed of the means that are available to relieve their suffering, including palliative care.

"Grievous and irremediable medical condition"

(2)   A person has a grievous and irremediable medical condition only if they meet all of the following criteria:

(a)   they have a serious and incurable illness, disease or disability;

(b)   they are in an advanced state of irreversible decline in capability; and

(c)   that illness, disease or disability or that state of decline causes them enduring physical or psychological suffering that is intolerable

to them and that cannot be relieved under conditions that they consider acceptable.

Criminal Code, ss. 241.2(1) and (2)), https:// laws-lois.justice.gc.ca/eng/acts/c-46/, Act current to 2023-02-22 and last amended on 2023-01-16. Reproduced with the permission of the Department of Justice Canada.

The original format of the MAiD legislation required that the person seeking MAiD have a reasonably foreseeable death. *Truchon v. c. Procureur général du Canada* was a 2019 Quebec case where the court was asked to review the constitutionality of the reasonably foreseeable death requirement for MAiD. The application involved two mentally competent persons (Truchon & Gladu), both completely incapacitated. Mr. Truchon suffered from spastic cerebral palsy and Mr. Gladu suffered from polio. They both faced the potential of living for years without any hope of recovery. Their applications for MAiD had been refused on the reasonably foreseeable death requirement. The court concluded that refusing them MAiD violated their right to equal treatment under section 7 of the Charter.

The *Truchon* decision compelled the federal government to take steps to consider changes to the MAiD legislation. They began an online consultation survey in early 2020 and received 300,000 responses within a 2-week period. The government subsequently introduced legislation to address the *Truchon* decision and other issues, and Parliament passed the revised legislation on March 17, 2021.

The revised law no longer requires that a person's death be reasonably foreseeable to be eligible for MAiD and now provides for a two-track approach (Table 8.1): (1) persons whose natural death is reasonably foreseeable and (2) persons whose natural death is not reasonably foreseeable. The safeguards have been relaxed for the first group, and stricter safeguards have been instituted for the second.

Division of Legislative Powers

Adding complexity to the implementation of this legislation is the division between federal and provincial jurisdictions. Jurisdiction over crime is a matter for the federal government, whereas provincial governments have authority over matters such as professional regulation and health. When initially enacted, the *Criminal Code* amendments allowed NPs to be exempt from the provisions related to aiding suicide,

TABLE 8.1

The Two-Track Approach of MAiD Legislation

Natural Death Reasonably Foreseeable	Natural Death Not Reasonably Foreseeable (All of the Safeguards for Persons Facing Natural Death Must Be Met)
The patient makes a MAiD request in writing after having been told that they have a "grievous and irremediable medical condition" (the written request is signed and dated by one independent witness).	The patient makes a MAiD request in writing after having been told that they have a "grievous and irremediable medical condition" (the written request is signed and dated by one independent witness).
Two independent doctors or nurse practitioners provide an assessment confirming that the MAiD eligibility criteria are satisfied.	Two independent doctors or nurse practitioners provide an assessment confirming that the MAiD eligibility criteria are satisfied.
Not required	If the practitioners who provide the assessment lack expertise in the medical condition causing the person's suffering, they must consult a practitioner with expertise in that condition.
Not required	The person must be advised of available and appropriate means to relieve their suffering, including counselling services, mental health and disability support services, community services, and palliative care; and the opportunity to consult with professionals who provide those services.
Not required	The practitioner must have discussed reasonable and available means to relieve the person's suffering and agree that the person has seriously considered those means.
Not required	The eligibility assessment should take at least 90 days unless the person is at risk of losing their capacity to make health care decisions and both assessments have been completed.
The person has been advised that they can withdraw the MAiD request at any time, in any manner.	The person has been advised that they can withdraw the MAiD request at any time, in any manner.
The person must confirm their consent immediately before receiving MAiD. This final confirmation of consent can be waived where the person is eligible for MAiD and is at risk of losing decision-making capacity before their preferred date to receive MAiD and has been told about that risk. A waiver of the final consent in writing is an arrangement made with their practitioner to administer MAiD on the preferred date if they have lost their capacity to provide final consent. This waiver of consent is invalid if the person demonstrates refusal or resistance to the administration of MAiD. Involuntary movements are not refusal.	The person must confirm their consent immediately before receiving MAiD. This final confirmation of consent can be waived where the person is eligible for MAiD and is at risk of losing decision-making capacity before their preferred date to receive MAiD and has been told about that risk. A waiver of the final consent in writing is an arrangement made with their practitioner to administer MAiD on the preferred date if they have lost their capacity to provide final consent. This waiver of consent is invalid if the person demonstrates refusal or resistance to the administration of MAiD. Involuntary movements are not refusal.
	Chart was prepared based on information from Justice.gc.ca MAID site regarding the 2021 amendments. https://www.justice.gc.ca/eng/cj-jp/ad-am/bk-di.html. Canada's medical assistance in dying (MAiD) law.

MAiD, Medical Assistance in Dying.

but the provincial legislation for NPs still had to be amended.

Due to this shared federal and provincial legal authority, clinicians involved in MAiD are advised to ensure that they do the following:

1. Comply strictly with the provisions of section 241.2 of the *Criminal Code*
2. Review and comply with any applicable provincial legislation (Each jurisdiction has slightly different processes for MAID. For example, British Columbia requires a regulated health professional to witness an eligibility assessment conducted via the Telehealth videoconferencing system, arranged by the doctor or nurse practitioner)
3. Review and ensure that their actions are within the scope of practice requirements of their regulatory body (Alberta does not require practitioners to make referrals for patients requesting MAiD; rather, the provincial health service makes such referrals or facilitates self-referrals [Steger, 2021])
4. Become familiar with and follow any relevant policies, guidelines, procedures, or processes their employer or agency has in place

5. Fully document all of the steps involved in patient care before, during, and after MAiD
6. Fully document the MAiD decision, as required by the *Criminal Code*, their regulatory body, and the provincial coroner or medical examiner's office
7. Be fully satisfied that the patient meets all the criteria for MAiD

Health Canada provides a framework that outlines the reporting expectations of clinicians in response to a MAiD request and for those who participate in its implementation (Health Canada, 2018).

Consent and Capacity

The ability of the person to consent to MAiD is assessed under the applicable provincial capacity standard. Persons are considered capable of making decisions about their care if they are able to understand the information that is relevant to making a specific decision and can appreciate the reasonably foreseeable consequences of a decision or lack of a decision. In the MAiD process, persons must be able to understand that death is the anticipated outcome and that they can withdraw the request for MAiD at any time.

Self-Administration

For self-administration of a substance to cause death, the same processes related to eligibility are followed. As previously discussed, non–extended class nurses are not permitted to administer medication to cause death. They are, however, permitted to assist a person to self-administer a substance prescribed as part of this protocol; however, they should "exercise extreme caution" because the decision and the action of taking medication to end life must be the person's own. Acceptable forms of assistance include:

1. Opening the bottle of medication
2. Lifting the glass of water to the person's mouth so that they can swallow the medication (for legislative background, see College of Nurses of Ontario [CNO], 2023).

There is no provision that family members, caregivers, or friends of the patient be advised that MAiD is being sought; however, the person should be encouraged to discuss this with them. With patient consent, discussions between the family and the clinicians can occur. Family members and/or other caregivers are legally able to help the patient self-administer the medication for MAiD, provided that the patient explicitly requests their help.

Where the decision has been made that the patient will self-administer the substance that will cause death, it is important to ensure that the patient or a responsible family member/caregiver can store the medication in a safe and secure manner so that it cannot be accessed by others. The MAiD team should develop a plan for the return of unused medication if the patient chooses not to proceed with MAiD or there is any left over. Patients and their family/caregivers should be educated and prepared for what to expect once the patient has ingested the lethal medication and death is imminent—for example, what to expect and what to do when the patient has died (i.e., instructions on notifying the clinician to attend at the location, reporting the death to the Office of the Chief Coroner, and so on).

Conscientious Objection

No person is obliged to participate in MAiD (*Criminal Code*, 1985, s. 241.2 (9)). The *Criminal Code* does not impose a duty on a clinician to participate in the process, and nurses have the right to conscientiously object to participating in the process for moral or religious reasons. However, as described in Chapter 7, nurses are subject to a pre-existing legal duty of care to patients, which prevents them from abandoning patients, and they must comply with the requirements, policies, and guidelines of their regulatory college. They also should review the advice provided by the CNPS (2021). Legal and policy decisions have highlighted the issue of how to balance the rights of individuals to access MAiD with the rights of health care providers to exercise conscience-based objections to participate in this process.

The CNO policy states that "conscientious objection must not be directly conveyed to the patient and no personal moral judgments about the beliefs, lifestyles, identity, or characteristics of the patient should be expressed" (CNO, 2021, p. 6).

Clinicians who have conscientious objections must respectfully inform their patients that they are unable to provide MAiD and refer them to another medical practitioner, NP, institution, or agency willing to provide MAiD. The referral must be made in a timely manner to ensure that patients are not subjected to unnecessary delays or adverse clinical outcomes (e.g., decline in capacity). Irrespective of a patient's desire to explore MAiD through another nonobjecting clinician, institution, or agency, clinicians must continue to provide ongoing care (excluding the provision of MAiD) and not abandon the patient. Nurses who object to participating in MAiD must transfer their care to another nurse or health care professional. However, ongoing care that is not related to MAiD must be provided until a new caregiver is identified. A chart outlining the management of MAiD requests and the obligations of clinicians who do not wish to participate appears in Fig. 8.2.

Agencies or organizations participating in MAiD should ensure that processes and policies are in place to support those health care professionals who do not want to participate in MAiD and to facilitate the reassignment process. Organizations that do not provide MAiD should also consider referrals to settings where this is offered. Government and health care organizations are encouraged to allocate appropriate resources to both MAiD and especially to high-quality palliative care, which may alter a person's decision. Careful planning should consider appropriate locations and settings for services, including protocols for facilitating assessment and treatment of patients at sites which do not offer MAiD (Carpenter & Vivas, 2020).

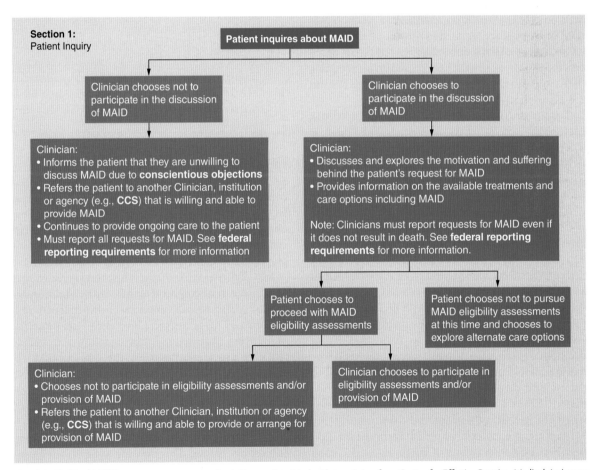

Fig. 8.2 ■ How MAiD requests are approached. *Source: Reprinted with permission from Centre for Effective Practice. Medical Assistance in Dying (MAiD): Ontario. Toronto: Centre for Effective Practice. https://tools.cep.health/tool/medical-assistance-in-dying-maid-in-ontario-track-one-natural-death-is-reasonably-foreseeable/*

Some clinicians argue that any obligation to make an effective referral is also a violation of their constitutional rights. Some who conscientiously object take the position that any referral to a clinician who offers MAiD is a violation of their religious or moral beliefs and that their duty to their patients is satisfied by advising them that they will not provide MAiD. In one case (*Christian Medical and Dental Society of Canada v. College of Physicians and Surgeons of Ontario,* 2019), the Ontario Court of Appeal considered the arguments of a Christian medical group that providing patients with effective referrals to MAiD resources impeded their religious freedom contrary to section 2(a) of the Charter. The court accepted that the law did infringe on the rights of the group under the Charter, but decided that this infringement was acceptable under section 1 of the Charter. The decision was confirmed on appeal. As a result, physicians in Ontario are required to provide effective referrals to patients seeking information about MAiD. Some provinces such as Alberta have passed laws exempting clinicians who conscientiously object to MAID from providing effective referrals.

Despite the right to refuse to participate in MAiD, some legal scholars have suggested that "there is a constitutional duty on publicly funded health care facilities to provide this service, regardless of the conscientious objection provision" in the *Criminal Code* (Robertson & Picard, 2018, p. 150).

Criticism of MAiD Legislation

Even among those who support MAiD, there are differing views on its application. The federal government has committed to continue studying issues related to access to MAiD for mature minors. Mature minors are those younger than the 18-year-old limit provided in the MAiD legislation but have the maturity to understand the nature and consequences of their health care decisions. Those who support access to MAiD by mature minors propose that they be fully assessed to determine if they have the capacity to consent to treatment. "[T]he capacity to make a decision is not tied strictly to age but is a function of maturity and ability of the patient to understand the nature of the decision to make and consequences of accepting or declining treatment" (CNPS, 2017). Apart from MAiD, mature minors are often able to consent or refuse treatment in relation to their own health care. In New Brunswick and Quebec, legislation specifically provides that minors

16 years old (New Brunswick) and 14 years old (Quebec) have the authority to consent to treatment within limitations. Therefore, if mature minors have the capacity to consent or refuse treatment, their exclusion from MAiD seems inconsistent.

Consultations with experts and then Parliament are ongoing about the issues and challenges associated with mature minors, advance requests, mental illness, palliative care, and the protection of Canadians living with disabilities. Of concern is the necessity to protect the vulnerable while ensuring individual autonomy.

Other issues that have been identified include:

- Whether families have the right to be informed when a family member makes a request for MAiD
- Whether a lack of access to palliative care is pushing some to MAiD when such interventions might alleviate their symptoms and improve the quality of their lives
- Whether some people with chronic illnesses and limited financial resources have applied for MAiD in the belief that the quality of their life is not sustainable because provincial disability supports are so limited (Alberga, 2022).

Early Experience With Assisted Dying

As noted, some critics of MAiD have expressed concern related to the influence of socioeconomic factors and lack of access to palliative care. One Ontario study undertaken in the early days of the legislation sought to describe the association of demographics and clinical factors on the decision to have MAiD (Downar et al., 2020). This study revealed that MAiD was most common among older, community-residing persons with cancer, neurodegenerative disease, or end-stage organ failure in the final months of life. They were frequently being followed by palliative care providers; therefore, the option of MAiD was unlikely due to inadequate access to palliative care. For many, the choice was influenced by their physical and psychological suffering. In this study, they were younger, wealthier, more likely to be married, and therefore less likely to live in an institution, suggesting that MAiD is unlikely to be driven by social or economic vulnerability (Downar et al., 2020). However, this study does not address the issue of awareness and access to MAiD, which may be limited by socioeconomic factors.

The Experience of Nurses

Nurses recognize the profound moral and legal implications of MAiD and appreciate the conflicting views of respect for the individual rights (autonomy) of persons that provides them with the dignified death they chose, versus that of sanctity of life and the need for better palliative care. In studies seeking input after the implementation of MAiD, nurses commented on the role of the nurse to advocate, not judge, and the extent to which MAiD aligned with the "heart," or "centre," of nursing, to provide person-centred, compassionate care (Pesut et al 2020a and 2020b). Some viewed MAiD, chosen by the person, as an extension of palliative, end-of-life care.

One study found that although most nurses intellectually supported MAiD, they acknowledged that the process was emotionally complex (Pesut et al., 2020a). Nurses described MAiD as an intense and sometimes surreal experience, noting that it was a different kind of death from what they had encountered before. They noted the experience of a planned death, where the time of death is known, versus a natural death. They also noted how the person was able to communicate right to the end and how the speed of the death did not fit the usual pattern of dying.

The central role nurses play in MAiD is not that different from other end-of-life care. Of primary importance is the relationship they build with the patient and family. Having patients express their wish to die is not new and involves a familiar conversation with the same questions. What is new are the options made available through MAiD. Nurses play a key role in relationship building, assisting in planning and organizing the event, and supporting the patient and family throughout the process. They assist by communicating to those involved what to expect, facilitating important end-of-life rituals, managing anxieties, and supporting those who do not understand or agree with the MAiD decision (McMechan et al., 2019; Pesut et al., 2019, 2020a, 2020b).

Typically, the team that provides MAiD would not have had a previous relationship with the patient and family, so the patient and family rely on the nurse to ensure continuity and to play an important coordinating role. As nurses accompany the patient along this journey, they humanize what could be a medicalized procedure focused event, creating a comfortable environment that conceals or camouflages the equipment and protocols required (Bruce & Beuthin, 2019).

Nurses have shared some of the reasons their patients chose MAiD (Pesut et al., 2020a). For many patients, the choice was based on actual or anticipated suffering, including pain, diminished mobility, and symptoms such as respiratory distress. Some did not want the "trade-offs" associated with palliative care, noting the effects of the sedation and pain management, and the uncertainty related to the time of death. Though some patients remained ambivalent about their decision, they wanted to take control or have a backup plan, just in case. Others were insistent that this was what they wanted (Pesut, 2020a).

According to Pesut et al. (2020a), nurses who had moral concerns regarding MAiD acknowledged these diverse views, but maintained a desire to be compassionate. They found that they were able to stay true to their convictions while staying true to their nursing role. They listened with compassion and empathy to the patient, and they were able to negotiate the challenging conversation while remaining aware of their own values and biases. However, some struggled with their exclusion from the patient's care once the MAiD decision was made.

Clearly, for nurses, the experience of MAiD, though rewarding, is complex and challenging emotionally. All nurses, whether they agree with MAiD or not, should be offered the opportunity to reflect on their values, beliefs, and biases, and any moral differences should be respected. To limit moral distress or residue, nurses should be provided with education, support, and the opportunity to debrief after these emotional experiences. The experience of nurses should lead to guidelines and best practices (Lamb et al., 2019).

ORGAN DONATION

The field of transplantation has grown tremendously in recent years. The long-term survival rates for lung, heart, kidney, and liver transplant recipients have improved remarkably. Patients who would have died without transplantation now may live much longer and have a good quality of life.

In Canada, organ donation is generally viewed as morally justified when treatment alternatives to transplantation are not readily available and when respect for the autonomy of donors and their families is maintained through appropriate legislation and guidelines.

The recent successes of organ transplantation, and improved management of rejection, have expanded the eligibility and need beyond the availability of donated organs. Not only is there a growing need, but advances in the neurosciences, compliance with seat-belt legislation, and a reduction in impaired driving have resulted in fewer traumatic brain related deaths and, thus, fewer opportunities for organ donation. Recent approaches have, therefore, focused on converting more potential donors to actual donors. Strategies explored to maximize the number of donors have included changes to the legislation with regard to the consent process, donor incentives, education, and hospital-based policy and resources. For more information, refer to provincial and territorial websites related to organ donation.

Consent for Donation

The system for consent across Canada is primarily framed as an opting-in system. This approach requires, in advance, the expressed consent of the donor or other specified individual at the time of death. Advance consent may be given through a provincial donor registry, such as BC Transplant or Ontario's Trillium Gift of Life Network, or may be indicated on a health card or a driver's licence. It can also be explicitly communicated by the person to a substitute decision maker or through an advance directive.

Low donor rates in relation to the growing number of patients who need organ transplants have raised questions about whether alternative systems for organ donation should be considered. The following is a brief overview of some possible approaches.

Recorded Consideration

The recorded consideration approach attempts to deal with the challenge health care professionals face in raising the topic of organ donation with family members (Youngner et al., 1985). It requires that health care staff routinely consider and document a dying or brain-dead patient's suitability for organ donation. If the patient's organs are suitable for donation, then the family is to be approached. The family's decision should also be documented in the patient's chart. (This is required by law, for example, in Prince Edward Island's *Human Tissue Donation Act* [1988].)

Required Request

With this system, all patients are asked about their position on organ donation when admitted to hospital or when they use the health care system in any way. Concerns have been raised about whether such questions are unduly stressful for patients, who hope to have their health care needs met in the hospital and, thus, may not wish to entertain the possibility of imminent death and organ donation (Youngner et al., 1985).

Presumed Consent

This approach is commonly referred to as the "opting out" approach. The approach is to presume that all persons would have chosen to donate their organs unless they had expressed otherwise beforehand. If the person has not opted out of the presumption, then their organs can be removed for transplantation. Those who favour this method reason that it would make it easier to approach the family about organ donation and would result in more organs being made available. They argue that autonomy is respected because individuals still have the right to refuse. Those who disagree with this approach say that asking bereaved family members not to opt out is unreasonable and undermines the notion of altruism. It has been noted that in countries where presumed consent is the law (e.g., France, Belgium, Singapore), organ donor rates improved for a while and then levelled off. This phenomenon was apparently related to the continuing reluctance of health care professionals to approach families in these circumstances (Youngner et al., 1985). Nova Scotia introduced a presumed consent law in 2019 (Nova Scotia Health, 2022). The *Human Organ and Tissue Donation Act (HOTDA)* was passed in 2019 and came into effect in 2021.

Under *HOTDA*, persons can register their decision to consent to organ donation or "opt out" of organ donation. If no decision is registered, consent to deceased donation is presumed. Children, non residents, and persons incapable of consenting are excluded from the presumption. The substitute decision maker for the deceased person can present evidence that the deceased would not have consented to deceased organ donation to overcome the presumed consent in *HOTDA*. The substitute decision maker can also present evidence that the deceased would have consented to overcome a registered "opt out." In a guide to the legislation, the options facing the substitute decision maker are provided:

5.2.1. If a consent or refusal is recorded in the Registry, and a substitute decision maker provides information that a reasonable person would conclude that the person would have made a different decision than what is recorded in the Registry, then the substitute decision maker may give consent (express consent) or refuse on behalf of the person, in accordance with that information. (Section 15 of the Act [HOTDA])

5.2.2. A substitute decision maker must provide the evidence they believe proves the person changed their mind.

5.2.3. The strength of various types of evidence ranges from the strongest evidence (a witnessed written document) to the least strong (oral, uncorroborated).

5.2.4. The information provided will be assessed to determine if a reasonable person would be satisfied with the evidence presented. (Nova Scotia Department of Health and Wellness, 2020, p. 3)

Other Canadian jurisdictions are studying the Nova Scotia experience with *HOTDA* to determine whether it is a model to follow (Horton, 2021).

Promotion of Organ Donation

Financial Incentives

Some suggest that organ donor rates would improve with an offer of a financial incentive, ranging from a lump-sum payment to coverage of the funeral expenses of the deceased. Again, there are concerns that this approach would not only undermine the notion of altruism but also might take advantage of those with financial challenges. As well, it would introduce a coercive element into the process (Irving et al., 2012; Youngner et al., 1985). At present, buying or selling human tissue or organs is prohibited by law in every Canadian province and territory. Penalties for breach of this prohibition vary from province to province but range from steep fines to several months' imprisonment.

Education

Education of public and health care professionals regarding organ donation has been encouraged. Further knowledge and better communication would ensure that "brain death" is understood, that individuals are aware of the donation options available to them, and that health care professionals understand and accept their role in the organ donation process. It is not adequate to educate only health care professionals working in hospitals. A significant role exists for nurses practising in the community to represent the interests of health care in general and to educate their patients about specific issues, such as organ donation (Youngner et al., 1985).

Ethical Issues Associated With Organ Donation

The ethical issues associated with organ donation include the determination of death, consent, donor management, and recipient responses. The organ donation process, if not managed properly, can be highly stressful for nurses, the interprofessional team, and, most important, the families of donors.

Nurses caring for a donor patient may experience moral distress during the donation process if the challenging transition from trying to save the life of the patient to managing that patient's organs for the benefit of others is not effectively managed. The nurse's focus shifts from recovery of the patient to advocating for that person's wishes and ensuring the well-being of the recipient in need of the transplant. A strong relationship between the nurse and the patients (both the donor and recipient), together with ethical management of the process by all members of the team, can make this a rewarding experience for all involved.

Case Scenario 8.4 illustrates some of the ethical and legal challenges of organ donation.

CASE SCENARIO 8.4

A GIFT OR AN OBLIGATION

M. R., a patient who has ingested a large quantity of barbiturates, is admitted to a critical care unit (CCU). The drugs have damaged M. R.'s brain to such a degree that M. R. has been declared brain dead.

M. R. remains on a ventilator and is presently hemodynamically stable. In the same hospital, another patient, J. S., is dying as a result of rejection of a heart transplant. J. S. has less than 24 hours to live unless another suitable heart is found.

Continued on following page

CASE SCENARIO 8.4 *(Continued)*

M. R. is judged by the CCU team to be a suitable donor for the urgently required heart. Furthermore, a signed organ donor card was found in M. R.'s wallet. As is the practice in most hospitals, and despite the existence of this card, the CCU team approaches M. R.'s parents and requests that they consent to donating their son's organs. The parents categorically refuse to give consent. They are not informed about J. S. for fear that this would constitute coercion. J. S. dies the next day.

Questions

1. What is the legal status of a signed organ donor card?
2. Is the consent of the donor's family required?
3. Could health care professionals be more aggressive in encouraging the donor's family to give consent? Should family be told about the recipient in need?
4. Might further legislation in the area of consent help? How?

Discussion

Across most of Canada the Canada's current approach to organ donation is a voluntary system of expressed consent. This is based on the principles of beneficence (doing good) and avoiding harm. Because society does not oblige us to help others or to be altruistic, the system is based on the notion of voluntarism and encourages organ donation through mechanisms such as a record on a driver's licence, health care card, or organ donor card, in which individuals can state which organs they are willing to donate upon death. Supporters of this system argue that procurement built on voluntarism promotes socially desirable virtues, such as altruism, while protecting the rights of persons who might refuse to donate (Task Force on Presumed Consent, 1994).

Certain problems have arisen with regard to this approach:

- For such reasons as superstition, individuals may choose not to sign a donor card, even when they support the concept.
- The donor card is not always available to health care professionals at the time of a patient's death.
- Whether or not a donor card is signed, families are approached, and, in practice, their decision takes precedence.

- Health care professionals are still reluctant to approach families about organ donation or to initiate a complex and time-consuming donation process (Task Force on Presumed Consent, 1994).

The last point raises some ethical issues with respect to the role of the health care team (especially nurses) as participants in the organ donation process. Some health care professionals cite grieving of the family as the reason for not approaching them about organ donation. Others claim that the cultural or religious perspectives of some patients preclude organ donation. The problem is that when health care professionals decide not to raise the issue with the family or fail to look for a signed organ donor card, then they are, in fact, making the decision for the patient not to donate, and this is disrespectful of the individual's autonomy.

Furthermore, we cannot make assumptions about the views of various cultural and religious groups. In fact, most world religions (including Christianity, Judaism, and Hinduism) support organ donation and transplantation. The Japanese Shinto religion and some sects of Tibetan Buddhism prohibit (or discourage) organ transplantation because of beliefs about the dead, taboos against injuring the body after death, and the extensive purifying rights required after death occurs (Task Force on Presumed Consent, 1994). In Korea, for example, many express aversion to organ donation, believing that the deceased person would be humiliated through the organ procurement process. Many Koreans have a strong belief in Confucianism, which requires that the body be intact for burial (Kim, 1998). Lack of knowledge and understanding of the concept and meaning of brain death is also a factor (Kim et al., 2004).

Nurses may experience emotional exhaustion in caring for organ donors and their families (Borozny, 1988; Hibbert, 1995). They may approach the care of the patient with mixed emotions and a sense of contradictions. Research suggests that health care professionals' attitudes, knowledge, and willingness to approach a family about organ donation can influence the bereaved family's decision-making process (Bidigare, 1991).

However, nurses are in the best position to raise the topic of organ donation with patients' families. The nurse caring for the patient has the best

CASE SCENARIO 8.4 *(Continued)*

opportunity to interact with the family throughout this difficult process. Nurses often develop a supportive relationship with patients' family members as they prepare them for the inevitable, and most have the communication skills to raise the subject of organ donation in a sensitive manner. Given the fact that families often forget about organ donation in the middle of a crisis, it is important that nurses ensure that this subject is raised.

Regardless of the decision, the nurse has represented the interests and wishes of the patient and family. Taking part in this process also eases the nurse's own transition from caring for the patient to maintaining that patient's organs for the benefit of future recipients. The relationship continues as the nurse ensures that the patient's wish to give to others is fulfilled.

The declaration of brain death remains a controversial process and continues to create emotional tension in health care professionals. It is difficult for families to accept that a person is dead when the chest continues to rise and fall and skin colour and body temperature seem normal. Some health facilities use particular rituals to acknowledge the occurrence of a death. For example, some operating room settings observe a moment of silence to respect the deceased and to acknowledge the emotions of family and staff. This observance can also ease the transition to the next phase of the donation process. Such rituals are significant, particularly for operating room nurses, who may be left alone with the patient after removal of the organs (Youngner et al., 1985). Hospitals should be sensitive to and support the needs of staff in such a situation.

Legislation

Legal Definition of Death

Removal of organ tissues from deceased donors is bound up with the legal and medical determination of death. Few jurisdictions in Canada or the United States provide a legislative definition of the moment of death. Historically, physicians have concurred that a person is dead when all vital signs (heartbeat, pulse, respiration) have ceased. In religious terms, death is seen as the moment when the soul leaves the body, generally at the time when the person's heart ceases to beat. Until well into the twentieth century, the courts recognized that a person was legally dead when the "vital functions [have] ceased to operate. The heart [has] always been regarded as a vital organ" in this determination (*R. v. Kitching and Adams*, 1976, p. 711, per O'Sullivan J.).

In the last half century, sophisticated medical technology has given physicians the tools to sustain the lives of seriously ill patients who, in the past, would have died. Patients who can no longer breathe on their own or whose heart function has ceased can now be kept alive with the aid of ventilators or various heart-lung machines that provide mechanical circulatory support for the heart and the lungs. As well, advances in transplantation technology have made it possible to transplant organs from donors with a non-beating heart.

It has become apparent that the traditional medical criteria for determining the fact of death have become inadequate. The question now is whether a person whose brain function has completely and irreversibly ceased but whose other bodily functions remain active can still be considered a living human being.

In 1975, Manitoba became the first province to enact a legal definition of the moment of death. *The Vital Statistics Act* provides that for all civil purposes (i.e., not for the purpose of criminal law), "the death of a person takes place at the time at which irreversible cessation of all that person's brain function occurs" (*The Vital Statistics Act*, C.C.S.M., c. V60, s. 2). This definition conforms to the accepted definition of death within the modern medical community. In arriving at a new medical definition of death, a committee of the Harvard Medical School suggested that brain death is established with the cessation of all brain function, that is, both brain and brainstem functions, and that the cessation of such brain function must be irreversible.

Manitoba's legislation provides specifically that death must be determined according to the definition set out in *The Vital Statistics Act*, with bodily circulation still intact as necessary for the purposes of a successful tissue transplantation, and that such determination must be made by at least two physicians (*The Human Tissue Gift Act*, C.C.S.M., c. H180, s. 8(1)).

With respect to human tissue donation, the laws of most of the provinces require that the death of a prospective donor be determined in the way stated above (see the Evolve site for the laws for each province and territory).

Consent

Legislation regarding organ donation is remarkably uniform across Canada except for the presumed consent approach introduced in Nova Scotia. The various statutes basically provide a mechanism for obtaining the consent of the donor (or others, if the donor is unable to consent) to the removal of tissue from the donor's body for transplantation into the body of another, for medical, education, or for purposes of scientific research.

There are two primary situations contemplated by the statutes:

1. The donor is living and has consented to the removal of nonregenerative tissue from their body for therapeutic use, such as a transplant to another person's body. This is legally referred to as an *inter vivos* (from Latin, meaning "among the living") *gift of tissue*; that is, the donor gives the tissue during their lifetime.

2. The donor (or another, if the donor has expressed no wishes on the matter) has directed that specified body parts be removed from their body for transplantation into another living person after the donor's death. This is legally known as a *postmortem gift of tissue*.

Redefining Death

Some health care professionals have responded to the shortage of organs by suggesting that the definition of death be extended to include cortical death, as in the case of the donor with anencephaly. This definition would include patients in a persistent vegetative state, who have no cortical activity although the brainstem is intact. Such persons can maintain their vital functions, and their body can be kept alive for years with appropriate nursing care. However, everything that makes the individual a person—the ability to communicate, to relate to others, to remember—is gone. These patients may live for years or may have treatment withdrawn and be allowed to die.

Those who seek to redefine death argue that we are losing a potential pool of organ donors who may have

previously expressed, while competent, the wish to donate organs at the time of death. Those who argue against this redefinition suggest that we cannot redefine death whenever it is convenient to do so. Furthermore, they argue that these questions should be raised not in the context of organ donation but out of a duty and responsibility to the patient in the persistent vegetative state (Keatings, 1990). To do otherwise would be to treat individuals, as Kant would say, as means and not as ends in and of themselves.

Redefining death to include cortical death would present procedural problems. Would this redefinition apply universally or only in cases in which organ donation is viable? In any case, when would biological life be deemed to end? Would this happen immediately after cortical death is declared? Or would it end when convenient—for example, when someone needs a transplant (Keatings, 1990)?

This definition allows for the maintenance of the dead-donor paradigm—that organ procurement cannot cause death. A well-known bioethicist has argued for the abandonment of the "dead-donor rule" (Koppelman, 2003). Elysa Koppelman suggested that individuals may be able to set up an advance directive to have their organs donated if cognitive function fails, even if death according to the technical definition has not occurred. This, she argues, could apply to persons who have suffered serious irreparable brain injury or to persons in persistent vegetative states. Others argue against abandoning the "dead-donor rule" and for redefining death to include persons with serious irreversible brain damage who have no functioning cerebral cortex (Campbell, 2004; Crowley-Matoka & Arnold, 2004; Dudzinski, 2003; Hester, 2003; Menikoff, 2002; Steinberg, 2003; Trachtman, 2003; Truog, 2000; Truog & Robinson, 2003; Veatch, 2003). Others call for a debate on what constitutes death in such circumstances, but not to have the need for organ donation as the impetus for this; rather, they propose a debate on the meaning of life itself and when it may not be worth sustaining (Koenig, 2003).

Non-heart-beating Organ Donation

In the early days of transplantation, before *brain death* was defined, organs were retrieved from the deceased person after cardiac death. Non-heart-beating organ donation (NHBOD) was abandoned because of the challenges of using nonperfused organs, those deprived of oxygen for a certain period. As the demand for donation grows and rejection technology improves, this approach is being reintroduced (Ethics Committee, American College of Critical Care Medicine [ACCCM], & Society of Critical Care Medicine, 2001).

The death of the NHBOD patient is determined by "traditional" or "cardiopulmonary" criteria: (1) unresponsiveness, (2) apnea, and (3) absent circulation. The "dead-donor rule," a recent security convention, states that it is unethical to cause death by procuring organs, which is why the notion of "brain death" was introduced. To ensure death has occurred with NHBOD, there must be a full 5-minute observation period after an onset of circulatory arrest, apnea, and unresponsiveness. Clearly, this approach to organ procurement requires a great deal of psychosocial support for patients and their families.

There are two situations in which NHBOD may occur. Organ donation may follow death occurring after planned withdrawal of life-sustaining therapy, such as when a patient refuses life-sustaining therapy, opts to withdraw life support, and offers organ donation after death. Other situations may arise when an unexpected cardiac arrest occurs and resuscitation is not successful (Bell, 2006).

Because it is legally and ethically justifiable to withhold or withdraw life-sustaining treatment in infants, children, and adolescents when the burdens of those treatments outweigh the benefits, then donation in these situations would be justified by using the same criteria, as long as the other special considerations regarding children are followed. Therefore, parental consent or consent of a competent adolescent would be required.

The following standards apply to all potential donors:

- Informed consent to withdraw treatment and informed consent to donate must be given.
- Organ procurement must not cause death.

- Death will be determined by using appropriate standards.
- End-of-life supportive care must continue to be provided to the patient, and special consideration of the family must be made (Ethics Committee, ACCCM, & Society of Critical Care Medicine, 2001).

Although aggressive treatment and care are being provided at this time, nurses focus on doing what is best for their patient. There may be ambivalence as the patient begins to die or as treatment is withdrawn and the patient proceeds toward death and organ donation. Some may view this as treating the organs, not the person, and see the person merely as a means to an end in organ donation. However, the care relationship the nurse has with the patient must be maintained even as the focus shifts to ensuring that the patient's wish to be an organ donor is realized (Day, 2001; Rassin et al., 2005).

Depending on the nature of the person's disease and the viability of their organs, it is now also possible to donate organs after MAiD. The person must satisfy the criteria for MAiD and also meet the criteria for organ donation. There are a number of legal and ethical issues that must be considered, especially ones that relate to consent (Yazdani et al., 2018)—that is, the decision must be voluntary and free of coercion. The situation is more complex when it involves a person receiving MAiD who wishes to donate to a relative or close friend. The team must be satisfied that the decision for MAiD is not made only for the purpose of organ donation, while also honouring the person's wish—that in death, they make a difference for someone they care about.

A challenge unique to NHBOD is that the patient who wishes to become a donor may, unlike a brain-dead donor, be conscious and aware of what is happening. Consider Case Scenario 8.5.

CASE SCENARIO 8.5

BRAD'S STORY

Brad Hoffman, 28 years of age, became a ventilator-dependent quadriplegic after a serious motor vehicle accident. Against the desires of his family and concerns of the health care team, Brad decided that he did not want to live in this state and asked that life

support be withdrawn. Moreover, he volunteered to be an organ donor. This case had numerous ethical and emotional challenges. Was Brad competent to make the decision to withdraw life support? Was he in a depressed state, and was this influencing his decision? Did he have enough time to appreciate that

Continued on following page

CASE SCENARIO 8.5 *(Continued)*

a good quality of life could still be sustained? Was his motivation to be a donor clearly separate from his wish to withdraw treatment? After much consultation among his family, the health care team, and an ethics consultant, life support was withdrawn and his organs donated. The team involved in his care experienced intense emotional issues in this case. But should it be more difficult or easier when a person's consent is clear and when that person is able to choose the nature of death and have family present

through that process? If the team had misgivings, what would that mean? Are there problematic moral issues that are not readily evident (Spike, 2000)?

What are your thoughts on this real-life situation? As a health care professional, what would your position be? What would the role of the nurse be in supporting Brad and his family? If you were in Brad's situation, what do you think you would do? What are your thoughts on the amount of time Brad should have to reflect on his decision in this situation?

Living Organ Donors

This form of organ donation involves a living person who donates a kidney, lung, or liver lobe to a family member or friend. The consent must be valid—that is, it must meet all of the criteria of an informed consent, as outlined in Chapter 6. The potential for living, that is, *inter vivos*, donation has expanded over the years. This approach began with related donors who were an identical match to the transplant recipient and expanded to include friends who also were a close match to the recipient. However, because not all potential transplant recipients can find a compatible donor from family or friends and as the evidence emerged that the success rate with unrelated donors was equivalent to transplants from identically matched siblings, the potential donor pool expanded to include persons with no relationship at all to the recipient. This led to the possibility of identifying sets of compatible donor–recipient pairs from a registry of incompatible pairs for possible multiple exchange combinations. For example, a family member or friend might wish to donate an organ but is incompatible with the recipient. Another pair may have the same issue. Consider then that an exchange is possible if the willing donor in pair A is compatible with the potential recipient in pair B, and the willing donor in pair B is compatible with the potential recipient in pair A (Saidman et al., 2006).

In most settings, additional counselling of the donor occurs, given the risks associated with this decision. Because of the many ethical issues, donor guidelines have been developed to ensure that the process is legally and ethically sound (Wright et al., 2004).

In all provinces and territories except Ontario, Prince Edward Island, and Quebec, only a person who has reached the age of majority may legally consent to an *inter vivos* gift of tissue. Ontario and Prince Edward Island allow persons below the age of majority but who are at least 16 years of age to give consent without the approval of a parent or guardian (see Ontario's *Trillium Gift of Life Network Act*, 1990, s. 3(1); Prince Edward Island's *Human Tissue Donation Act*, 1988, s. 6(1)).

In Quebec, a minor (a person who has not yet reached the age of majority) may consent to an *inter vivos* donation of regenerative tissue only with consent of a parent or tutor (in Quebec, the equivalent of a child's legal guardian) and with permission of the court, provided that the procedure does not result in serious risk to the health of the minor (*Civil Code of Québec*, art. 19, para. 2). However, common law would likely permit such transfers if the donor were an adult, mentally competent, and making a free and fully informed decision.

Apart from being of the requisite age, a person in Alberta, British Columbia, Newfoundland and Labrador, Nova Scotia, Ontario, Saskatchewan, or the Yukon must be mentally competent to consent and must make a free and informed decision (see Alberta's *Personal Directives Act*, 2000, s. 3(1); British Columbia's *Human Tissue Gift Act*, 1996, s. 3(1); Newfoundland and Labrador's *Human Tissue Act*, 1990, s. 4(1); Nova Scotia's *Human Organ and Tissue Donation Act*, 2019, s. 1 and 5; Ontario's *Trillium Gift of Life Network Act*, 1990, s. 3(1); Saskatchewan's *The Human Tissue Gift Act*, 2015, s. 3

and 4; and the Yukon's *Human Tissue Gift Act*, 2002, s. 3(1)). A "free and informed decision" (as discussed in Chapter 6) follows the common law requirements for fully informed consent to medical treatment set out by the Supreme Court of Canada in *Reibl v. Hughes* (1980). The physician must inform the donor of all potential and material risks inherent in the procedure that would be reasonably likely to affect the donor's decision.

For their consent to be valid, Prince Edward Islanders must specifically be able to understand the consequences and nature of transplanting tissue from their body during their lifetime (*Human Tissue Donation Act*, 1988, s. 6(1)). If there is any doubt on this point, a physician must determine through an independent assessment whether the transplantation should be carried out (ss. 6(2), (8)).

Living Organ Donors: The Vulnerable and the Incapable

Situations in which the prospective donor is a minor, is mentally incompetent, or is otherwise unable to make an informed decision because of not understanding the nature and consequences of the procedure pose a special problem. Such a situation might arise, for example, if the health risk to the donor (a minor) is minimal and, therefore, perfectly acceptable, and the tissue is urgently required to save the life of that person's sibling.

As mentioned above, the Prince Edward Island statute provides for an independent assessment in a situation in which the donor appears to not understand the nature and consequences of the transplantation and yet consents to it. The assessors must consider whether:

- The transplant is the treatment of choice
- The donor has been coerced or induced to give consent
- Removal of the tissue will create a substantial health or other risk to the donor
- The Act and its regulations have been complied with (*Human Tissue Donation Act*, 1988, s. 8(6))

In Prince Edward Island, this requirement for assessment also applies in the case of donors under age 16 years, even if they understand the nature and consequences of the transplant (*Human Tissue Donation*

Act, 1988, ss. 7(1), (4)). In the case of a minor under age 16 years, parental consent is also required for an *inter vivos* gift of regenerative tissue (e.g., bone marrow). An additional requirement for *inter vivos* donors under age 16 years in Prince Edward Island is that all other members of the donor's family must be eliminated as potential donors for medical or other reasons. The assessors must give written reasons for their decision and must indicate in their assessment that the transplantation should be carried out.

The Prince Edward Island statute further provides that a person may appeal the decision to the Supreme Court of Prince Edward Island within 3 days (*Human Tissue Donation Act*, 1988, s. 9(1)). The Court may confirm, vary, or quash (cancel) the assessors' decision, or return the matter to the assessors for further action. Pending the decision of the appeal, the transplantation cannot proceed.

Manitoba's *The Human Tissue Gift Act* (C.C.S.M., c. H180) and Ontario's *Trillium Gift of Life Network Act* (1990) permit persons under age 18 years but at least 16 years of age to consent to the donation of tissue while living. However, a physician who is not and never has been associated with the proposed recipient must certify in writing that they believe such person is capable of understanding and does understand the nature and effect of the transplantation. Furthermore, in Manitoba, a parent must consent, and the donor must be a member of the recipient's immediate family (*The Human Tissue Gift Act*, ss. 10(1), (2)). The physician who makes the certificate cannot participate in the transplantation. This provision addresses concerns over potential conflicts of interest.

In Manitoba, persons under age 16 years may donate tissue while living only if these conditions are met:

- The proposed recipient is a member of the donor's immediate family.
- Only regenerative tissue will be given.
- The recipient would likely die without the tissue.
- The life and health risks to the donor are minimal.
- The donor consents to the transplantation.
- The donor's parent or legal guardian consents.
- The transplantation is recommended by a physician who is not and never has been involved in

any way with the recipient and will not be involved in the transplantation.

■ Court approval is obtained.

Alberta, British Columbia, Newfoundland, Nova Scotia, Ontario, Saskatchewan, and Yukon do not require an assessment procedure in the case of a minor or mentally incompetent *inter vivos* donor. Ontario's *Health Care Consent Act, 1996* (s. 6, para. 3), for instance, specifically states that its provisions do not affect the law with respect to, among other matters, the removal of regenerative or nonregenerative tissue for implantation in another person's body.

The human tissue donation statutes of most of these provinces are virtually identical. However, they do provide that if the donor giving consent is a minor, is mentally incompetent to consent, or is unable to give a free and informed decision, the consent is still legally valid if the person acting on that consent (presumably, the physician who will perform the transplantation) has no reason to believe that the donor is a minor, is mentally incompetent, or is unable to make a free and informed decision. There is, thus, a requirement of good faith on the part of the person performing the transplantation and a duty upon them to ensure that a prospective donor is, indeed, a mentally competent adult who is giving a free and informed consent.

In most cases, this provision does not pose a problem. Most physicians and nurses are competent to assess the general mental capabilities of their patients. A careful review with the patient of all material risks inherent in the transplantation, within the criteria stated in *Reibl v. Hughes* (1980), would likely address the problem of a free and informed consent. The case of the minor poses a slightly different problem when that person appears much older than they actually are. The level of maturity disclosed in the conversation between the health care professional and the minor cannot be considered conclusive. The statute protects health care professionals acting in good faith in such a situation.

Apart from this, such prospective donors would require some sort of court authorization according to common law. This has been the traditional route in jurisdictions lacking procedures, such as those required in Prince Edward Island, or explicit provisions for court authorization, such as those in Quebec's Civil Code. A court reviewing such a case would likely consider factors

such as those mentioned in the Prince Edward Island Act and, further, would consider the impact of the procedure on the donor.

In the case of a minor, some courts have relied on the "competent minor" rule. This rule holds that a person under the age of majority may be sufficiently mature to comprehend fully the nature and consequences of the transplantation. Because the donor in these cases is not receiving a direct health benefit from the transplantation, in some American states, the courts have considered that the infant donor still derives future emotional benefit from the survival of their sibling. The family is, thus, relieved from the potential stress of the death of one of its members and can provide full emotional support to the donor. Furthermore, especially in cases in which the donor is old enough to have expressed even a rudimentary wish to help the sibling (although not fully comprehending the nature and consequences of the transplantation), that child is spared the emotional guilt that may develop later in life from not having had an opportunity to save the sibling's life (Sneiderman et al., 1989).

Postmortem Donation

Consent to donation of tissue after the donor's death is somewhat different. The policy behind the law in such cases is to encourage the donation of organs after death because there is always a large pool of recipients who urgently need them. Thus, the requirements for lawful consent are more relaxed and flexible.

In all provinces and territories, a person over the age of majority (age over 16 years in Ontario and Prince Edward Island) may consent in writing to the removal of any and all tissue for therapeutic, medical educational, or medical research purposes. Except in Quebec, the written document containing the consent may be part of a will or other testamentary instrument (e.g., organ donor card, driver's licence), regardless of whether such will is legally valid.

In Manitoba and Ontario, persons under age 18 years but at least 16 years of age may consent to such removal, but only with the consent of their parent or guardian, unless the parent or guardian is unavailable (e.g., dead, physically or mentally ill, or otherwise absent) (see Manitoba's *The Human Tissue Gift Act*, C.C.S.M., c. H180, ss. 2(1), 2(2); and Ontario's *Trillium Gift of Life Network Act*, 1990, s. 3). These provisions permit flexibility and promote the availability of organs. Consent given by a person under age 16 years is deemed valid if the person who acted on it had no reason to believe that the postmortem donor was in fact under age 16 years. This mirrors the provisions of *inter vivos* donations in most provinces and imposes a requirement of good faith on the part of physicians acting upon the donor's directive.

In Quebec, a minor 14 years of age or older may authorize the removal of organs or tissue or give their body for medical or scientific purposes. A minor under age 14 years may also do so with the written consent of a parent or guardian (*Civil Code of Québec,* art. 43).

Most provinces allow consent to be made orally by the donor in the presence of two witnesses during the donor's last illness. Manitoba and Prince Edward Island do not specify whether the consent must be given in written form. The statutes of those two provinces speak of the removal of tissue "as may be specified in the consent," which implies requirement for written consent. However, in a case in which a clear, unequivocal oral consent is given in the presence of two or more witnesses, it is possible that such consent would be permissible as clear evidence of the donor's last wishes. In all cases, the donor may revoke (cancel) their consent at any time prior to death, when consent becomes effective.

Postmortem Donations Lacking the Deceased's Consent

What of situations in which the deceased expressed no wishes regarding donation of tissues or organs after death, or was incapable of giving consent? This is different from specifically refusing consent because the law requires that such refusal, however unfortunate for the prospective recipient, be respected. Yet, organs or tissue may be urgently needed to save the life of another. In such cases (i.e., the prospective donor has expressed no wishes and death is imminent in the opinion of a physician), the law in all jurisdictions allows other specific persons to make the decision regarding the removal of tissue or organs from the body of the deceased.

There is a hierarchy of persons who may be approached to make this decision:

1. The spouse of the donor
2. If there is no spouse, any of the donor's children over age 18 years

3. If there are no children, either of the donor's parents (or legal guardian, in some provinces; in Prince Edward Island, the person's guardian ranks above their spouse)
4. Any of the donor's siblings
5. The donor's next of kin
6. If none of the above is available, anyone who is in lawful possession of the body

The statutes make clear that the sixth category excludes the coroner, the medical examiner, the embalmer, and the funeral director. It might conceivably include the executor or administrator of the donor's estate because such a person is responsible for the proper and respectful disposal of the deceased's remains, either by burial or cremation.

Sometimes, relatives of the deceased will disagree over permitting the removal of organs or tissue. For example, the spouse of a patient, N. S., whose death is imminent, might refuse a physician's request for removal of the patient's kidneys, whereas the patient's parent may be in favour of such a request. The law in most provinces and territories provides a resolution to such a conflict: no person may act on a consent given on behalf of a dying or deceased donor if such person knows of an objection to it by anyone having the same or closer relationship to the donor than the one who gave the consent. Thus, in our case scenario, the wishes of the donor's spouse would overrule those of the donor's parent. Similarly, in a case in which the donor's sibling gave consent and the donor's other sibling objected, that objection would void the consent and end the matter unless another relative closer in relationship to the donor consented. Manitoba's legislation does not provide a mechanism for resolving such disputes, but it is likely that a health care professional in that province faced with a similar conflict could resolve it in this manner.

In Quebec, the Civil Code permits the deceased's heirs or successors to give or refuse consent (*Civil Code of Québec,* art. 42). There is no mechanism for conflict resolution in the Civil Code. However, a person qualified to give consent to care for the donor (when living) may also consent to the removal of tissue or organs from the deceased's body (*Civil Code of Québec,* art. 45, para. 1). In Quebec, a physician may proceed with the transplantation of an organ or tissues from a deceased person if two physicians certify that they were unable to obtain such consent in due time and that the operation was urgently required to save a human life or to significantly improve the quality of a life (*Civil Code of Québec*, art. 45, para. 2).

Finally, the law, as always, respects the wishes of the deceased or dying donor. If health care professionals acting on the consent of a donor's spouse or other relative has reason to believe that the donor would object to the removal, or, as in Manitoba, that such removal would be contrary to the donor's religion (*The Human Tissue Gift Act,* C.C.S.M., c. H180, s. 4(3)(a)), they cannot proceed on the basis of the consent. Similarly, if the health care professional in charge of the case believes that death occurred in circumstances requiring an inquest by a coroner or medical examiner (i.e., the deceased did not die of natural causes and an inquest into the cause of death is required), that professional cannot proceed on the basis of the consent unless the coroner or the medical examiner agrees. This requirement preserves the evidentiary value of a postmortem examination of the body.

Legislative Strategies to Promote Organ Retrieval

Manitoba and Ontario have tried, in their organ donation legislation, to encourage physicians and other health care professionals to identify potential organ donors. The Manitoba Act requires the last physician who attended the deceased to consider, upon the death of one who has given no direction as to organ donation (or whose direction is invalid because the person was incompetent), whether it is appropriate to request permission of the donor's proxy or other relative to remove tissue or use the body for therapeutic purposes (*The Human Tissue Gift Act*, C.C.S.M., c. H180, s. 4(1)). Ontario's Act requires a designated health care facility to notify the Trillium Gift of Life Network of the death or imminent death of a patient in its care (*Trillium Gift of Life Network Act*, 1990, s. 8.1(1)). The Network, established under the Act, is then required to determine, based on the viability of the organs, whether the health care facility should contact the patient or the patient's substitute decision maker concerning consent for tissue donation. This is to ensure that in every instance where viable organs might be retrieved, the patient or patient's substitute decision maker is proactively given an opportunity to consider organ donation.

Prince Edward Island law requires an attending physician or other person to record whether they discussed tissue donation with any of those authorized to provide consent on behalf of the patient to removal of organs or tissue. If no such discussion has taken place, the reason that it has not must be recorded (*Human Tissue Donation Act*, 1988, s. 4). This is as far as the Prince Edward Island legislation goes. It does not demand that such consultation take place. As mentioned earlier, Nova Scotia introduced a presumed consent law, *Human Organ and Tissue Donation Act (HOTDA)*, in 2019. Statistics from Nova Scotia Health, published in January 2022, indicate that there has been a significant increase in tissue donations (a 40% increase in 2021 over 2020) and the availability of organs for transplantation.

CASE SCENARIO 8.4A

APPLICATION TO A GIFT OR AN OBLIGATION

The misconceptions and misinformation surrounding organ tissue laws in Canada have regrettably contributed to a low rate of organ retrieval across the country. The case scenario of M. R. and J. S. raises the issue of whether the critical care unit (CCU) team ought to have been more persuasive with M. R.'s family. This would have been an appropriate role for the nurses in M. R.'s team. With the valid organ donor card, the team could have proceeded despite the parents' wishes. Unfortunately, however, in practice, most hospitals do not contravene the wishes of the next of kin of the deceased, even with a valid consent from the deceased, possibly because the attempt to persuade the family to consent might be deemed coercive. However, if the team approaches the family in a gentle, diplomatic, and sensitive way, the request need not be coercive; in fact, a request made in such a manner might garner earnest support from families. Many more lives could be saved if this situation were expressly addressed in each province's legislation.

SUMMARY

Nurses today belong to a health care culture that constantly strives to solve the mysteries of life and death. This chapter has explored the many complex ethical, legal, and emotional issues that are associated with transitions at the end of a person's life.

The historical emphasis on the principle of sanctity of life in health care has driven the development of treatment modalities and technologies that can cure many previously terminal diseases and save lives but that can also simply prolong the process of dying or compromise the quality of those lives saved. The fear of dying in isolation or in pain and suffering has driven society to seek other options to protect people from this unfortunate possibility.

Nurses play a vital role during this significant journey by providing compassionate care and comfort to the patient, supporting the family, and ultimately ensuring that the process of dying is dignified and respectful of all involved.

Nurses have a significant role in ensuring that patients' rights and dignity are respected throughout the process of dying. In the delivery of compassionate care, the goal of nursing is that patients are made comfortable, are kept free of pain and suffering, and remain in control of their lives and the nature of their deaths. When permitted by law, persons are able to make decisions about where and how they die and who should accompany them during this transition. Nurses support the wishes of patients at the end of life by ensuring that their cultural and religious beliefs are respected, their advance directives are followed, influencing a respectful organ donation process when that is the person's wish, and being sensitive to the needs of the dying, across the life continuum from premature neonates to older persons.

CRITICAL THINKING

The following scenarios are provided to stimulate reflection, discussion, and analysis. As you review each case, consider the following questions as well as those specific to the case:

1. Have the nurses in these cases violated any ethical or legal standards?
2. If so, what are these standards?
3. Is there risk of any civil or criminal liability?
4. How could these situations have been prevented?

Discussion Points

1. What are your views on Medical Assistance in Dying (MAiD)? Are you comfortable with the guidelines and the safeguards that have been put in place to prevent abuse? What are your thoughts on expanding the legislation to include minors and the mentally ill, and to permit advance directives? What role should nurses play in these deliberations?
2. Consider a team debate where one team argues for MAiD and the other team argues against it. Apply the theories described in Chapter 2 to the discussion.
3. What guidelines are in place in your facility to ensure that a person has a peaceful and dignified death? Can these guidelines be improved?
4. Does your facility have any policies or rules that limit family access to patients? Can these rules or policies be supported ethically?

CASE SCENARIO 8.6

IN WHOSE BEST INTERESTS?

A 29-year-old sustained a major head injury in a car accident 7 years ago and is presently living in a long-term care facility. The patient cannot communicate in any way, requires total care, and is incontinent of urine and stool. The patient is believed to be in a persistent vegetative state, and the team thinks the patient's prognosis is hopeless. The patient has a gastrostomy tube through which they receive regular feedings.

The patient's parents believe that their child would not wish to be maintained in this way and have requested that the feeding tube be removed. They have made this request several times in past years. However, the hospital's policy does not allow discontinuation of enteral feeding. As the patient's his gastrostomy tube is replaced at regular intervals, the family is now asking that it not be replaced in the event that it accidentally falls out.

Questions

1. What are your views on this hospital's policy regarding withdrawal of treatment?
2. As a nurse, how would you support this family?
3. Do you agree with the family's plan?
4. In this situation, what would be the legal requirements for organ donation in your home province?
5. What criteria does your hospital use for determining death?

CASE SCENARIO 8.7

WHO DO I WANT BESIDE ME?

A 74-year-old patient, who suffered a serious heart attack causing a small hole in her ventricular septum, is in critical condition. The only option is to provide mechanical cardiac support and perform immediate surgery.

The patient's family remain in the waiting room of the critical care unit (CCU) during the surgery, which takes about 6 hours. They are relieved when the surgery is completed and the patient returns to the ICU. They have been told they will be able to visit within a few minutes after the patient is settled but when they inquire about visiting, they are told they will have to wait because it is the change of shift. A half hour passes, and the family asks again. This time, they are told that the nurses are still organizing care; so they must wait a bit longer. What is happening, in fact, is that the patient is still bleeding from the surgery. The nurses are in the process of administering transfusions, and the patient is being assessed by the surgeon and a hematologist. An hour and a half later, the family has still not been allowed into her room. Upon asking again, they are allowed a 5-minute visit.

Questions

1. What are the nurses' responsibilities to this patient and family? Did they meet these responsibilities? Was their approach nurse- or patient-centred?
2. What policies in hospitals and CCUs might restrict nurses from meeting the needs of patients and families?
3. How might nurses and nursing leaders ensure that policies and rules reflect high ethical and professional standards?
4. Can you think of similar situations in your own practice experience?

CASE SCENARIO 8.8

THE COST OF COMFORT?

A case manager in the home care setting is currently coordinating the care of a patient with cancer, who is dying at home. The patient is expected to die within the next few days. Community nurses visit daily, but the patient's family are providing most of her care. Although the patient receives morphine on a regular basis, the patient is still in great discomfort and is emaciated; the skin over the coccyx has broken down, and the cancer has metastasized to the bones. The family informs the case manager that during a recent hospital admission, the nurses provided a special mattress that relieved the patient's discomfort considerably. The case manager explains that this mattress is not a resource that is covered and instead offers the services of special-duty nurses for the next few nights. Because the patient's death is imminent, the case manager is concerned that the family will need their rest. The family refuses the offer of assistance of additional nurses because they want to remain present with their parent during the final hours. They make arrangements to rent the mattress themselves at their own cost.

Questions

1. What responsibilities does the case manager have to ensure that this patient's care needs are met?
2. Does it make sense that a more cost-effective and practical intervention (the mattress) be denied? How can nurses change agency policies in order to introduce guidelines that focus on individual needs? (Or should all patients be treated the same way?)

CASE SCENARIO 8.9

A LITTLE MORE TIME

O. W. is pregnant with their first child. Things have been going very well with the pregnancy, and O. W. and their partner are looking forward to meeting their baby. O. W. is 24 weeks into their pregnancy when O. W. suddenly experiences severe abdominal pain. O. W.'s partner rushes O. W. to the hospital, where O. W. is found to be in active labour. The health care team attempts to slow down O. W.'s labour, but they are not successful. Meanwhile, they do an emergency ultrasonography to evaluate the baby's condition. They find that the baby has significant cardiac problems that, if not addressed immediately after birth, will result in death soon after. It is possible for the nearest pediatric centre that performs cardiac surgery to send a team to the hospital to resuscitate the baby and transport it immediately to the pediatric facil-ity. For this option to be successful, O. W. will have to undergo a Caesarean section. The potential out-comes for the baby are not known.

The parents are presented with another option. The baby can be delivered vaginally and receive pal-liative care.

Because 1 hour has passed since O. W. started to have abdominal pain, they have to make an immedi-ate decision.

Questions

1. What are the ethical issues associated with this scenario?
2. How can the health care team support the parents?
3. Who should be involved in the decision?
4. How might this decision be made? What are the factors to consider?

REFERENCES

Statutes

An Act respecting end-of-life care, SQ 2014, c. 2 (Quebec).

Canadian Charter of Rights and Freedoms, Part I of the *Constitution Act, 1982,* being Schedule B to the *Canada Act 1982* (UK), 1982, c. 11.

Christian Medical and Dental Society of Canada v. College of Physicians and Surgeons of Ontario, 2019 ONCA 393.

Civil Code of Québec, CQLR c. CCQ-1991 (Quebec).

Criminal Code, R.S.C. 1985, c. C-46 (Canada).

Criminal Law Amendment Act, S.C. 1972, c. 13 (Canada).

Health Care Consent Act, 1996, S.O. 1996, c. 2, Sch. A (Ontario).

The Health Care Directives Act, C.C.S.M., c. H27 (Manitoba).

Human Organ and Tissue Donation Act, SNS 2019, c 6 (Nova Scotia).

Human Tissue Act, R.S.N.L. 1990, c. H-15 (Newfoundland and Labrador).

Human Tissue Act, R.S.N.W.T. 1988, c. H-6 (Northwest Territories and Nunavut).

Human Tissue Donation Act, R.S.P.E.I. 1988, c. H-12.1 (Prince Edward Island).

The Human Tissue Gift Act, C.C.S.M., c. H180 (Manitoba).

Human Tissue Gift Act, R.S.B.C. 1996, c. 211 (British Columbia).

Human Tissue Gift Act, S.N.B. 2004, c. H-12.5 (New Brunswick).

The Human Tissue Gift Act, SS 2015, c. H-15.1 (Saskatchewan).

Human Tissue Gift Act, R.S.Y. 2002, c. 117 (Yukon).

Personal Directives Act, R.S.A. 2000, c. P-6 (Alberta).

Representation Agreement Act, R.S.B.C. 1996, c. 405 (British Columbia).

Substitute Decisions Act, 1992, S.O. 1992, c. 30 (Ontario).

Trillium Gift of Life Network Act, R.S.O. 1990, c. H.20 (Ontario).

The Vital Statistics Act, C.C.S.M. c. V60 (Manitoba).

Case Law

Carter v. Canada (Attorney General) [2015] SCC 5, [2015] 1 S.C.R. 331.

Cuthbertson v. Rasouli [2013] SCC 53.

Golubchuk v. Salvation Army Grace General Hospital et al. [2008] MBQB 49 (CanLII).

Nancy B. v. Hôtel-Dieu de Québec [1992] RJQ 361; (1992), 86 DLR (4th) 385; (1992), 69 CCC (3d) 450 (SC).

R. v. Kitching and Adams [1976] 6 WWR 697, at p. 711 (Man. CA).

R. v. Latimer [1995] CanLII 3921 (SK CA).

R. v. Latimer [1997] 1 SCR 217; 152 Sask. R. 1 (SCC). Sentence fol-lowing second trial ordered by Supreme Court of Canada: (1998), 121 CCC. (3d) 326; 172 Sask. R. 161, 185 W.A.C. 161, 22 C.R. (5th) 380, [1999] 6 W.W.R. 118, [1998] S.J. No. 731 (QL); aff'd.

R. v. Latimer [2001] 1 S.C.R. 3; (2001), 193 D.L.R. (4th) 577; [2001] 6 W.W.R. 409; (2001), 150 C.C.C. (3d) 129; (2001), 39 C.R. (5th) 1; (2001), 80 C.R.R. (2d) 189; (2001), 203 Sask. R. 1.

Re Quinlan 137 NJ Super. 227; 348 A.2d. 801 (Ch. Div. 1975), In re Quinlan, 70 NJ 10, 355 A.2d. 647 (SC 1976).

Reibl v. Hughes [1980] 2 SCR 880; (1980) 14 CCLT 1; 114 DLR (3d) 1; 33 NR 361 (SCC).

Rodriguez v. British Columbia (Attorney General) [1993] 3 SCR 519, 1993 CanLII 75 (SCC) [1993] BCWLD 347; (1992), 18 WCB (2d) 279 (SC), aff'd. (1993), 76 BCLR (2d) 145; 22 BCAC 266; 38 WAC 266; 14 CRR (2d) 34; 79 CCC (3d) 1; [1993] 3 WWR 553, aff'd. [1993] 3 SCR 519.

Truchon c. Procureur général du Canada, 2019 QCCS 3792.

Texts and Articles

Aboriginal Justice Implementation Commission. (1999). Ab-original concepts of justice: Aboriginal people and the role of elders. In *Report of the Aboriginal Justice Inquiry of Manitoba.* http://www.ajic.mb.ca/volumel/chapter2.html

Adams, J. A., Bailey, D. E., Jr., Anderson, R. A., et al. (2011). Nursing roles and strategies in end-of-life decision making in acute care: A systematic review of the literature. *Nursing Research and Practice, 2011,* 527834.

Alberga, H. (2022). Ontario woman enduring effects of long COVID begins process for medically assisted death. *CTV News.* https://toronto.ctvnews.ca/ontario-woman-enduring-effects-of-long-covid-begins-process-for-medically-assisted-death-1.5976944

Andershed, B. (2006). Relatives in end-of-life care—Part 1: A systematic review of the literature the five last years, January 1999–February 2004. *Journal of Clinical Nursing, 15*(9), 1158–1169.

Anderson, I. (2002). *Indigenous perspectives on death and dying.* Ian Anderson Continuing Education Program in End-of-Life Care. University of Toronto. https://www.cpd.utoronto.ca/endoflife/Slides/PPT%20Indigenous%20Perspectives.pdf

Baumann-Hölzle, R., Maffezzoni, M., & Bucher, H. U. (2005). A framework for ethical decision making in neonatal intensive care. *Acta Paediatrica, 94*(12), 1777–1783.

Bell, M. D. D. (2006). Emergency medicine, organ donation and the *Human Tissue Act. Emergency Medicine Journal, 23*(11), 824–827.

Bidigare, S. A. (1991). Attitudes and knowledge of nurses regarding organ procurement. *Heart & Lung, 20*(1), 20–25.

Bigham, B. L., Koprowicz, K., Rea, T., et al. (2011). Cardiac arrest survival did not increase in the Resuscitation Outcomes Consortium after implementation of the 2005 AHA CPR and ECC guidelines. *Resuscitation, 82*(8), 979–983.

Booth, M. (2006). Ethical issues in resuscitation and intensive care medicine. *Anaesthesia and Intensive Care Medicine, 8*(1), 36–39.

Borozny, M. L. (1988). Brain death and critical care nurses. *The Canadian Nurse, 84*(1), 24–27.

Bremer, A., & Sandman, L. (2011). Futile cardiopulmonary resuscitation for the benefit of others: An ethical analysis. *Nursing Ethics, 18*(4), 495–504.

Browne, A., & Sullivan, B. (2006). Advance directives in Canada. *Cambridge Quarterly of Healthcare Ethics, 15*(3), 256–260.

Bruce, A., & Beuthin, R. (2019). Medically assisted dying in Canada: "Beautiful death" is transforming nurses' experiences of suffering. *Canadian Journal of Nursing Research, 52*(4), 268–277.

Bruce, A., & Boston, P. (2011). Relieving existential suffering through palliative sedation: Discussion of an uneasy practice. *Journal of Advanced Nursing, 67*(12), 2732–2740.

Campbell, C. S. (2004). Harvesting the living? Separating "brain death" and organ transplantation. *Kennedy Institute of Ethics Journal, 14*(3), 301–318.

Canadian Armed Forces, 4th Canadian Division Joint Task Force (Central). (2020). *Operation LASER—JTFC observations in long term care facilities in Ontario.* https://www.macleans.ca/wp-content/uploads/2020/05/JTFC-Observations-in-LTCF-in-ON.pdf

Canadian Institute for Health Information. (2021). *Long-term care and COVID-19: The first six months.* https://www.cihi.ca/en/long-term-care-and-covid-19-the-first-6-months

Canadian Nurses Association. (2017). *Code of ethics for registered nurses.*

Canadian Nurses Protective Society. (2017). *Ask a lawyer: Mature minor.* https://cnps.ca/article/mature-minor/

Canadian Nurses Protective Society. (2021). *Medical assistance in dying: What every nurse should know.*

Canadian Paediatric Society. (2004). Treatment decisions regarding infants, children and adolescents. *Paediatric & Child Health, 9*(2), 99–103.

Cantor, M. D., Braddock, C. H., III., Derse, A. R., et al. (2003). Do-not-resuscitate orders and medical futility. *Archives of Internal Medicine, 163,* 2689–2694.

Carlet, J., Thijs, L. G., Antonelli, M., et al. (2004). Challenges in end-of-life care in the ICU. *Intensive Care Medicine, 30*(5), 770–784.

Carpenter, T., & Vivas, L. (2020). Ethical arguments against coercing provider participation in MAiD (medical assistance in dying) in Ontario, Canada. *BMC Medical Ethics, 21*(46). https://bmcmedethics.biomedcentral.com/articles/10.1186/s12910-020-00486-2

Centre for Effective Practice. (2017). *Medical Assistance in Dying (MAiD): Ontario.* https://thewellhealth.ca/MAiD/

Chittick, W. C. (1992). "Your sight today is piercing": The Muslim understanding of death and afterlife. In H. Obayashi (Ed.), *Death and afterlife: Perspectives of world religions* (pp. 125–139). New York: Greenwood Press.

Cohen, R. W. (2004). A tale of two conversations. *Hastings Center Report, 34*(3), 49.

College of Nurses of Ontario. (2021). *CNO guidance on nurses' roles in medical assistance in dying.* https://www.cno.org/globalassets/docs/prac/41056-guidance-on-nurses-roles-in-maid.pdf

College of Nurses of Ontario. (2023). *Medical assistance in dying—General FAQs.* https://www.cno.org/en/trending-topics/medical-assistance-in-dying/medical-assistance-in-dying--faqs/

College of Registered Nurses of Manitoba. (2021). *Medical assistance in dying: Guidelines for Manitoba nurses.* https://www.crnm.mb.ca/wp-content/uploads/2022/01/MAID-guideline-July142021.pdf

Committee on Fetus and Newborn (American Academy of Pediatrics). (2007). Noninitiation or withdrawal of intensive care for high-risk newborns. *Pediatrics, 119*(2), 401–403.

Crowley-Matoka, M., & Arnold, R. M. (2004, September). The dead donor rule: How much does the public care…and how much should we care? *Kennedy Institute of Ethics Journal, 14*(3), 319–332.

CTV. (2008). Orthodox Jew to remain on life support, trial next. *CTV News.* https://www.ctvnews.ca/orthodox-jew-to-remain-on-life-support-trial-next-1.276306

Day, L. (2001). How nurses shift from care of a brain injured patient to maintenance of a brain dead organ donor. *American Journal of Critical Care, 19,* 306–403.

Downar, J., Fowler, F. A., Halko, R., et al. (2020). Early experience with medical assistance in dying in Ontario, Canada: A cohort study. *CMAJ, 192*(8), E173–E181.

Dudzinski, D. M. (2003, Winter). Does the respect for donor rule respect the donor? *The American Journal of Bioethics, 3*(1), 23–24.

Epstein, E. (2007). *Moral obligations of NICU healthcare providers at the end of palliative life.* Unpublished abstract, University of Virginia School of Nursing.

Ethics Committee, American College of Critical Care Medicine, & Society of Critical Care Medicine. (2001, September). Recommendations for nonheartbeating organ donation: A position paper by the Ethics Committee, American College of Critical Care

Medicine, Society of Critical Care Medicine. *Critical Care Medicine, 29*(9), 1826–1831.

Hayes, C. (2004, January/March). Ethics in end-of-life care. *Journal of Hospice and Palliative Nursing, 6*(1), 36–45.

Health Canada. (2018). *MAiD at a glance.*

Heino, L., Stolt, M., & Haavisto, E. (2022). The practices of nurses about palliative sedation on palliative care wards: A qualitative study. *Journal of Advanced Nursing, 78*(11), 3733–3744.

Hester, D. M. (2003). "Dead donor" versus "respect for donor" rule: Putting the cart before the horse. *The American Journal of Bioethics, 3*(1), 24–26.

Heyland, D. K., Allan, D. E., Rocker, G., et al. (2009). Discussing prognosis with patients and their families near the end of life: Impact on satisfaction with end-of-life care. *Open Medicine, 3*(2), e101–e110.

Hibbert, M. (1995). Stressors experienced by nurses while caring for organ donors and their families. *Heart & Lung, 24*(5), 399–407.

Historica Canada. (2018). *Robert latimer case.* http://www.thecanadianencyclopedia.ca/en/article/robert-latimer-case/

Horton, R. (2021). *New Nova Scotia law makes it easier to be an organ and tissue donor.* https://www.blood.ca/en/research/our-research-stories/research-education-discovery/nova-scotia-presumed-consent-organ-donation

Irving, M. J., Tong, A., Jan, S., et al. (2012). Factors that influence the decision to be an organ donor: A systematic review of the qualitative literature. *Nephrology Dialysis Transplantation, 27*(6), 2526–2533.

Ives-Baine, L. (2007). A lasting and meaningful difference: Bereavement care. The Hospital for Sick Children. *Nursing Matters, 8*(3), 3–6.

Janvier, A., & Barrington, K. J. (2005). The ethics of neonatal resuscitation at the margins of viability: Informed consent and outcomes. *Journal of Pediatrics, 147*, 579–585.

Jezewski, M., & Finnell, D. (1998). The meaning of DNR status: Oncology nurses' experiences with patients and families. *Cancer Nursing, 21*(3), 212–221.

Johnston, G., Vukic, A., & Parker, S. (2013). Cultural understanding in the provision of supportive and palliative care: Perspectives in relation to an Indigenous population. *BMJ Supportive & Palliative Care, 3*(1), 61–68.

Jordan, M., Keefer, P. M., Lee, Y. A., et al. (2018). Top ten tips palliative care clinicians should know about caring for children. *Journal of Palliative Medicine, 21*(12), 1783–1789.

Keatings, M. (1990). The biology of the persistent vegetative state, legal and ethical implications for transplantation: Viewpoints from nursing. *Transplantation Proceedings, 2*(3), 997–999.

Kelly, L., & Minty, A. (2007). End-of-life issues for Aboriginal patients: A literature review. *Canadian Family Physician, 53*(9), 1459–1465.

Keown, D. (2005). End of life: the Buddhist view. *Lancet, 366*, 952–953.

Kim, J. R., Elliott, D., & Hyde, C. (2004, March). Korean health professionals' attitudes and knowledge toward organ donation and transplantation. *International Journal of Nursing Studies, 41*(3), 299–307.

Kim, Y. S. (1998). *Organ transplantation: Principles and practice.* Huny-Mon Pub.

Kirsch, R. E., Balit, C. R., Carnevale, F. A., et al. (2018). Ethical, cultural, social, and individual considerations prior to transition to limitation or withdrawal of life-sustaining therapies. *Pediatric Critical Care Medicine, 19*(8), S10–S18.

Koenig, B. A. (2003, Winter). Dead donors and the "shortage" of human organs: Are we missing the point? *The American Journal of Bioethics, 3*(1), 26–27.

Kolarik, R. C., Arnold, R. M., Fischer, G. S., et al. (2002). Advance care planning: A comparison of values statements and treatment preferences. *Journal of General Internal Medicine, 17*(8), 618–624.

Koppelman, E. R. (2003). The dead donor rule and the concept of death: Severing the ties that bind them. *The American Journal of Bioethics, 3*(1), 1–9.

Kowalski, W. J., Leef, K. H., Mackley, A., et al. (2005). Communicating with parents of premature infants: Who is the informant? *Journal of Perinatology, 26*(1), 44–48.

Kramer, K. P. (1988). *The sacred art of dying: How world religions understand death.* Paulist Press.

Lamb, C., Babenko-Mould, Y., Evans, M., et al. (2019). Conscientious objection and nurses: Results of an interpretive phenomenological study. *Nursing Ethics, 26*(5), 1337–1349.

Lang, F., & Quill, T. (2004). Making decisions with families at the end of life. *American Family Physician, 70*(4), 719–723.

Law Reform Commission of Canada. (1980). *Medical treatment and criminal law. Working paper No. 26.*

Law Reform Commission of Canada. (1983). *Euthanasia, aiding suicide and cessation of treatment.* Report No. 20.

McAllister, M., & Dionne, K. (2006). Partnering with parents: Establishing effective long-term relationships with parents in the NICU. *Neonatal Network: The Journal of Neonatal Nursing, 25*(5), 329–337.

McMechan C., Bruce, A., & Beuthin, R. (2019). Canadian nursing students' experiences with medical assistance in dying. *Quality Advancement in Nursing Education, 5*(1), 2.

Meadow, W. (2006, June). 500-gram infants—and 800-pound gorillas—in the delivery room. *Pediatrics, 117*(6), 2276.

Meier, E. A., Gallegos, J. V., Thomas, L. P., et al. (2016). Defining a good death (successful dying): Literature review and a call for research and public dialogue. *The American Journal of Geriatric Psychiatry, 24*(4), 261–271.

Meller, S., & Barclay, S. (2011). Mediation: An approach to intractable disputes between parents and paediatricians. *Archives of Disease in Childhood, 96*(7), 619–621.

Menikoff, J. (2002, Summer). The importance of being dead: Non-heart-beating organ donation. *Issues in Law & Medicine, 18*(1), 3–20.

Mills, M., & Cortezzo, D. E. (2020). Moral distress in the neonatal intensive care unit: What is it, why it happens, and how we can address it. *Frontiers in Pediatrics, 8*, 581.

Molloy, D. W., Guyatt, G. H., Russo, R., et al. (2000). Systematic implementation of an advance directive program in nursing homes: A randomized controlled trial. *JAMA, 283*(11), 1437–1444.

Murray, S. A., Kendall, M., Boyd, K., et al. (2005). Illness trajectories and palliative care. *British Medical Journal, 330*(7498), 1007–1011.

Nova Scotia Department of Health and Wellness. (2020). *Human organ and tissue donation act information guide.* https://beta.novascotia.

ca/sites/default/files/documents/1-2403/human-organ-and-tissue-donation-act-information-guide-en.pdf

Nova Scotia Health. (2022). *Progressive donation legislation saves lives, inspires innovation.* https://www.nshealth.ca/news/progressive-dona-tion-legislation-saves-lives-inspires-innovation#:~:text5Since%20December%202020%2C%20547%2C245%20Nova,of%20the%20eligible%20donor%20population

Paris, J. J., Graham, N., Schreiber, M. D., et al. (2006). Approaches to end-of-life decision-making in the NICU: Insights from Dos-toevsky's *The grand inquisitor. Journal of Perinatology, 26*(7), 389–391.

Pesut, B., Thorne, S., Schiller, C., et al. (2020a). Constructing good nursing practice for medical assistance in dying in Canada: An in-terpretive descriptive study. *Global Qualitative Nursing Research, 7.* https://doi.org/10.1177/2333393620938686

Pesut, B., Thorne, S., Schiller, C., et al. (2020b). The rocks and hard places of MAiD: A qualitative study of nursing practice in the con-text of legislated assisted death. *BMC Nursing, 19,* 12.

Pesut, B., Thorne, S., Stager, M. L., et al. (2019). Medical assistance in dying: A review of Canadian nursing regulatory documents. *Policy Politics & Nursing Practice, 20*(3), 113–130.

Physician-assisted suicide and the right to die with assistance. (1992). *Harvard Law Review, 105*(Note), 2021.

Porteri, C. (2018). Advance directives as a tool to respect patients' values and preferences: Discussion on the case of Alzheimer's dis-ease. *BMC Medical Ethics, 19,* 9.

Rassin, M., Lowenthal, M., & Silner, D. (2005). Fear, ambivalence, and liminality: Key concepts in refusal to donate an organ after brain death. *JONA's Healthcare Laws Ethics and Regulation, 7*(3), 79–85.

Robb, N. (1997). Death in a Halifax hospital: A murder case highlights a profession's divisions. *Canadian Medical Association Journal, 157,* 757–762.

Robb, N. (1998). The Morrison ruling: The case may be closed but the issues it raised are not. *Canadian Medical Association Journal, 158,* 1071–1072.

Robertson, G., & Picard, E. (2018). *Legal liability of doctors and hos-pitals in Canada* (5th ed.). Carswell.

Ross, H. M. (2001, April). Islamic tradition at the end of life. *MEDSURG Nursing, 10*(2), 83–87.

Saidman, S. L., Roth, A. E., Sönmez, R., et al. (2006). Increasing the opportunity to live kidney donation by matching for two- and three-way exchanges. *Transplantation, 81*(5), 773–782.

Singer, P. A., Robertson, G., & Roy, D. J. (1996). Bioethics for cli-nicians: 6. Advance care planning. *Canadian Medical Association Journal, 155*(12), 1689–1692.

Sneiderman, B., Irvine, J. C., & Osborne, P. H. (1989). *Canadian medical law: An introduction for physicians and other health care professionals* (pp. 220–223). Carswell.

Solomon, C. M., & Schell, M. S. (2009). *Seven keys to doing business with a global mindset.* McGraw-Hill.

Solomon, M. Z., O'Donnell, L., Jennings, B., et al. (1993, January). Decisions near the end of life: Professional views on life-sustaining treatments. *American Journal of Public Health, 83*(1), 14–23.

Solomon, M. Z., Sellers, D. E., Heller, K. S., et al. (2005, October). New and lingering controversies in pediatric end-of-life care. *Pediatrics, 116*(4), 872–883.

Spike, J. (2000). Controlled NHBD protocol for a fully conscious person: When death is intended as an end in itself and it has its own end. *The Journal of Clinical Ethics, 11*(1), 72–76.

Steger, M. (2021, September 7). *Update on Medical Assistance in Dying in Canada.* https://www.bcli.org/update-on-medical-assistance-in-dying-in-canada/

Steinberg, D. (2003, March). Eliminating death. *The American Journal of Bioethics, 3*(1), 17–18.

Tang, V. T. N. (2002). *Buddhist view on death and rebirth.* https://www.urbandharma.org/udharma5/viewdeath.html

Task Force on Presumed Consent. (1994). *Organ procurement strate-gies. A review of ethical issues and challenges* (p. 7). Multiple Organ Retrieval & Exchange Program of Ontario.

Trachtman, H. (2003, Winter). Death be not political. *The American Journal of Bioethics, 3*(1), 31–32.

Truog, R. D. (2000, September). Organ transplantation without brain death. *Annals of New York Academy of Sciences, 913*(1), 229–239.

Truog, R. D., & Robinson, W. M. (2003, September). Role of brain death and the dead-donor rule in the ethics of organ transplanta-tion. *Critical Care Medicine, 31*(5), 2391–2396.

Veatch, R. M. (2003, Winter). The dead donor rule: True by defini-tion. *The American Journal of Bioethics, 3*(1), 10–11.

Venneman, S. S., Narnor-Harris, P., Perish, M., et al. (2008). "Allow natural death" versus "do not resuscitate": Three words that can change a life. *Journal of Medical Ethics, 34,* 2–6.

Webster, B. (2022). *Palliative care in the pandemic* [General meeting presentation]. Hospice Peterborough.

Wright, L., Faith, K., Richardson, R., et al. (2004). Ethical guidelines for the evaluation of living organ donors. *Canadian Journal of Surgery, 47*(6), 408–413.

Yazdani, S., Buchman, D. Z., Wright, L., et al. (2018). Organ dona-tion and medical assistance in dying: Ethical and legal issues fac-ing Canada. *McGill Journal of Law and Health, 11*(2), 59–85.

Youngner, S. J., Allen, M., Bartlett, E. T., et al. (1985, August). Psy-chosocial and ethical implications of organ retrieval. *New England Journal of Medicine, 5*(313), 321–324.

9 ETHICAL AND LEGAL ISSUES RELATED TO ADVANCING SCIENCE AND TECHNOLOGY

LEARNING OBJECTIVES

The purpose of this chapter is to provide an overview of:

- The legal, social, and ethical dimensions that arise out of scientific innovation, including molecular and DNA technology
- Advances in genetics and genomics and their influence on existing and future generations
- Developments in reproductive science and technology
- The role of nursing in supporting those affected by these technologies

INTRODUCTION

Extraordinary advancements in health care, science, and technology have had a strong influence on the nurses' role. Advancements include pharmaceutical development, digital communication, telehealth, robots used to treat patients in remote areas, and technology that improves patient care and safety. In medical science, there have been advancements in genetic reproductive technologies, stem cell research, **personalized medicine**, and the development of vaccines using mRNA technology.

The use of these technologies raises many ethical questions as to whether it is:

- Right to use science to predict our future state of health and life expectancy
- Appropriate to manipulate genes to save lives and eliminate disease from future generations
- The right of every human being to have a child
- Right to control the characteristics and attributes of children yet to be born

Science and technology enable us to extend life, overcome infertility, eliminate genetic anomalies, manipulate and control the characteristics of potential human beings, predict the risk of future diseases, find cures, and identify strategies for prevention. With the assistance of science, we can connect with previously unknown relatives anywhere in the world and learn about our ancestral origins. This power to manipulate the creation and experience of life may ultimately reshape society and redefine future generations.

Nurses who work in settings where these technologies are used face profound social, psychological, and emotional challenges and are confronted by questions about their own values and beliefs concerning life and its potential. As advanced technologies are introduced, nurses may struggle with the consequences of these technologies when the quality of the outcomes and future life of patients, and the effect on their families, is uncertain. Genetic counsellors, many of whom are nurses, face daily ethical challenges as they support individuals and families to make complex decisions not faced by previous generations. Nurses should be aware of the clinical utility of genetic testing as its relevance grows and becomes more applicable to nursing practice. Genetic information impacts not only the patients involved but also their immediate and extended family and possibly future generations. The knowledge revealed from genetic and genomic assessments can result in significant ethical dilemmas.

It is important that nurses understand the implications and far-reaching consequences.

This chapter will examine the complex ethical and legal issues related to science and technology, including the rapidly advancing areas of genetics, personalized medicine, reproductive science, and in utero intervention.

THE EMERGING WORLD OF GENETICS AND GENOMICS

In 1997, scientists in the United Kingdom were able to clone a sheep known as "Dolly." Scientists transplanted the nucleus from a mammary gland cell of a sheep into the enucleated egg of a ewe, and then electric currents were used to stimulate fusion and cell division. The resulting embryo was implanted into the uterus of another ewe, and Dolly (genetically identical to her genetic parent, the adult sheep) was born months later (Freudenrich, 2001; Gibson, 1998).

To date, a human clone has not been created yet it is becoming clear that questions no longer exist as to whether these technologies will advance but, rather, when and in what ways (Phelan, 2022). Controversy about the possibility continues, with many countries explicitly banning attempts at human cloning. With each development in genetics, more ethical questions are raised.

Today it is possible to:

- Select embryos based on gender (Ethics Committee of the American Society for Reproductive Medicine, 2015)
- Diagnose and treat a fetus in utero for cardiac anomalies or other congenital conditions
- Screen for conditions and deficiencies including congenital adrenal hyperplasia, congenital hyperthyroidism, sickle cell disease, thalassemia, cystic fibrosis (CF), and Tay-Sachs disease (American College of Obstetricians and Gynecologists [ACOG], 2017; Canadian Organization for Rare Disorders [CORD], 2006)
- Predict whether an individual is a genetic carrier of conditions, such as mitochondrial dysfunction, Huntington's disease, or is predisposed to cancer or cardiovascular illnesses
- Manipulate or change genes to alter their influence on that person and future generations
- Predict one's response to various interventions, enabling the identification of the treatment with the best likelihood for success

Deoxyribonucleic acid (DNA), the carrier of genetic information, is the main component of chromosomes and is present in all living organisms. The scientific discovery of DNA and its role in heredity began in the nineteenth century and culminated in a series of peer-reviewed articles published in the scientific journal *Nature* in 1953. The potential uses of DNA have been pursued since then. DNA evidence was first used in 1988 to secure a murder conviction in a British criminal case. Since then, DNA evidence has become widespread in criminal investigations, with multiple convictions being overturned as a result of new or more accurate DNA evidence (Anderson, 2015).

The Difference Between Genetics and Genomics

The main focus of genetics is the study of the function and composition of a single gene, a specific sequence of DNA that exists on a single chromosome (Genome Canada, 2022). One gene encodes a specific product or trait, such as hair, eye, or skin colour, and it can also indicate the genetic markers for certain diseases and disorders. The study of genetics deals primarily with how one trait gets passed along from parent to child, and through generations. This trait or gene can be traced back through ancestors to see how it was passed down and who was affected by it (Difference Between, n.d.).

Genomics, on the other hand, is the study of all genes and their interrelationships to better understand their combined influence on the organism. The study of genomics deals with the sequencing and analysis of an organism's genome. The genome, then, is the sum total of genetic information of an individual, encoded in the structure of their DNA (Difference Between, n.d.; World Health Assembly [WHA], 2004; World Health Organization [WHO], 2002). It includes all of an organism's DNA, that is, all of its genes. Containing all of the information needed to develop and support an organism, the entire genome is present in all cells within the nucleus (U.S. National Library of Medicine, 2018a, 2018b). In genomics, the entire genome of the organism is mapped to distinguish between the genetic markers and identify which ones are linked to specific traits. This information can then be used to understand how genes are linked to certain diseases, how they are passed on genetically, and their impact and whether, in fact, they always cause that disease (Difference Between, n.d.).

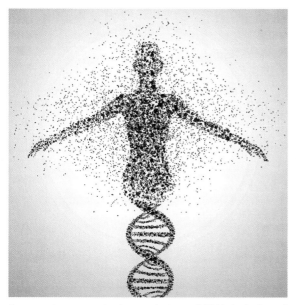

A *genome* is an organism's complete set of DNA, including all of its genes *and* all of the information needed to build and maintain that organism. It is the sum total of genetic information of an individual, encoded in the structure of their DNA. *Source: istockphoto.com/Lonely_*

Genetic testing focuses on the detailed analysis of a single gene or a specific part of the genome, whereas *genomic sequencing* refers to analyzing the entire genetic information that is stored in the chromosomes or the entire DNA content that is present within the cell of a person (Difference Between, n.d.; U.S. National Library of Medicine, 2018a, 2018b).

Genetic Testing

Variations, changes, or mutations can be observed in DNA, genes, chromosomes, and cell proteins. These mutations can occur randomly or be influenced by environmental factors. Mutations include missing (deleted) or extra (insertion) genes, or the rearrangement of genetic material (National Human Genome Research Institute [NHGRI], 2016b). Genetic disorders

are caused by these mutations, and some can be passed from generation to generation. Inherited mutations are known to cause disorders such as sickle cell disease, CF, and Tay-Sachs disease. In most cases, these are recessive genes, so both parents must carry the same gene to have an affected child.

Most mutations are meaningless; however, some can be pathogenic and, therefore, have major health implications for individuals and families. Pathogenic variations cause diseases, some of which are actionable, and some that are not. A known pathogenic variation is linked to Huntington's chorea, which currently has no cure (NHGRI, 2016b).

Other mutations make one predisposed to diseases such as cancer, cardiovascular disease, and certain psychiatric conditions. The mutations do not specifically cause these diseases, but the onset of these diseases is more likely to be influenced by lifestyle and environmental factors. Individuals who know of these predispositions have the opportunity to introduce mitigation and prevention strategies. Other mutations have uncertain significance at this time, and others are known to be benign.

Some variations have a positive influence and respond and adapt to risks or exposures over time. For example, a mutation that resists or protects against human immunodeficiency virus (HIV) has been identified, and individuals with sickle cell trait (carriers for the recessive gene for sickle cell) are less likely to die of malaria (NHGRI, 2016b).

Genetic testing seeks to identify variations in chromosomes, genes, or proteins to confirm or rule out an existing genetic condition or the risk of developing or passing on (to offspring) a genetic disorder (U.S. Department of Energy Office of Science, n.d.). There are three types of genetic tests—molecular, chromosomal, and biochemical. Molecular genetic tests study single genes to identify variations or mutations. Chromosomal tests analyze whole chromosomes to determine whether there are large changes, such as an extra copy of a chromosome, that can cause a genetic condition. Biochemical genetic tests study abnormalities in proteins and can indicate changes to the DNA (Canadian Cancer Society, n.d.).

Genetic testing is the technology of choice for determining specific genetic disorders, particularly in children (Szego, 2016). It is a component of the diagnostic process and targets genes related to the areas of concern, permitting differential diagnoses that need to be confirmed or ruled out. The results can also guide medical management and determine whether others are at risk, such as siblings or extended family members (Normand et al., 2017).

The testing process targets a primary variant or alteration in a disease-causing gene that is thought to play a role in causing the individual's health problem. It can also identify a secondary variant in a disease-causing gene that is not related to the individual's health issue but may be related to other health risks in the present or in the future.

Specific genetic testing can also be triggered by a person's family history, for example, to determine the risk of developing certain cancers. These include cancers such as breast, ovarian, and colon cancers, which are more prevalent in some families. Because findings of these types of gene variations only predict the risk of cancer, a positive result does not mean that the cancer will occur—other influential factors, such as lifestyle and the environment, also contribute to the overall risk. The reverse is also true; if the result is negative, it does not mean that cancer will not develop, as all of the genetic links have not been determined (Canadian Cancer Society, n.d.). As mentioned, some findings may be medically actionable, while others may not. For example, changes to one of the two *BRCA* genes (tumour suppressors that control the way cells grow in certain tissues of the body) are associated with an increased chance of developing breast and ovarian cancers. In this situation, interventions such as having a double mastectomy and the removal of the ovaries could mitigate or prevent the disease from occurring ("BRCA," 2008; Canadian Cancer Society, n.d.).

Genetic testing is also key to "precision medicine," enabling the practice of proactive care by identifying potential diseases in advance and treating them with targeted therapies tailored to an individual's unique genome. For example, genetics in cancer care is transforming approaches to treatment and early diagnosis. In some cancers, it is helping to identify the most effective chemotherapy and may predict how well the treatment will be tolerated. For example, research has demonstrated that women with a specific type of breast cancer (cell type HER2t) have a much better outcome when treated with a particular chemotherapy protocol (Nahta & Esteva, 2006).

Genetic testing has benefits as well as limitations and risks; therefore, the decision about getting tested is an emotional and complex one. Genetic counsellors and nurses caring for these individuals and their families are key in ensuring they receive the support and advice they need to make these important decisions.

Prenatal Testing

Preconception and prenatal genetic screening and testing are available for a limited number of severe child-onset diseases to identify whether a potential offspring is at risk. There are four categories of testing in these circumstances—carrier, preimplantation, in utero, and newborn screening (ACOG, 2017).

Carrier Screening

Potential parents can be screened to determine whether they each carry a gene for a serious recessive disease which would put their potential children at risk. This testing can be undertaken before or during pregnancy (Government of Canada, 2013b). Testing before conception provides individuals with the chance to pursue assisted reproductive technologies to avoid having an affected child.

Preimplantation Screening

This type of screening occurs within the context of in vitro fertilization (IVF). Embryos created using in vitro fertilization are tested before implantation to determine whether any gene variants are present.

In Utero Screening

In utero screening is undertaken on cell samples obtained through amniocentesis or chorionic villus (placenta) sampling. Genetic testing of the fetus offers both opportunities and ethical challenges. The information could result in a choice to terminate a pregnancy or to prepare for the birth of a child with ongoing challenges. Testing may also help to detect and facilitate treatment of a fetal condition in utero (ACOG, 2017).

Newborn Screening

In this circumstance, a newborn is tested when issues of concern are identified, and the presence of a genetic disease needs to be confirmed or ruled out.

There are many potential benefits to undertaking genetic testing when the focus is on a specific concern. However, along with the opportunities to improve the future life of these children, ethical questions arise regarding the long-term consequences of these interventions and issues associated with the right to life and who decides whose life is worth living. Ethically challenging is the question of the extent to which preimplantation genetics should be used in pursuit of the "genetically ideal" child. In the situation of IVF, parents can not only choose the gender of their child, but also potentially test embryos for a number of factors, such as level of cognition and intelligence, longevity, and traits such as hair colour and body stature.

Also debated is the appropriateness of testing the fetus for adult-onset disorders, such as the identification of the *BRCA* gene; or for a disease with no known therapeutic or preventive treatment, such as Huntington's chorea; and whether the decision to undertake these tests should be reserved for the child to make upon reaching adulthood (NHGRI, 2016b).

Genetic testing provides only one piece of information about a person's health; other genetic and environmental factors, lifestyle choices, and family medical history also affect a person's risk of developing many disorders. These factors are discussed during consultation with genetic counsellors or with the health care team.

Genetic Molecular Biology: Advancements in the Development of Vaccines

The emergence of vaccines to respond to the COVID-19 virus introduced the public to a field of scientific technology previously unknown to most. Messenger ribonucleic acid (mRNA) technology is situated in the field of genetic molecular biology. This science is concerned with the structure and function of genes at the molecular level. mRNA is situated in every cell of the body. Its main function is to transport messages from DNA, located in the nucleus of the cell, to the cytoplasm, where the messages it carries are translated into the production of proteins (Mascola, 2020, Pardi, 2020). After successful translation of its message, the mRNA molecule self-destructs.

During the COVID-19 pandemic, despite extensive clinical trials, the safety of the mRNA vaccine was challenged by those who questioned its seeming rapid development. In fact, this science had been explored and developed for about 30 years, and vaccines using the technology were already being tested. When the COVID-19 virus emerged, mRNA science had advanced to the point that vaccines could be developed quickly. Traditional vaccines use a small live or dead sample of the virus or a similar virus to stimulate the immune system to react to the actual virus. Traditional vaccine development takes time to establish the material that will be used to stimulate the immune system. With mRNA technology, genetic instructions, via the mRNA, are delivered to the cells to produce a copy of a protein found on the surface of the virus, a spike protein. This spike protein stimulates the immune response (Mascola & Fauci, 2020; Pardi et al., 2020).

Messenger RNA technology allows new vaccine therapies to be tailored quickly in response to new threats by simply identifying the genetic sequence of the pathogen. As this technology advances, there is great potential for the development of therapies for other illnesses or disorders, including vaccines to boost the immune system to fight against cancer and prevent infectious disease (Pilkington et al., 2021; Szabó et al., 2022). Research is currently underway to develop a vaccine that protects against all known influenza strains and would not need to be adjusted each flu season (Arevalo et al., 2022). The review process undertaken by the Public Health Agency of Canada demonstrated to Canadians the ethical and scientific rigour undertaken to ensure the efficacy and safety of new treatments prior to their approval for use in this country. Despite this, skepticism about the safety of vaccines continues to be a serious threat to public health.

The Human Genome Project

The Human Genome Project (HGP), launched in 1990 and completed in 2003, identified the approximately 20,500 genes in human DNA. Included in the goals of this collaboration was the urgency of addressing the ethical, legal, and social issues that arise from this technology (NHGRI, 2016a; U.S. Department of Energy Office of Science, n.d.).

The outcomes of this project provided scientists with the knowledge to identify genetic diseases and the opportunity to create strategies for their cure and prevention. This work paved the way for research and analysis in this area. It advanced the technique of determining the exact sequences of bases in the DNA molecule, creating a better understanding of the function of genes. Of note was the discovery that 99.9% of our DNA is similar—that is, only 0.01% of our genes differentiate us from each another (NHGRI, 2016a, 2016b).

Knowledge gained from an understanding of the human genome will likely foster innovations in health care for many years to come. This knowledge of the human genome has the potential to influence the prevention, diagnosis, and treatment of communicable and genetic diseases; chronic illnesses, such as cardiovascular disease, cancer, diabetes, major psychoses, and dementia; rheumatic disease, asthma, and much more (WHO, 2002).

Personal Genome Project Canada

Scientists in Canada undertook their own genome initiative. The Personal Genome Project Canada was launched in 2007 to establish a publicly accessible dataset of genomic information and to connect this information with human traits and characteristics. The main goals of the project were to create a readily accessible online database for use by researchers and to determine approaches to the application of genetic knowledge into clinical practice. Canadians were invited to have their genetic information included in this database, and the response was overwhelming (Reuter et al., 2018).

A sample of participants agreed to be part of a focused study to correlate personal details about their lifestyles, traits, and health history to their whole genome sequence. Self-reported baseline trait data included the person's date of birth, medication use, allergies, previous vaccinations, personal health history, ethnicity/ancestry, and indicators such as blood pressure, height, and weight (Reuter et al., 2018; Scherer et al., 2017).

Because this database and the information collected were to be shared publicly, a rigorous informed consent process was undertaken. Participants had to be over age 18 years and were required to pass an examination to validate their understanding of the wide range of risks and benefits. This was to ensure that they had a clear understanding of the implications of the study (Scherer et al., 2017).

For example, as part of the informed consent process, some of the information shared with potential participants included:

- A caution that research results should not substitute for clinical evaluation and care
- The potential that they could lose the ability to obtain life insurance or employment
- The risk of discovering that they were not biologically related to their families
- The risk that others might use the database to identify biological relationships with them (sperm donors)
- That gene variants might be identified that may be benign, pathogenic, or, of as yet unknown significance
- That findings would also have implications for immediate and extended family who may or may not want to know the results (Scherer et al., 2017)

The study identified gene variations that were known to be pathogenic and had health implications, some that had uncertain significance at this time, and others that were known to be benign. Though the study suggested that whole genome sequencing will likely become part of mainstream health care, it also revealed limitations with the current understanding of the genome. For example, some of the participants carry mutated genes that, based on current knowledge, should indicate that they have a disease associated with that variant, but, in fact, they do not. These findings support the conclusion that there is much more to be revealed about the genetic influences of disease (Reuter et al., 2018).

Whole Genome Sequencing

Traditionally, genetic testing assumed a focused diagnostic inquiry targeting a known and specific gene. Whole genome sequencing (WGS) offers new challenges and opportunities as the data identified in this analysis may generate additional findings, such as the prediction of a future disease that the person being tested, or their family, may or may not want to know about. The ethical challenges associated with WGS are compounded in the context of pediatrics, many arguing for deferring genetic testing for adult-onset disorders until the child is able to consent (Anderson et al., 2017; Szego et al., 2014).

In situations where changes in the *BRCA* (tumour suppressing) genes are detected, the potential interventions to avoid breast and ovarian cancers involve life-changing surgeries, creating dilemmas for those faced with such choices ("BRCA," 2008). Also, scientists have identified three genes that are linked to early-onset Alzheimer's disease. Would a person want to know this information, given that, currently, nothing can be done to prevent the onset of this disease (Mayo Clinic Staff, 2016)?

Experts suggest that genomic analysis will become a standard component of proactive health care, given its potential to identify a person's predisposition to medically actionable conditions, guide their management of these conditions, explain uncharacterized disease, reveal carriers for recessive disorders, and provide predictors of medication safety and response (Lionel et al., 2018; Normand et al., 2017; Reuter et al., 2018; Szego, 2016; Szego et al., 2014). For example, recent advances in the understanding of the genomic architecture of diabetes and its complications have provided the framework for development of precision medicine to personalize diabetes prevention and management (Xie et al., 2018).

Direct-to-Consumer Genetic Testing

Historically, genetic testing was available only through health care providers, such as physicians, nurse practitioners, and genetic counsellors, who can identify the most appropriate testing and interpret the test results. Direct-to-consumer genetic testing markets directly to consumers, giving people access to genetic information without necessarily involving a health care professional (Su, 2013; U.S. National Library of Medicine, 2018c). The pricing for some types of at-home genetic testing can be very expensive, posing the risk of intensifying health inequality. While some of the information provided can be of social interest, other genetic data may be more problematic. One feature offered by some of the at-home test kits is the identification of relatives who are open to being contacted, resulting in the offspring of sperm donors unexpectedly finding that they have multiple half-siblings.

There are advantages to this growing market as it may promote awareness of genetic diseases, allow consumers to take a more proactive role in their health care, and offer a means for people to learn

about their ancestral origins. However, there are significant risks and limitations. For example, individuals may be misled by the results without guidance from a health care professional who is experienced in the interpretation and communication of genetic information. Therefore, there is the risk of making important decisions based on inaccurate, incomplete, or misunderstood information about one's health (Ries & Einsiedel, 2010). Consumers may also experience an invasion of genetic privacy if testing companies use their genetic information in an unauthorized way (Office of the Privacy Commissioner of Canada, 2017).

To illustrate the power of these open-source databases, consider how genetic genealogy analysis was used to identify the accused in two Ontario cold cases. In 2020, the process helped identify the murderer of a young girl, Christine Jessop, who died in 1984 (Christine Jessop cold case). In 2022, this analysis identified the accused in the murder of two women in 1983. This technology requires the presence of DNA secured either from the victim's body or the crime scene. These DNA samples undergo full genome testing, and the results are then compared with data uploaded from open-sourced databases to identify genetically related people.

Through this analysis, more distant genetic matches and family relationships may be identified. The process then makes connections to family trees to narrow down a pool of genetically related people, and then other information (such as sex, age, and unusual disease strains) can be used to narrow the search.

The final step requires the DNA of the suspect or suspects, which if not available may require a DNA warrant. This process is also used to identify family when the identity of a victim is not known (de Groot et al., 2021; Ortenzi, 2018, Powers, 2022).

Ethical Challenges With Genetic Testing

Although ethical questions related to genetic testing have been recognized for some time, the issues have gained greater urgency as the science advances. The rapid advances in this field are best understood when considering that what took 8 months to sequence (one gene in a roundworm) 30 years ago would now take 8 hours. Also, the 10-year journey to identify the CF gene would now take 10 weeks. The ethical challenges posed by this technology include those related to consent, privacy and confidentiality, protection of the vulnerable, and health equity. Adding an additional layer of complexity is the impact on others, such as extended family, beyond those of the individual undertaking this testing.

With respect to consent, some suggest that genetics should be treated as a unique class and be subject to a more rigorous consent process, as demonstrated by the process used for Personal Genome Project Canada. Genes do not merely inform individuals and their health care providers about the diagnosis of an existing illness—they can predict future health and may have consequences not only for that person but also for others genetically related to them. Genetic information is different from other kinds of personal health information, in that it is not unique to the individual being tested and has implications for an entire biological family. This familial nature of genetic information raises ethical dilemmas with regard to obligations to protect the confidentiality of the individual who has consented to a test on the one hand and the duty to protect the health of a different individual on the other. Individuals should be made aware of these challenges in advance to help them plan and respond to the test results, including the disclosure of the intent to undergo such testing to their biological family, since this knowledge could potentially benefit family members (e.g., allow them to influence their own health outcomes) or expose unknown kinship. These ethical complexities reinforce the importance of ensuring that those undertaking genetic testing be educated about the implications of the findings on others and why such disclosure should, in many circumstances, be encouraged to provide others with the option of being informed, or not, of the results (ACOG, 2008).

The results of testing might have important consequences or require difficult choices for persons regarding their current or future health, career, marriage, or reproductive options. Do all persons undergoing testing want to be informed that genetic testing has identified a predisposition to a certain disease when it cannot be treated or prevented? Do they want to know if the testing reveals that they have or are carriers of a specific disease? Adding to the complexity of securing consent are the many uncertainties attached to the results of genetic testing (i.e., the reliability of tests and the unavailability of effective interventions to treat or prevent many genetic diseases).

There are ethical concerns about the extent to which persons may be subject to discrimination based on the existence of a variant gene. Individuals can be screened to determine their susceptibility to conditions, some of which may be prevented and others that may not, raising many questions about the burdens and benefits of screening, how privacy rights are affected, and whether this increases the potential for discrimination (Chadwick, 2008; Office of the Privacy Commissioner of Canada, 2017). For example, what if an insurance company imposed mandatory genetic screening and denied insurance to individuals based on their future risk of disease (Chadwick, 2008)? What if employers did the same and individuals were denied employment or the opportunity to advance in their careers because of future potential illnesses?

In 2017, the *Genetic Non-Discrimination Act* became law in Canada. The Act prohibits anyone from requiring a person to undergo or reveal the results of a genetic test as a condition of employment or before selling that person a good or service, such as life or disability insurance. The constitutionality of this law was challenged because jurisdiction over health, employment, and insurance belongs to the provinces and not to the federal government (*Reference re Genetic Non-Discrimination Act*, 2020). In a split decision (5–4), a majority of the Supreme Court of Canada held that the legislation was within federal jurisdiction and was valid. Legislation making genetic testing a prohibited ground of discrimination was introduced in Ontario but has not become law. No other provinces have passed such legislation. However, current protections against discrimination on the grounds of disability in the *Canadian Charter of Rights and Freedoms* (1982, s. 15, "Equality") may include genetic predispositions.

With the introductions of these technologies, there is the need to protect those most vulnerable. Genetic testing in children poses particular ethical challenges. For example, is it right to screen children for adult-onset disorders that are not preventable? Should such results be revealed to children? To adolescents? How should consent be determined? Some suggest that when the focus of testing is on genetic evaluation of an adult-onset disease, testing should not be undertaken until the person is 18 years of age and can make that decision for themselves (Canadian Cancer Society, n.d.). It is a different circumstance, however, if the disease might manifest itself in childhood or if there is an opportunity for prevention.

The same is true of sharing the results of the genetic tests of family members with a child. It is argued that disclosure should wait until the child is able to understand the information and make these decisions, though there are more complex challenges when the testing reveals information that may require more immediate attention (Anderson et al, 2017; Szego, 2016; Szego et al., 2014; Wright et al., 2018).

There are also ethical questions about the most appropriate use of these technologies. Should people be screened only for conditions that are preventable or where a cure is possible? Genetic testing may predict the risk or possibility of conditions that may be incurable, others that may be curable or prevented, and conditions that today are incurable but may become curable in the future.

There are pros and cons to predictive testing. On the positive side, if persons believe they are at risk for a condition, knowing one way or the other may lessen the anxieties and uncertainties associated with not knowing. Knowing allows one to prepare for the future; for example, the knowledge that the early onset of an incurable disease is possible may alter how that person leads their life and may allow them to make lifestyle changes that could prevent or delay the onset of the illness. There might even be treatment interventions that minimize the risk of getting the disease, and related individuals who may also be susceptible may be identified.

On the negative side, individual reactions may vary and be unpredictable. For example, knowing one is possibly destined for a future plagued by serious illness or disability may produce emotional breakdowns, depression, anxiety, and the risk of suicide. Some people may experience guilt, knowing their offspring may also be at risk. Alternatively, they may deny themselves having children (Shuman, 2008). As noted, when an

individual chooses to seek genetic information, the data may also have implications for family members. Should that information be shared? Does the individual who chooses to have the testing done have the right to maintain the confidentiality of that information? Does the health care team doing the testing have a duty to warn others who may be at risk? Consider a woman who tests positive for the *BRCA* gene but does not want this information shared with her siblings.

Other concerns relate to issues of social justice and the fair distribution of resources. Because it is currently not covered by the health care system, access to whole genome sequencing is influenced by one's ability to pay. Who should pay for this very expensive technology? Can only those who can afford it have access to this screening, thereby excluding those who cannot afford to pay?

Should testing become public policy, or should it be an individual choice? How is privacy protected? Do individuals have the right to confidentiality when they are found to be susceptible to a disorder that may also affect their siblings or other members of their family? What if a person refuses to have this information disclosed when others may also be at risk? Do health care professionals have a duty to warn others? What if the testing reveals information that may be of significance to others? Under what circumstances can confidentiality be breached (Shuman, 2008)?

It has recently been suggested that each person's entire genome may be available for diagnostic and therapeutic purposes in the not-too-distant future. The ethical issues related to the field of genetics and genomics are extremely challenging. There will be more challenges in the future because this science has the potential to create profound changes and to open up new possibilities, including gene therapy and genome editing technologies (Elliot et al., 2014).

CASE SCENARIO 9.1

IS IT OUR BUSINESS?

The parents of a newborn baby, who has been diagnosed with cystic fibrosis (CF), are referred for genetic counselling and DNA testing for common mutations of the CF gene.

The initial report from the molecular laboratory shows that only one CF gene mutation has been

identified in the baby, and this mutation has been inherited from the mother. So far, a second mutation in the father remains unidentified. They are called and given the results.

Several months later, an updated report is received from the laboratory indicating that both CF gene mutations have now been identified in the baby

Continued on following page

CASE SCENARIO 9.1 *(Continued)*

but that the father is not the carrier of the other mutation. Because he does not carry either mutation, it is clear that he is not the father of this child.

Questions

1. Should you reveal the outcome of this testing? To whom?

2. Are there possible future outcomes for the child?

3. Who are your patients in this situation? Can you ensure that all of their rights are respected?

CASE SCENARIO 9.2

WHOSE RIGHT TO KNOW?

A 17-year-old teenager with Down syndrome lives with her family and functions well, but she has the intellectual and emotional levels of a 10-year-old. She works part time at a local store where she has met a young man of 19 who is developmentally challenged. They have developed a romantic relationship, and the young woman is now pregnant. By the time her condition is noted and confirmed, she is in her second trimester. She is excited about the prospect of being a mother, but her parents are concerned about the baby's health and want genetic testing undertaken on the fetus.

Questions

1. Who has rights in this situation? Who should decide whether testing should be done? Who decides what action should be taken if the fetus's test result is positive for Down syndrome?

2. What are the best interests of the parties involved?

3. How would you counsel this family?

CASE SCENARIO 9.3

HOW MUCH SHOULD BE KNOWN?

A 17-year-old woman is worried about her father, who has been demonstrating changes in personality over the past few years. She has just been told that her father, who is 42 has Huntington's disease. Huntington's disease is a degenerative brain disorder that usually manifests between the ages of 30 and 50 years. There is no cure. Death usually occurs 15 to 20 years after its onset. Behavioural, emotional, and physical symptoms occur. The person displays involuntary movements and a drunken gait, may become depressed and irritable, and may exhibit aggressive outbursts, social withdrawal, and short-term memory loss.

The daughter is aware that her grandmother also had this disease but does not know if anyone else in the family had it. Her mother has just told her that an available genetic test could inform her, with 100% accuracy, whether she will develop the symptoms. She thinks her mother wants her to have the test, but she is not sure if she wants to.

Questions

1. Do children have a right to privacy and confidentiality, even from their parents?

2. Can parents demand testing?

3. When is a child's dissent determinative?

4. Who has, or should have, a say when genetic information will have implications for other individuals?

5. What are the ethical implications if this woman wants to have children?

Gene Modification Technologies

Existing and potential genetic technologies are capable of modifying variant genes and, thus, curing and preventing disease and preventing the transfer of faulty genes to future generations. Some technologies target germline or reproductive cells, such as sperm and ova, where the modifications are passed down through generations. Other technologies target somatic cells, those that only affect the individual, such as the treatment of disease or the manipulation of personal traits (NHGRI, 2016b; U.S. National Library of Medicine, 2018d).

Gene Therapy

Gene therapy has the potential to treat many diseases—those acquired, for example, HIV infection or certain cancers; or those inherited through a faulty gene. In gene therapy, a variant gene is identified (facilitated through a greater understanding of gene sequencing), modified, replaced, or augmented with a healthy gene so that it can function normally (Government of Canada, 2005; Guo & Huang, 2012).

Effective gene therapy requires the efficient delivery of the healthy gene to the target cells of the recipient. The transfer of the healthy gene is undertaken in two ways. In one scenario, the genes of a virus are removed and replaced with the new gene. When the virus infects the recipient cell, it leaves behind the healthy genetic material, which then replicates and modifies the faulty gene. Other approaches to gene transfer involve the use of liposomes (synthetic, cationic lipids or polymers) that are modified to target specific tissue, loaded with healthy DNA, and delivered to the recipient cells either in a laboratory setting (ex vivo) or directly to the patient (in vivo) (Government of Canada, 2005; Guo & Huang, 2012).

In the laboratory, healthy genes are transferred into the patient's cells, grown, and then returned to the patient. The in vivo approach delivers the carrier (virus or liposome) directly to the patient, where the transfer occurs within the targeted cells (Government of Canada, 2005; Guo & Huang, 2012; Torchilin, 2005).

Animal-to-Human Organ Transplantation

Advancements in genetic technology have also contributed to developments in animal-to-human transplantation. The possibility to genetically modify an animal's donor organ minimizes the risk of rejection. Therefore, xenotransplantation from one species to another is viewed as a possible solution to the shortage of donor organs; however, this technology has significant ethical consequences. These include the pressure to consent when there are so many unknown future consequences, quality of life considerations, and the cost–benefit analysis, including the risk of animal-to-human infection. For example, the recipient may be required to quarantine for extended periods to minimize transfer of animal borne diseases to other humans. There are also questions of animal rights and placing the well-being of the human above the animal, since this approach requires the death of the animal (Krishna & Lepping, 2011).

Gene Replacement Therapy

Gene replacement therapy includes mitochondrial replacement in women who carry a pathogenic mitochondrial gene mutation. The mitochondrion is the energy production engine for the cell, and mutations of the mitochondrial gene can cause a number of serious diseases in the offspring of female carriers. The offspring might experience developmental delays, seizures, muscle weakness, dementia, cramping and low tonicity, balance and vision issues, and problems with the function of organs, such as the kidney, heart, and more (Mitochondrial, 2008). Individuals with mitochondrial disease are more likely to have a short life expectancy because at this point there is only symptom management and no cure. The technology is currently available, but the ethical issues associated with it are the focus of great debate, and it currently contravenes the *Assisted Human Reproduction Act* (Szego, 2011). The Act prohibits genetic alterations that are capable of being passed on to offspring and the creation of "an embryo that consists of cells of more than one embryo, fetus, or human being" (*Assisted Human Reproduction Act*, 2004, s. 3). In spite of these concerns, in 2017 the United Kingdom became the first country to license the clinical use of mitochondrial replacement therapy after the first baby born through mitochondrial replacement therapy had been revealed to the world in 2016 (Bredenoord & Appleby, 2017).

The process involves organelle (structures with specialized functions within a cell, such as mitochondria) transplantation, that is the transfer of the nucleus of the carrier's (the mother) egg to the enucleated egg of a healthy person. The resulting egg, therefore, has the nucleus of the mother without the disease-causing mitochondria. This egg is then fertilized and, if successful, results in the birth of a healthy child, free of mitochondrial disease. This child would no longer carry the mutated gene and, therefore, would not pass it on to future generations. This child, however, would have the genetic material of three individuals: the donor, the mother, and the father. However, the genetic component of mitochondria is only responsible for driving the energy-producing function of the cell, and the nucleus of the mother contains the morally relevant DNA that shapes the traits and characteristics of the offspring. Some argue this is not different from organ transplantation, and therefore it should be treated as such and legalized in Canada (Szego, 2011). The fact that mitochondrial replacement therapy has been permitted in the United Kingdom and the Netherlands suggests that it may happen in Canada as well. However, as mentioned earlier, the *Assisted Human Reproduction Act* prohibits genetic changes that could be passed on to offspring, and mitochondrial replacement therapy specifically facilitates this (Szego, 2011).

Genome Editing

Genome editing is an evolving science that involves making specific changes to the DNA of a cell or organism. Gene editing differs from previously described gene therapy in that the technology enables a gene sequence to be cut, moved, and replaced at very specific areas in the genome.

In most approaches, specific enzymes are used to cut the DNA, which is then repaired by the cell but results in a change, or "edit," in the DNA sequence. Genome editing has the potential to add, remove, or alter DNA in the genome, thus changing the characteristics of a cell or an organism and modifying the influence that gene has on a particular disease or its treatment.

There are two categories of gene editing, somatic and germline. Germline therapies target reproductive cells and somatic therapies target non reproductive cells. Changes to reproductive cells can be passed down through generations, whereas somatic cell editing only affects the individual. Somatic genome editing has been used to alter human blood cells that are then put

back into the body to treat such conditions as leukemia (NHGRI, 2017).

Because germline editing can affect future generations, there is a moratorium on this technology as its safety and accuracy has not been established. However, in 2018, a Chinese scientist used clustered regularly interspaced short palindromic repeats (CRISPR) technology to successfully edit the embryos of twin girls to make them resistant to HIV.

CRISPR, an evolving technology, is revolutionizing gene editing. Considered a more efficient system, it has adopted a bacterial defence system that can be programmed to target specific stretches of the genetic code and to edit DNA at precise locations. With these systems, researchers can permanently modify genes in living cells and organisms and, in the future, may make it possible to correct mutations at precise locations in the human genome in an effort to treat genetic diseases (The Broad Institute, 2018; Carroll, 2017; Cribbs & Perera, 2017; Ratan et al., 2018; Shin & Lee, 2018).

The Chinese government and many of their scientists renounced the use of this technology, and since the experiment violated Chinese laws and regulations, the scientist was charged and sentenced to 3 years in prison. China subsequently introduced additional laws to limit this research without strict guidelines and approvals (Global Gene Editing Regulation Tracker, 2020). Although in their infancy, germline editing strategies are being investigated to treat not only leukemia but also several other blood cancers as well as genetic conditions, such as CF and Duchenne muscular dystrophy.

Proponents of gene editing are excited about the potential to learn more about the influence of genes on conditions such as cancer and to eliminate genetic diseases, such as Huntington's disease and CF. But critics say that the process could go wrong or be misused in so many ways that it is best left alone.

Ethical Issues With Gene Editing

The ethical debate around gene editing is more heated with respect to human germline manipulation. In this context, the intervention is targeted to egg and sperm cells (germ cells), which would allow the change to be passed on to future generations. Because gene therapy involves making changes to the body's basic foundation, that which drives all components of that person, the science raises very unique and complex ethical challenges.

Less controversial is somatic gene editing, where the process targets a disease-causing gene in an individual, an edit that will not be passed on to future generations. The questions in relation to somatic gene editing focus on whether this technology should be used beyond the treatment or prevention of an illness for enhancements of human traits, such as a person's stature, physical strength, and ability or increasing intellectual capacity. This capability raises questions about how one decides what is normal and what is not. For example, persons with autism have some abilities that surpass those who do not (U.S. National Library of Medicine, 2018a).

Many questions remain with regard to gene editing; for example, how does one decide what a moral intervention is and what is not? Is it acceptable to make changes that eliminate that person's disease but not to make changes that will eliminate a disease-causing variant for generations to come? Supporters of gene editing argue that the potential benefits of this technology override any concerns about abuse, which could be mitigated with legislation and regulations, as is the case with other technologies. Banning this practice, they argue, would limit knowledge generation that could lead to a healthier society. They propose that there are some good moral arguments in favour of germline genetic intervention, whose goal is to prevent or alleviate disease or disability in humans in the future. Such interventions are more efficient than repeating gene therapy generation after generation (Walters, 1999).

Others argue that regardless of the benefits, it is wrong to interfere with the human germline and the evolution of genes from one generation to another. They express concerns about the safety of gene manipulation when the long-term implications for future generations are unknown. There are concerns that modifying the body's plan, or programming, might result in unforeseen alterations and irreversible effects that could have serious consequences for persons in the future; first and foremost, genome editing must be safe before it is used to treat patients (Cribbs & Perera, 2017; Gene Therapy Net.com, 2018; NHGRI, 2017; Walters, 1999).

Other ethical questions that must be considered are those related to consent and health equity; concerns about access and affordability that may lead to serious health disparities.

The people who would be most affected by germline gene therapy are not yet born. Therefore, they cannot choose whether to have treatment or not. So is it moral for persons living today to make such decisions for future generations? Do they appreciate the unknown consequences of these interventions? At the same time, are these considerations any different from when parents are expected to act in the best interests of their children?

Most agree that scientists should not engage in germline manipulation at this time because the safety and accuracy of genome editing has not yet been established. Scientific communities across the world are approaching germline therapy research with caution because the implication for future generations is not yet predictable (Cribbs & Perera, 2017; Gene Therapy Net.com, 2018; NHGRI, 2017; Walters, 1999).

STEM CELL TECHNOLOGIES

What Are Stem Cells?

Stem cells are unspecialized, undifferentiated cells that renew themselves through cell division to produce multiple cells, and when certain biological conditions are met, they can be induced to differentiate and become specialized cells with special functions, such as blood, muscle, and brain cells. With such regeneration, cells, tissue, and damaged organs can be repaired and function restored, whether loss was related to congenital anomalies, disease, trauma, or aging (Greenwood & Daar, 2008). For example, cardiac cells may be stimulated to regenerate, thereby healing damaged tissues after a myocardial infarction. The focus of current research in this area is to control cell differentiation in order to create tissue or organs, such as those of the heart, liver, kidneys, eyes, or even parts of the brain, from a single stem cell. In the future, this technology may be used to repair damaged tissue associated with such conditions as Alzheimer's disease, Parkinson's disease, diabetes, Huntington's chorea, multiple sclerosis, amyotrophic lateral sclerosis, and acute leukemia, as well as spinal cord and other traumatic injuries (Alison et al., 2002; Government of Canada, 2006).

Embryonic stem cells exist in the human embryo and differentiate to become a fetus and then a human being. The 3-to-5-day-old human embryo develops multiple cell types that evolve to become the heart, skin, lungs, and other organs. Embryonic cells exist not only in the fetus but also in the blood of an umbilical cord (cord blood). Human stem cells (somatic cells) exist in such tissues as bone marrow, where they differentiate and replicate to produce red and white blood cells. Somatic cells also exist in muscle, skin, intestine, and brain cells, where they generate replacement cells that supplant those damaged through injury and disease (Alison et al., 2002; Kern et al., 2006; National Institutes of Health, 2016).

Stem cell research has the potential not only to regenerate tissue but also to advance pharmacogenetics and "personalized medicine." It is possible to predict a person's response to particular treatments and, based on the genetic makeup of that person, identify which medications and therapies are the most appropriate (ScienceDaily, 2012; Shuman, 2008).

Genetic modification of stem cells enables the production of insulin (Vegas et al., 2016). Stem cells are also being modified to resist infection; for example, stem cells that repopulate the immune system of patients with HIV infection once they are implanted (Hutter, 2016).

Adult somatic stem cells are being used to evaluate the safety of new drugs and the potential of cancer chemotherapy. The potential application of autologous stem cells (generated from that person) in the generation of organs and tissue offers the possibility of replacement of cells and tissue, eliminating the challenge of organ donation, transplantation, and the risk of rejection. Also possible is the treatment of macular degeneration, spinal cord injury, stroke, burns, heart disease, diabetes, osteoarthritis, and rheumatoid arthritis (Trounson & McDonald, 2015).

Ethical Challenges

The use of stem cells for the treatment of the conditions noted earlier has been controversial, primarily because the major focus of earlier research involved the use of fetal tissue and human embryos (Volarevic et al., 2018). Embryonic tissue, found in the fetus and in the human embryo, is highly suited to stem cell technology because of the lack of differentiation of these stem cells and their ability to regenerate into specialized cells with specific functions. The debate was

fuelled by the fact that the tissue mainly came from elective abortions or unused embryos, and concerns about the potential exploitation of pregnant women and the possibility of embryos being created for this purpose alone (Mahowald, 1996). The question over when life begins was at the heart of the debate over the use of embryonic tissue for stem cell transplantation. The debate focused on whether the embryo or fetus is simply tissue or a human being and whether the fact that it has the potential for life matters (Childress, 1997, p. 302; EuroStem Cell, 2018).

Those who believe that the fetus is simply tissue have no serious moral concerns about its use in the generation of stem cells, but those who support the second and third perspectives argue that the fetus has some moral standing given its potential for life or that life already exists (Childress, 1997, p. 302; EuroStem Cell, 2018).

If one objects to abortion, then it would follow that deriving gain from such a process would be considered wrong. Those with these views, however, might accept their use if it is separate from the act of abortion (i.e., the decision to abort is separate from the decision to donate). In this case, they would expect that fetal tissue should be afforded the same respect as cadaveric tissue from human donors (Childress, 1997, p. 302).

There is also the argument that across the world, there are thousands of embryos that are either destroyed or frozen on a long-term basis and that will never realize life. Therefore, as long as this tissue is treated with the same respect that is given to other tissues or organs donated, then their use in this context is justified (EuroStem Cell, 2018).

The ethical arguments essentially focus on whether the embryo or fetus has moral status or not and whether respect for sanctity of life in this circumstance outweighs the potential benefits and our duty to those already living and suffering from incurable diseases (EuroStem Cell, 2018).

Additional concerns associated with fetal transplantation relate to consent. Consent for fetal tissue donation is provided by the parent and is similar to consents provided in other circumstances, such as organ donation. Some suggest that the parent, in choosing abortion, has relinquished the right to make decisions about the tissue or product of the abortion (Childress, 1997). The assumption that parents have the best interests of their child in mind is the basis for their right to make choices on their child's behalf. When a person chooses to abort a fetus, the validity of this consent on behalf of the fetus is, therefore, in question (Childress, 1997, p. 302; Mahowald, 1996). There are other consent questions related to the role of the biological father.

This argument would not apply to embryos, however, because they were created for the purpose of procreation, to create life. The parents, in this circumstance, might view that their embryos would be making a difference to others when they cannot exist for their initial intent.

There are numerous arguments in favour of the use of embryonic tissue, given the potential benefits of treating and curing diseases that reduce lifespan and result in severe morbidity, as well as the associated perceived benefits of reduction in the cost of care, reduction of ongoing physical and psychological suffering, and the ability to save lives (Childress, 1997, p. 302; Mahowald, 1996; ThoughtCo., 2019).

The recent advances in the application and knowledge regarding somatic stems cells offers a potential alternative to the use of embryonic tissue, reducing some of the major ethical challenges associated with its use (Alison et al., 2002; Volarevic, 2018).

Legislative Responses

At present, there is somewhat of a legislative void on the issue of stem cell transplantation. Parliament enacted federal legislation in 2004 (the *Assisted Human Reproduction Act*) dealing with assisted human reproduction. This statute (discussed in more detail under "Gestational Surrogacy") specifically governs and regulates the use of technology in the creation of human life. It does not, however, purport to regulate the use of human reproductive tissue for therapeutic purposes. Nevertheless, this statute does regulate the use of embryos to an extent. Under the Act, an embryo is defined as:

> *a human organism during the first 56 days of its development following fertilization or creation, excluding any time during which its development has been suspended, and includes any cell derived from such an organism that is used for the purpose of creating a human being. (Assisted Human Reproduction Act, 2004, s. 3, "embryo")*

The Act defines the *fetus* as

> *a human organism during the period of its development beginning on the fifty-seventh day following fertilization or creation, excluding any time during which its development has been suspended, and ending at birth. (Assisted Human Reproduction Act, s. 3, "foetus")*

The use of such reproductive tissue for the purpose of creating human life is heavily regulated, and certain activities are prohibited by this statute. It should be noted, however, that parts of this Act were struck down as being unconstitutional by the Supreme Court of Canada *Reference re the Assisted Human Reproduction* (2010). The court ruled that the parts of the Act that involved efforts to manage reproductive technologies were not an area that the federal government could regulate. The Act was limited to the creation of offences in relation to human reproduction as part of the federal jurisdiction over crime. In 2012, the *Assisted Human Reproduction Act* was substantially amended to bring it in line with the Supreme Court decision. The Act now defines certain human reproductive practices that are illegal and prohibits the sale of human reproductive material.

Apart from the *Assisted Human Reproduction Act*, most provinces would likely treat fetal tissue as any other human remains. Human tissue gift legislation governs donations of tissues from living donors in all provinces and territories. The statutes explicitly exclude the donation of embryos or fetal tissue in some cases (see, for example, Manitoba's *The Human Tissue Gift Act*, CCSM c. H180; Prince Edward Island's *Human Tissue Donation Act*, 1988; and Ontario's *Trillium Gift of Life Network Act*, 1990, "tissue," which explicitly "does not include . . . spermatozoa, an ovum, an embryo, a foetus . . ."). The statutes in other provinces and territories are not clear and may or may not address fetal tissue donation (von Tigerstrom, 2015).

In common law, there are no property rights attached to a deceased's body. A deceased person's executor has a limited right to possession of the body for the purposes of arranging a funeral and the burial, but this is clearly not applicable in cases involving fetal tissue.

REPRODUCTIVE TECHNOLOGIES

Significant scientific and technological advances have been made in the area of reproductive science. In fact, many technologies, including fertility control, labour and childbirth management, and screening procedures to monitor fetal development have been available for decades (Deech & Smajdor, 2007; Stanworth, 1987).

In recent decades, the management of labour and childbirth moved from the home to the hospital setting. Giving birth, once a family-oriented process in which the mother was assisted by female relatives, friends, or midwives, has evolved into a medical procedure within a hospital environment (Public Health Agency of Canada, 2021). Many hospitals now attempt to balance the safety of the baby with the creation of family-centred, home-like environments and by encouraging the presence of midwives and labour coaches. Also, with the introduction of professional midwives, some parents are once again opting for home deliveries.

With advancing technology, fetal development can now be monitored from the very early stages of pregnancy. A majority of women now undergo ultrasonography at many points during their pregnancy; high-risk and older pregnant women often undergo amniocentesis to assess for problems with the fetus early in development, either to facilitate a decision regarding the termination of a pregnancy or to take action to correct problems and prevent complications (Chokr, 1992; Stanworth, 1987). These procedures also provide parents with the choice of knowing the gender of their baby in advance (Perinatal Services BC, 2010).

Advances in reproductive science are successfully managing infertility in men and women, and the same technologies are also facilitating parenthood for single men and women and same-sex couples.

Advancing Science and the Challenge of Infertility

Once controversial, but now less so, **new reproductive technologies** aim to overcome the many causes of infertility. Although many with infertility have embraced these options, these technologies raise profound social, legal, ethical, and emotional questions. They have thrust us into uncharted territory related to the creation of life itself.

The need for these technologies stems from the basic human desire—or powerful cultural pressures—to procreate (Patel et al, 2018a, 2018b; Stanworth, 1987). Having children is viewed by society as the progression of relationships and is influenced by society's expectations of parenting as an important social role. Involuntary childlessness can be a threat to one's self-esteem, relationships, and family dynamics. When associated with loss, for example, failed procedures or spontaneous abortions, this can result in profound grief and emotional distress (Patel et al., 2018a, 2018b). Many couples or individuals are prepared to accept the physical, psychological, and emotional risks associated with these technologies for the sake of having a child, even when the outcome is uncertain (Robertson, 1995).

There are varying views on whether infertility is a disease (and, therefore, a medical condition) or whether its influences are primarily social in nature.

Infertility as a Medical Condition

Infertility is considered by some to be a medical problem related to a dysfunction of the body, specifically, the reproductive system. There are several factors that influence fertility in men and women. In men, they include endocrine or testicular disorders, issues with the transport of sperm (motility and lifespan), and other unknown factors (American Pregnancy Association, n.d.-b).

Some of the factors associated with female infertility include problems with ovulation, endocrine disorders, and structural damage to the fallopian tubes, uterus, and cervix (American Pregnancy Association, n.d.-a).

From this perspective, infertility is an important health issue requiring medical solutions (e.g., infertility treatments) to "fix" the problem. This position is promoted by those who believe, from a health equity perspective, that such treatments should be covered under provincial health care insurance plans. Some provinces fund IVF in certain circumstances. In 2015, Ontario introduced a policy (fertility program) of funding for one round of IVF for residents (Motluck, 2016). Some other provinces have set up partial funding through tax credits or grants, and several have not provided any support. In the 2017 federal budget, a measure was introduced allowing taxpayers to claim, as medical expenses, the costs related to IVF treatments going back up to 10 years before the year the tax credit is claimed (Thompson, 2017).

Infertility as a Social Condition

Persons with infertility seeking assisted reproduction have a strong desire to have a child as genetically closely related to them as possible (Schiedermayer, 1988). Some argue that this desire or need to have biological children is socially constructed or influenced. The stigma and emotional distress experienced by couples or individuals often results from the strong pressure placed on them to bear children (Chokr, 1992; Government of Canada, 1996; Lie & Lykke, 2017; Patel et al., 2018a, 2018b).

Reproductive Innovation

The birth of the first "test tube" baby in 1978, Louise Brown, heralded the beginning of the proliferation of reproductive innovations, including **assisted insemination** (AI), **donor insemination** (DI), in vitro fertilization (IVF), cryopreservation, ovum/egg donation, embryo donation, and gestational **surrogacy**. Advanced genetic technologies that provide the opportunity for sex selection, prenatal diagnosis, and, as discussed, genetic screening have also been introduced.

Assisted Insemination

Assisted insemination, the first reproductive technology to be introduced, involves the insertion of sperm into the uterus at the time of ovulation. This option is available to couples when the male partner has issues such as a low sperm count or poor sperm motility. This approach may also occur in concert with hormonal treatment to facilitate sperm or ovum production, control the timing of ovulation, or improve the receptivity of the uterus to the sperm. It is also an option for single women or lesbian couples when the sperm is provided by a donor known to the recipient, or for a homosexual male with a female surrogate.

Anonymous Therapeutic Donor Insemination

Therapeutic donor insemination (TDI) involves the insertion of sperm from a healthy donor into a fertile uterus. This approach is used with heterosexual couples when the male partner is infertile or with single women

and lesbian couples. Sperm donors are required to undergo extensive screening for infection and genetic diseases. Donor semen can be obtained from a registered sperm bank.

Donor insemination (DI) technologies raise ethical questions concerning screening, confidentiality, disclosure, and the nature of relationships with future offspring. Presently, donations to sperm banks are anonymous, but donors can elect to have their identity released to offspring when a specific age is reached, usually 18 years (Gruben & Cameron, 2017). The collection of data related to the donation is limited to certain statistical information and protected by provincial privacy legislation. Advocates for this approach suggest that the number of donors would decrease if donors' identities were to be revealed to the recipients and their children. However, this has not been the case in other jurisdictions where donor privacy is more limited (Gruben & Cameron, 2017). The United Kingdom, the Netherlands, Sweden, and some of the Australian states have reduced or limited donor anonymity, but no material change in the number of donors has been observed (Gruben & Cameron, 2017). The Australian state of Victoria, as of March 2017, removed gamete-donor anonymity, despite assuring donors of ongoing anonymity at the time of donation (Czarnowski, 2020).

Ethical challenges arise regarding the disclosure to the child of the nature of the conception and the identity of the biological father, especially if the child experiences medical problems of a hereditary nature. The status of a donor's confidentiality is at risk as these offspring become adults and assert their right to know the background of their biological parent.

The argument against anonymous donors is based on three concepts: (1) children conceived through TDI should have access to the health information about donors on a continuing basis; (2) these children should have the knowledge that would help them avoid sexual relationships with genetically related individuals; and (3) these children should know their genetic origins for security and peace of mind (Gruben & Cameron, 2017).

Consider the circumstance where a child develops leukemia and needs bone marrow transplantation. Would breaking rules of confidentiality be justified if the biological father might be a potential bone marrow donor (Gruben & Cameron, 2017)? Arguments for disclosure arise when the offspring of a confidential sperm donor experiences medical problems of a hereditary nature. The anonymity of donors is also being challenged by offspring who are asserting their right to know the background of their biological parent (Gruben & Cameron, 2017). With advances in genetic testing and the introduction of public databases that include a person's genome (e.g., Personal Genome Project Canada), there is the growing potential that sperm donors will be identified, whether disclosure is voluntary or not.

In Canada, legislation on donor identification is divided between the federal and provincial/territorial governments. Provincial family law, in most provinces, did not recognize third-party reproduction and did not clarify the place of the donor in the life of the child. This placed donors and parents in a difficult position regarding the rights of donors as parents under family law. In some jurisdictions, there was an incentive for parents to keep donor information confidential because it could undermine their parental rights if donors were known and chose to assert their rights. Anonymity made this a less risky proposition. Quebec, Ontario, and British Columbia have introduced amendments to their laws to recognize assisted human reproduction and clarify that donors of sperm and eggs do not have parental rights unless specifically intended (*Children's Law Reform Act, 1990,* Part 1; *Family Law Act*, 2011). Donor identification was not addressed in the British Columbia and Ontario legislation. In the *Civil Code of Québec* (1991):

> *Personal information relating to medically assisted procreation is confidential. However, where the health of a person born of medically assisted procreation could be harmed if the person were deprived of the information requested, the court may allow the information to be transmitted confidentially to the medical authorities concerned. (art. 542)*

In a British Columbia case, a child conceived through TDI sued the province on the grounds that the Charter rights of such children would be violated if identifying information were not made available to them (*Pratten v. British Columbia (Attorney General)*, 2012, relying on ss. 7 and 15). The case was successful

on the grounds of section 15 of the Charter (Equality) at trial but was overturned on appeal. At trial, the court accepted that children conceived through TDI were analogous to adopted children and that, as adopted children, were entitled to information about their parents under the provincial adoption legislation. As such, TDI-conceived children were considered to be entitled to information about the donor. However, the British Columbia Court of Appeal (BCCA) found that the rights created for adopted children did not extend to TDI-conceived children and dismissed the case.

Under the *Assisted Human Reproduction Act* (2004), donor-identifying information was intended to be collected under the auspices of the federal government. The Supreme Court of Canada struck down major parts of the legislation, and the information-gathering process was dismantled and left up to the provinces. Most of the provinces and territories have not addressed the issue of donor anonymity. Donor information is confidential medical information and subject to the strict rules of confidentiality and non disclosure of all such information. In the provincial legislation regarding IVF funding, the presumption appears to be that donation will be an anonymous process and does not address the issue of donor disclosure.

Quebec, British Columbia, and Ontario have legislation regarding the status of donors and parents under family law. Donors are presently not treated as parents in most circumstances, although three- or four-parent families are also possible under the legislation. For example, under Ontario's *Children's Law Reform Act* (1990), a three-parent family could consist of a biological mother, a nonbiological mother (surrogate), and a sperm donor who was acting as a de facto parent (*A.A. v. B.B.*, 2007).

Although the official channels for donor identification remain limited, public disclosure of genetic data is making it easier to track down donors regardless of their desire for anonymity. For example, databases such as AncestryDNA and 23andMe can be used to track down family members. Also, as the popularity of home DNA tests has spread, people often unexpectedly find unknown relatives, siblings, donors, and illegitimate children, among others. The days of anonymity for donors may be coming to an end (CBC, 2016; Chung et al., 2018; Fetters, 2018).

In Vitro Fertilization

In vitro fertilization (IVF) was developed to overcome conditions associated with infertility that traditional forms of artificial insemination could not address. These conditions include mechanical obstructions resulting from damaged or absent fallopian tubes, endometriosis, intractable ovulatory problems, unexplained infertility, and some forms of male infertility resulting in low sperm count (Fluker & Tuffin, 1996). The success rate of this technology has improved over time (Gunby et al., 2011; Wade et al., 2015).

IVF is a process whereby fertilization of the egg and conception occur outside of the female's body in a laboratory setting. The procedure involves a series of interventions that begin with the use of drugs to hyperstimulate the ovaries to produce excess eggs, followed by ultrasound-guided laparoscopic aspiration of these eggs. The retrieved eggs are then mixed with the partner's (or donor's) sperm in a petri dish. After approximately 48 hours, about three of the successfully fertilized eggs (embryos) are transferred into the woman's uterus (Reynolds & Schieve, 2006). The remaining embryos may be cryopreserved and, if necessary, implanted at a later date, although this practice raises questions about what to do with any unused embryos (Fluker & Tuffin, 1996). Questions about who owns the embryos and what happens if one of the partners dies (i.e., should the embryos be destroyed or does the remaining partner have rights to use them) become relevant. Custody debates over frozen embryos have also arisen in divorce proceedings. There is an instance of this in an Oregon case, where the state's Court of Appeal declared that a divorced wife had the right to dispose of frozen embryos that had been created with her husband's sperm during their marriage (see *Re Dahl and Angle*, 2008). In that case, the agreement between the clinic that provided the storage and retrieval service for the embryos and the couple stipulated that if the spouses could not agree, the wife would have the right to decide on proper disposal. The Court of Appeal confirmed the ruling, and the wife was given the right to destroy the genetic material (Chapman & Zhang, 2014).

In Canada, cases related to frozen sperm and eggs have concluded that this material is "property" and is subject to the usual division of property rules in family law. In a British Columbia case, a husband asked that the court release to him 13 straws of semen that remained from a quantity the couple had purchased during their marriage and used for the conception of their two children. The husband was in a new relationship and wanted the children from his new partner to be related to his existing children, but the ex-wife wanted to dispose of the sperm. The court held that property was to be divided equally and that the husband could have half the frozen sperm (*J.C.M. v. A.N.A.*, 2012). However, if the provisions of the AHRA apply, the Act supersedes the property rights of the parties.

In *S.H. v. D.H.* (2018), an Ontario court considered the ownership of a donated egg and sperm purchased by the couple during their marriage. The trial court reviewed the agreements made between the husband, wife, and the clinic providing the donated material. Based on the review, the court ordered that the donated egg and sperm be turned over to the wife for her use and that she pay the husband for the value of his share in the property. On appeal, the decision was set aside. The Appeal judges found that the federal *Assisted Human Reproduction Act* applied and that use of the donated embryo required the consent of the doner. The genetic material was not related to either spouse but to donors to the clinic that sold the genetic material to the couple. Under the *Assisted Human Reproduction Act* (2004), the couple were the doners of the material, and the use of the genetic material required the consent of both. As the husband had withdrawn his consent, the genetic material could not be used. The law invalidated the contract between the couple. There is great debate about these challenging questions but little consensus on their resolution.

Cryopreservation

The number of embryos transplanted into the uterus is based on the balance between maximizing the rate of success (implantation) and limiting the risk of multiple births, especially in high-risk pregnancies (The Practice Committee, 2013). Any additional embryos may be maintained in liquid nitrogen for future use, if necessary, in a process known as **cryopreservation**. This minimizes the need for further invasive and costly procedures to retrieve eggs. The survival rate of embryos after thawing is about 90%, and they can be stored for decades (IVF Canada, n.d.).

Ovum/Egg Donation

A variation of IVF, egg donation is used to enable pregnancies in women who have a normal uterus but nonfunctioning ovaries. The eggs are donated from healthy donors who undergo ovarian stimulation, or from women with normal functioning ovaries who are already participating in the IVF program. Embryos are created from the donor's egg that is fertilized by either the partner's or a donor's sperm, which is then implanted into the recipient's uterus (Cobo et al., 2015; Fluker & Tuffin, 1996). The donor may be known to the recipient or be a participant of an anonymous donor program.

Embryo Donation

With cryopreservation, embryos can be frozen indefinitely for use in the future. Questions have arisen about what to do with them when they are no longer needed or wanted by the couple or individual. The options are to destroy them, to use them for research purposes, or to donate them to other couples (Robertson, 1995).

The option of **embryo donation** may be desirable when neither partner is fertile but the woman has sufficient uterine capacity for pregnancy and childbirth. It may also be an option for older, single women who are no longer producing eggs, for lesbian couples for whom sperm donation has not worked, and for couples who cannot afford IVF or egg donation (Robertson, 1995). This is also a cost-effective option, as the recipient is not burdened with the costs associated with IVF. In 2022, healthy twins were born after the donation of embryos that had been cryopreserved over 30 years previously. The embryos, donated by an anonymous couple, were created by the husband's sperm and a donated egg (Christensen, 2022).

Many ethical questions arise out of embryo donation (Huele et al., 2019; Lovering, 2020; Widdows & MacCallum, 2002), including whether embryo donation should be treated like adoption, with similar legal processes, screening, and rules (Hallich, 2019; Huele

et al., 2019). For example, should recipients undergo the same social and psychological testing to ensure they are fit parents (Robertson, 1995)? Further questions relate to whether the donor couple should be informed about the outcome (positive or negative) of the donation and whether their anonymity should be maintained (Robertson, 1995).

Gestational Surrogacy

Surrogacy involves a woman who bears a child for another couple or individual. The gestational "mother" may be the biological parent (through sperm donation of either the male partner or a donor) or may carry the embryo of the couple, an embryo donated by another couple, or one created from a donor egg and donor sperm. This approach may be considered by couples who are infertile and have experienced multiple failures with IVF; by women who have health conditions that limit the completion of a pregnancy or an anatomical condition that causes repeated spontaneous abortions; or women who have had hysterectomies (Robertson, 1995). It is also an option for homosexual couples. There are varying rules and regulations regarding surrogacy around the world (Armour, 2012). The Canadian approach to surrogacy will be discussed later in this chapter.

The many approaches to surrogacy raise complex ethical, emotional, and relational issues. These arise, in part, from the sheer number of parties involved (the infant, the surrogate mother, the couple or individual seeking a surrogate, and society as a whole). Other issues related to surrogacy involve concerns regarding the surrogates' own reproductive future; their production of offspring with whom they will not be involved; the appropriateness of the recipients to raise the child; the process of informed consent; and the possibility of coercion, especially when financial remuneration is a factor (Sherwin, 1992).

Case Scenario 9.4 highlights only a few of the complex ethical issues associated with reproductive technologies.

CASE SCENARIO 9.4

PARENTHOOD—A RIGHT OR A PRIVILEGE?

A 30-year-old woman, M. D., who has cystic fibrosis (CF), is involved in a lesbian relationship with S. P., 15 years her senior. They would like to have a child,

and S. P. has been tested and determined to be infertile. Although M. D. is fertile, her medical condition places her at high risk during pregnancy and delivery. The couple can afford IVF, so they set up a meeting

CASE SCENARIO 9.4 *(Continued)*

at an infertility clinic, where they are interviewed by a nurse and an infertility specialist.

The couple say that they are interested in IVF and would like eggs from M. D.'s ovaries to be retrieved and fertilized by donor semen. Once there is successful fertilization, they would like the embryos transplanted into S. P.'s healthy uterus. Because M. D. is worried about passing on the genes for CF, they also request genetic testing on the embryos, and the destruction of those with the CF gene.

Issues

1. Reflecting on your values, what is your response to this situation? Should your response influence your approach to supporting and counselling this couple?
2. What ethical and social questions does this case raise?
3. What are the rights of the various parties: the couple, the nurse and the physician, the potential donor, and the offspring?
4. How do you think these emerging technologies influence the future of society?
5. How might various cultures view this scenario and the opportunities this technology offers?
6. What is the nursing role, and what should be the nature of the nursing relationship with this couple?

Discussion

This case scenario highlights the extent of ethical challenges associated with this advancing science. On the surface, it would appear that only good can result from this couple's request. They would meet their goals of parenthood, and the resulting child or children would have the opportunity of a good life. Yet several questions persist.

What are the rights of the two women in this case scenario? Is procreation a right or a privilege? If it is a privilege, should it be granted only to those who are physically able to procreate? What constitutes "good" parents? What are the rights of the potential child? Should criteria be established to screen potential parents? Should this couple's status as lesbians be a factor? What about the fact that one parent is older and the other is likely to have a short life expectancy because of her disease? Should the donor have any say relative to potential recipients of his sperm? What should this couple disclose to their child, or children, when asked about the biological father? Should the donor process remain private and anonymous? Is it fair that this technology is available only to affluent people? Should health care professionals be using genetic technology to screen for abnormalities, such as CF, or, further, to manipulate physical characteristics, such as sex or hair or eye colour? (People with even minor disabilities are concerned about the negative social attitudes that may emerge in attempts to create "perfect" humans.) Is it right to destroy "imperfect" embryos? Who would be the legal mother of the potential child? Who should have custody if the two women separate? What should be done with the surplus embryos? If the couple choose to donate them, should the recipients be told about the potential for the CF variant? If the donated embryos produce a child with medical or genetic issues, would M. D. and the medical team bear any legal liability?

The issues that arise from these technologies are numerous, and the answers are not clear. The potential impact on future generations is daunting.

Legislative Perspectives

To respond to the legislative and regulatory void in this rapidly evolving area of biotechnology, Parliament enacted the *Assisted Human Reproduction Act* in 2004. However, portions of the Act were declared unconstitutional by the courts, and the scope of the Act has been reduced to prohibiting the sale of genetic

material for reproductive purposes and to prohibiting some forms of manipulation of reproductive material. This federal statute, as amended, recognized and declared the following:

(a) The health and well-being of children born through the application of assisted human

reproductive technologies must be given priority in all decisions respecting their use.

(b) The benefits of assisted human reproductive technologies and related research for individuals, for families and for society in general can be most effectively secured by taking appropriate measures for the protection and promotion of human health, safety, dignity, and rights in the use of these technologies and in related research.

(c) Although all persons are affected by these technologies, women, more than men, are directly and significantly affected by their application, and the health and well-being of women must be protected in the application of these technologies.

(d) The principle of free and informed consent must be promoted and applied as a fundamental condition of the use of human reproductive technologies.

(e) Persons who seek to undergo assisted reproduction procedures must not be discriminated against, including on the basis of their sexual orientation or marital status.

(f) Trade in the reproductive capabilities of women and men and the exploitation of children, women and men for commercial ends raise health and ethical concerns that justify their prohibition.

(g) Human individuality and diversity, and the integrity of the human genome, must be preserved and protected. (Assisted Human Reproduction Act, 2004, s. 2)

The Act makes it illegal to clone a human being or to create any life form that is a hybrid of a human and another animal species. It also bans, among other things, the use of assisted reproductive technologies for the purpose of **sex selection** or the transplanting of human genetic material or an embryo that was previously transplanted into a nonhuman life form.

The Act also bans the payment of money to any woman for a surrogacy arrangement or to arrange for the services of a surrogate mother. Compensation for reasonable expenses is permitted to surrogates for living expenses during the pregnancy. It is also illegal to counsel a woman under 21 years old to become a surrogate mother or to perform a procedure on such a

person for the purposes of assisting her to become a surrogate mother (*Assisted Human Reproduction Act,* 2004, s. 6). The Act also makes it illegal to purchase, sell, or advertise for purchase or sale human cells, genes, in vitro embryos, sperm, or ova for the purpose of reproduction (*Assisted Human Reproduction Act,* 2004, s. 7).

Special Considerations Regarding Fertility Preservation in Persons with Cancer

The situation of persons with cancer deserves discussion, as the treatment of cancer poses a serious threat to fertility (Government of Canada, 2013a).

Male fertility can be affected by:

- The specific cancer itself
- Anatomical problems related to the cancer or to treatment interventions, for example, surgery related to the reproductive system (i.e., removal of testes)
- Primary or secondary hormonal insufficiency
- Damage to or depletion of the germinal stem cells

Female fertility can be affected by:

- Treatment that causes a reduction in the primordial follicles
- Hormonal imbalance
- Interference in the functioning of the ovaries, related to surgery involving the fallopian tubes, uterus, or cervix
- The early onset of menopause

The evidence demonstrates that cancer survivors have an increased risk of emotional distress related to infertility (Canadian Cancer Society, 2014). Although adoption is a consideration, if possible, some would prefer to have their own biological offspring. Therefore, to prevent infertility, some young women with cancer may choose a less toxic regimen of chemotherapy, even though the risk of a recurrence may increase (Goodwin et al., 2007; Jemal et al., 2003).

Finding ways to restore fertility in men, women, and prepubescent males and females with cancer is a factor in helping them cope emotionally with their cancer diagnosis and treatment (European Society of Human Reproduction and Embryology Task Force on Ethics and Law, 2004; Poirot et al., 2007). In the meantime, sperm, egg, and embryo cryopreservation is an option available to those who can afford it. The biggest challenges, however, relate to finding methods to preserve fertility in prepubescent males and females.

Unique Challenges for Children With Cancer

Today, the majority of children with cancer have a high cure rate and are expected to be long-term survivors (Goodwin et al., 2007; Jemal et al., 2003). With the advanced reproductive technologies of today, parents are able to influence the extent to which their children's fertility may be preserved, possible through the cryopreservation of sperm or eggs for future use. The following options are available for their consideration; however, these options are not without ethical challenges.

Sperm Cryopreservation

Sperm cryopreservation in adolescent boys and young men is an option, since sperm production begins at age 13 or 14 years. However, this poses challenges for the adolescent, as this option of sperm collection requires masturbation. Depending on their developmental stage, some may be reluctant to proceed if they lack an appreciation of the purpose or find the process embarrassing. These factors may influence a valid informed consent. Obtaining parental consent in addition to the child's consent or assent is the standard in these circumstances. Given the sensitivities associated with this process, the health care provider's approach to these children needs to be respectful and responsive to their stage of development. If ejaculation is not possible, then sperm extraction or aspiration via testicular biopsy may be an option, as is the case with prepubescent boys. These options, however, raise other challenges with respect to the child's understanding of the issues and the extent to which consent is given free of coercion and influence from others (Bahadur, 2004; Robertson, 2005).

Oophorectomy and Ovarian Cryopreservation

Oophorectomy and ovarian cryopreservation can be offered to premenarcheal girls in advance of cancer treatments that cause ovarian failure (Hamish et al., 2014; Weintraub et al., 2007). Ovarian tissue must be retrieved before treatment, cryopreserved, and grafted after treatment is completed or at an appropriate age. Strips of the ovarian cortex are obtained via laparoscopic surgery

and frozen. Later, they may be grafted into tissue in the forearm, where the eggs mature. The eggs are then frozen and later, IVF is necessary to achieve conception. Alternatively, the tissue may be grafted to the remaining ovary or into the adjacent peritoneum, and eggs may be released later, allowing pregnancy to occur spontaneously.

However, these options raise many challenging and complex questions around consent regarding future unknowns, especially when young children are involved. After the eggs in the graft mature, what if the child dies before these eggs can be used? What are the options for donation? If donation takes place and is effective, what of the welfare of resulting offspring (Lee et al., 2006)?

Challenges Regarding Consent

Considerations related to future fertility are challenging for the child and the parents. At a time when they are responding to a cancer diagnosis, parents must also deal with the challenge of deciding what is in their child's best interests about future fertility and procreation. In this context, the "best interests" of the child include the successful treatment of cancer, minimizing additional risks associated with fertility preservation, and their future interest in procreation. There are some risks, although minimal, associated with fertility-preservation procedures, so parents must balance these with ensuring their child has options available to them in the future. For all procedures, parents' consent is required; however, depending on the age and level of maturity of the child, assent or consent is required. There would need to be clarification of the risks associated with the procedure itself and details regarding future risks and benefits as part of the consent discussion. An important consideration is the actual risk of sterilization associated with cancer treatment. Obtaining the child's agreement to such procedures may be challenging because young children may not be comfortable with or totally understand the discussion and options present and may not appreciate the future consequences of the decision (Grundy et al., 2001).

The consent process in these circumstances has two phases. In the first phase, by electing to have the child undergo fertility-preservation treatments, the parents are making a decision to ensure their child's future right to decide whether to have children is held in trust. In the second phase, the grown-up child can exercise the right to have children, or not (Grundy et al., 2001).

Regulating New Reproductive and Genetic Technologies: Setting Boundaries, Enhancing Health

The Royal Commission on New Reproductive Technologies was created in 1989 to examine the social, medical, legal, ethical, economic, and research implications of these new technologies (Government of Canada, 1996). The mandate of the Royal Commission, which issued its final report in November 1993, was to recommend policies and safeguards and to direct special attention to the implications for women's reproductive health and well-being and the prevention of infertility (Government of Canada, 1996). The Royal Commission made 293 recommendations that focused on the prevention of infertility, the management of assisted reproduction, sex selection for nonmedical reasons, prenatal diagnosis techniques and gene therapy, judicial interventions in pregnancy and birth, and the use of fetal tissue (Government of Canada, 1996).

In response, in 1995 the federal government called for a moratorium on the use of specific practices, established an advisory committee, and proposed a legislative framework intended to "protect the health and safety of Canadians, ensure the appropriate treatment of human reproductive materials and... protect the dignity and security of all persons, especially women and children" (Government of Canada, 1996). The intention was to manage reproductive and genetic technologies through a plan that would prohibit unacceptable technologies and develop a legislated regulatory process to manage technologies deemed acceptable.

It was proposed that the following practices be prohibited:

- Sex selection for nonmedical purposes
- Buying and selling of eggs, sperm, and embryos
- Germline genetic alterations
- **Ectogenesis** (maintaining an embryo in an artificial womb)
- Cloning of human embryos
- Creation of animal–human hybrids
- Retrieval of sperm or eggs from cadavers or fetuses for fertilization and implantation, or research

involving the maturation of sperm or eggs outside the body
- Commercial preconception or surrogacy arrangements egg donation in exchange for in vitro fertilization services

In the proposed legislative framework, which eventually became the *Assisted Human Reproduction Act*, additional practices were added (Government of Canada, 1996):

- Transfer of embryos between humans and other species
- Use of human sperm, eggs, or embryos for assisted reproduction or research without the informed consent of the donors
- Research on human embryos 14 days or more after conception
- Creation of embryos for research
- Offering to provide or to pay for prohibited services

Under the *Assisted Human Reproduction Act* (2004), all the activities listed are prohibited. The regulation of human reproductive activities was found to be beyond the legislative powers of the federal government and has been removed from the legislation. The Act is now limited to prohibiting certain activities related to reproductive technologies and limiting the sale and distribution of genetic material for reproduction. The use and regulation of human tissues is regulated by provincial and territorial legislation on tissue donation and transplantation (e.g., the Alberta *Human Tissue and Organ Donation Act,* 2006).

Ethical Perspectives

Implications for Women: Feminist Perspectives

Reproductive technologies are primarily applied on women's bodies and have implications for women's reproductive autonomy; thus, they are of strong interest to feminist thinkers. Feminist thinkers offer varying views, ranging from the perspective that these technologies are a step toward the liberalization of women (i.e., they help to overcome biological limits) (Chokr, 1992; Lie & Lykke, 2019; Throsby, 2004, Ch. 1), to challenging the assumption that they are beneficial for women (i.e., they are a means toward more social control, exploitation, and coercion of women) (Deech

& Smajdor, 2007). There is greater consensus that women must be at the centre of all discourse and policy development and define what is best for them. Some argue that the focus of the related ethical discussions has been too narrow, avoiding the broader social implications of these technologies' introduction (Dickenson, 2016; Sherwin, 1992). According to Dr. Susan Sherwin, a Canadian feminist, these practices must be evaluated within the context of broader social structures that can be oppressive to women. (Sherwin, 1992). She argued for the need to explore the possibility that new approaches to reproduction will bring about "profound cultural change" and that their social, political, and economic effects also need to be evaluated (Sherwin, 1992). The lower social and economic status of many women may make them susceptible to the risks associated with reproductive technologies (especially the high risk of failure and the unknown long-term effects of the drugs used to hyper-stimulate the ovaries). There is also a need to evaluate those social influences that contribute to the expectations placed on people, especially women, to procreate (Dickenson, 2016). Although the intention of these technologies is to give persons the right to reproductive choices, including that of legitimizing alternative forms of family and social structures (Chokr, 1992), some feminists are concerned that in practice, the actual control will belong to others, specifically the male-dominated medical profession (Sherwin, 1992).

Additional concerns arise from the potential for the commercialization of the technology and, therefore, commodification of women's reproduction (McIlroy, 1996). Of further concern is how older women are treated differently than older men in regard to fertility and reproduction (Lie & Lykke, 2017). Finally, strategies to understand and prevent infertility, provide good prenatal care, and explore alternatives such as adoption should not be overlooked (Chokr, 1992).

Implications for Offspring

Several known and unknown risks exist for the children who are produced through reproductive technologies. Thirty percent of IVF deliveries are multiple births; thus, these babies are at high risk for low birth weight or problems during delivery (Government of Canada, 1996). Furthermore, little is known about the long-term effects of the drugs used throughout the procedure on the resulting children.

Legal uncertainties regarding family relationships may result in the future because in some situations, the legal parenthood of the child may be unclear or challenged. Inheritance, custody, access, and support issues may be raised in future years.

Some parents choose to keep their use of donor insemination secret from family members, friends, and the child, who is usually presented as their biological offspring. This practice has been encouraged in the past by many infertility programs. This conspiracy of silence means that many children born through assisted reproduction do not know the circumstances of their birth (Schiedermayer, 1988; Sherwin, 1992).

With regard to sperm donors, unless they agree to disclosure, the present practice is to maintain the anonymity of the donor (Government of Canada, 1996). Thus, if children conceived in this manner were made aware of the circumstances of their birth, they would not (as is the case with adoption) be able to demand that their biological fathers be identified (Gruben & Cameron, 2017). As mentioned earlier, this is changing, with growing public access to genome sequencing (Fetters, 2018).

Consent

As described in Chapter 6, informed consent requires that persons—in the case of donor insemination, the recipient and the donor—be fully informed of all material risks, uncertainties, and benefits, and that the process be free of coercion. The last issue is especially important when surrogates or donors are friends or relatives who may be subjected to personal pressure to participate. Factors influencing consent around reproductive technologies include the emotional nature of the process and the psychological effects on both recipients and donors.

Exploitation Versus Appropriate Remuneration: Financial Incentives

A major concern, as expressed by feminist thinkers, is the potential exploitation of poor and middle-class women as breeders for the upper class (Zipper & Sevenhuijsen, 1987). Feminists note that although women now can make their own reproductive choices, they are still forced to make these decisions under social conditions that remain controlled by men and that stress the importance of female fertility.

Presently, there is no payment to egg donors, although, typically, they are not required to bear the costs of the procedure. Since 2004, payment for sperm donation has been banned. Before 2004, men had long been paid for semen donation—a far less invasive procedure. Defenders of this practice claim that payment only covers expenses and that without such payment, the rate of donation would decrease.

Many current reproductive technologies are expensive and, as noted earlier, are not consistently funded across Canada. Thus, their availability is limited to those who are able to pay, creating inequity of access. Furthermore, concerns arise in embryo donation when the decision to donate may be influenced by the prohibitive costs associated with cryopreservation.

Social Justice

As discussed earlier, the cost of these programs is not covered by most provincial and territorial health systems. The high cost of this technology is prohibitive to many, resulting in serious inequities across the system. The issue becomes more profound when one considers infertility resulting from cancer and its treatment.

Psychological Impact

Reproductive technologies are recent, evolving, and imperfect. Although success rates are improving (Gunby et al., 2011; Wade et al., 2015), failure of the technology can leave potential parents at risk of feelings of extreme loss and grief. Nurses must help their patients deal with potential grief and mourning, as well as the psychological effects arising from the technological processes on themselves (Patel et al., 2018a).

These processes place a great burden on the relationships among the people involved. The drugs used to stimulate ovum production can cause emotional lability. The regimentation of the process and the coldness of the environment for procreation are the extreme opposite of a normally private and intimate experience. Fear of failure adds further strain. Nurses must consider all these factors in the care that they provide. They need to understand the issues and be prepared to support and guide their patients through a difficult, emotionally charged process.

With the introduction of each new technology in this field, more possibilities, as well as more ethical questions, emerge.

CASE SCENARIO 9.5

CONFLICT IN VALUES

One evening, a nurse working on a busy gynecology unit is caring for two patients who have recently experienced abortions. P. A., a 24-year-old single woman, has had a saline abortion, as she and her boyfriend decided late (at 16 weeks) that they did not wish to proceed with the pregnancy. The process was painful, and the patient found it disturbing to see the dead fetus. Afterward, she was tearful and unable to sleep.

The nurse's other patient, A. B., spontaneously aborted at 24 weeks. She has just returned from having a dilatation and curettage (D&C) procedure. She and her partner were part of the in vitro fertilization (IVF) program at the hospital. This was her third pregnancy, and she had aborted each time. Because there are no embryos left, she and her partner will have to begin the process again, and her obstetrician does not recommend this. She is very upset and unable to sleep.

The nurse has limited time on the shift. Now, she wonders which patient needs her most.

Questions

1. What would you do in this nurse's situation? What principles would guide your actions?
2. Should both these patients be on the same unit? Should both have been assigned to the same nurse? Might this circumstance contribute to moral distress for the nurse?
3. What responsibilities do nursing leaders have to ensure that hospital environments and structures minimize ethical conflicts for nursing staff?

SUMMARY

In this chapter, some of the complex technologies in health care today were described and the associated legal and ethical challenges explored. These technologies have the ability to influence not only the creation of life but also the nature of future generations, and they have the potential to eliminate illness and disease.

There have been significant advances in the areas of reproductive technologies, stem cell technology, genetics, and genomics.

In a diverse society such as Canada's, patients and their families come from many religious and cultural backgrounds and may view the meaning of life from varying perspectives. Nurses must be sensitive to these differences and respectful of the values and beliefs of others.

Nurses must be aware of new technologies because these technologies may influence practice and policy in many settings; for example, the field of reproductive sciences is no longer limited to clinical arenas that focus on reproduction. Nurses in oncology may now be exposed to these interventions and will be able to support their patients through fertility-related processes.

CRITICAL THINKING

The following case scenarios are intended to facilitate further reflection, discussion, and analysis.

Discussion Points

1. What are the major challenges related to genetics? Have you been exposed to genetics-related challenges in your practice?
2. Should society pay for all genetic screening? Should society pay for some? What kind?
3. Reflect on your views of gene editing and its potential. Engage in a debate with yourself or others regarding the pros and cons of this technology.
4. Identify the key arguments in favour of new reproductive technologies. In your opinion, are these arguments valid? What are the opposing arguments?
5. How can the exploitation of women be prevented as new reproductive technologies emerge? What concerns in this regard have been expressed by feminist thinkers?

CASE SCENARIO 9.6

I AM AFRAID: YES, I WANT TO HAVE BABIES WHEN I GROW UP

A 9-year-old girl has just been diagnosed with leukemia. Indications are that she will likely be cured. However, the chemotherapy will make her infertile.

The team offers her parents the opportunity to have her ovarian tissue cryopreserved to ensure that her eggs develop to enable in vitro fertilization (IVF) in the future. Her parents have different opinions about this. Her mother, knowing that her daughter often talks about having babies, thinks this should be done. Her father disagrees, believing their daughter is going through enough.

They agree to discuss the options with their daughter, who agrees she wants to have children when she grows up but cries when the procedure is described to her. She does not understand what a lot of this means but says she is afraid and does not want the surgery.

Questions

1. What are the competing ethical issues in the scenario?
2. How can the parents decide what is in their daughter's best interests?
3. How would you as the nurse support this young woman and her parents through this highly emotional process so that they can make the best choice for their child?

CASE SCENARIO 9.7

THE PERFECT CHILD

A couple tried for some time to conceive before trying IVF and were successful in the first attempt, obtaining five healthy embryos. They have asked the health care team to test the embryos for positive traits and characteristics they might have inherited from the family. They would like a male embryo to be implanted first and a female frozen for later use. Red hair is a recessive gene in the family, and,

if possible, they would like a girl with red hair. They ask whether it is possible to predict the intelligence of their future children, as they would like to take that into consideration.

Questions

1. Do you think these choices should be made available to these parents?
2. Do you think new reproductive technologies have the possibility of influencing future generations?

REFERENCES

Statutes

Assisted Human Reproduction Act, S.C. 2004, c. 2 (Canada).
Canadian Charter of Rights and Freedoms, Part I of the *Constitution Act, 1982*, being Schedule B to the *Canada Act 1982* (UK), 1982, c. 11.
Children's Law Reform Act, RSO 1990, c. C.12, (Ontario).
Civil Code of Québec, CQLR c. CCQ-1991 (Quebec).
Family Law Act, SBC 2011, c. 25 (British Columbia).
Genetic Non-Discrimination Act, S.C. 2017, c. 3 (Canada).
The Human Tissue Gift Act, CCSM c. H180 (Manitoba).
Human Tissue and Organ Donation Act, SA 2006, c H-14.5 (Alberta).
Human Tissue Donation Act, RSPEI 1988, c. H-12.1 (Prince Edward Island).
Trillium Gift of Life Network Act, R.S.O. 1990, c. H.20 (Ontario).

Case Law

A.A. v. B.B. [2007] ONCA 2.
https://www.cbc.ca/radio/thecurrent/the-current-for-oct-19-2020-1.5767530/genetic-genealogy-technique-used-in-christine-jessop-cold-case-comes-with-privacy-concerns-warns-expert-1.5767904
J.C.M. v. A.N.A. [2012] BCSC 584 (CanLII). http://canlii.ca/t/fr3z5
Pratten v. British Columbia (Attorney General), 2012 BCCA 480 (CanLII).
Re Dahl and Angle, Doc. DR04090713 A133697, Oct. 8, 2008.
Reference re Assisted Human Reproduction Act, 2010 SCC 61 (CanLII).
Reference re Genetic Non-Discrimination Act, 2020 SCC 17.
S.H. v. D.H. [2018] ONSC 4506 (CanLII). http://canlii.ca/t/ht5kw

Texts and Articles

Alison, M. R., Poulson, R., Forbes, S., et al. (2002). An introduction to stem cells. *The Journal of Pathology, 297*(4), 419–423.
American College of Obstetricians and Gynecologists. (2008). Ethical issues in genetic testing. ACOG Committee Opinion no. 410. *Obstetrics and Gynecology, 111*, 1495–1502.
American College of Obstetricians and Gynaecologists. (2017). *Prenatal genetic screening.* https://www.acog.org/Patients/FAQs/Prenatal-Genetic-Screening-Tests
American Pregnancy Association. (n.d.-a). *Female infertility.* http://americanpregnancy.org/infertility/male-infertility/

American Pregnancy Association. (n.d.-b). *Male infertility.* http://americanpregnancy.org/infertility/male-infertility/
Anderson, A. S. (2015). Wrongful convictions and the avenues of redress: The post-conviction review process in Canada. *Appeal: Review of Current Law and Law Reform, 20*(5). https://canlii.ca/t/6sr
Anderson, J. A., Meyn, M. S., & Shuman, C. (2017). Parents perspectives on whole genome sequencing for their children: Qualified enthusiasm? *Journal of Medical Ethics, 43*, 535–539.
Arevalo, C. P., Bolton, M. J., Le Sage, V. et al. (2022). A multivalent nucleoside-modified mRNA vaccine against all known influenza virus subtypes. Science, 378(6622), 899–904. doi:10.1126/science.abm0271
Armour, K. L. (2012). An overview of surrogacy around the world: Trends, questions and ethical issues. *Nursing for Women's Health, 16*(3), 231–236.
Bahadur, G. (2004). Ethics of testicular stem cell medicine. *Human Reproduction, 19*(12), 2702–2710.
BRCA. (2008). http://inthefamily.kartemquin.com/content/brca-101.
Bredenoord, A. L., & Appleby, J. B. (2017). Mitochondrial replacement techniques: Remaining ethical challenges. *Cell Stem Cell, 21*(3), 301–304. https://www.sciencedirect.com/science/article/pii/S1934590917303272
The Broad Institute. (2018). *Questions and answers about CRISPR.* https://www.broadinstitute.org/what-broad/areas-focus/project-spotlight/questions-and-answers-about-crispr
Canadian Cancer Society. (n.d.). *Genetic testing.* http://www.cancer.ca/en/cancer-information/cancer-101/what-is-cancer/genes-and-cancer/genetic-testing/?region5on
Canadian Cancer Society. (2014). *Fertility after cancer treatment.* http://www.cancer.ca/en/about-us/for-media/media-releases/national/2014/fertility-after-cancer-treatment/?region5on
Canadian Organization for Rare Disorders. (2006). *Newborn screening in Canada status report.* https://www.raredisorders.ca/content/uploads/Canada-NBS-status-updated-Sept.-3-2015.pdf
Carroll, D. (2017). Genome editing: Past, present, and future. *Yale Journal of Biology and Medicine, 90*, 653–659.
CBC. (2016, September 13). I always wanted a sister: 3 half siblings of same sperm donor meet for the first time. The Current. https://www.cbc.ca/radio/thecurrent/the-current-for-september-13-2016-1.3759566/i-always-wanted-a-sister-offspring-with-same-sperm-donor-meet-for-first-time-1.3759573

Chadwick, R. (2008). Genetic testing and screening. In P. A. Singer & A. M. Viens (Eds.), *The Cambridge textbook of bioethics*. Cambridge University Press.

Chapman, J. E., & Zhang, M. (2014). In the matter of the marriage of Dahl and Angle (2008). In *The Embryo Project Encyclopedia*. https://embryo.asu.edu/pages/matter-marriage-dahl-and-angle-2008

Childress, J. F. (1997). *Practical reasoning in bioethics*. Indiana University Press.

Chokr, N. (1992). Feminist perspectives on reproductive technologies: The politics of motherhood. *Technology in Society, 14*, 317–333.

Christensen, J. (2022, November 21). Parents welcome twins from embryos frozen 30 years ago. *CNN*. https://www.cnn.com/2022/11/21/health/30-year-old-embryos-twins/index.html

Chung, E., Glanz, M., & Adhopia, V. (2018, January 25). Donor-conceived people are tracking down their biological fathers, even if they want to hide. *CBC News*. https://www.cbc.ca/news/science/sperm-donor-dna-testing-1.4500517

Cobo, A., Garrido, N., Pellicer, A., et al. (2015). Six years' experience in ovum donation using vitrified oocytes: Report of cumulative outcomes, impact of storage time, and development of a predictive model for oocyte survival rate. *Fertility and Sterility, 104*(6), 1426–1434.

Cribbs, A. P., & Perera, S. M. W. (2017). Science and bioethics of CRISPR-Cas9 gene editing: An analysis towards separating facts and fiction. *Yale Journal of Biology and Medicine, 90*, 625–634.

Czarnowski, A. (2020). Retrospective removal of gamete donor anonymity: Policy recommendations for Ontario based on the Victorian experience. *Canadian Journal of Family Law, 33*(2), 251.

de Groot, N. F., van Beers, B. C., & Meynen, G. (2021). Commercial DNA tests and police investigations: A broad bioethical perspective. *Journal of Medical Ethics, 47*, 788–795.

Deech, R., & Smajdor, A. (2007). Fertility is a feminist issue. In R. Deech & A. Smajdor (Eds.), *From IVF to immortality: Controversy in the era of reproductive technology*. Oxford Scholarship Online.

Dickenson, D. (2016). *Feminist perspectives on human genetics and reproductive technologies*. John Wiley & Sons Ltd.

Difference Between. (n.d.). Difference between genetics and genomics. *Differences Between*. http://www.differencebetween.info/difference-between-genetics-and-genomics.

Elliot, R. L., Jiang, X. P., & Head, J. F. (2014). Mitochondria organelle transplantation: The mitochondrion, "an intracellular organelle for cell-based therapy." *International Journal of Applied Science and Technology, 4*(5), 158–162.

Ethics Committee of the American Society for Reproductive Medicine. (2015). Use of reproductive technology for sex selection for nonmedical reasons, *Fertility and Sterility, 103*, 1418–1422.

European Society of Human Reproduction and Embryology Task Force on Ethics and Law. (2004). Ethical considerations for the cryopreservation of gametes and reproductive tissues for self-use. *Human Reproduction, 19*(2), 460–462.

EuroStem Cell. (2018). *Embryonic stem cell research: An ethical dilemma*. https://www.eurostemcell.org/embryonic-stem-cell-research-ethical-dilemma

Fetters, A. (2018, May 18). Finding the lost generation of sperm donors. *The Atlantic*. https://www.theatlantic.com/family/archive/2018/05/sperm-donation-anonymous/560588/

Fluker, M. R., & Tuffin, G. J. (1996). Assisted reproductive technologies: A primer for Canadian physicians. *Journal of the Society of Obstetrics and Gynecology Canada, 18*, 451–465.

Freudenrich, C. (2001). How cloning works. *How Stuff Works*. https://science.howstuffworks.com/life/genetic/cloning.htm

Gene Therapy Net.com. (2018). *Ethical and social issues in gene therapy*. Retrieved from http://www.genetherapynet.com/ethical-and-social-issues-in-gene-therapy.html

Genome Canada. (2022). *Canada's genomics ecosystem leader*. https://www.nature.com/scitable/definition/genome-43/

Gibson, J. P. (1998, February/March). Cloning Daisy: The genetic future? *Info Holstein Newsletter*. University of Guelph.

Global Gene Editing Regulation Tracker. (2020). *China: Germline/embrionics*. https://crispr-gene-editing-regs-tracker.geneticliteracyproject.org/china-germline-embryonic/

Goodwin, T., Oosterhuis, E. B., Kiernan, M., et al. (2007). Attitudes and practices of pediatric oncology providers regarding fertility issues. *Pediatric Blood & Cancer, 48*(1), 80–85.

Government of Canada. (1996). *New reproductive and genetic technologies: Setting boundaries, enhancing health*.

Government of Canada. (2005). *Gene therapy*. https://www.canada.ca/en/health-canada/services/science-research/emerging-technology/biotechnology/about-biotechnology/gene-therapy.html

Government of Canada. (2006). *Stem cells*. https://www.canada.ca/en/health-canada/services/science-research/emerging-technology/biotechnology/about-biotechnology/stem-cells-biotechnology-science-research.html

Government of Canada. (2013a). *Cancer and fertility*. https://www.canada.ca/en/public-health/services/fertility/cancer-fertility.html.

Government of Canada. (2013b). *Genetic testing and screening*. https://www.canada.ca/en/public-health/services/fertility/genetic-testing-screening.html

Greenwood, H. L., & Daar, A. S. (2008). Regenerative medicine. In P. A. Singer & A. M. Viens (Eds.), *The Cambridge textbook of bioethics* (p. 153). Cambridge University Press.

Gruben, V., & Cameron, A. (2017). Donor anonymity in Canada: Assessing the obstacles to openness and considering a way forward. *Alberta Law Review, 54*(3), 665–680.

Grundy, R., Larcher, V., Gosden, R. G., et al. (2001). Fertility preservation for children treated for cancer (2): Ethics of consent for gamete storage and experimentation. *Archives of Disease in Childhood, 84*(4), 360–362.

Gunby, J., Bissonnette, F., Librach, C., et al. (2011). Assisted reproductive technologies (ART) in Canada: 2007 results from the Canadian ART Register. *Fertility & Sterility, 95*(2), 542–547.

Guo, X., & Huang, L. (2012). Recent advances in nonviral vectors for gene delivery. *Accounts of Chemical Research, 45*(7), 971–979.

Hallich, O. (2019). Embryo donation or embryo adoption? Conceptual and normative issues. *Bioethics, 33*(6), 653–660.

Hamish, W. L., Smith, A. G., Kelsey, T. W., et al. (2014). Fertility preservation for girls and young women with cancer: Population-based validation of criteria for ovarian tissue cryopreservation. *Lancet Oncology, 5*(10), 1129–1136.

Huele, E. H., Kool, E. M., Bos, A. M. E., et al. (2019). The ethics of embryo donation: What are the moral similarities and differences of surplus embryo donation and double gamete donation? *Human Reproduction, 35*(10), 2171–2178.

Hutter, G. (2016). Stem cell transplantation in strategies for curing HIV/AIDS. *AIDS Research and Therapy, 13*(1), 31.

IVF Canada. (n.d.). *Fertility preservation.* https://ivfcanada.com/services/fertility-preservation/

Jemal, A., Murray, T., Samuels, A., et al. (2003). Cancer statistics. *A Cancer Journal for Clinicians, 53*, 5–26.

Kern, S., Eichler, H., Stoeve, J., et al. (2006). Comparative analysis of mesenchymal stem cells from bone marrow, umbilical cord blood, or adipose tissue. *Stem Cells, 24*(5), 1294–1301.

Krishna, M., & Lepping, M. (2011). Ethical debate: Ethics of Xenotransplantation. *BJMP, 4*(3), a425.

Lee, S. J., Schover, L. R., Partridge, A. H., et al. (2006). American Society of Clinical Oncology recommendations on fertility preservation in cancer patients. *Journal of Clinical Oncology, 24*(18), 2917–2931.

Lie, M., & Lykke, N. (2017). *Assisted reproduction across borders: Feminist perspectives on normalization, disruptions and transmissions.* Routledge.

Lionel, A. C., Costain, G., Monfared, N., et al. (2018). Improved diagnostic yield compared with targeted gene sequencing panels suggests a role for whole-genome sequencing as a first-tier genetic test. *Genetics in Medicine, 20*, 435–443.

Lovering, R. (2020). A moral argument for frozen human embryo adoption. *Bioethics, 34*(3), 242–251.

Mahowald, M. B. (1996). The brain and the I: Neurodevelopment and personal identity. *Journal of Social Philosophy, 27*(3), 49–60.

Mascola, J. R., & Fauci, A. S. (2020). Novel vaccine technologies for the 21st century. *Nature Reviews Immunology, 20*(2), 87–88.

Mayo Clinic Staff. (2016). *Alzheimer's genes: Are you at risk?* https://www.mayoclinic.org/diseases-conditions/alzheimers-disease/in-depth/alzheimers-genes/art-20046552

McIlroy, A. (1996, April 8). Ottawa to regulate baby trade. *The Globe and Mail,* A1.

Mitochondrial transplant for human embryos. (2008, February 14). https://hplusbiopolitics.wordpress.com/2008/02/14/mitochondrial-transplant-for-human-embryos/

Motluck, A. (2016 September 30). Ottawa couple says Ontario's-fertility-funding program is discriminatory. *The Globe and Mail.*

Nahta, R., & Esteva, F. J. (2006). HER2 therapy: Molecular mechanisms of trastuzumab resistance. *Breast Cancer Research, 8*(6), 215.

National Human Genome Research Institute. (2016a). *An overview of the human genome project.* https://www.genome.gov/12011238/an-overview-of-the-human-genome-project/

National Human Genome Research Institute. (2016b). *Genetic variation. National DNA Day, April 28, 2008.* [PowerPoint]. https://www.genome.gov/pages/education/modules/geneticvariation.pdf

National Human Genome Research Institute. (2017). *Genome editing.* https://www.genome.gov/27569222/genome-editing/

National Institutes of Health. (2016). *Stem cell information home page: Stem cell basics.* https://stemcells.nih.gov/info/basics/stc-basics

Normand, E. A., Alaimo, J. T., & Van den Veyver, I. B. (2017). Exome and genome sequencing in reproductive medicine. *Fertility and Sterility, 199*(2), 213–220.

Office of the Privacy Commissioner of Canada. (2017). *Direct-to-consumer testing and privacy.* https://www.priv.gc.ca/en/privacy-topics/health-genetic-and-other-body-information/02_05_d_69_gen/

Ortenzi, T. J. (2018, June 2). Hunt for Golden State Killer led detectives to Hobby Lobby for DNA sample. *Washington Post.*

Pardi, N., Hogan, M. J., & Weissman, D. (2020). Recent advances in mRNA vaccine technology. *Current Opinion in Immunology, 65,* 14–20.

Patel, A., Sharma, P. S. V. N., & Kumar, P. (2018a). "In cycles of dreams, despair, and desperation": Research perspectives on infertility specific distress in patients undergoing fertility treatments. *Journal of Human Reproductive Science, 11*(4), 320–328.

Patel, A., Sharma, P. S. V. N., & Kumar, P. (2018b). Role of mental health practitioner in infertility clinics: A review on past, present and future directions. *Journal of Human Reproductive Sciences, 11*(3), 219–228.

Perinatal Services BC. (2010). *BCPHP obstetric guideline 19: Maternity care pathway.* http://www.perinatalservicesbc.ca/Documents/Guidelines-Standards/Maternal/MaternityCarePathway.pdf

Phelan, J. (2022, May 9). Why haven't we cloned a human yet? *Live Science.* https://www.livescience.com/why-no-human-cloning

Pilkington, E. H., Suys, E. J., Trevaskis, N. L., et al. (2021). From influenza to COVID-19: Lipid nanoparticle mRNA vaccines at the frontiers of infectious diseases. *Acta Biomaterialia, 131*, 16–40.

Poirot, C. J., Martelli, H., Genestie, C., et al. (2007). Feasibility of ovarian tissue cryopreservation for prepubertal females with cancer. *Pediatric Blood & Cancer, 49*(1), 74–78.

Powers, L. (2022, November 28). Man arrested and charged in grisly 1983 killings of 2 women in Toronto, police say. *CBC News.* https://www.cbc.ca/news/canada/toronto/tice-gilmour-cold-case-murders-arrest-1.6666333

The Practice Committee of the American Society for Reproductive Medicine and the Practice Committee of the Society for Assisted Reproductive Technology. (2013). Criteria for number of embryos to transfer: A committee opinion. *Fertility and Sterility, 99*(1), 44–46.

Public Health Agency of Canada. (2021, April 26). *Chapter 4 Infographic: Labour and birth in Canada.* https://www.canada.ca/en/public-health/services/publications/healthy-living/labour-birth-infographic.html

Ratan, Z. A., Son, Y. F., Haidere, M. F., et al. (2018). CRISPR-Cas9: A promising genetic engineering approach in cancer research. *Therapeutic Advances in Medical Oncology, 10.* https://doi:10.1177/1758834018755089.

Reuter, M. S., Walker, S., Thiruvahindrapuram, B., et al. (2018). The Personal Genome Project Canada: Findings from whole genome sequences of the inaugural 56 participants. *CMAJ, 190*(5), E126–E136.

Reynolds, M. A., & Schieve, L. A. (2006). Trends in embryo transfer practices and multiple gestation for IVF procedures in the USA, 1996–2002. *Human Reproduction, 21*(3), 694–700.

Ries, N. M., & Einsiedel, E. (2010). *Online direct-to-consumer genetic testing: Issues and policy options.* Policy Brief No. 3. Genome Canada. https://www.genomecanada.ca/sites/default/files/pdf/en/GPS-Policy-brief-June2010.pdf

Robertson, J. A. (1995). Ethical and legal issues in human embryo donation. *Fertility and Sterility, 64*, 885–894.

Robertson, J. A. (2005). Cancer and fertility: Ethical and legal challenges. *Journal of the National Cancer Institute Monographs, 34,* 104–106.

Scherer, S., Brudno, M., Church, G., et al. (2017). *Personal Genome Project Canada: Full consent form.* The Hospital for Sick Children.

Schiedermayer, D. L. (1988, Fall). Babies made the American way: Ethics and interests of surrogate motherhood. *The Pharos of Alpha Omega Alpha-Honor Medical Society, 51*(4), 2–7.

ScienceDaily. (2012). *Use of stem cells in personalized medicine.* https://www.sciencedaily.com/releases/2012/11/121126151021.htm

Sherwin, S. (1992). *No longer patient: Feminist ethics and health care.* Temple University Press.

Shin, J. W., & Lee, J. (2018). The prospects of CRISPR-based genome engineering in the treatment of neurodegenerative disorders. *Therapeutic Advances in Neurological Disorders, 1,* 1–11.

Shuman, C. (2008, April). *Genetic counselling—Translating genetic information for patients and their families. In* Symposium conducted at the Canadian Medical Hall of Fame/Pfizer Canada Discovery Day in Health Sciences, University of Toronto, Toronto, ON.

Stanworth, M. (1987). Reproductive technologies and the deconstruction of motherhood. In M. Stanworth (Ed.), *Reproductive technologies: Gender, motherhood and medicine* (pp. 11–35). University of Minnesota Press.

Su, P. (2013). Direct-to-consumer genetic testing: A comprehensive view. *The Yale Journal of Biology and Medicine, 86*(3), 359–365.

Szabó, G. T., Mahiny, A. J., & Vlatkovic, I. (2022). COVID-19 mRNA vaccines: Platforms and current developments. *Molecular Therapy, 30*(5), 1850–1868.

Szego, M. J. (2011). Organelle transplantation should be legalized in Canada [Editorial]. *Journal of Obstetrics and Gynaecology Canada, 33*(4), 329.

Szego, M. J. (2016). Whole genome sequencing as a genetic test for autism spectrum disorder: From bench to bedside and then back again. *Journal of the Canadian Academy of Child and Adolescent Psychiatry, 25*(2), 116–121.

Szego, M. J., Meyn, M. S., Anderson, J. A., et al. (2014). Predictive genomic testing of children for adult onset disorders: A Canadian perspective. *American Journal of Bioethics, 14*(3), 19–21.

Thompson, E. (2017, March 23). Access to tax credit for fertility treatments expanded in budget. *CBC News.*

ThoughtCo. (2019). *Pros and cons of embryonic stem cell research.* https://www.thoughtco.com/pros-cons-of-embryonic-stem-cell-research-3325609

Throsby, K. (2004). *When IVF fails.* Palgrave Macmillan.

Torchilin, V. P. (2005). Recent advances with liposomes as pharmaceutical carriers. *Nature Reviews Drug Discovery, 4,* 145–160.

Trounson, A., & McDonald, C. (2015). Stem cell therapies in clinical trials: Progress and challenges. *Cell Stem Cell, 17*(1), 11–22.

U.S. Department of Energy Office of Science. (n.d.). *Human genome project information.* http://www.ornl.gov/hgmis

U.S. National Library of Medicine. (2018a). *What are the ethical issues surrounding gene therapy?* https://ghr.nlm.nih.gov/primer/therapy/ethics

U.S. National Library of Medicine. (2018b). *What is direct to consumer testing?* https://ghr.nlm.nih.gov/primer/dtcgenetictesting/directtoconsumer

U.S. National Library of Medicine. (2018c). *What is genetic testing?* https://ghr.nlm.nih.gov/primer/testing/genetictesting

U.S. National Library of Medicine. (2018d). *Your guide to understanding genetic conditions.* https://ghr.nlm.nih.gov/primer/hgp/genome

Vegas, A. J., Veiseh, O., Gürtler, M., et al. (2016). Long-term glycemic control using polymer-encapsulated human stem cell–derived beta cells in immune-competent mice. *Nature Medicine, 22*(3), 306–311.

Volarevic, V., Markovic, B. S., Gazdic, M., et al. (2018). Ethical and safety issues of stem cell-based therapy. *International Journal of Medical Sciences, 15*(1), 36–45.

von Tigerstrom, B. (2015). Human tissue legislation and a new medical paradigm: Governing tissue engineering in Canada. *McGill Journal of Law and Health,* 8(2), S1–S56.

Wade, J. J., MacLachlan, V., & Kovacs, G. (2015). The success rate of IVF has significantly improved over the last decade. *Australian and New Zealand Journal of Obstetrics and Gynaecology, 55*(5), 473–476.

Walters, L. (1999, February). *Ethical issues in human gene therapy. Human Genome News, 10*(1-2). https://web.ornl.gov/sci/techresources/Human_Genome/publicat/hgn/v10n1/16walter.shtml

Weintraub, M., Gross, E., Kadari, A., et al. (2007). Should ovarian cryopreservation be offered to girls with cancer? *Pediatric Blood & Cancer, 48*(1), 4–9.

Widdows, H., & MacCallum, F. (2002). Disparities in parenting criteria: An exploration of the issues, focusing on adoption and embryo donation. *Journal of Medical Ethics, 28*(3), 139–142.

World Health Assembly. (2004). *Genomics and World Health. Fifty seventh World Health Assembly, resolution.* https://apps.who.int/gb/ebwha/pdf_files/WHA57/A57_R13-en.pdf

World Health Organization. (2002). *Genomics and world health: Report of the Advisory Committee on Health Research.*

Wright, C. F., Fitzpatrick, D. R., & Firth, H. V. (2018). Paediatric genomics: Diagnosing rare disease in children. *Nature Reviews Genetics, 19,* 253–268.

Xie, F., Chan, J., & Ma, R. C. W. (2018). Precision medicine in diabetes prevention, classification and management. *Journal of Diabetes Investigation, 9*(5), 998–1015. https://doi.org/10.1111/jdi.12830.

Zipper, J., & Sevenhuijsen, S. (1987). Surrogacy and feminist notions of motherhood. In M. Stanworth (Ed.), *Reproductive technologies: Gender, motherhood and medicine* (pp. 118–138). University of Minnesota Press.

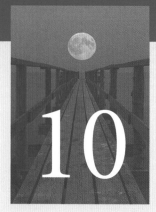

10 SAFEGUARDING PATIENT RIGHTS

LEARNING OBJECTIVES

The purpose of this chapter is to enable you to understand:

- The rights of patients and the corresponding obligations of health care professionals
- A patient's right to information, respect, and to be treated with dignity
- A person's right to be treated without prejudice or discrimination
- The unique needs of those most vulnerable and their right to protection
- A person's right to privacy and confidentiality and the conditions under which disclosure is permitted
- A patient's right to safe care within the health care environment

INTRODUCTION

A *right* is a claim or privilege to which one is justly entitled, either legally or morally. Persons in Canada have rights guaranteed under the *Canadian Charter of Rights and Freedoms* (1982, s. 2). Persons using Canada's health care system have specific legal rights to privacy and confidentiality, to an informed consent, to establish an advance directive, and to identify a substitute decision maker. Further, they have moral rights to be treated with dignity and respect without discrimination, to be told the truth, to receive safe care, and to choose the extent to which family members are engaged in their care. Competent persons have the legal and moral right to refuse treatment (or to request that it be withdrawn), and to die with dignity. Frequently, there is an interplay between moral and legal rights.

When an individual has a right, then others have an obligation to ensure that right is protected. These obligations are clearly expressed in nursing codes of ethics and in many health care settings through the posting of a patient rights and responsibilities framework or through their mission statement and values. Frequently expressed in an organizational code of ethics, these standards impose an obligation on health care professionals to provide a minimum standard of respectful, safe, and competent care.

Rights also come with responsibilities. Patients have moral responsibilities to themselves, the professionals caring for them, and the health care organization, which includes treating others with respect, respecting the privacy of other persons receiving care, and disclosing information necessary for their own care. Though patients have a right to safe health care, that right cannot be guaranteed if they fail to disclose information relevant to that care.

In this chapter, the relationship between rights and obligations is clarified, and the important rights of patients within the health care system are clarified. The rights of those most vulnerable, specifically older persons, the Two-Spirit, Lesbian, Gay, Bisexual, Transgender, Queer, Intersex, Plus (2SLGBTQI+) communities, and the Indigenous peoples in Canada will be highlighted.

302

WHAT ARE RIGHTS AND OBLIGATIONS?

Rights

Though they may overlap, rights fall into three major categories: human rights, legal rights, and moral rights.

Human Rights

Human rights are rights that all people across the globe should expect. In 1948, the United Nations created the Universal Declaration of Human Rights (UDHR) as a standard for nations worldwide. It asserts the following:

> Human rights are rights inherent to all human beings, regardless of race, sex, nationality, ethnicity, language, religion, or any other status. Human rights include the right to life and liberty, freedom from slavery and torture, freedom of opinion and expression, the right to work and education . . . Everyone is entitled to these rights without discrimination. (United Nations, n.d.)

These rights are frequently established by individual countries in their laws, and through their constitutions, statutes, and international treaties. How governments protect these rights varies across the world.

Legal Rights

Legal rights are those privileges, liberties, or protections granted through legislation to persons within a specific country, usually based on what is considered the common good. They can change over time or be repealed. Legal rights make explicit an individual's claim to such entitlement. For example, one explicit right under the Charter is the freedom of persons to think, say, write, or otherwise act in accordance with their beliefs (Canadian Charter of Rights and Freedoms, 1982, s. 2). This legal right is based on the moral right to autonomy, or the right to act on one's own, free of interference or control by the state or others. However, this right is not absolute. Laws also regulate the behaviour of citizens, and there are limits to the freedom of persons to do as they please. With individual freedom comes a responsibility to others. That is, there are reasonable limits on individual rights relative to the collective good of society. For example, during the COVID-19 pandemic, this collective good to protect society led to lockdowns and

mask mandates. Those who refused to comply with these requirements risked fines and potentially more serious legal consequences. In some settings, including health care settings, vaccine mandates were imposed. Individuals were free to choose not to comply with vaccine mandates, but with this choice came consequences that limited their mobility and employment status. The UDHR, while strongly advocating for human rights, upholds reasonable limits on individual freedoms and individual responsibility to others (United Nations, 1948).

The rights of patients in a publicly funded health care system are clearly stated in the *Canada Health Act* (1985). The primary objective of this federal legislation is to ensure publicly funded health care has the ability "to protect, promote and restore the physical and mental well-being of residents of Canada and to facilitate reasonable access to health services without financial or other barriers" (*Canada Health Act*, 1985, s. 3). The Act's main objective is to ensure that all eligible residents of Canada have reasonable access to health services on a prepaid basis, without direct charges at the point of service for such care. Since rights carry corresponding obligations, in this context the state has the corresponding obligation to provide that care. Otherwise, the right becomes meaningless.

Legal rights can be enforced by individuals through court action—that is, through the coercive power of the state to compel individuals, organizations, or the state itself to act or refrain from acting in particular ways. Chapter 4 describes the basic legal and political rights and freedoms held by Canadians under the Charter, and federal and provincial/territorial legislation.

There are special rights granted to the Indigenous peoples in Canada. These are enshrined in legislation, the Constitution, and the treaties and agreements entered between Canada and the First Nations, Inuit, and Métis.

Moral Rights

Moral rights are those that all humans should expect and are based on what is considered just and good within a society. They are not all formally recognized in law, but they are acknowledged as the societal norms and values within a culture. Moral rights are frequently the foundation of human rights and legal rights.

For example, in health care it has been generally accepted practice that one ought to respect a person's moral right to autonomy, privacy, and confidentiality. These rights are now established in law. Historically within health care there were protocols regarding confidentiality and the privacy of health care information. Now this right is embedded in legislation, and there are consequences if it is breached.

Moral rights evolve from ethical principles and values. In health care they are frequently based on the principles of autonomy, beneficence, justice, and nonmaleficence (as discussed in Chapter 2). In the health care setting, these rights are enforced, not necessarily through the courts but through practice standards and the ethical values and codes of ethics of the profession. However, if necessary, these rights could be enforced through court action in civil negligence or criminal proceedings, should their breach bring harm to the patient.

However, not even moral rights are absolute. Though people have the right to choose the direction of their own health care, these choices have limits. For example, when a patient with coronary artery disease wishes to have cardiac surgery versus a less invasive and safer angioplasty that is known to have better outcomes, the patient may find it hard to secure a willing clinician.

Obligations

As noted, rights carry corresponding obligations for others to protect those rights. An **obligation** is anything that a person must do, or refrain from doing, to permit the full exercise of the rights of another. For example, for a patient to exercise the right to give informed consent, the health care professional charged with that person's care is obliged to ensure that all relevant information has been provided, that the patient has been told of all relevant material risks and consequences inherent in the procedure, and that the patient's questions and concerns have been answered to the best of the health care professional's ability.

Nurses have these obligations. As they fulfill their responsibilities, nurses advocate on behalf of their patients, especially those who are unable to act or speak on their own behalf. If patients have the moral right to be treated with dignity, then nurses have the obligation to provide care that corresponds to that expectation. If patients have the right to competent care, then nurses

must observe all applicable standards of practice and are obliged to be current with the latest developments in their area of practice.

Significant Rights in Health Care

Respect and Dignity

Moral rights include the right to be treated with dignity. Dignity can be described as the relationship between one's sense of self and the respect given to them by others.

Health care professionals have an obligation to treat all patients with respect and dignity and to treat them as persons in their own right. Nurses respect the dignity of others when they treat them as worthy persons, especially when they are most vulnerable (Haddock, 1996). In other words, treating patients as human beings worthy of respect—or "as persons of moral value". Respect also includes the right to be treated courteously, to privacy, and to be addressed by one's preferred name or title, with the corresponding obligation of health care providers to introduce themselves by name to those in their care. It is important for nurses to listen carefully, to focus on patients' perceptions and needs, and to respect their culture, religion, values, and relationships with friends and family. For example, talking about patients without engaging them, as if they were not present, diminishes their humanity and is disrespectful, even in situations where the patient is not in a conscious state or is cognitively impaired.

Nurses who fail to keep patients as the focus of their care violate their ethical responsibilities. It is important to remember that there is more to the very ill person in the critical care unit (CCU) or the older person with cognitive impairment in a long-term care setting. They have a story, a history, family, and friends who care for them. Simply put, nurses should treat all patients as they would want to be treated. We would all want to maintain our independence and integrity of self if possible and in all circumstances. Certain aspects of the right to respect finds formal recognition in the law. For example, all patients have the right to equal access to health care resources and facilities without regard to gender, colour, mental or physical disabilities, ethnicity, creed, or religion. These rights are enshrined in provincial and territorial human rights codes and in the *Canadian Charter of Rights and Freedoms.*

Informed Consent

In the health care context, patients not only have the moral right to the information they need for the purposes of granting or refusing informed consent, but also have the right to more general information as to what the facility and its caregivers can and cannot do. This information would also include educational material about their condition, access to reliable resources, role descriptions of the health professionals involved in their care, the proposed treatment plan, and the plan of care after discharge. Of course, this also includes the patient's right to refuse or otherwise control the information provided.

The right to informed consent was discussed at length in Chapter 6. This is not only a legal right but also a moral right based on the ethical principles of autonomy, individual respect, respect for self-determination, and the right of individuals to make decisions about the course of their lives. To exercise these rights, patients must be fully informed about their health condition, prognosis, and treatment options, together with the consequences and risks of acting or not acting. Lack of information, or the giving of incorrect or insufficient information, deprives the patient of the right to make a truly informed decision about the course of treatment. Patients or their substitute decision makers also have the responsibility to disclose information relevant to the decision and to ask questions and seek clarification as necessary. As discussed in previous chapters, the provision of treatment without fully informed consent can lead to legal liability for negligence—even battery, if no consent was given.

CASE SCENARIO 10.1

A LEARNER'S RIGHT?

M. P. has consented to have vaginal polyps removed. Her gynecologist has explained the procedure in detail. M. P. is also aware that while under anaesthesia, she will undergo a thorough pelvic examination. However, the gynecologist has not told her specifically that there will be nursing and medical students present during the procedure. This is a teaching hospital, and all patients are expected to be informed, when they are admitted, of the role of students.

Third-year medical students are present during M. P.'s procedure. To give them experience in conducting pelvic examinations, the gynecologist allows three of them to undertake separate examinations. The circulating nurse expresses concerns about this to the gynecologist, who claims that M. P. has consented to the examination and that there is nothing wrong with giving the students some experience. How else are they going to learn?

Issues

1. Who do you agree with?
2. In the circumstances, is M. P.'s consent to this examination legally and morally valid?
3. Were any of M. P.'s rights violated?
4. What action should the circulating nurse take?
5. What is the hospital's responsibility?

6. How may appropriate learning experiences for students be ensured?

Discussion

Chapter 6 explores the elements and aspects of a truly informed consent.

As part of the obligation to provide general information, the health care team should provide to the patient, upon admission to a health care facility, an orientation to the roles of the health care team, their functions, the physical layout of the unit, and the unit's routines, procedures, and schedules. This orientation should include information about promoting health and preventing disease.

In the case of teaching hospitals, patients should be made aware of the role of students within the facility and the nature of their relationships within the health care team. However, a general overview of the involvement of students (e.g., interns, residents, student nurses) does not fulfill the additional obligation to provide more explicit information in particular circumstances in which the patient may be at greater risk (e.g., a medical student performing thoracentesis for the first time or a nursing student establishing their first intravenous line) or the invasion of privacy when students are present during a

Continued on following page

CASE SCENARIO 10.1 *(Continued)*

(vaginal examination). For example, patients should be informed when surgical residents are to play a primary role during an operative procedure. In our case scenario, the gynecologist had an obligation to

inform this patient and to obtain consent to allow the students this learning opportunity. Teaching settings should ensure that processes are in place to meet this obligation.

Access to Health Information and Teaching

Nurses throughout the system are expected to facilitate smooth, safe, effective transitions across the continuum of care for the patient and family (e.g., nursing standards require nurses to inform patients of community resources). Furthermore, nurses are expected to provide patients with the knowledge and skills to care for themselves (to the extent that they are able) prior to discharge. This is a significant component of safe care. When patients are not able to provide self-care, they may choose to have family members or friends involved. This knowledge might include information about nutrition, the proper use and maintenance of medical equipment, or the proper administration of medication and how to seek further information from reliable sources.

Knowledge about how persons gain access to the health care system is invaluable. Nurses contribute by providing education about the workings of the system, providing information on treatment alternatives and facilities, responding to requests regarding alternatives or complements to traditional health care, and so forth. When the patient is incompetent, the nurse should discuss these matters with the family or substitute decision maker(s).

Patients have the right to know and understand their diagnosis. A challenge for nurses occurs when patients ask them about their diagnosis prior to the diagnosis being disclosed by the physician. In such a situation, nurses must proceed carefully. In Ontario, for example, under the *Regulated Health Professions Act, 1991* (s. 27(2), p. 1), "communicating to the individual or his or her personal representative a diagnosis identifying a disease or disorder as the cause of symptoms ... in circumstances in which it is reasonably foreseeable that the individual or his or her personal representative will rely on the diagnosis" is a **controlled act** specifically restricted to physicians and nurse practitioners. A nurse would be permitted to

make a diagnosis according to the rules and regulations governing the delegation of controlled acts only if authorized to do so under the *Nursing Act, 1991*, as the holder of an extended certificate in primary health, pediatrics, adult care, and anaesthesia (*Expanded Nursing Services for Patients Act, 1997*). Other provinces may or may not legally restrict the making of a diagnosis, for example, in their medical professional statutes.

In most cases, while responding to such questions, the nurse need not communicate the diagnosis but simply confirm that which is self-evident to the patient. For example, suppose that a female patient was previously told that she may have breast cancer. Surgery is performed to explore the extent of the tumour and to remove it, if necessary. The patient, once awake in the post-anaesthesia care area, asks the attending nurse whether a tumour was found and whether any of her breast tissue was removed. She already feels some pain from the incision and knows that her breast does not feel right. The patient's physician has left for the day without having had a chance to speak with her about the results of the surgery. Should the patient be left in limbo while awaiting the physician's return? To ease the patient anxiety, the nurse, while exercising professional judgement, could properly confirm the patient's suspicions that more extensive surgery other than a biopsy was undertaken, while reassuring her that the surgeon would explain the rationale and the biopsy results as soon as possible. The nurse should be prudent, exercise judgement, and consider all the alternatives, including paging the physician to return to discuss the situation with the patient.

Ethical challenges for nurses arise when physicians fail to communicate a diagnosis to a patient, for example, to protect the patient from emotional harm. In this circumstance, if nurses are aware of the diagnosis, if asked, should they share this with the patient? In such a case, nurses, as a patient advocate, should stress to the physician the patient's right to be informed.

If this approach is not effective, the nurse may have to turn to the physician's superiors or higher authorities in the health care facility.

Advance Directives

Advance directives, including "no cardiopulmonary resuscitation (CPR)" decisions, are discussed in Chapter 8. In the last few decades, the documentation of do not resuscitate (DNR) decisions have become standard in health care settings. These documents provide clear instructions to the team in the event of a sudden cardiac arrest. These documents can accompany a person being transferred between settings, such as from a hospital to a long-term care setting. Even though persons may state their wish to have CPR in such a directive, ethically there is debate as to whether the team is obliged to proceed with CPR when it is clear that CPR would not be appropriate and would be futile (Kon et al., 2016; Luce, 1995; Weijer et al., 1998). If it is determined that CPR would be futile, there is an obligation to communicate this to the patient or family if the patient is incapable.

Special challenges occur in the community where individuals on the scene may not be aware of a person's wishes and proceed with CPR during an emergency situation. There are particular struggles for first responders whose main purpose is to perform life-saving interventions in an emergency and to stabilize the person prior to transfer to hospital. There have been challenges in circumstances where a person has chosen to receive palliative care at home and does not wish CPR. Frequently, family members call for help when their family member experiences distressing symptoms, such as severe pain or shortness of breath. In the past, the policy has been that first responders cannot follow an advance directive in these circumstances without a clear understanding of the person's end-of-life plan. To address this concern, some provinces (Ontario, British Columbia, and Nova Scotia) have introduced a process to ensure that the patient's or the family's wish not to have CPR is understood, documented, and communicated to first responders (BC Emergency Health Services, n.d.; Emergency Health Services Branch, Ontario Ministry of Health and Long-Term Care, 2007, 2017; End of Life Planning Canada, 2016). In Ontario, a medical directive, signed by a physician or nurse practitioner, confirms the existence of a signed DNR order and is accepted by emergency responders. This process also allows paramedics to provide palliative care, for example, pain management and oxygen administration for shortness of breath, thus supporting a peaceful death without CPR. These processes are important in eliminating any confusion and misunderstanding and in avoiding additional distress for the patient, the family, and the first responders (Trottier, 2015). Consider Case Scenario 10.2.

CASE SCENARIO 10.2

A DIGNIFIED DEATH—WHOSE CHOICE?

G. V., 18 years of age, is dying of lymphoma and has expressed a wish to die at home. All aggressive treatments attempted so far have failed, and for the past few weeks, G. V. has been receiving palliative care at home.

One night, G. V. experiences sudden shortness of breath, and the family responds by calling 911. By the time the ambulance team arrives, G. V.'s condition has stabilized, but the attendants insist that G. V. be taken to the closest emergency department. G. V. is admitted to a medical unit while the physician on call attempts to locate the primary physician.

Meanwhile, two of the nurses notice that G. V. has stopped breathing. The nurses, aware of G. V.'s history, are faced with a dilemma. The family is outside in the waiting room, and since the nurses have not heard from the primary physician, they do not have a no-CPR order. They have two choices: they can call a code and perform CPR, or they can invite the family into the room and give them some privacy.

Issues

1. What are G. V.'s rights in this situation?
2. How would the policy in your institution (if applicable) guide you in this scenario?
3. What is the role of policy in assisting nurses to make the right decision?
4. What is the right decision in this case, legally and ethically?

Continued on following page

CASE SCENARIO 10.2 *(Continued)*

Discussion

A distinction should be made between "no CPR" and "DNR." The latter is a broader concept that includes any treatment given to sustain life (e.g., blood transfusion, artificial ventilation, dialysis, antibiotic therapy). CPR is limited to the technique of compressing the patient's chest without applying artificial ventilation. It is important to carefully document the precise nature of the patient's wishes (or those of the substitute decision maker) in this respect. The order withholding CPR in no way limits the administration of other treatments to which the patient has not denied consent.

Some caregivers may feel that honouring the patient's wishes regarding resuscitation conflicts with the principles of beneficence and nonmaleficence—that is, to promote the patient's well-being and prevent harm. Certain guidelines have been developed to resolve such conflicts. These guidelines are like those followed in other treatment situations and outlined, for example, in Saskatchewan's *Health Care Directives and Substitute Health Care Decision Makers Act* (1997) and Ontario's *Substitute Decisions Act, 1992*.

In a situation like this, first, the patient should be assessed to determine whether CPR would be effective in prolonging life with a quality acceptable to the patient. When possible, the results of the assessment should be disclosed to the patient, whose wishes should be obtained and respected. The course of action to be followed, and any discussions held among caregivers, the patient, and the patient's family with respect to

the decision, should be carefully documented in the patient's chart. Furthermore, the reasons for the decision should be documented and communicated directly to the health care team. The no-CPR decision should be reviewed at regular intervals decided by the decision maker, either the patient or their substitute. It should also be communicated to the health care team of any other unit to which the patient is subsequently transferred.

In cases in which patients are incompetent, their advance directive should be respected, subject to any changes expressed by the patient after making it. Such changes should be documented and made known to the attending physician. If there is no advance directive and no substitute decision maker has been appointed, the decision to implement or withhold CPR will be made by others on the basis of their knowledge of the patient's values and wishes.

In this case scenario, the information available to the nurses indicates that G. V. and the family had accepted that death was imminent. They chose a course of action inconsistent with aggressive medical intervention. Clearly, G. V. had chosen to die at home, surrounded by family and friends. In the absence of a written directive, the expressed consent of the patient and family ought to be obtained, documented, and respected. Policies are meant to guide action. The application of Rigid "rules" to every circumstance may, in fact, contradict good judgement and conflict with individual choice.

Confidentiality

The confidentiality of a person's health information is considered a significant right. However, it is not absolute, and in some circumstances a patient's right to confidentiality may conflict with the health care professional's broader obligations to provide care to others and to prevent harm.

Statutory Duty of Disclosure

In many provinces, statute law establishes requirements or conditions for the disclosure of certain health information. For example, many public health laws

require health care professionals to disclose to their local medical officer of health (usually employed in the municipality by a local board of health or other such authority) the identity of anyone diagnosed with certain communicable or sexually transmitted infections (e.g., gonorrhoea and human immunodeficiency virus/acquired immunodeficiency syndrome [HIV/AIDS], among others). (See the Evolve site for a list of laws with respect to HIV/AIDS.) Such disclosures help prevent the potential spread of diseases that can be controlled to some extent. The virulence and seriousness of these illnesses are deemed sufficient to justify the infringement on the patient's right to confidentiality. For example, in Case Scenario 10.3, it would be unlawful for the physician at the clinic not to divulge the fact that Jim is HIV-positive (and may, in fact, have full-blown AIDS) to the local medical officer of health. Also during the COVID-19 pandemic, the reporting of positive tests was required to ensure tracking of patterns and rates of infection in order to develop public health guidelines and policy related to the appropriate management of the pandemic emergency.

CASE SCENARIO 10.3

CONFLICTING OBLIGATIONS

J. S. is a 34-year-old man who is well known to the community health centre that he and his family have attended for several years. He is married has two young children and his wife is now 8 months pregnant. He is a computer salesman and spends much time away from home meeting with clients across the country.

A few weeks ago, J. S. presented to the clinic complaining of generalized fatigue and lethargy. He had recently lost 5 kg of body weight and had noticed some unusual lesions on his inner thighs. As part of the blood screening done at that time, an HIV test was undertaken, but without his knowledge. The test turned out to be positive. Given his clinical picture, it was likely that AIDS had already developed.

J. S.'s primary care nurse is present when the physician relays the bad news to him. Clearly distraught, J. S. admits that he has had sexual encounters with several women during his business trips and, on several occasions, did not bother to use a condom. Fearful of the effects that this revelation would have on both his family and his business contacts, J. S. pleads with his caregivers to keep the diagnosis confidential. Given his wife's pregnancy, he feels this knowledge might cause her undue distress and harm. He assures them that he and his wife have not had intercourse since she became pregnant. He refuses any treatment for his AIDS-related symptoms because it would reveal the diagnosis to everyone. Instead, he asks that his family, including his wife, be told that he has terminal and incurable cancer. The physician (who is also his friend) is willing to go along with this for now.

Issues

1. Did the clinic have the right to test J. S. for HIV without his knowledge or consent?
2. Should the health care team keep J. S.'s diagnosis confidential from his wife?
3. Should the fact that Jim's wife is also the clinic's patient influence their actions and decisions?
4. Does the team have an obligation to follow J. S.'s instructions and misrepresent this diagnosis to others?
5. If the primary care nurse disagrees with the decision of the physician, what action can this nurse take?

Discussion

The patient has the right to know the extent of any assessments and tests that the agency is performing. In some provinces, public health laws require that a health care agency obtain consent for HIV testing.

The primary legal rule with respect to any information that the health care practitioner obtains from the patient during their professional relationship is that such information is confidential and may not be disclosed to anyone who has no valid purpose for requesting it. There are exceptions to this rule, both in common law and as provided by statute. But, as discussed in Chapter 5, in many provinces, the improper disclosure of confidential information about a patient constitutes professional misconduct.

For example, it may be necessary for one health care professional to share selected information contained in the patient's health records with another provider for consultative purposes. A health care practitioner who has become involved in a patient's treatment may need to know what treatment has been provided thus far and the progress of the patient's recovery. This is a normal part of obtaining a complete history, which the patient should expect upon being admitted to a health care facility. No specific consent need be obtained in such a case because it is clearly implied that all persons involved in the patient's treatment have a valid reason for reviewing that patient's records. Nevertheless, the patient always has the right to expect that any information

Continued on following page

CASE SCENARIO 10.3 *(Continued)*

divulged to a nurse or other health care practitioner will remain confidential until and unless another professional has a valid need for it.

In this scenario, the nurse and physician are faced with a decision that could compromise their professional relationship with J. S. They should provide support and allow J. S. time to digest and understand the situation, including why his wife should be informed. If he agrees, they can guide him in the process of disclosure. Since there is still the risk of harm to his wife and their unborn child, the team has a moral and professional obligation to inform her. Certainly, the clinic owes her an equal duty of care as she, too, is their patient.

The nurse should discuss these points carefully with the physician. If the physician still refuses to manage this situation as required, it would be appropriate for the nurse to appeal to the next level of authority until satisfied that action will be taken. The nurse should not simply let the matter drop. Furthermore, the nurse and the physician must disclose that they have a legal obligation to inform the local medical officer of health about this infection. This is required by law in all provinces and territories.

In *Pittman Estate v. Bain* (1994), the negligence of a family physician was considered in relation to his failure to disclose to a patient that he had been exposed to HIV-contaminated blood products during surgery. Dr. Bain had learned through the communicable disease network that his patient, Mr. Pittman, may have been exposed to an HIV-contaminated blood product he had received during heart surgery 4 years earlier. Dr. Bain believed that his patient was in poor health as a result of his heart condition, that he was depressed, and that he had a limited sexual relationship with his wife. He decided not to inform Mr. Pittman and not to ask him to be tested. It was subsequently discovered that, unfortunately, Mr. Pittman had AIDS and had infected his wife as well. Dr. Bain was sanctioned by the College of Physicians and Surgeons, and in a civil trial undertaken by Mrs. Pittman, he was found negligent. His failure to communicate the risk of AIDS to his patient fell below the duty of care he owed his patient and shortened Mr. Pittman's life. The court did not address any duty to notify Mrs. Pittman because it was satisfied that if Mr. Pittman had been informed, he would, in turn, have informed his wife.

Gunshot wounds and suspicions about child abuse are two other types of statutory obligations that require the disclosure of information about patients. However, the disclosure of confidential information should only occur where the obligation is clear. Referring to the policies of the agency, the regulatory college, and legal counsel is always advisable.

Similarly, there is a recognized exception to confidentiality where a person has knowledge of potential risk to others or the patient in the future. The duty to warn has been incorporated into the Ontario *Personal Health Information Protection Act, 2004*, which permits disclosure when it is "necessary for the purpose of eliminating or reducing a significant risk of serious bodily harm to a person or group of persons" (s. 40(1)). When a patient discloses an intention to hurt or kill another person, this remark may be a manifestation of a patient's illness; nevertheless, if the nurse forms the opinion, in good faith, that the patient poses "a signifi-

cant risk of serious bodily harm" to a person, then the nurse should report to the authorities in the institution and to the police.

Recently, the issue of the duty to warn was part of public discussion in relation to the case of former Ontario nurse, Elizabeth Wettlaufer. Wettlaufer killed and attempted to kill several older residents under her care. Wettlaufer was an inpatient at the Centre for Addiction and Mental Health (CAMH) in Toronto when she confessed her crimes to several people. She wrote a detailed list of her victims, which was passed on to the Toronto Police, and an investigation began. Subsequently, Wettlaufer was convicted and sentenced to life in prison (Lancaster, 2017).

Determining how to deal with information about a crime that is part of the personal health information of a patient is a complex process involving the balancing of the duty of confidentiality with concern for public safety.

DUTY OF CONFIDENTIALITY. Unless required by law, disclosure of personal health information without consent is inappropriate and can lead to civil liability, professional discipline, and employment issues. Under privacy legislation, such as Ontario's *Personal Health Information Protection Act, 2004* or Alberta's *Health Information Act* (2000), the person who is authorized to make decisions about disclosing personal health information is the "custodian/trustee" of the information—usually a privacy officer or manager. Nurses who are not custodians/trustees need to consult with the person who holds the position of custodian/trustee of personal health information in their organization before making any disclosure to the police.

EXCEPTIONS TO DUTY OF CONFIDENTIALITY. As mentioned, nurses who are not custodians/trustees of personal health information should consult the proper authority before relying on these exceptions. These exceptions include:

1. *Court orders:* These include search warrants or subpoenas, which are written orders issued by a judge. A warrant permits a search and seizure of the information detailed in the warrant. A *subpoena* is an order for a witness to attend a legal proceeding and to bring certain evidence with them.
2. *Public safety:* This is a reference to the duty to warn and the statutory equivalents. In the legislated versions of the duty, such as Ontario's *Personal Health Information Protection Act, 2004* or Alberta's *Health Information Act* (2000), the authority to disclose the personal health information belongs to the custodian/trustee and not the nurse unless the nurse has been appointed as the custodian/trustee as well. Determining whether the standard in the legislation is met, such as clear and imminent threat of serious bodily harm or death (Alberta's *Health Information Act*) is complex, and if there is time, the nurse should defer to the custodian/trustee and any relevant institutional policies.

In circumstances similar to that in the *Wettlaufer* case, nurses who become aware of a patient's confession to a crime should first consult their immediate supervisor and engage the custodian/trustee of personal health

information (or equivalent) about disclosing this information to the police. If the risk is immediate, the nurse would have to weigh the potential danger against the delay in consulting appropriately. Where the nurse had a "good faith" belief that the danger was imminent, then consideration should be given to informing the police immediately. The information disclosed should be limited to only what is necessary to address the imminent danger and should not include the person's whole health file.

The right to confidentiality may be limited in cases in which there is a legal obligation to disclose the information, such as in a health disciplinary hearing, a civil or criminal trial, or a coroner's or other government-authorized inquiry. In practice, however, most courts will not readily violate patient–professional confidentiality without a strong or compelling reason to do so.

If required by a court, the health care professional must answer all questions. Failure to do so would place the practitioner in danger of being found in contempt of court and liable to a heavy fine or possible imprisonment.

A patient's confession of prior illegal activity (e.g., use of illegal drugs) made to a health care professional, especially when related to their treatment, may not have to be disclosed (consider the exceptions discussed earlier). But it is possible that at some point, a court may compel the practitioner to disclose such a fact. The only professional who would be exempt from disclosing such facts would be a lawyer (yet, even a lawyer would have to guard against being an accessory to a patient's crime). Although the health care professional is under no obligation to aid the police, concealing the whereabouts of a fugitive could be construed as aiding and abetting such a person. This is especially likely in light of the *Criminal Code* offence of being an accessory to a crime after the fact (*Criminal Code,* 1985, s. 23(1)). One is an accessory when one, "knowing that a person has been a party to the offence, receives, comforts or assists that person for the purpose of enabling that person to escape" (*Criminal Code,* 1985, s. 23(1)). By not divulging the information, with the intent that the patient should avoid detection by the police, the health care practitioner may be subject to criminal charges.

Another instance in which provincial law requires disclosure is in cases of suspected child abuse. Many provinces have set up child abuse registries. The laws that establish these are intended to encourage the reporting of situations in which a child has been sexually or physically abused. Indeed, these laws require child care workers, physicians, nurses, and other health care professionals to report suspected cases of child abuse, either to the police or to the local Children's Aid Society (CAS) for further action. In most cases, it is an offence punishable by fine or imprisonment for a health care practitioner to fail to report an instance of suspected child abuse encountered during practice (see, for example, *Child, Youth and Family Services Act*, 2017, s. 125).

Abuse of residents of long-term care homes and retirement homes also must be reported. The law requires reporting by anyone who knows or has reasonable grounds to suspect that a resident has been, or might be, harmed (e.g., see Ontario's *Long-Term Care Homes Act, 2007*, s. 24; see also *Retirement Homes Act, 2010*). Similar legislation exists across Canada. This obligation includes family members of residents; staff and owners of long-term care homes; doctors, nurses, and other health care professionals under the *Regulated Health Professions Act, 1991;* drugless practitioners; and/or social workers. Professionals have a duty to report even if the report is based on information that is confidential or private.

In 2020, the obligation to disclose was applied on a large scale when military personnel issued a report detailing the neglect they observed while assisting in long-term care homes in Ontario during the COVID-19 pandemic. Some of their observations included failure to meet palliative care standards, aggressive behaviour toward the residents, and poor communication and care planning (Canadian Armed Forces, 4th Canadian Division Joint Task Force [Central], 2020).

Chapter 5 discusses the obligation of health care professionals to disclose incidents of sexual abuse of patients by other health care practitioners. Indeed, even in provinces that have no such explicit requirement with respect to abuse by health care professionals, such behaviour is a reportable criminal offence and constitutes professional misconduct.

Disclosure of Confidential Information in Court Testimony

There will be occasions, such as in a malpractice action or an inquest into a death, when the nurse must disclose information in court testimony. Most provincial nursing statutes and regulations permit such disclosure. However, even when lawfully disclosing patient information, the nurse should be prudent. Only those details that are relevant to the issues in the hearing, trial, or inquiry should be disclosed. The nurse should not give a "blanket" disclosure of all possible information, which may not be relevant to the issues under inquiry. The nurse must use discretion and common sense. Even when serving as a witness, a nurse may retain a lawyer to advise on what information may be disclosed and what information should remain private. This type of legal advice may be available from the employer, the union, or a professional liability insurer, such as the Canadian Nurses Protective Society (CNPS).

Ensuring Confidentiality in the Treatment Setting

Inadvertent disclosure of confidential information can occur in casual conversations with colleagues, friends, or relatives who have no valid right to such details. Therefore, nurses must always take care not to divulge confidential patient information when engaged in casual conversation in social settings unconnected to their work and duties.

Likewise, the old saying "the walls have ears" applies to hospitals and other health care facilities. For example, care should be taken when discussing details of a patient's condition in hallways, stairways, and elevators. There are other instances in which confidential information may inadvertently be disclosed, such as when a patient is being seen by a nurse in an emergency department in the presence of other people. The best way to address such a situation is by simply closing a door or drawing a curtain around the patient's bed and speaking in a low voice.

Legal Protection of the Patient's Right to the Privacy of Health Information

Canada is an open society where concepts and issues that were once taboo (e.g., sex and issues of sexuality, euthanasia, and the right to die with dignity) are publicly addressed. Along with this openness, and the fast pace of technological advances, there has been an increase in society's expectations with respect to the protection and promotion of personal privacy, especially in matters of personal health and finances. In response, all provinces and territories have passed privacy legislation to protect individuals' rights to control the disclosure of such information.

Most provinces have enacted legislation regulating access to personal health information. See, for example, Alberta's *Freedom of Information and Protection of Privacy Act* (2000); British Columbia's *Personal Information Protection Act* (2003); Manitoba's *Personal Health Information Act* (C.C.S.M., c. P-33.5); Newfoundland and Labrador's *Personal Health Information Act* (2008); Ontario's *Personal Health Information Protection Act, 2004*; and Saskatchewan's *Health Information Protection Act* (1999). In general, these statutes focus on the rules for the collection and disclosure of personal health information to protect the privacy and confidentiality of individuals, while ensuring the effective provision of health care (*Personal Health Information Protection Act, 2004*, s. 1(a)).

Such statutes generally make it an offence to disclose any personal health information about an individual without that person's written or implied consent.

The range of what is considered "health information" is broad and should be carefully considered by nurses in possession of any personal information about a person in their care.

Under Ontario's Act, a health information custodian (usually the management of the health care institution) is responsible for protecting the privacy, accuracy, and confidentiality of personal health information and must have appropriate policies and practices. Nurses must follow their agencies' policies concerning the compiling, storage, use, retention, sharing, and disclosure of such information. Violation of privacy can be grounds for termination of employment.

The disclosure of health information can only be done legally with either the express or the implied consent of the person to whom the information pertains. *Express consent* must be made by that specific individual, must be an informed consent, and must not be obtained through fraud, deception, or coercion. *Implied consent* would include situations in which a health care professional involved in the person's care discloses health information about that patient to another professional who is part of the health care team (or "circle of care") treating the patient. For example, consent would be implied by a patient for a nurse to disclose treatment orders to a physician who is consulted by the patient's treating physician or to other nurses involved in the patient's care. Where the disclosure is to be made to a non–health care professional, however, the patient must give express and informed, or "knowledgeable," consent. It cannot be implied. A patient's consent is considered knowledgeable when the patient knows the reason the information is being collected or disclosed, the specific information being sought, and that they can give or withhold consent. Consent can be given conditionally, for example, if information is to be disclosed only in the case of certain events or circumstances.

In the absence of consent, there must be legal authority for the disclosure referenced in the applicable privacy legislation that allows for disclosure in the absence of consent. The police may approach health care providers for information obtained while providing health care, which the police believe is relevant to an investigation. With reference to police requests for information, the authority to disclose confidential health information about an individual is usually based on a court order, warrant, or subpoena in a criminal proceeding, which the legislation recognizes as an authorized disclosure without consent.

Privacy Breaches

When nurses access information about a patient that they are not entitled to—that is, when they access information about a person when they are not part of that person's circle of care—they can face serious consequences, including discipline and termination of employment. Such terminations have been considered appropriate by many arbitrators, who have cited the seriousness of deliberate breaches of patient privacy. Such breaches fail to comply with privacy laws and constitute professional misconduct. See, for example, the discipline decision, *College of Nurses of Ontario v. Brutzki* (2016), where the staff member was found to have committed professional misconduct by improperly accessing 24 electronic records on 29 occasions. She was suspended for 2 months, reprimanded, and ordered to undergo additional training. She was also terminated by her employer after 13 years of service.

In *North Bay Health Centre v. Ontario Nurses' Association* (2012), an experienced nurse with a good record was terminated for accessing 5,804 patient records and making over 12,000 inappropriate inquiries over a 7-year period. In *Timmins & District Hospital v. O.N.A. (Peever)* (2011), a nurse with 22 years of experience accessed the mental health records of a patient who was her son's former partner and involved in a child custody dispute with him. The nurse was terminated from her position. The arbitrator concluded, "[I]n practicing his or her profession, a registered nurse is ethically bound to respect and ensure the confidentiality and privacy of patients' health care information as a fundamental, internalized precept of the exercise of all professional duties and responsibilities. That being the case, the grievor, a registered nurse, cannot have been unaware that in accessing the patient's health care information . . . she was violating her Code of Ethics." However, in *Vancouver Coastal Health Authority v. Health Sciences Association of British Columbia* (2014), citing mitigating circumstances related to extreme stress in the nurse's life, an arbitrator substituted a 3-month unpaid suspension for termination. The number of records accessed, the reasons for accessing them, the use made of the information, the remorse expressed, and the experience and employment history of the nurse are all factors that have been considered in disciplining nurses for breach of confidentiality. Sanctions include suspension from work for several months or termination of employment.

There are further potential legal consequences of privacy breaches, as illustrated in a case involving the Peterborough Regional Health Centre (PRHC; see *Hopkins et al. v. Kay et al.,* 2015). This case demonstrated that organizations can be held liable for significant civil damages, even when they take a zero-tolerance approach to privacy breaches and respond appropriately. In 2011, the PRHC terminated several employees who had inappropriately accessed the health information of up to 280 patients. The PRHC undertook a hospital-wide privacy education and awareness campaign, and, as required by Ontario's *Personal Health Information Protection Act, 2004* (PHIPA), notified the affected patients. The Information and Privacy Commissioner of Ontario conducted an investigation and found that the PRHC had "responded reasonably" and that "no further action was warranted." However, a group of affected patients launched a class action suit, seeking over $5 million in damages. The Ontario Court of Appeal held that it was permissible to bring a class action proceeding for civil damages, even though the Commissioner had already conducted an investigation under PHIPA (*Hopkins et al. v. Kay et al.,* 2015). The court reached this conclusion on the basis that the legal framework of PHIPA did not exclude the right to proceed against the hospital in negligence and tort. In June 2023, a proposed settlement was submitted to the court for approval that provided for PRHC to pay compensation of up to $988,000 ($650 per patient). PRHC Press Release June 15, 2023.

In a serious violation of privacy, employees of Rouge Valley Health System and Scarborough Hospital including an RN sold patient information about new mothers to a person interested in selling them Registered Education Savings Plans (RESPs). This situation led to charges under privacy legislation and the province's *Securities Act* (the salesperson was licensed under the securities legislation). The actions of the employees had violated the *Personal Information Protection and Electronic Documents Act* (2000). The employees were terminated for cause. The RN resigned her registration and was convicted criminally and sentenced to 6 months conditional, house arrest, probation and community service. (CNO V Cruz, 2017).

Inappropriate Use of Social Media

The impact of social media today is powerful and raises many ethical and legal issues and challenges. There are many positive aspects to social media, including the efficient and timely sharing of information and the ability to maintain relationships over wide geographical areas. During the COVID-19 pandemic, social media offered nurses the opportunity to share information regarding best practices, support one another, provide education to the public, and engage in advocacy related to the improvements necessary to manage the pandemic effectively (Glasdam et al., 2022; O'Leary et al., 2022). However, there are risks associated with the use of social media in relation to personal privacy. Other effects of social media are becoming apparent (Ngai et al., 2015). Easy access to Facebook, Twitter, and other social media puts employees at risk of unintentionally breaching patient confidentiality when uploading innocuous posts. Examples of potential breaches through social media include:

- Posting information about a patient—even if the person's name is not included, details may allow others to infer who the person is, especially if it is a media story
- Posting pictures of patients and families
- Discussing patients with other colleagues over social media, even if names are not included (Hicks, 2017)

The British Columbia College of Nurses and Midwives (BCCNM, 2022) has shared scenarios depicting social media privacy breaches and boundary violations that, though hypothetical, represent the types of complaints/reports it receives. The following is a summary of these scenarios:

- A pediatric nurse posted photographs and information about patients on Instagram and Facebook, and although the children were not named, they were identifiable to colleagues, other patients, and families. This nurse also maintained Facebook friendships with parents. The college's investigation found that this nurse failed to respect and maintain professional boundaries and was required to undertake remedial action, including education and sessions with the BCCNM's Regulatory Practice Consultant, and to disclose the investigation's findings to existing and future employers.
- A nurse working in a primary care setting was found to have breached professional boundaries by seeking out a patient on Facebook with the intent of establishing a personal relationship. The college imposed sanctions similar to those in the above scenario.
- A nurse in a small town posted disrespectful, derogatory, and unprofessional comments about patients whose life choices the nurse did not agree with. Again, no names were included, but given it was a small town, colleagues and others would have been able to identify the patients. In addition to the actions taken by the college in the above scenarios, this nurse received a 4-week suspension from the college.

Regulatory colleges take these breaches seriously, and the results of these actions can have consequences for the future careers of nurses who fail to respect persons' rights to privacy and confidentiality.

To protect employees from inadvertently breaching confidentiality and privacy rules, it is important that regular communication and education be provided by the employer. The Canadian Nurses Association (CNA) *Code of Ethics* (2017) addresses this issue to ensure that nurses always protect the privacy rights of their patients.

The College of Nurses of Ontario and the BCCNM are members of an international group of nursing regulators who have developed guidelines for social media. *Social Media Use: Common Expectations for Nurses* (International Nurse Regulator Collaborative, 2017) includes the "6 P's of Social Media Use":

- Professional—Act professionally at all times.
- Positive—Keep posts positive.
- Patient/Person-free—Keep posts patient and person free.
- Protect yourself—Protect your professionalism, your reputation, and yourself
- Privacy—Keep your personal and professional life separate; respect privacy of others.
- Pause before you post—Consider implications; avoid posting in haste or anger.

There are also risks when nurses post inappropriate or critical comments about their employer and other colleagues, as these comments may have a negative influence on public perception (Borden Ladner Gervais, 2018). In *Strom v. Saskatchewan Registered Nurses' Association* (2018), Strom, a nurse, appealed a fine imposed on her by her regulator for statements posted on social media. The nurse had posted critical comments about nursing and other health care professionals about the care a family member had received. Strom was found guilty of professional misconduct. The nursing regulator held that although Strom had a constitutional right to freedom of expression, she had failed to follow proper channels in making her complaints, had identified herself as a nurse while making her complaints, had used the title of nurse for private purposes, and had made her comments without having made sufficient effort to obtain complete information about the circumstances. She was fined and ordered to pay $25,000 in costs. The decision was set aside by the Saskatchewan Court of Appeal (*Strom v. Saskatchewan Registered Nurses' Association*, 2020). The Court of Appeal held that the regulator was obliged to consider the posts in context and did not recognize that many of Strom's comments were both critical and laudatory and intended to contribute to public awareness and discourse. There must be a link between the off-duty conduct and the profession that showed a sufficiently negative impact on the profession or the public interest.

Computer Records and Confidentiality

Many hospitals and other health care settings have introduced electronic health and employee records.

Consequently, there is wider access to information by a potentially greater number of people. Access in most cases is controlled by means of magnetized cards and passwords. It is important for nurses to use their own passwords and not to use others' means of access because the use of passwords and access cards is the nurse's electronic signature. Thus, if nurses were to share their access codes with another care provider, any action or documentation undertaken on the system would be attributed to the nurse who "owns" the code.

Many computer systems have a record of which person gained access to a particular patient's record. The date and time of such access will also be noted. Regular audits of access are carried out and improper access is often discovered in this way.

Personal Privacy

Not only does the right to privacy include the choice to keep information about oneself private from others—confidentiality—it also means freedom from intrusion and the right to be left alone. Freedom from intrusion—personal privacy—includes one's choice not to be observed by others, and this is applicable to the every-day practice of nursing and how care is provided. For example, when patients are bathing, they should be assured as much privacy as possible. This right extends to treatment situations and examinations. Thus, care should be taken when examining a patient to ensure that unauthorized persons are not present and that pictures only be taken with the patient's permission, even if done for educational purposes. If a room is fitted with mirrored windows, the curtains or blinds should be drawn unless students or other members of the team are observing in the adjacent room behind the window. If that is the case, this should be disclosed to the patient.

Discharge From Hospital

Competent patients have the right to leave the hospital. When this choice is against medical advice (AMA) and the team is unable to dissuade the patient, the patient must sign a waiver acknowledging the advice that leaving is not recommended at this time. If a competent patient refuses to sign the waiver, this should be carefully documented in the chart.

In cases involving a person with a mental illness, the mental health statutes of most provinces may permit such persons to be prevented from leaving if they pose a threat or danger to themselves or to others.

When patients are discharged, the hospital has an obligation to ensure that a plan is in place to ensure they arrive home safely. For example, in cases involving same-day surgery, a patient should not be sent home if the sedative has not worn off. Usually, prior to such surgery, patients are required to arrange for someone to transport them home or be prepared to take a taxi. In many hospitals and health care agencies, patients who have been sedated are required to wait for a specified period and to be accompanied by another person when they leave the institution.

There are instances where patients have been discharged prematurely. An inquest was held into the death of a 68-year-old woman in Manitoba, Heather Brenan, who collapsed in the doorway of her house after being sent home via taxi at 2235 in the evening (Re Brenan, 2015). She had spent 3 days in the emergency department, having presented with several health concerns and was not admitted to an inpatient unit. After being discovered in her doorway, she was resuscitated, transferred to the critical care unit, but died the following morning. The cause of Brenan's death was a pulmonary embolus. A component of the inquest's mandate was "to examine the hospital policy regarding the discharge of patients at night, particularly those elderly, frail and who reside alone" (s. III(1)(b) p. 9).

At the time of Brenan's death, there was no safe discharge policy, though one was implemented after her death. Recommendations from this inquest included:

- The implementation of an Emergency Program Guideline for Safe Discharge in order to:
    - Provide better guidance and criteria for discharge planning
    - Ensure that patients are discharged only when it is safe and reasonable to do so
    - Assist the team in ensuring the discharge plan is appropriate and safe
- The need to maintain a culture of patient safety in the emergency department, regardless of the pressure to maintain patient flow
- The establishment of programs to ensure that compliance with these guidelines is monitored on a continuing basis (Re Brenan, pp. 106–108)

SPECIAL CONSIDERATION FOR THOSE MOST VULNERABLE

There are individuals and groups at greater risk for the abuse or disregard of their rights. It is important for nurses to be aware of these vulnerable populations to ensure that their rights are honoured and be prepared to advocate on their behalf in all contexts. Those at risk include older persons, members of 2SLGBTQI+ communities and Indigenous communities, and persons with a mental illness.

In 2015, the United Nations promulgated the 2030 Agenda for Sustainable Development, with the commitment to eliminate poverty in all its forms, end discrimination and exclusion, and reduce the inequalities and vulnerabilities that leave people behind and undermine the potential of individuals (United Nations, 2015).

The Rights of Older Persons

The United Nations pledge is relevant to older persons who are vulnerable to finding themselves discriminated against and shunned. The UN Convention on the Rights of Persons with Disabilities (CRPD) also applies to older persons, describing those with "... long-term physical, mental, intellectual or sensory impairments which in interaction with various barriers may hinder their full and effective participation in society on an equal basis with others" (United Nations, 2006, Art. 1).

Older persons, especially those with cognitive impairment, are at risk for disrespectful treatment, even when this is unintentional. Older persons have a life story and deserve to be treated in a manner that recognizes their contributions in life and acknowledges the wisdom they have acquired (Galik et al., 2009). The Indigenous peoples in Canada are admirable role models in this regard, as they recognize and value the wisdom and life story of their Elders.

Several themes have emerged in the literature regarding what is most important to older persons. Being treated with dignity is important to all age groups, but especially to older persons, because it enhances their sense of self and their well-being. This means being treated with respect and being recognized as persons who deserve to maintain their independence as much as and where possible. Dignity includes being allowed to participate in their own care and in any decision-making processes that are about them (Bayer et al., 2005). The complex issues of consent related to older persons are discussed in Chapter 6. The care requirements of older persons are often complex and challenging to meet in a system not always designed to effectively respond to their needs. Consider the structures and processes in long-term care settings where residents are awoken early to ensure everyone is present at the same time for breakfast in the dining room. This practice does not meet the needs of those who prefer to sleep longer and would choose a lighter breakfast later. There are changes in some settings where the care is more resident-centred and residents have more choices, including when to get up in the morning and when to eat (CBC, 2022).

Caring for older persons with cognitive impairment creates complex nursing care challenges. These persons require patience and understanding as their disease progresses, while nurses caring for them must also care for themselves and avoid or minimize moral distress. The ethical principles of beneficence, nonmaleficence, and an ethic of care are fundamental to providing quality nursing care to this vulnerable community. While providing care, nurses are encouraged to:

- Communicate in a way that will not cause distress, without making assumptions about a person's ability to communicate and comprehend
- Treat them with kindness and support, and
  - Maintain eye contact and direct one-on-one interaction
  - Be patient and offer assurance when they make mistakes or feel embarrassment
  - Ask clear and simple questions requiring yes or no answers to minimize confusion
  - Do not interrupt or argue
  - Engage in conversations in quiet spaces without distractions
  - Be in their world (McGilton, 2004)
- Establish a routine with a daily care plan
- Incorporate activities that also respond to the stress-reduction needs of the staff, such as listening to music or taking a walk
- Assess safety issues and avoid risk of injury due to disorientation or confusion
- Use best practices to manage responsive behaviours, anxiety, and anger (Cohen-Mansfield, 2001; Dupuis & Luh, 2005)
- Encourage time for the person to socialize with family and friends

Care in the Community

Many people want to stay in their home for as long as possible and choose how they live and how and where they die. Community resources are expanding to support older persons and persons with self-care challenges at home. Alternative options, such as integrated care communities and retirement facilities, are growing in number and provide a greater choice. There are larger challenges for older persons whose home is the street and for those with a long history of mental illness. Nurses in the community play a strong and significant role, not only in coordinating and providing their care but also in addressing their many other needs, such as maintenance of function and social support, for example, by listening and engaging in conversations with those who want to share their story. Nurses also play an important role in preventing social isolation, another issue during the COVID-19 pandemic, as older persons in the community were at a greater risk of being further marginalized.

A further contributor to social isolation in older persons occurs when they are excluded from engaging in social networks they identify with, partly due to unmet community mobility needs. Health equity is a consideration when describing the community needs of older persons. Their community mobility needs are influenced by a complex set of factors that are both external and internal. These factors represent the multifactorial interaction between the person and their environment. External factors include societal attitudes and environmental and structural factors such as access challenges, poor maintenance of sidewalks, and service availability, such as age-friendly public transport and snow clearing. Internal factors include finances, personal fear and apprehension, and personal functional limitations. Nurses practising in public health and in the community play an important role in identifying these factors and in lobbying and advocating for change on behalf of older persons living in the community (Biljon et al., 2022).

In response to the World Health Organization (WHO, 2018) launch of age-friendly cities and communities, there is a movement to create a similar approach to recognize enhancements that improve the lives of older persons within the health care system. These would create care and systems that encompass the living environment of older persons with a focus on the social determinants of health and a prevention-focused public health system (Fulmer et al., 2020).

Dignity and Respect in Long-Term Care

Long-term care homes provide the support of interprofessional teams that include dietitians, pharmacists, physiotherapists, occupational therapists, social workers, and recreational therapists, who focus on patients' social needs. In many settings, clinical nurse specialists and nurse practitioners (NPs) with a specialty in geriatrics are available for consultation and to help avoid emergency department visits as much as possible. Evidence is emerging that supports the value of having permanent NPs in clinical leadership and direct care roles in long-term care.

Older persons in long-term care can be particularly vulnerable, especially when there are inconsistencies and lack of continuity with the care provided to them. This is especially so for those with cognitive impairment who are not able to advocate for themselves. This is of greater concern when most staff providing direct care are unregulated care providers and when staffing ratios are high. Nurses must play an active role in monitoring the care that residents receive and in ensuring the appropriate supervision of unregulated care providers. They should be active in developing (in collaboration with the resident and family) an appropriate plan of care that is evaluated on an ongoing basis. They should also support and engage family members to share the advocacy and monitoring role. Essentially nurses must play a strong leadership role in these settings. For example, is it inappropriate to infantilize older persons by encouraging the use of adult incontinence products when other nursing interventions, such as regular toileting, can be used to manage incontinence? Is it respectful when the staff, or even family and friends, have personal conversations with each other while ignoring the older person?

Nurses should be aware of and respond when residents are not being treated with dignity and respect, which occurs in the following instances:

- They are addressed in a disrespectful manner, for example being called "Mamma" or "Pappa" instead of how they would like to be addressed. Older persons should be asked how they would prefer to be addressed.

- They are subjected to embarrassment and humiliation when denied privacy during toileting or bathing.
- They are left to die alone when their decline is not recognized, and the family is not informed in time.
- The care plan is not followed, and the person is put at risk as a result.
- There is inadequate pain management, especially when they are being mobilized. Many older persons have co-morbidities that cause pain such as arthritis, complications from previous fractures, and metastatic cancers.
- Visual aids are not used to communicate intended actions to a hearing-impaired person.
- A caregiver fails to introduce themselves when entering the room of a visually impaired person.
- The person is infantilized through the language used, such as use of the term *diaper* instead of *brief*.
- They are not given choices about or engaged in acts of daily living.
- Toileting protocols are not utilized to prevent or manage incontinence.
- Personal grooming is neglected, such as failing to shave a male resident on a regular basis.

Sleep Deprivation

When staffing resources are limited, there can be great pressure on the team to focus on tasks and getting things done on time, to the detriment of the resident. For example, in long-term care, residents' sleep may be disrupted by being woken up at an early hour because of a fixed breakfast time. Sleep complaints among patients in hospitals include insomnia, interrupted sleep, and difficulty maintaining sleep. Adequate sleep is considered a necessary component of healing and recovery; however, the environment of hospitals and long-term care homes are not conducive to this. These settings, especially hospitals, have high levels of ambient noise and light, which cause sleep disturbance as care is provided around-the-clock. The hospital and long-term care settings set sleep times arbitrarily, often based on the shift schedules of the staff. Nurses are also required to deliver care, such as assessments, delivery of medications, and so on to patients and residents during all hours of the day and night (Maggio et al., 2013; Missildine et al., 2010).

It is understood that cognition deteriorates in older persons because of many factors, including hormonal changes. These changes are influenced by various stressors, such as sleep deprivation (Maggio et al., 2013). Hospitals and long-term care facilities should take this into consideration and make structural changes to ensure that the sleep of an older person is not interrupted, especially because this can contribute to further deterioration in cognition. Ensuring an uninterrupted sleep could mitigate problems related to confusion and agitation, which can influence the quality of life and safety of older persons.

The Dilemma of Restraint Use

A significant ethical dilemma faced by nurses is the use of both physical and chemical restraints. Dilemmas arise relative to the conflict between autonomy and nonmaleficence, the person's right to choose freedom from restrictions versus the risk of harm associated with falls. The challenge is that the majority of the time, restraints are being considered in relation to persons who are not competent to appreciate the risks. Historically, physical restraints were frequently used in long-term care and hospital settings. They were not proven to be beneficial but were associated with many safety concerns as well as anxiety and stress for the person being restrained, and moral distress for the staff imposing them. Standards across the system now focus on least-restraint alternatives. Nurses' attitudes toward the use of physical restraints has been described as ambivalent, with concern and respect for a person's dignity on the one hand and anxiety and responsibility related to the resident's safety on the other. Nurses experience feelings of frustration and guilt when using physical restraints against a patient's will and primarily justify their decision based on the expected benefits related to the safety of the patient when they believe that the physical restraints will be effective in preventing falls or injuries. There is a strong relationship between the use of restraints and the dependency needs of the person, mobility limitations, cognitive impairment, and staff ratios (Hofmann et al., 2015; Möhler & Meyer, 2014; Möhler et al., 2012).

There is a difference when restraints are used for the purpose of managing wandering residents versus protecting persons with mobility issues who may not remember that their safety requires remaining in a wheelchair. More strategies need to be designed and implemented to manage these risks and to address the challenges nurses face in these circumstances. Alternatives, such as chair and bed alarms, are available but require timely attention, which is not always possible. Other options that focus on distraction, management of anxiety, and a physical infrastructure that facilitates observation are worth considering. The challenge is creating a plan that focuses on the least and safest restraint possible and that is individualized to the needs of each person, while balancing respect for the person's dignity and the principle of nonmaleficence and the individual's safety. Nurses need to balance the harms associated with the use of restraints versus, in some situations, no immediate harm to any person.

When there is no choice but to use a restraint, protocols related to the safe use of restraints, constant monitoring, and emotional support for the person should be strictly followed. Person-centred structures and processes that greatly value the persons and their needs should be in place.

Challenges in Long-Term Care Settings

COVID-19 exposed the suboptimal working conditions and approaches to care in long-term care settings. These challenges have existed for some time but were revealed to the broader population in Canada during the pandemic. During that period, the CNA delivered key messages regarding those living in long-term care, noting that even before the pandemic, long-term care residents had greater and more complex needs. The CNA identified that most residents were over 85 years of age, and that dementia was a major reason for moving to these settings. In spite of this complexity, there were fewer regulated nurses and other health disciplines working in long-term care, and the workload of those employed in these settings was unsustainable and unsafe for residents (CNA, 2020).

The COVID-19 pandemic compromised the care of these residents further and revealed many opportunities for improvement (Thompson et al., 2022).

The Role of Essential Family Members

In many settings—the home, hospital, and long-term care—key family members become primary caregivers and, in this role, provide a variety of important crucial care functions. An essential family member may participate in care delivery, simply be present, or be involved in planning and coordinating care. They are more able to articulate the needs and challenges of their family member and identify early changes in their condition. Vulnerable older persons and those with disabilities often receive support from family members prior to their transition to a care home setting. Frequently, family members continue to be engaged in care in the long-term care setting.

In long-term care settings, families play an important role as advocates by ensuring that the best interests of the residents are sought and maintained. This is especially important for persons with cognitive impairment, decreased function, and or multiple comorbidities. Resident safety is enhanced when family members effectively assist in caregiving and ongoing monitoring of care.

The meaningful engagement of a resident's family in care is essential to the provision of quality of care, and it ensures a person- and relationship-centred approach. Evidence-informed models of family- and person-centred care respect the knowledge and expertise that families contribute to the care and safety of those who are most vulnerable (Gallant et al., 2022).

Unfortunately, this evidence-informed approach was compromised early in the COVID-19 pandemic, with across-the-board visiting restrictions that failed to recognize the *essential* role that families play in ensuring the safety of those in long-term care settings (Johnston et al., 2022).

Across-the-board visiting restrictions added to the risks faced by some of the most vulnerable in Canadian society. Visiting restrictions, though necessary as an infection control measure to protect residents early in the pandemic, limited those persons most *essential* to the safety and well-being of residents in these settings—caring family members (Gallant et al., 2022; Johnston et al., 2022). Family members are not visitors, and an outright ban on family presence, rather than identifying an essential family partner, exposed residents to a greater risk of dying from COVID-19 and other complications associated with reductions in care. During this crisis, residents in long-term care were at a greater risk of falling, dehydration, skin breakdown, and acquiring infections other than

COVID-19. Residents were more predisposed to responsive behaviours, triggered by fear and anxiety, largely a result of social isolation and the lack of family presence. In one study by Chu et al. (2022), essential care partners described the trauma from prolonged powerlessness and helplessness, due to separation from their family member and the inability to provide care. They also described situations where they perceived a lack of compassion from staff and administrators, also experiencing great distress.

Residents in long-term care were disproportionally affected by the COVID-19 pandemic. During the first wave of the pandemic, 80% of COVID deaths across the Canadian population occurred in long-term care (Canadian Institute for Health Information, 2020). Other deaths in long-term care resulted from the consequences of being isolated from essential family members and the influence of a greater staff workload. These circumstances had a significant emotional and psychological impact on providers and families and demonstrated the need for more nursing expertise (Akhtar-Danesh et al., 2022; Jones, 2022).

Advance Planning

Older persons want to retain independent control over their lives for as long as possible. Nurses can help support them in thinking about their future needs and wishes (Vellani et al., 2022a, 2022b). Advance directives related to health care are as important as advance planning for their living needs while they remain in control and can make the choices that are important to them. Transitions might include moving to a more accessible home, such as a single-level house or a condo apartment, exploring potential retirement facilities or, depending on other needs, the most preferred long-term care facility (Calnan et al., 2005; McGilton et al., 2018; Stratton & Tadd, 2005).

The issue of advance directives regarding Medical Assistance in Dying (MAiD) is discussed in detail in Chapter 8. This is an important issue for older persons who may want to indicate in advance their wish to pursue this option, in circumstances where they become cognitively impaired and are no longer able to make such decisions.

Human Rights and Older Persons

Two human rights concerns that have gained prominence in recent years relate to ageism and elder abuse.

Ageism

Ageism can be defined as a way of treating older persons based on negative stereotypes and attitudes, resulting in a lack of sensitivity to their abilities and needs. Ageism focuses on the person's age versus their abilities and totally disregards their acquired wisdom and potential. It is a person's human right to be treated as an equal, regardless of age.

The *Ontario Human Rights Code,* section 1, prohibits age discrimination in employment, housing accommodation; goods, services, and facilities; and contracts and membership in trade and vocational associations. Age discrimination is often not taken as seriously as other forms of discrimination. However, it can have economic, social, and psychological impacts that are just as profound as any other form of discrimination (Ontario Human Rights Commission, n.d.-a). The *Canadian Charter of Rights and Freedoms* (1982), section 15, mandates equal treatment of all, before and under the law, without discrimination based on age. Age is a prohibited ground of discrimination in every province and territory, as well as at the federal level (Chun & Gallagher-Louisy, 2018).

Aging is a highly individual experience, so it is not possible to generalize about the skills and abilities of an older person. Human rights principles require individuals to be assessed on their own merits and abilities and not based on age, generalizations, and stereotypes. For example, a 77-year-old person might have serious medical issues, limited functional ability, and frailty, which would result in a higher risk of harm during surgery (Bethell et al., 2019). A strong, healthy 88-year-old with the ability to walk 10 km a day would be a strong candidate for even a complex surgical intervention.

The Supreme Court of Canada has recently made it clear that it is no longer acceptable to structure systems in a way that disregards the needs of all age groups and place a special focus on the young. Rather, the age diversity that exists in society should be reflected in the design stages of policies, programs, services, facilities, and so forth so that physical, attitudinal, and systemic barriers are not created (Ontario Human Rights Commission, n.d.-a).

Elder Abuse and Neglect

Older persons are entitled to respect and have the right to feel safe and secure. *Elder abuse* is defined as any action, by someone in a relationship of trust, resulting in harm or distress to an older person (Wong et al., 2020). It can be a single incident or a pattern of behaviour. Neglect is lack of action, which can result in physical, psychological, or financial harm (Government of Canada, 2012). This is now recognized as a significant problem, with studies demonstrating that 5% to 10% of older persons report such abuse (Acierno et al., 2010; Cooper et al., 2008). It is more prevalent among those who are cognitively impaired, socially isolated, and within complicated and dependent relationships with their abusers (Wang et al., 2015).

Elder abuse often occurs because the abuser is in a position of power and control over the older person. The aggressor can be a family member, friend, caregiver, or health care professional, and elder abuse occurs among people of all backgrounds and diversity. See, for example, *College of Nurses of Ontario v. Leclair* (2011), where a staff member was found to have abused her position as a caregiver for the patient. She had received numerous gifts from the patient during the time he was a resident and failed to maintain appropriate boundaries with the patient, had solicited gifts, and had an inappropriate relationship with him. She was held to have committed professional misconduct. In *Danilova v. Nikityuk* (2017), the court considered the relationship between a Russian couple who had immigrated to Canada and their parents who had joined them at a later date. The court found that after the relationship broke down, a situation of elder abuse had developed, and the Nikityuks had been deprived of their property and were physically and emotionally abused. Damages of nearly $400,000, including $25,000 in punitive damages, were awarded.

Nurses, especially those in the community or emergency departments, can play a strong role in assessing for elder abuse (Wang et al., 2015). They are able to observe symptoms or signs of abuse or neglect, which may include the following

- *fear, anxiety, depression or passiveness in relation to [the abuser];*
- *unexplained physical injuries [that may result in repeated visits to the emergency department];*
- *dehydration, poor nutrition or poor hygiene;*
- *Improper use of medication;*
- *confusion about new legal documents, such as a new will or a new mortgage;*

- *sudden drop in cash flow or financial holdings; and*
- *reluctance to speak about the situation. (Government of Canada, 2012)*

Psychological abuse of older persons includes actions that decrease their sense of self-worth and dignity and may include bullying behaviour, such as insults, threats, intimidation, and harassment. Other examples include keeping them isolated or treating them like children, as in the examples described earlier.

Financial abuse is the most common form of abuse and involves actions that decrease the financial worth of the person, for example, misusing or stealing an older person's assets, property, or money.

Neglect includes inactions that may result in harm to an older person and may include a caregiver or family member not providing food, shelter, and medications. Those most vulnerable are socially isolated and have complex health conditions.

Older persons, as with many victims of abuse, may feel ashamed or too embarrassed to tell anyone. They may fear retaliation or punishment, or they may have concerns about having to move from their home or community. They may also feel a sense of family loyalty. They may not know how to seek help. Nurses in the community and in family practice settings who have developed long-term trusting relationships are able to observe for concerns and to encourage dialogue (Wang et al., 2015).

In 2012, amendments to section 718.2 of the *Criminal Code* made it an "aggravating factor" influencing sentencing if there is "evidence that the offence had a significant impact on the victim, considering their age and other personal circumstances, including their health and financial situation." The effect of this change is that, in sentencing a person convicted of a *Criminal Code* offence, the court should impose a harsher sentence on the person when the victim's description falls within the wording of the legislation. This factor had already been considered by judges during sentencing, but the amendment imposed an obligation on judges to consider this factor (Echenberg & Kirkby, 2012).

2SLGBTQI+ Communities

Discrimination, even laws, against the 2SLGBTQI+ community exists across the globe. Even in Canada, before 1969, same-sex behaviours between consenting adults were considered crimes that resulted in imprisonment.

In 1996, the *Canadian Human Rights Act* was amended to specifically include sexual orientation as one of the prohibited grounds for discrimination, ensuring that individuals "make for themselves the lives that they are able and wish to have." (*Canadian Human Rights Act*, 1985, s. 2). The Act has been amended by the addition of "without being hindered in or prevented from doing so by discriminatory practices based on race, national or ethnic origin, colour, religion, age, sex, sexual orientation, gender identity or expression, marital status, family status, genetic characteristics, disability or conviction for an offence for which a pardon has been granted" (s. 2).

Within the *Canadian Charter of Rights and Freedoms* (1982), section 15 states that every individual is to be considered equal regardless of religion, race, national or ethnic origin, colour, sex, age, and mental or physical disability.

In 2000, Canada took the lead internationally with the introduction of Bill C-23, which gave same-sex couples the same social and tax benefits as heterosexuals in common-law relationships. Again, in 2005, the Canadian Parliament enacted the *Civil Marriage Act,* marking a milestone by allowing same-sex couples to be married anywhere in Canada (*Civil Marriage Act*, 2005).

All members of the 2SLGBTQI+ community are at risk of experiencing harassment and discrimination.

Nurses must understand the diverse expression of gender and sexuality in order to respond to their unique needs and ensure that their rights are respected within the health care system.

Gender identity, each person's internal experience of gender, is a person's sense of self as a woman, a man, both, or neither along the gender spectrum. A person's identity may be the same or different than that assigned at birth. *Gender expression* is how a person expresses their gender, including their behaviour, appearance, choice of name, and pronouns. A person's gender identity is not related to their sexual orientation.

Gender nonconforming persons do not follow gender stereotypes based on the sex they were assigned at birth and may or may not identify as trans.

Transgender is often used to refer to people who chose not to accept the more traditional conceptions of gender and identify with a gender other than the one assigned to them at birth. *Transgender* is sometimes used as an umbrella term to include transsexuals, drag queens and kings, some butch lesbians, and (heterosexual) male cross-dressers. The term *transsexual* applies to persons who self-identify and live as the sex "opposite" to the one assigned to them at birth. This would also include those who use hormonal and/or surgical interventions to alter their bodies to fit with their identified gender (Ontario Human Rights Commission, n.d.-b; Stanford Encyclopedia of Philosophy, 2014).

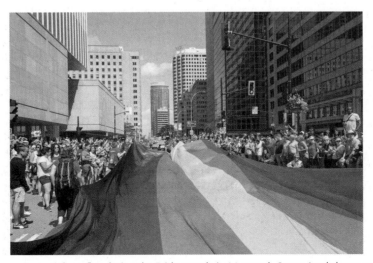

People holding a giant rainbow flag during the Pride parade in Montreal. *Source: istockphoto.com/Marc Bruxelle.*

The Unique Challenges of Transgender and Transsexual Persons

Transgender persons, who do not identify with the gender they were assigned at birth, and transsexual persons, who chose to alter their bodies to conform with their gender of choice, are at a particular risk of experiencing barriers to culturally and medically appropriate health care. These barriers may be socio-cultural, institutional, and financial because the treatments they need may not always be funded by the system. The physical and emotional transitioning process is complex and challenging, the person potentially choosing such treatments as hormone therapy or surgery. It is important that nurses acquire knowledge about the unique issues these individuals face and be sensitive to these complexities. Knowledgeable and sensitive nurses ensure that their care is safe, inclusive, and supportive. Nursing leaders and health care organizations should ensure that the systems and processes, such as building questions related to gender into nursing and health assessments, are in place to support the health care team and to ensure a better experience for the transgender person (Hein & Levitt, 2014).

To practise ethically, nurses must be sensitive to the unique needs of these patients in relation to privacy; access to washroom facilities; room assignments; and the need for a sensitive, welcoming environment. Co-gendering is becoming more common across the country, where males and females share the same room to facilitate the admission of patients when a room with a person of the same gender is not available.

Transsexual persons may require feminizing/masculinizing interventions or those for any other medical needs. As with any other patients, rather than making assumptions about their needs, it is important that nurses listen to what is most important to them and provide respectful, person-centred care. This includes asking them about preferred names or pronouns and mirroring their language when referring to themselves, their partners, and their bodies. It is important to learn from them who they are by hearing and understanding their stories (Lambda Legal, 2013).

To ensure that the ethical and legal rights of transgender persons are understood and respected, it is important that health care settings include education and awareness about the 2SLGBTQI+ community as a component of an ongoing education program, especially programs that focus on cultural sensitivity. As with all patients, the right care is person centred.

Respect for Differences

Considering the diversity of the Canadian population, it is imperative that nurses have the knowledge to provide culturally competent and culturally safe care. Whether in patients' homes or in the community, hospitals, or long-term care settings, nurses form professional relationships with patients from multiple backgrounds and cultures. They engage with people and communities who may live in and interpret their worlds in many ways (Arnold & Bruce, 2006).

Because individuals and groups use their basic beliefs and values to guide their actions (Andrews & Boyle, 2002), it is important for nurses to be aware of these to understand the culture within the context of health and illness. For many cultures, ethical decisions are grounded in both religious beliefs and cultural values. It is also important to be cautious about the assumptions that the dominant cultural values of Western society might impose on the various perspectives of other cultures (Andrews & Boyle, 2002). Various cultures view their reality or world from many different perspectives. This is known as a culture's **world view**, which is a comprehensive framework of basic beliefs and values that individuals, groups, and communities use to guide their actions (Uys & Smit, 1994). In a sense, it is the lens through which they interpret and clarify the reality of their everyday lives. Without an understanding that these various views exist, nurses and other team members may not be aware of these differences and therefore may not be able to address the needs of that patient and family. When the unique cultural perspectives of patients and families are not understood or addressed, those with different world views can be left feeling frustrated, dominated, and oppressed (Uys & Smit, 1994).

Box 10.1 provides illustrations of various world views, especially with respect to health care. They are offered as examples of how values and the interpretation of these values influence perspectives. These illustrations demonstrate the importance of undertaking individual cultural assessments because it is not possible for nurses to know the complexities of every culture. Through a cultural assessment, nurses can learn and understand the values and beliefs of each patient or family.

BOX 10.1
WORLD VIEWS: CULTURAL PERSPECTIVES

CHINESE HEALTH CARE CULTURE

Within the Chinese culture, holism and caring permeate every aspect of health care. Illness is viewed as a state of disharmony between the individual and the natural and social environment. Traditionalists believe that both caring and curative processes are necessary to enable the restorations of a person's harmony, and the way a person is cared for is important to a therapeutic climate. It is considered the moral duty of the family to provide care for family members who are unwell. The family is the basic social unit through which people learn appropriate ways of relating to others. How they treat one another within the family is an important indication of their integrity (Wong & Pang, 2000). Consider the following norms within traditional Chinese culture and how they might influence health care:

- Children are required to obey their parents, protect them, bear their burdens, and try their best to help them lead a good long life.
- Families (not the individual) take charge of treatment decisions.
- Family members accept a moral duty to take care of their sick relatives. This is grounded in the Confucian ethical system of role relationships.

INDIGENOUS COMMUNITIES

In Indigenous languages, there is no direct translation corresponding to the Western concept of *health*. Instead, there are the concepts of the individual living in harmony with nature and of a complex, dynamic process that has to do with social relationships, land, and the identity of the individual and their role within the community.

Through the oral tradition of Indigenous cultures, stories are passed across generations, enabling a transfer of cultural experiences that embed values and beliefs. These stories have major significance because they reflect the entire historical range of Indigenous human experience and provide an orientation to life and reality. They are often shared through fables that have animals as characters. Within the fables, metaphors are used to illustrate the values and norms of the culture and hence to influence thinking and ways of knowing and being.

Indigenous people traditionally view themselves in terms of "self in society" rather than "self and society." They place a stronger focus on the family and the community, which has implications for their views of informed consent and decision making regarding care. An individual would want to consult with family members or community Elders before making a decision regarding their course of treatment (Arnold & Bruce, 2006; Uys & Smit, 1994).

HINDUISM AND SIKHISM

Though unique in many ways, Hindu and Sikh cultures traditionally approach morality similarly, emphasizing duty over

rights. They also share a belief in rebirth (reincarnation) and the concept of karma, in which actions of past lives influence the experience of present and future lives. The fundamental idea of karma is that each person is repeatedly reborn so that the soul may be purified and ultimately join the divine cosmic consciousness. The moment of conception marks the rebirth of a fully developed person who has lived many previous lives.

Though different from one another in many respects, these cultures share values related to purity and have a holistic view of the person that affirms the importance of family, culture, the environment, and the spiritual dimensions of life (Coward & Sidhu, 2000). Both cultures share the belief that for each person, "birth and death are repeated in a continuous cycle" (Coward & Sidhu, 2000, p. 168). For example, in this belief system, the termination of a fetus would send that "soul" back into the karmic cycle of rebirth. This belief is significant, as it may influence decision making and the application of ethical principles in these circumstances. For instance, the issues that may challenge an expectant mother from a Western society may not be at play in these cultures, as they would be assured that the soul would have the opportunity for future rebirth. These beliefs would also influence views on end-of-life choices, such as withdrawal of treatment and Medical Assistance in Dying.

Questions for Discussion

1. How would these cultural differences influence your nursing practice? Should they influence practice?
2. What have you observed in practice when families from various cultures have views on consent that differ from the Canadian "norm"?
3. When a conflict of values exists and there are risks to the patient because of them, how should this conflict be resolved?

These scenarios are shared to provide some examples of the various cultural approaches/values related to health care. However, though a patient may be from one of these cultures, one should not assume that they share these perspectives. In all contexts, and as with all patients, nurses should undertake a cultural assessment to determine a patient's values, beliefs, and preferences.

Arnold, O. F., & Bruce, A. (2006). Nursing practice with Aboriginal communities: Expanding worldviews. *Nursing Science Quarterly, 18*(3), 259–263; Coward, H., & Sidhu, T. (2000). Bioethics for clinicians: 19. Hinduism and Sikhism. *Canadian Medical Association Journal, 163*(9), 1167–1170; Uys, L. R., & Smit, J. H. (1994). Writing a philosophy of nursing? *Journal of Advanced Nursing, 20*(2), 239–244; and Wong, T. K. S., & Pang, S. M. C. (2000). Holism and caring: Nursing in the Chinese health care culture. *Holistic Nursing Practice, 15*(1), 12–21.

In many cultures, the ethical agent may be neither the patient nor the family, but the leader of the community. Individuals may not be seen as autonomous but, rather, as integrated within their extended family, cultural group, and environment. In some cultures, males are dominant, whereas in others, the matriarchs lead the family. Nurses need to be respectful of these varied values and cultures to ensure optimal, ethical decision making that is not imposed on by dominant Western thinking. Nurses in all circumstances must:

- Understand the concepts that are important to a person's culture
- Involve the family and the community with the consent of the patient
- Respect modesty and purity concepts
- Use interpreters who understand the culture and the health care issues
- Consider traditional medicine (of that culture) as a complement to Western medicine
- Understand when cultures use a duty-based versus rights-based approach (as discussed in Chapter 2) to ethical decision making
- Be respectful of diverse cultural and religious assumptions regarding human nature, purity, health and illness, life and death, and the status of the individual

Patients and families who come from diverse cultural backgrounds are at greater risk not only when there are language barriers, but when there is not a shared understanding of what is meaningful and most important to them. Illness and associated stressors compound these challenges of language and comprehension (Andrews & Boyle, 2002). To ensure culturally safe care, there needs to be a balance of power between providers and patients, as well as an acknowledgement of the social, political, and economic factors that influence and shape individual responses and trusting relationships.

Indigenous Rights

Indigenous history in Canada is complex, complicated, and replete with many ethical and legal challenges. The experience of Indigenous peoples in Canada carries a legacy of oppression and colonization. This section highlights aspects of this history to enlighten nurses about the abuses experienced by the Indigenous peoples in Canada that should influence their nursing practice and the care provided to these communities.

Government oversight of Indigenous peoples in Canada is provided by Indigenous Services Canada, the Crown, and Indigenous and Northern Affairs Canada. Nurses are encouraged to seek more information from sources such as the Canadian Indigenous Nurses Association.

Important Aspects of History

Colonization

Colonialism, also discussed in Chapter 2, occurs when one nation takes control over another, conquering and exploiting its population, and frequently forcing its own language and cultural values upon its people.

The concept of colonialism is linked to imperialism, where a nation extends its power and influence over another through diplomacy or force. This sense of entitlement of European nations was achieved at the expense of Indigenous peoples. Invading Europeans brought with them new illnesses and epidemics, forcibly removing Indigenous peoples from their lands and causing the near extinction of native species of animals and plants that had historically been used by Indigenous peoples for food and clothing. Resistance resulted in warfare where they were labelled as "savages." Focused on "civilizing" Indigenous peoples, the Europeans ignored their spiritual and cultural traditions and outlawed their spiritual and cultural traditions and ceremonies. Over time, children were removed from their families and taken to boarding schools or placed with non-Indigenous families and separated from their cultural traditions.

Doctrine of Discovery

Papal bulls, public decrees issued by the Popes in the fifteenth and sixteenth centuries, guided and legitimized the colonization and evangelization of lands not inhabited by Christians. These edicts were intended to avoid conflict between the Catholic nations during their colonial expansion. The Doctrine of Discovery has been used by European nations to justify further colonization.

The Doctrine is now condemned as unjust, racist, and in violation of the human rights of Indigenous People. The Truth and Reconciliation Commission of Canada (TRC, 2015) refers to the Doctrine in Number 45 of its Calls to Action and asks the federal government to "[r]epudiate concepts used to justify European sovereignty over Indigenous lands and peoples such as the Doctrine of Discovery and *terra nullius*." In 2023, following decades of advocacy by Indigenous groups, members of the Catholic Church and governments and others including the TRC Call to Action, the Vatican repudiated the Doctrine of Discovery, affirming that using it to justify colonization and the subjugation of Indigenous peoples is against the teachings of the Church and explicitly endorsed the United Nations Declaration on the Rights of Indigenous Peoples. In Canada, British law related to colonization has had much more ongoing significance than the Doctrine of Discovery.

The Indian Act
The *Indian Act* was introduced in 1867 and has been amended several times since then. The original intent of the Act, the primary statute governing Indigenous communities in Canada, was paternalistic. The Act has narrow jurisdiction, covering First Nations on reserves (land held by the Crown and granted exclusive use of a band, or nation) and Inuit living in their traditional lands. The Act controls those who are entitled to be an "Indian" and is thus entitled to be registered and granted legal status as an "Indian." Over the past few decades, the federal government has transferred some authority over to specific Indigenous communities (Fryer & Leblanc-Laurendeau, 2019; King, 2012; Lawrence, 2016). Further detail on the *Indian Act* is provided in Chapter 4.

The Act prescribes federal government funding for many services such as health care, which are normally covered by provincial, territorial, or municipal governments (Government of Canada, n.d.).

Residential Schools
The *Indian Act* led, in 1883, to the establishment of "Indian schools," which through education, had as an objective the "civilization" and "assimilation" of Indigenous children. Indigenous children, many removed from their homes and communities, were taught with the same curriculum as that provided to children across the country; however, given the culture of abuse in these settings, learning was challenging. Students were forbidden from practising their cultural traditions and from speaking their own languages. Their traditional languages, religion, and lifestyle were repressed. More than 150,000 children attended these schools between 1879 and 1996. The

trauma associated with being taken away from their families and communities, and the consequences of abuse, continues to be felt experienced across generations today. Though nurses could never hope to understand the impact this has had on Indigenous peoples, it is important for nurses to be sensitive to the consequences of this history and the impact it has on Indigenous families and communities today while they care for Indigenous patients (Chartrand et al., 2006; Government of Canada, n.d.).

The Indian Residential Schools Settlement Agreement and the Truth and Reconciliation Commission
In response to the harms resulting from residential schools on multiple generations, a class action settlement, the Indian Residential Schools Settlement Agreement (Government of Canada, 2021), awarded $2.8 billion of dollars to former students and others impacted by this legacy (The Canadian Press, 2023). An important outcome of this settlement was the establishment of the Truth and Reconciliation Commission (active from 2008 to 2015), which documented the history and lasting impacts of the residential schools on survivors and their families. The Commission listened to the testimony of approximately 7,000 witnesses and recommended 94 Calls to Action. The Commission concluded that thousands of children died in these schools of disease, suicide, while attempting escape, and malnutrition. In many instances, their families were not informed, and they were buried on or near school grounds, often in unmarked graves, some of which are now being discovered. Two prime ministers have apologized on behalf of the Canadian people, Prime Minister Stephen Harper in 2008 and Prime Minister Justin Trudeau in 2017. Leaders of the churches who participated in operating the schools for the government have also apologized. The path to reconciliation has begun, but there is much more to do (TRC, 2021).

INDIAN HOSPITALS. Another historical injustice toward Indigenous peoples was the establishment of "Indian hospitals." This hospital system was established in the 1930s and expanded in the late 1940s and 1950s with the last facility closing in the 1980s. The hospitals were understaffed and overcrowded, and they utilized less educated and non-regulated staff (Geddes, 2017; Indigenous Corporate Training, 2017; Lux, 2016).

In the beginning, these hospitals segregated "Indians" in response to perceptions that they were a threat to public health and to the non-Indigenous population. Specifically, they were introduced to control the spread of infectious diseases such as tuberculosis (TB) (ironically, introduced by European settlers), which, due to factors such as poverty and living conditions, were more prevalent in Indigenous communities. Invasive treatment for TB continued in these hospitals, even when more advanced treatments were being provided in other settings. People were removed from their communities, some taken thousands of kilometres away, kept against their will, denied access to the higher level of care provided in other hospitals, and subjected to experimentation without or with inadequate consent. As well, a number of Indigenous women were subjected to forced sterilizations, agreeing to these procedures while in labour or when physically and emotionally vulnerable. Tragically, this practice has continued in recent years.

INDIGENOUS WOMEN AND FORCED STERILIZATION. A Senate report released in 2022 noted that coercive sterilization continues to happen in Canada and that the precise number of cases is unknown (Standing Senate Committee on Human Rights, 2022).

Various government policies governed forced sterilization, for example, *Alberta's Sexual Sterilization Act*, in force from 1928 until 1972. Though Indigenous women only represented 2.5% of the province during this time, they constituted 25% of those sterilized. Even after these policies were abolished, the practice continued.

The findings of a study exploring allegations of forced tubal ligation of Indigenous female, patients within the Saskatoon Health Region found that these women felt coerced into having a tubal ligation post-delivery, most believing this to be a type of birth control that was reversible. The women shared that the team, including nurses, social workers, and physicians, pressured them when they were most vulnerable. They stated they felt powerless to resist and have suffered serious consequences as a result (Boyer & Bartlett, 2017).

A study undertaken by the Université du Québec en Abitibi-Témiscamingue revealed that there had been at least 22 incidents of forced sterilization of First Nations and Inuit women in Quebec since 1980 and as recently as 2019. Many of those who participated in the study were not aware of their sterilization until years later, when they sought treatment for fertility. According to Boyer et al. (2017), "Ingrained problems of racism and discrimination will not be solved until

the system is changed so that health care is delivered in a way that is culturally competent and inclusive of an Indigenous model" (p. E1408).

Boyer (2017) suggested that the current model of health care delivery fails either to appreciate or address the subset of health determinants that affect Indigenous patients. Systemic and structural change requires leadership from health care and government, and the creation of new policies, structures, and resources to address racism and discrimination against not only Indigenous people, but also other racialized and marginalized communities.

The Canadian Constitution and Indigenous Rights

The Canadian Constitution was repatriated in 1982 and included the *Canadian Charter of Rights and Freedoms*. Initially, specific Indigenous and treaty rights were excluded from the Constitution. However, after extensive lobbying by First Nations, Inuit, and Métis organizations, section 35 of the Constitution was amended to recognize and protect existing Indigenous and treaty rights (including Indigenous practices, traditions, and customs):

35 (1) *The existing aboriginal and treaty rights of the aboriginal peoples of Canada are hereby recognized and affirmed.*
   (2) *In this Act, "aboriginal peoples of Canada" includes the Indian, Inuit, and Métis peoples of Canada.*
   (3) *For greater certainty, in subsection (1) "treaty rights" includes rights that now exist by way of land claims agreements or may be so acquired.*
   (4) *Notwithstanding any other provision of this Act, the aboriginal and treaty rights referred to in subsection (1) are guaranteed equally to male and female persons. (Constitution Act, 1982)*

There has been a lack of consensus on the definition of these rights; hence, the responsibility to define, interpret, and protect them has been left to the courts. More details on the Constitution as it relates to Indigenous rights are provided in Chapter 4.

Two complex cases in Ontario highlight the challenges in interpreting the *Canadian Charter of Rights and Freedoms* with respect to Indigenous rights as outlined in the *Constitution Act*. In both cases, First Nations children were diagnosed with acute lymphoblastic leukemia (ALL), and the parents of both children exercised their rights to opt for Indigenous medicine and to withdraw consent for chemotherapy for their children.

The first case, early in 2014, involved 10-year-old Makayla Sault. After she experienced complications associated with the chemotherapy she was receiving, at Makayla's request, her mother withdrew her consent for this treatment and elected for traditional healing and alternative therapies instead. The hospital made an appeal to the local Children's Aid Society (CAS) because it was believed that Makayla was a child in need of protection. After an investigation, the agency refused the hospital's appeal, citing sections 72 and 40 of the *Child and Family Services Act* (*Ontario Ministry of the Attorney General, 2018*). The agency concluded that Makayla was not a child in need of protection and therefore would not force her to return for chemotherapy. Makayla died in 2015.

The second case occurred later in 2014 and involved an 11-year-old child (referred to as *J. J.*), where, again, consent for chemotherapy was withdrawn. The hospital filed a report with the CAS, and again the agency refused to intervene. This time, the hospital brought forward an application under the *Child and Family Services Act* to ask the court to compel the CAS to intervene to restart the child's treatment as soon as possible. In a landmark ruling by the Ontario Court of Justice (*Hamilton Health Sciences Corp. v. D.H.*, 2014), the court upheld the right of J. J.'s parents to decline chemotherapy and to pursue Indigenous medicine for her. The court held that the family had rights under section 35 of the *Constitution Act*, which guarantees the treaty rights of Indigenous peoples in Canada. These rights entitled them to pursue Indigenous health care if they chose to do so. The court then refused the order requested by the hospital (*Hamilton Health Sciences Corp. v. D.H.*, 2014). A First Nations person (as was this child) is protected by section 35 of the *Constitution Act*. The key question in this case was whether the practice of Indigenous medicine is one of the rights guaranteed in the Constitution, and the court decided that it was.

In a follow-up decision, the court amended its original ruling to include the following:

[83a] But, implicit in this decision is that recognition and implementation of the right to use traditional medicines must remain consistent with the principle that the best interests of the child remain paramount.

The aboriginal right to use traditional medicine must be respected, and must be considered, among other factors, in any analysis of the best interests of the child, and whether the child is in need of protection. Taking into account the aboriginal right, and the constitutional objective of reconciliation and considering carefully the facts of this case, I concluded that this child was not in need of protection.
[83b] In law as well as in practice, then, the Haudenosaunee have both an aboriginal right to use their own traditional medicines and health practices, and the same right as other people in Ontario to use the medicines and health practices available to those people. This provides Haudenosaunee culture and knowledge with protection, but it also gives the people unique access to the best we have to offer. Facing an unrelenting enemy, such as cancer, we all hope for and need the very best, especially for our children. For the Haudenosaunee, the two sets of rights mentioned above fulfill the aspirations of the United Nations Declaration on the Rights of Indigenous Peoples, which states in article 24, that "Indigenous peoples have the right to their traditional medicines and to maintain their health practices . . . Indigenous individuals also have the right to access, without any discrimination, to all social and health services." (*Hamilton Health Sciences Corp. v. D.H.*, 2015)

This ruling clarified that the law remains unchanged and that with respect to any issue involving the health of a child that the child's best interests are the priority. It also clarified that although the right to use traditional medicine is protected by the Constitution, it is not absolute, especially with respect to children. The decision further suggested that the best option for treatment is the integration of Indigenous and Western medical systems. (Note that non-Indigenous persons may also choose a holistic approach to treatment that may include Indigenous medicine or other complimentary therapies.) In the first ruling, the judge believed that the mother would bring the child back for chemotherapy, if necessary. This did, in fact, occur, and when J. J.'s disease relapsed, she was readmitted for an integrated program of chemotherapy and Indigenous healing. So, it continues to be the case for all children that if a physician or the team believes that the decisions of a parent or substitute decision maker put a child at risk and in need of protection, there is an obligation to report this to the CAS, which will undertake an investigation and determine the child's need for protection. An appeal of its decision can always be brought before the court, as deemed appropriate (Borden Ladner Gervais, 2015).

Under the *Child, Youth and Family Services Act* (which replaced the *Child and Family Services Act* in 2017), taking a child into custody to protect that child's safety is permitted when a child protection worker believes, on reasonable grounds, that the child is at risk of harm. The precedent is that when a child requires medical treatment to cure, prevent, or alleviate physical harm or suffering, and the parent or guardian declines or is unable to provide consent for that treatment, then in the best interests of the child, that child would be considered to be in need of protection. In the case of an Indigenous child, the courts have indicated that in evaluating best interests, the uniqueness of Indigenous culture, heritage, and traditions and preservation of the child's cultural identity needed to be considered as well (Hamilton Health Sciences 2015).

Although the Indigenous person's right to use traditional medicine must be respected, the best interests of the child, some argue, are most likely to be achieved by a treatment plan that combines the best that both systems have to offer.

In cases where parents belonging to the Jehovah's Witnesses faith refuse blood transfusion, on religious grounds, the opinion of the court is that although parents have the right to choose among equally effective types of medical treatment for their children, they do not have the right to deny a child a medical treatment that has been deemed necessary by a medical professional and for which there is no legitimate alternative. A parent's freedom of religion, guaranteed by section 2 of the Charter, does not include the imposition of religious practices that threaten the safety, health, or life of a child and that limiting the constitutional rights of parents, to promote a child's welfare, is fully consistent with the principle of fundamental and natural justice. The difference between these cases; and unlike the parents of the First Nations children, as described earlier, the right of parents who are Jehovah's Witnesses to refuse a blood transfusion, on behalf of their children, is not enshrined in a constitutionally grounded treaty right (see *A.C. v. Manitoba (Director of Child and Family Services)*, [2009], involving a mature minor aged 16; and *B. (R.) v. Children's Aid Society of Metropolitan Toronto*, [1995], involving an infant).

Control Over Resources

Despite colonization and the diligent efforts of politicians and bureaucrats for at least the last 200 years, the culture and identity of the Indigenous peoples in Canada has survived. In the twentieth century, Indigenous people moved from being an inconvenience that would eventually disappear to being an indelible part of everyday decisions in Canada. Part of this change emerged because of Indigenous involvement in resource development decisions. The Mackenzie Valley Pipeline Inquiry (1974–1977), also known as the Berger Inquiry, widely consulted Dene, Inuit, and Métis peoples about a major pipeline development in the Yukon and Northwest Territories. The report concluded that the project should not go ahead, in part because of the potentially devastating impact on the Indigenous people of the Mackenzie Valley area.

In 1975, the Quebec and Canadian governments, the Cree and Inuit of Northern Quebec, and several other parties settled numerous land claims and established a framework for the development of a very large hydroelectric project in the James Bay region of Northern Quebec. The agreement arose from litigation over the rights of the Cree and Inuit and the refusal of the Quebec government to recognize those rights. These two situations clearly indicated to many Canadians, for the first time, that Indigenous peoples were going to assert their rights and force their inclusion in discussions about the economic development of Canada. The process has been gradual and grudging, but progress has been made.

Indigenous Rights and Health Care

There are challenges in determining which level of government is responsible for a particular health care program or service for Indigenous people because some are covered by the "*Indian Act*" and others are not. With respect to health care for Indigenous peoples, the federal, provincial, and territorial levels of government share jurisdiction. Indigenous peoples are included in the per capita allocations of funding from the federal fiscal transfer and are entitled to provincial and territorial health care services as residents of a province or territory. Indigenous Services Canada funds or directly provides services for First Nations and Inuit that supplement those provided by provinces and territories. For example, during the pandemic, the federal government provided additional public health funding to Indigenous communities to provide them with the flexibility to design and implement strategies to prevent and respond to COVID-19 within their communities (Fryer & Leblanc-Laurendeau, 2019; Indigenous Services Canada, 2022).

According to the Government of Canada (2023):

A coordinated approach to address the health needs of First Nations, Inuit and Métis, and health care delivery among all levels of government including Indigenous governments, remains an ongoing challenge. Improved clarity and a shared understanding of the role of various levels of government is needed, including for Métis, off-reserve First Nations and urban Inuit populations.

Jordan's story, shared in Case Scenario 2.7 in Chapter 2, highlights these challenges.

Considerations for Nurses

The experience of Indigenous peoples in Canada carries a legacy of oppression and colonization. The devastating impacts of residential schools, Indian hospitals, the child welfare system, and other colonial experiences have created deep losses for Indigenous peoples. Nurses must be aware of this history, and given Indigenous peoples' position in Canada, nurses must understand and respect Indigenous peoples' values, culture, and moral traditions.

It is clear that the Indigenous peoples in Canada have suffered abuse and discrimination over the past centuries. Though improving, today they sadly continue to face discrimination, systemic racism, and abuse in the health care system, as demonstrated by the stories described in this book, for example Joyce Echaquan (Chapters 2 and 5) and Brian Sinclair (Chapter 2). The effects of this discrimination, especially the consequences of residential schools, Indian hospitals, and the missing and murdered Indigenous women and girls, have left a legacy of pain and suffering for many generations. Nurses must understand this history and its consequences as they care for Indigenous people, and especially respect Indigenous people's lack of trust in the health care system. As advocates, nurses must shift this paradigm and create an environment of trust and mutual respect.

This journey includes the creation of a culturally safe environment. Cultural safety exists when there is mutually respectful engagement, freedom from discrimination and racism, and when power imbalances are replaced with equality in relationships—essentially an environment where persons feel safe when receiving care. This begins with humility, and by nurses engaging in self-refection to better understand their own biases and systemic biases. It also involves listening and learning from the wisdom and experience of Indigenous persons entrusted to their care (Beagan, 2018; Curtis et al., 2019; First Nations Health Authority, 2022; Wesp, 2018).

The Rights of Persons With a Mental Illness

Background

Mental illness has been misunderstood for centuries, leading to all forms of abuse and inhumane treatments. In the past, members of this vulnerable population were hidden by families or treated as outcasts in the community. In recent centuries, abandoned by their families, many were lodged in warehouses or asylums, which, as history shows, were notorious for deplorable and inhumane living conditions, where persons were exposed to a lifetime of abuse (Foerschner, 2010).

Over time, individuals with mental illnesses were subjected to "treatments" such as purging, bloodletting, and hot and cold shock therapy. Approaches started to evolve somewhat from the late 1800s to the mid-1900s, with attempts at treatment through interventions such as psychoanalysis, psychosurgery (lobotomies), insulin shock treatment, and electroconvulsive therapy (ECT). These measures often resulted in minimal or no benefit and, in some cases, caused further harm to the person. In recent decades, research has provided greater insights into mental illnesses, and their treatment (especially pharmacological) has resulted in better outcomes (Foerschner, 2010). However, there remains considerable opportunity for improvement. Persons with mental illness still face stigmatization and misunderstanding and have a greater risk for drug dependency and homelessness. Over time, legislation has been introduced to ensure that they receive the care they need while safeguarding their rights and protecting them from abuse.

All provinces and territories have legislation—that is, mental health legislation—in place to protect persons with serious mental health problems so that they receive the treatment they need while ensuring their rights under the *Canadian Charter of Rights and Freedoms* are protected. This legislation is intended to protect both the person with mental illness and the public from harm. (See the Evolve site for the specific legislation in each province and territory.)

As a rule, if a person's state of mental health is such that it poses a threat to themselves or others, such a person may be committed to a mental health facility for treatment upon the order of an examining physician. In most provinces, the determination that such a state of mind exists must be made by a physician (see, for example, Ontario's *Mental Health Act* (1990, s. 15(1)). In British Columbia, under the *Mental Health Act*, a single physician can issue a certificate for involuntary detention for up to 48 hours. Detention beyond 48 hours requires a second medical certificate from another physician. In Newfoundland and Labrador, a person may be detained in such a treatment facility only if two physicians certify that the patient is a danger to self or others by reason of a mental disorder (*Mental Health Care and Treatment Act*, 2006, s. 17).

Generally, there are two categories under which a person suffering a mental illness is admitted to a mental health facility: (1) the person is not a threat to self or others and (2) the person poses a threat to self or others. The first category usually comprises voluntary patients, and they cannot be detained without their consent. Persons in the second category generally may be admitted to a facility on an involuntary basis and may be detained without their consent. However, the matter does not end there. There are procedural safeguards in place to provide for a review of the detention of involuntary patients and to ensure they are not detained arbitrarily or without proper grounds. If they cease to pose a danger to themselves or others, the law generally requires that they be released when they wish.

Involuntary Admissions

Most people with a mental illness seek assistance voluntarily. However, others, because of the nature of their illness, will not accept or recognize that they are ill. Therefore, they refuse treatment, which may result in additional suffering, disruptions, and harm to that person and to others. The provisions within the mental health legislation across the country ensure that patients with mental illness receive the care they require by granting authority and establishing strict

criteria and procedures for involuntary admissions to psychiatric care facilities. For example, in British Columbia, a physician must find that the person meets the following criteria (British Columbia Ministry of Health, 2005; *Mental Health Act*, 1996, s. 22). The person:

- Is suffering from a mental disorder that seriously impairs the person's ability to react appropriately to their environment or to associate with others
- Requires psychiatric treatment in or through a designated facility
- Requires care, supervision, and control in or through a designated facility to prevent the person's substantial mental or physical deterioration or for the person's own protection or the protection of others
- Is not suitable as a voluntary patient

If these conditions are satisfied, then the physician completes the appropriate documentation, which is a medical certificate in British Columbia, providing the legal authority for that person to be admitted for a 48-hour period. The certificate authorizes others, the police, paramedics, and family to bring that person to a psychiatric facility. In certain circumstances persons can be brought to a facility by the police or ordered there by a judge, where the physician is required to assess the person on the basis of this criteria.

The patients must be reassessed within 48 hours by a second physician, and this second review permits additional detention for up to 1 month. Patients are subjected to frequent reassessments within structured timelines and are discharged when they have recovered (British Columbia Ministry of Health, 2005).

In *McCorkell v. Director of Riverview Hospital* (1993), a challenge to the constitutionality of the British Columbia *Mental Health Act* was made on the basis that involuntary committal and detention of mentally ill persons violated section 7 ("liberty") of the Charter. The court considered the safeguards within the legislation that had to be met for committal and the review process of committals and determined that section 7 of the Charter was not violated.

The approach described in the British Columbia legislation is the same model used across Canada, with minor variations. Involuntary admissions must be supported by medical evidence, and in most cases, confinement for any length of time will require the opinion of two doctors. The patient is entitled to a hearing, almost immediately, to determine whether involuntary admission is justified. The continuation of an involuntary admission is subject to regular reviews, and further opportunities for hearings are available to patients.

Rights Under the Act

The mental health acts also ensure safeguards and protections for the involuntarily admitted patient. These include the right to notification. This ensures that these patients are informed about procedures, the findings, and their rights throughout the entire process. They can also expect that their condition will be reviewed on a regular basis and that they are updated on those findings. They are entitled to a second opinion and have the right to access and appeal, to a review panel, and/or to the courts (British Columbia Ministry of Health, 2005).

The *Mental Health Act* of the Yukon, for example, articulates the rights of persons with a mental illness. As in many provinces, only minimal physical restraints may be used on such patients—that is, only what is reasonable and necessary, considering the person's physical and mental condition (*Mental Health Act*, 2002). Other patient rights in the Yukon include the right to receive and make phone calls (*Mental Health Act*, 2002, s. 40(4)(a)); to have reasonable access to visitors (s. 40(4)(b)); to have access at any time to the person's legal representative, guardian, or other authorized person (s. 40(4)(c)); to send and receive correspondence (s. 40(4)(d)); to vote (s. 40(5)(c)); to wear clothing of the person's choice (s. 40(5)(b)); to security of the person (s. 40(6)); to confidentiality (s. 40(7)); and to be informed (if detained) of the reasons for detention (s. 41). In the other Canadian jurisdictions, similar rights exist.

Voluntary Admissions

As mentioned, most people present to a mental health facility on a voluntary basis. However, under the British Columbia *Mental Health Act*, (1996) there is a requirement that these patients officially authorize their consent to treatment. If they are younger than 16 years of age, the consent of a parent or guardian is required. These patients are granted the same rights as any other patient with a condition other than mental illness. However, even persons who present voluntarily may be admitted on an involuntary basis if it is determined that they are not capable of providing consent, and if they meet the above criteria.

Considerations for Informed Consent

Consent is a central factor in decisions related to privacy and confidentiality. It becomes more complicated when the persons involved have an illness that affects their ability to give consent. As with all other patients, patients detained under mental health legislation have to consent to treatment unless they are incapable of doing so. *Capacity* is defined as the ability to understand what form of consent is being requested (the subject matter or the request) and the ability to appreciate the consequences of withholding or giving consent. In Ontario, the *Health Care Consent Act, 1996* deals with defining patients as being either capable or incapable regarding consenting to treatment (or refusing treatment).

In Ontario, and in most other provinces when a patient who can make an informed treatment decision refuses treatment, and they may do so at any time, the psychiatric facility must respect that refusal. It does not matter whether the committal is voluntary, involuntary, or informal. The only issue is whether the patient is deemed capable.

The attending physician may decide that the individual is incapable of making treatment decisions. In this case, substitute consent can be given by the proper substitute consent giver. Under the *Mental Health Act, 1990*, a patient can appeal the finding of incapacity by filling out Form A under the *Health Care Consent Act, 1996*, requesting that the Consent and Capacity Board review the finding of incapacity.

The Consent and Capacity Board is an independent body, and its members are appointed by the provincial government. When the case involves involuntary committal, there must be one lawyer, one psychiatrist, and one member who is neither a lawyer nor a psychiatrist on the hearing panel. One member must be an expert in evaluating capacity when that is the issue. The board can be convened either at the request of the patient, at the request of the psychiatric facility's officer-in-charge, or because an automatic review is required under the *Mental Health Act, 1990.*

The right to treat patients without their consent differs from province to province. For example, there are differences between Ontario and British Columbia. In Ontario, involuntary patients can refuse treatment unless the attending physician certifies that the patient is not mentally competent under the *Health Care Consent Act, 1996.* Where the patient is not competent, the *Health Care Consent Act* provides a framework for the designation of substitute decision makers. In addition, the *Health Care Consent Act* provides for giving emergency treatment without consent to both capable and incapable patients (s. 25). According to the Act, "there is an emergency if the person for whom the treatment is proposed is apparently experiencing severe suffering or is at risk, if the treatment is not administered promptly, of sustaining serious bodily harm" (s. 25(1)). Where the patient is incapable, treatment can be provided if the delay in obtaining consent, or a refusal, will prolong the suffering of the person or will put the person at risk of sustaining serious bodily harm. Treatment may be administered in situations where the person is capable, but consent or refusal cannot be ascertained because of a language barrier or "a disability"; where because there is no evidence the person does not want the treatment; or where efforts have been made to communicate and further delay would make the situation worse.

The British Columbia *Mental Health Act* (1996) authorizes compulsory treatment of all involuntary patients if the assessment has established that these patients are mentally incapable of giving their consent for treatment. Regarding treatment of involuntary patients, the appropriate procedures and documentation must be followed.

As with all consent processes, the physician must inform patients of the nature of their condition, as well as the rationale and consequences of treatment. During this process, the physician assesses the extent to which a person can give or refuse consent.

Where a patient is deemed capable of consenting, then treatment may begin after the person signs the consent form, witnessed by another person and the physician. Where a patient is deemed capable of consenting but refuses, or where the patient is found to be incapable of giving a valid consent, the director of the facility or designate has the power to consent on behalf of that person.

In contrast to the *legislation* of all other Canadian jurisdictions, once someone is involuntarily admitted, the British Columbia *Mental Health Act* (1996) deems the patient to have consented to any psychiatric treatment chosen by the treating physician. In other words, a person's consent is not required for a particular treatment. As noted earlier, a constitutional challenge to the legislation was initiated in 2016 on the grounds that the provisions of the British Columbia *Mental Health Act* violate the *Canadian Charter of Rights and Freedoms* (1982, s. 7, "security of the person") (Canadian Mental Health Association–British Columbia Division, 2017). Unfortunately, the application was dismissed in 2018 on the basis that the plaintiff, as an advocacy group, lacked the status to pursue the matter. The individuals with status had withdrawn from the application (*MacLaren v. British Columbia (Attorney General)*, 2018).

As provided in other legislation, treatment can be provided in an urgent or emergency manner prior to the formal consent process to prevent death, serious harm, or injury when the person is not able to consent (unconscious, under the influence of drugs or alcohol) and when a substitute decision maker is not available.

Similar to the provision in the Ontario *Health Care Consent Act, 1996*, the British Columbia Ministry of Health (2005) takes the following position: "Common law also recognizes that, in an emergency, where a person's life is at risk or where there may be serious harm to the person's health and where the individual is incapable of consenting to treatment, emergency treatment may be provided to a person of any age without that person's consent" (p. 20). The use of restraints is very controversial, but the use of restraints, where they would represent the most minimal level of intervention, may be a suitable response during an emergency. The use must only be for the protection of the patient or others and cannot be used as a punishment or disciplinary measure (College of Nurses of Ontario, 2017).

For many patients, mental illness is a lifelong process. They understand the nature of their illness well and appreciate that their illness may cause them to refuse treatment that, while in a healthy state, they know they need. If a person expresses a preference regarding treatment while capable, those wishes are considered and followed if they are consistent with the caregiver's obligation to provide the most appropriate care required to manage the specific condition. The Ontario *Health Care Consent Act, 1996* and *Mental Health Act, 1996* (1990) make provisions for respecting the express health care wishes of patients.

Access to Medical Assistance in Dying (MAiD) for Persons With a Mental Illness

Currently, people whose sole medical condition is having a diagnosis of a mental illness are not eligible for MAiD in Canada. Legislation to change this continues to be under review. However, persons with a mental illness may be eligible for MAiD if they also have a 'grievous and irremediable' physical health condition. Proponents of changes to the legislation argue that MAiD would be justifiable as a last resort for competent persons suffering from an intractable psychiatric illness when all treatments have been exhausted, and that they should not be treated differently from other persons. Others raise concerns regarding the vulnerability of this population, issues related to competency, and the need for greater access to treatment (Bahji & Delva, 2021; Konder & Christie, 2019; Tanner, 2018; Ventura & Austin, 2017).

A survey of Canadian psychiatrists revealed that the majority of respondents, though in support of MAiD in general, did not support the legalization of MAiD for persons with a mental illness. Their objections were based upon concern for this vulnerable patient community, personal moral objections, lack of resources and the availability of effective treatments, and concern for the effect it would have on the therapeutic relationship (Rousseau et al., 2017). Those who support having access to MAiD agree that it ought to be an option of last resort, when all treatments options are exhausted, and that additional rigour be involved in the approval process.

THE RIGHT TO SAFE CARE

Patients who engage with the health care system have the right to expect competent, quality care. They trust that the system and those who care for them focus on their best interests and protect them from unnecessary harm. Since the time of Florence Nightingale, quality has been a core value of the nursing profession and

continues to be paramount to the societal obligations and commitments of the profession. Over the past few decades, the focus on quality and patient safety has strengthened in health care. As a result, the knowledge base regarding quality and safety has advanced, and various theories and methodologies have evolved. It is essential that nurses not only be experts in this area but also contribute to the advancement of this knowledge and to a deeper understanding of quality and safety in health care (LaSala, 2009; McGaffigan, 2019; Tye, 2020).

Over the last few decades, there has been greater recognition of how a consistent focus on quality improvement enhances patient safety and prevents harm. The shift in thinking about patient safety has resulted in a greater recognition of the human and system factors that contribute to errors. This understanding led to organizational transformation to a "just culture," where nurses (and all health care professionals) are obliged to disclose any errors or near misses, without fear of criticism or discipline. A system-oriented focus evaluates the structures and processes that might have led to mistakes, rather than instantly attributing blame to an individual. Further, there is an acknowledgement of the role of patients and families in patient safety, the importance of transparency, and the healing factors associated with acknowledging and disclosing errors.

Key research studies revealed serious concerns about patient safety and reinforced the urgency of ensuring greater accountability for quality and safety across the health care system. In 2000, a landmark report by the US Institute of Medicine (IoM), *To Err Is Human: Building a Safer Health System*, revealed alarming data that 98,000 deaths/year in the United States were related to medical errors and were among the top 10 causes of death in the country (Institute of Medicine [US] Committee on Quality of Health Care in America, 2000). In Canada in 2004, Baker and colleagues undertook a similar study to determine the extent of errors occurring in Canadian hospitals. This study, of 20 hospitals in five provinces, found that 1 in 13 patients experienced an adverse event while in hospital. The greatest number of these adverse events occurred in teaching hospitals, where patient care is generally more complex and acute. Furthermore, Baker et al. (2004) reported that of the 185,000 adverse events that occur in Canadian hospitals each year,

70,000 are preventable. Since the publication of these reports, quality in health care has steadily become a top priority for health care providers (Berwick, 2002; Corrigon, 2005; de Jonge et al., 2011).

A follow-up study undertaken in 2016 by the Canadian Institute for Health Information (CIHI) and the Patient Safety Institute (CPSI) revealed that between 2014 and 2015, out of 138,000 hospitalizations, one in five involved more than one occurrence of harm and estimated that, in any given day, over 1,600 hospital beds in Canada were occupied by patients whose hospital stay was extended as a result of an error. Beyond the effects of harm experienced by the patient and family, these extended hospital stays resulted in increased costs to the system and limited access to other patients requiring admission (CIHI & CPSI, 2016).

These studies identified many factors that account for errors, including:

- Communication breakdowns
- Poor team collaboration
- Fatigue
- Workload
- Multiple distractions and interruptions
- Complexity of processes
- Reliance on memory
- Limited orientation and transitions to new roles
- Staffing models

Though the focus of these studies was on hospital care, one can assume that the same risks apply to other settings, including the community.

In 2002, a National Steering Committee on Patient Safety published *Building a Safer System,* a report that proposed a strategy for improving patient safety in Canada. An important recommendation, implemented by Health Canada, was the establishment of the Canadian Patient Safety Institute (CPSI). Established in 2003, the CPSI collaborates with health care professionals, the government, and health care organizations to advance the quality and safety of patient care. The CPSI offers a number of programs, including tools and resources, designed to promote patient safety (CPSI, 2016).

The health care system is a human endeavour, and humans are imperfect—they make mistakes. Many reasons account for human errors. Therefore, it is so important that highly effective systems exist to compensate for such human limitations. For example, tools such as checklists mitigate a person's reliance on memory alone.

Errors in health care are most often the result of systemic problems—layered failures in the system (Reason, 2000)—rather than of individual acts. James Reason compares these systems to layers of Swiss cheese that line up temporarily and provide opportunities for accidents to happen. Consider the first layer as the physician who makes the wrong calculation and orders the wrong dose of an antibiotic. Once the order is received in pharmacy, the second layer, the technician, distracted at the time, dispenses the antibiotic without checking. When the antibiotic arrives on the unit, it is administered by a novice nurse, the third layer, who, unfamiliar with the normal dosage ranges, fails to look them up and administers the drug (the fourth layer), and the holes in the cheese line up. A system approach recognizes these failures and puts safeguards in place to prevent future errors. Electronic order entry and documentation systems have such safeguards.

Yet, historically, the tendency has been to blame individuals for errors and adverse events (Rankin, 2004). Not surprisingly, health care professionals are instinctively defensive when it comes to being questioned or talking openly about medical errors and disclosure of errors. However, when error is not acknowledged, there is a missed opportunity to learn and to improve patient safety. Across the country, there is a growing focus on changing the systems and processes that contribute to or influence the occurrence of errors and adverse events.

This attention has led to governments taking leadership in the introduction of policies and legislation to support patient safety and high-quality care.

Provincial governments have introduced legislation with the intention of improving the systems surrounding health care and reducing avoidable errors. For example, in Newfoundland and Labrador, the *Patient Safety Act* (2001) was enacted to create systems for the reporting, investigation, and communication of information about patient safety indicators. In Ontario, the *Excellent Care for All Act, 2010* was passed with the intention of improving outcomes for Ontario patients by strengthening the health care sector's organizational focus and accountability to deliver high-quality patient care. This Act imposed requirements on hospitals to improve quality assurance, gather data, and develop quality improvement plans.

The success of these initiatives has been limited. In 2014, Baker reviewed his 2004 study and concluded that even after 10 years of effort and expense, "Canadian health care is still not reliably safe" (Baker, 2014, p. 1). In a 2017 review of progress on patient safety, Hardcastle concluded that legislative progress has been fragmented and that some provinces lag behind others. Lack of data on the link between scientific governance reforms and patient outcomes in Canada limits any assessment of the effectiveness of the measures that have been taken. Hardcastle (2017) argued that patient safety can be improved but that hospitals must step forward; take responsibility for the work of all of health care professionals, including physicians; take responsibility for reducing errors out of the hands of physicians; and develop systems to reduce errors.

A Patient's and Family's Right to Know: Disclosure of Error

After an error occurs, the health team needs to be open and transparent with the patient and family. Disclosure of error is the process by which health care professionals communicate adverse events to patients or families. This process acknowledges the right of patients and families to be informed and facilitates the healing process of all concerned. Legislation regarding reporting and disclosure now exists across the country; the moral thing to do is now enshrined in law.

In patient safety literature, **harm** is defined as "an outcome that negatively affects a patient's health and/ or quality of life" (Disclosure Working Group, 2008, p. 8). It is an adverse event related to the care or services provided to the patient, rather than to the patient's underlying problem or illness. When harm occurs, the ethically responsible action is full disclosure of that harm to the patient or family. **Disclosure** is the process by which health care professionals communicate an adverse event to the patient (Disclosure Working Group, 2008). In the legislation regarding patient safety, the communication of errors and adverse outcomes to patients is often specifically required. See, for example, section 17 of Newfoundland and Labrador's *Patient Safety Act* (2001): "Every regional health authority shall establish a policy for ensuring that an adverse health event is disclosed to the affected patient."

As discussed, patients are entitled to information about themselves, so when errors are made and harm results, patients and families have the right to be informed about them. Ethical and professional obligations to be open and honest are consistent with professional codes

of ethics and patients' rights. When harm results because of error, not only the patient but also others connected to them suffer. The health care professionals involved can experience serious guilt and remorse. For the healing of all concerned, disclosure to the patient and/or the family is necessary to begin the healing process.

Sadly, sometimes a patient dies as the result of error. Understandably, families hope for some acknowledgement of the error and its role in the death of the family member, especially when the death was unforeseen. Such acknowledgement is important for a family in dealing with their loss and provides them with some assurance that such errors will not be repeated, thereby preventing another family from suffering a similar tragedy. A family wants clear and honest answers as to what happened to their loved one, and hospitals have an ethical and spiritual obligation to sit down with the family and, with compassion and grace, disclose the truth.

The disclosure process needs to be open and transparent. With the patient's or family's consent, the physicians, nurses, and other relevant members of the team involved in the patient's care should be present. The process may not be completed in only a single conversation—several meetings may be necessary to ensure that all of the patient's or family's issues, concerns, and questions are addressed (Disclosure Working Group, 2008, p. 16; Keatings et al., 2006; Morath, 2006). The disclosure of errors may lead to litigation. However, in practice, patients who are told about adverse events are much less likely to bring legal actions. Furthermore, many provinces and territories have created legislative exceptions, which exclude quality assurance information and error reports from being admissible as evidence in litigation. This protection encourages open reporting and disclosure (Bélanger-Hardy & Quesnel, 2016).

The absence of full disclosure of medical errors means the loss of one of the most effective tools for improving systems and patient safety and inevitably results in the same errors being repeated (Box 10.2).

Health care professionals need to approach the question of full and open disclosure of adverse events with the same commitment and hold it to the same standard of practice applied to any other treatment or decision. When this does not happen, they betray the trust of patients, families, and one another. Health care organizations have to introduce practices and

BOX 10.2
THE CLAIRE LEWIS STORY

On October 14, 2001, 3 days after undergoing surgery to remove a craniopharyngioma, 11-year-old Claire Lewis died in the critical care unit (CCU) of a Canadian hospital. The reason for her sudden death was believed by the CCU staff to be postoperative complications. The real reason may have been overlooked had it not been for her father, John Lewis, and his certainty that his daughter's death could have been prevented.

When Claire died, the health care team that had cared for her for 3 days in the CCU believed the most appropriate care had been provided. However, even if the team had believed that serious errors had been made, there was no system in place for reporting a critical event such as this error and alerting the hospital's senior leadership to the concern.

Claire's father, John, was himself a registered nurse working at the hospital where his daughter died and had been at her bedside for most of the 3 days after her surgery. He was present when she died. After her death, he reviewed Claire's medical records and arrived at a clear understanding of the errors that had been made and the system failings that had contributed to his daughter's preventable death.

It was almost 4 months, however, before the hospital's senior leaders became aware of the issues surrounding Claire's death. The silence on the part of the hospital staff after Claire's death, coupled with a coroner's report that found nothing untoward in her care, infuriated the grieving father. Understandably, the family had hoped for some form of acknowledgement from the hospital in terms of its role in Claire's death. Disclosure of adverse events that lead to morbidity and mortality is important for the families involved as they struggle to deal with their losses.

Immediately after Claire's death, an initial review of her care was conducted. Led by physicians and the risk management staff, the review failed to address the critical aspects identified by her father. Furthermore, the hospital's legal advisors edited the report that was sent to the family. Failing to answer many of the family's questions, the report served only to deepen feelings of distrust and anger.

A meeting between the family and the hospital about 4 months after Claire's death resulted in her family feeling an even greater sense of alienation. They were upset about the report; the team who met with them was unprepared for the meeting; and too many people, including a physician whom the family had specifically requested not attend, were in attendance. According to Claire's father, "the meeting was a disaster, as middle management, with wagons in a circle and with a wall of white coats present designed specifically to intimidate two devastated parents, tried to chalk Claire's death up to complications of surgery." Understandably, the family felt offended by the seemingly insincere efforts on the part of the hospital to address their concerns.

Subsequently, a second review identified the errors in Claire's care. However, the debate about what to disclose continued. The executive team and the legal advisors had differing perspectives and concerns. Finally, once the question about disclosure made its way to the hospital's senior leaders, the decision was quickly made by them that there would be full disclosure.

The review of Claire's care in the CCU, the admission of error, and the full disclosure of those errors set the stage for those involved to begin a process that produced 19 recommendations for change to address both system and competency issues.

A letter was sent to the family, along with the conclusions of the second review and a list of recommendations for changes at the hospital. The family, however, was so deeply hurt by the hospital's failure to make this disclosure earlier and the previous failed attempt at dialogue that they refused to meet with the hospital leaders. Despite this refusal, the senior leaders persisted in maintaining contact with the family and continued to make offers to meet and engage in open discussion.

It was almost 3 years after Claire's death that the family was finally able to accept the hospital's invitation to work together to set the stage for helping everyone to start to heal and move forward. According to Claire's father, "the hospital's disclosure brought with it unforeseen and unimaginable benefits for the family, the hospital, physicians, and nurses alike." The silence that followed Claire's death had felt like a cover-up to the family and led to the feeling that there had been some intent to harm. "The apology melted this horrific feeling away, slowly opening the door to a meaningful dialogue between the family and the hospital staff" (Keatings et al., 2006, p. 1085).

The bereaved need to find meaning in the seemingly senseless deaths of their loved ones, but when medical errors occur, there are many victims. A number of the staff who had cared for Claire were deeply affected by her death, the review, and the subsequent disclosure process. The disclosure provided staff, as well as the family, the opportunity to "make sense" of Claire's death, to begin to heal and move forward, and to become part of the process of change that would improve patient safety.

MORE THAN ONE VICTIM

Not only did Claire and her family suffer the consequences associated with her death; nurses and physicians were also affected, both personally and professionally. Throughout this sad journey, two of Claire's nurses repeated their desire to meet with her family. They wanted the opportunity to apologize for what they may or may not have done that might have contributed to Claire's death and to acknowledge the family's loss and grief. But their legal advisors cautioned against this. When they did meet with the family, it was their decision, taken despite legal advice not to do so.

BOX 10.2—cont'd
THE CLAIRE LEWIS STORY

When John, Claire's father, met with the nurses, he was accompanied by his eldest daughter Jessie, who did not have a clear understanding of what had happened to her sister the day she died. During the meeting, she became aware of the complexity of factors that had led to Claire's death. Both she and John came to understand the pain and heartache experienced by these nurses. The nurses simply said how sorry they were to John and Jessie, who, not feeling the need for further explanation, gave them a hug (Keatings

et al., 2006). These professionals, through disclosure and forgiveness, were then able to move on with their professional careers, richer for the experience.

Hicock, L. & Lewis, J. (2004). *Beware the grieving warrior: A child's preventable death, a father's fight for justice.* ECW Press; Keatings, M., Martin, M., McCallum, A., et al. (2006). Medical errors: Understanding the parent's perspective. *Pediatric Clinics of North America, 53*(6), 1079-1089.

---

processes to consistently and accurately recognize the occurrence of adverse events. It is essential that such recognition of adverse events be inextricably tied to full and open disclosure. Simply put, it is the right thing to do.

SUMMARY

This chapter has dealt with the rights and responsibilities of patients within the health care system, and the obligations of health care professionals to ensure that patients' rights are respected. A health care professional's obligations to respect patients' rights are not always clear; in fact, they may conflict with equal obligations to respect the rights of others. These rights and obligations evolve from the ethical theories and principles described in earlier chapters.

Nurses are obliged to ensure that patient rights are respected and upheld. The pressures of diminishing resources, workload, and other factors in today's health care settings may impose barriers to providing even such basic patient rights as privacy and dignity. Regardless, nurses should always be mindful of their duty and obligation to ensure the rights of patients, especially those most vulnerable, while ensuring that they are themselves treated with respect. Most important, in today's complex health care environment, health care professionals have a responsibility to ensure the safety of patients and a duty to inform them when mistakes

are made. Professional codes of ethics and patient bills of rights help make certain that patients are informed of their rights and nurses' obligations to protect them.

CRITICAL THINKING

The following case scenarios offer an opportunity for reflection, discussion, and analysis.

Discussion Points

1. Does your work setting or the settings where you have had clinical placements have a bill of rights and responsibilities? How is this statement communicated? Do you believe it is the nurse's responsibility to ensure that patients know their rights?
2. Can you think of situations in which the rights discussed in this chapter might potentially conflict with the rights of the institution? Of the nurse? Of other patients and families? How do we balance these rights?
3. Do visiting hours in your facility support the rights of patients? What processes are in place to support families of the terminally or seriously ill?
4. What procedures and policies need to be in place to guard against sexual harassment of patients by staff?

CASE SCENARIO 10.4

TO INTERVENE OR NOT TO INTERVENE?

M. B., a registered nurse, is visiting their parent, a resident in a long-term care facility. Upon hearing raised voices in the next room, M. B. goes to investigate and witnesses a nurse shouting at a resident who was not cooperating when the nurse was trying to turn them. When the nurse leaves the room obviously frustrated, M. B. goes in to see if the resident is okay.

The resident is 60 years old and has Guillain-Barré syndrome. The resident has total paralysis in the lower extremities with and minimal function in the upper body. The resident reveals that "everything is okay" and that this incident should not be shared with anyone else, and states that, "It's easier this way. I'm totally dependent on the staff here, and the nurse didn't hurt me and is just overworked."

Questions

1. Is there a violation of ethical or legal standards?
2. Is there risk of any civil or criminal liability?
3. What are the resident's rights in this situation? Are there conflicting rights here?
4. As a nurse, does M. B. have any obligation in this situation even though M. B. is not an employee of this facility?
5. What action do you recommend?

CASE SCENARIO 10.5

ACCESS AND DISCLOSURE

K. K. is a registered nurse in the emergency department of a local community hospital. One evening, a neighbour presents with abdominal pain of unknown origin and is admitted to the surgical unit.

Some days later, another neighbour asks K. K. how their neighbour is doing. K. K. accesses the neighbour's chart via the electronic record and discovers that this neighbour has not been informed of a diagnosis of advanced liver cancer. The attending surgeon is well known for having a paternalistic approach. K. K. recognizes that this information should not be shared with anyone else but is concerned that this neighbour is being kept in the dark.

Questions

1. Is there a violation of ethical or legal standards?
2. Is there risk of any civil or criminal liability?
3. As an employee of the hospital, did K. K. have the right to access this chart?
4. What should a hospital policy state with respect to employee access to health records?
5. What dilemma is K. K. now facing, and how can it be resolved?

REFERENCES

Statutes

Canada Health Act, RSC 1985, c. C-6.

Canadian Charter of Rights and Freedoms, Part I of the *Constitution Act*, 1982, being Schedule B to the Canada Act 1982 (U.K.), 1982, c. 11.

Canadian Human Rights Act, R.S.C., 1985, c. H-6.

Child, Youth and Family Services Act, 2017, S.O. 2017, c. 14, Sch. 1 (Ontario).

Civil Marriage Act, SC 2005, c. 33 (Canada).

Constitution Act, 1982, being Schedule B to the *Canada Act* 1982 (U.K.), 1982, c. 11.

Criminal Code, R.S.C. 1985, c. C-46 (Canada).

Excellent Care for All Act, 2010, SO 2010, c. 14, (Ontario).

Expanded Nursing Services for Patients Act, 1997, S.O. 1997, c. 9 (Ontario).

Freedom of Information and Protection of Privacy Act, R.S.A. 2000, c. F-25 (Alberta).

Health Care Consent Act, 1996, S.O. 1996, c. 2, Sch. A (Ontario).

Health Care Directives and Substitute Health Care Decision Makers Act, S.S. 1997, c. H-0.0001 (Saskatchewan).

Health Information Act, R.S.A. 2000, c. H-5 (Alberta).

Health Information Protection Act, S.S. 1999, c. H-0.021 (Saskatchewan).

Long-Term Care Homes Act, 2007, S.O. 2007, c. 8 (Ontario).

Mental Health Act, R.S.B.C. 1996, c. 288 (British Columbia).

Mental Health Act, R.S.O. 1990, c. M.7 (Ontario).

Mental Health Act, R.S.Y. 2002, c. 150 (Yukon)

Mental Health Care and Treatment Act, SNL 2006, c. M-9.1 Newfoundland and Labrador.

Nursing Act, 1991, S.O. 1991, c. 32 (Ontario).

Patient Safety Act, SNL 2001, c. P-3.01, (Newfoundland and Labrador).

Personal Health Information Act, C.C.S.M., c. P-33.5 (Manitoba).

Personal Health Information Act, S.N.L. 2008, c. P-7.01 (Newfoundland and Labrador).

Personal Health Information Protection Act, 2004, S.O. 2004, c. 3, Schedule A (Ontario).

Personal Information Protection Act, S.B.C., 2003, c. 63 (British Columbia).

Personal Information Protection and Electronic Documents Act, SC 2000, c. 5 (Canada).

Regulated Health Professions Act, 1991, S.O. 1991, c. 18 (Ontario).

Retirement Homes Act, 2010, S.O. 2010, c. 11 (Ontario).

Substitute Decisions Act, 1992, S.O. 1992, c. 30 (Ontario).

Case Law

A.C. v. Manitoba (Director of Child and Family Services) [2009] SCC 30 (CanLII).

B. (R.) v. Children's Aid Society of Metropolitan Toronto [1995] SCC 115 (CanLII).

College of Nurses of Ontario v. Brutzki [2016] CanLII 104252 (ON CNO). http://canlii.ca/t/h3s7v

College of Nurses of Ontario v. Cruz [2017] CanLII 49268 (ON CNO), https://canlii.ca/t/h546j.

College of Nurses of Ontario v. Leclair [2011] CanLII 100585 (ON CNO).

Danilova v. Nikityuk [2017] ONSC 4016 (CanLII). http://canlii.ca/t/h4k55

Hamilton Health Sciences Corp. v. D.H. [2014] ONCJ 603 (CanLII).

Hamilton Health Sciences Corp. v. D.H. [2015] ONCJ 229 (CanLII).

Hopkins et al. v. Kay et al. [2015] ONCA 112 (CanLII).

MacLaren v. British Columbia (Attorney General) [2018] BCSC 1753 (CanLII).

McCorkell v. Director of Riverview Hospital [1993] CanLII 1200 (BC SC). http://canlii.ca/t/1dk2g

North Bay Health Centre v. Ontario Nurses' Association [2012] CanLII 97626 (ON LA).

Pittman Estate v. Bain [1994] CanLII 7489 (ON SC). http://canlii.ca/t/1wc23

Strom v. Saskatchewan Registered Nurses' Association [2018] SKQB 110 (CanLII).

Strom v. Saskatchewan Registered Nurses' Association [2020] SKCA 112 (CanLII)

Timmins & District Hospital v. O.N.A. (Peever) [2011] 208 LAC (4d) 43.

Vancouver Coastal Health Authority v. Health Sciences Association of British Columbia [2014] CanLII 15539 (BC LA).

Texts and Articles

Acierno, R., Hernandez, M. A., Amstadter, A. B., et al. (2010). Prevalence of and correlates of emotional, physical, sexual, and financial abuse and potential neglect in the United States: The National Elder Mistreatment Study. *American Journal of Public Health, 100,* 292–297.

Akhtar-Danesh, N., Baumann, A., Crea-Arsenio, M., et al. (2022). COVID-19 excess mortality among long-term care residents in Ontario, Canada. *PLoS One, 17,* 0262807.

Andrews, M. M., & Boyle, J. S. (2002). Transcultural concepts in nursing care. *Journal of Transcultural Nursing, 13*(3), 178–180.

Arnold, O. F., & Bruce, A. (2006). Nursing practice with Aboriginal communities: Expanding worldviews. *Nursing Science Quarterly, 18*(3), 259–263.

Bahji, A., & Delva, N. (2021). Making a case for the inclusion of refractory and severe mental illness as a sole criterion for Canadians requesting Medical Assistance in Dying (MAiD): A review. *Journal of Medical Ethics, 48*(11), 929–934.

Baker, G. R. (2014). An opportunity for reflection. *Healthcare Quarterly, 17,* 1.

Baker, G. R., Norton, P. G., Flintoft, V., et al. (2004). The Canadian adverse events study: The incidence of adverse events among hospital patients in Canada. *Canadian Medical Association Journal, 170*(11), 1678–1686.

Bayer, T., Tadd, W., & Krajcik, S. (2005). Dignity: The voice of older people. *Quality in Ageing and Older Adults, 6*(1), 22–29.

BC Emergency Health Services. (n.d.). *No cardiopulmonary resuscitation—Medical order.* https://www2.gov.bc.ca/assets/gov/health/forms/302fil.pdf

Beagan, B. L. (2018). Chapter 6—A critique of cultural competence: Assumptions, limitations, and alternatives. In C. Frisby & W. O'Donohue (Eds.), *Cultural competence in applied psychology: An evaluation of current status and future directions* (pp. 123–138). Springer.

Bélanger-Hardy, L., & Quesnel, C. (2016). Patient safety incidents and protection of quality assurance activities: Legislative and jurisprudential responses in Canada. *McGill Journal of Law and Health, 9*(1), 69.

Berwick, D. M. (2002). A user's manual for the IOM's "Quality Chasm" report. *Health Affairs, 21*(3), 80–90.

Bethell, J., Puts, M. T. E., Sattar, S., et al. (2019). The Canadian frailty priority setting partnership: Priorities for older adults living with frailty. *Canadian Geriatric Journal, 22*(1), 22–33.

Biljon, H., Niekerk, L., Margot-Cattin, I., et al. (2022). The health equity characteristics of research exploring the unmet community mobility needs of older adults: A scoping review. *BMC Geriatrics, 22,* 808.

Borden Ladner Gervais. (2015). *Update: Recent case regarding parent refusing chemotherapy for First Nation child in favour of traditional medicine: What are the implications for health care providers?* http://blg.com/en/News-And-Publications/Documents/Publication_4105.pdf

Borden Ladner Gervais. (2018). *Nurse disciplined for unprofessional posts on social media loses appeal.* Mondaq. https://www.mondaq.com/canada/healthcare/706338/nurse-disciplined-for-unprofessional-posts-on-social-media-loses-appeal

Boyer, Y. (2017). Healing racism in Canadian health care. *CMAJ, 189*(46), E1408–E1409.

Boyer, Y., & Bartlett, J. (2017). *Tubal ligation in the Saskatoon health region: The lived experience of Aboriginal women.* https://www.saskatoonhealthregion.ca/DocumentsInternal/Tubal_Ligation_intheSaskatoonHealthRegion_the_Lived_Experience_of_Aboriginal_Women_BoyerandBartlett_July_22_2017.pdf

British Columbia College of Nurses and Midwives. (2022). *Social media scenarios.* https://www.bccnm.ca/RPN/learning/socialmedia/Pages/Social_media_scenarios.aspx

British Columbia Ministry of Health. (2005). *Guide to the Mental Health Act.* http://www.health.gov.bc.ca/library/publications/year/2005/MentalHealthGuide.pdf

Calnan, M., Woolhead, G., Dieppe, P., et al. (2005). Views on dignity in providing health care for older people. *Nursing Times, 101*(33), 38–41.

Canadian Armed Forces, 4th Canadian Division Joint Task Force (Central). (2020). *Operation LASER—JTFC observations in long term care facilities in Ontario*. https://www.macleans.ca/wp-content/uploads/2020/05/JTFC-Observations-in-LTCF-in-ON.pdf

Canadian Institute for Health Information. (2020). *Pandemic experience in the long-term care sector how does Canada compare with other countries?* https://www.cihi.ca/sites/default/files/document/covid-19-rapid-response-long-term-care-snapshot-en.pdf

Canadian Institute for Health Information, & Canadian Patient Safety Institute. (2016). Measuring patient harm in Canadian hospitals. With what can be done to improve patient safety? Authored by Chan, B., & Cochrane, D. Canadian Institute for Health Information.

Canadian Mental Health Association–British Columbia Division. (2017). *Policy perspective: Charter challenge of the BC Mental Health Act—Involuntary treatment (section 31).* https://cmha.bc.ca/documents/policy-perspective-charter-challenge-of-the-bc-mental-health-act-involuntary-treatment-section-31/

Canadian Nurses Association. (2017). Code of ethics for registered nurses.

Canadian Nurses Association. (2020, October 1). *CNA's key messages on COVID-19 and long-term care.* https://hl-prod-ca-oc-download.s3-ca-central-1.amazonaws.com/CNA/2f975e7e-4a40-45ca-863c-5ebf0a138d5e/UploadedImages/documents/Covid-19_Key-Messages-on-Long-Term-Care_e.pdf

Canadian Patient Safety Institute. (2016). *About CPSI.* http://www.patientsafetyinstitute.ca/en/Pages/default

The Canadian Press. (2023, March 9). "Historic" $2.8B class-action Indigenous court settlement approved. *CBC News.* https://www.cbc.ca/news/canada/british-columbia/indigenous-class-action-settlement-approved-1.6774186

CBC.ca (2001) Natives Speak Out: Native people air long-held grievances at the Berger Commission. *Canada – A peoples history* https://www.cbc.ca/history/EPISCONTENTSE1EP17CH2PA1LE.html

CBC. (2022). *This long-term care home radically changed the way it operates. Residents say it's working.* https://www.cbc.ca/news/canada/toronto/long-term-care-resident-centred-1.6659458

Chartrand, L. N., Logan, T. E., & Daniels, J. D. (2006). *Métis history and experience and residential schools in Canada.* The Aboriginal Healing Foundation.

Chu, C. H., Yee, A. V., & Stamatopoulos, V. (2022). "It's the worst thing I've ever been put through in my life": The trauma experienced by essential family caregivers of loved ones in long-term care during the COVID-19 pandemic in Canada. *International Journal of Qualitative Studies on Health and Well-Being, 17*(1), 2075532.

Chun, J., & Gallagher-Louisy, C. (2018). *Overview of human rights codes by province and territory in Canada.* Canadian Centre for Diversity and Inclusion. https://ccdi.ca/media/1414/20171102-publications-overview-of-hr-codes-by-province-final-en.pdf

Cohen-Mansfield, J. (2001). Nonpharmacologic interventions for inappropriate behaviors in dementia: A review, summary, and critique. *American Journal of Geriatric Psychiatry, 9*(4), 361–381.

College of Nurses of Ontario. (2017). *Practice standard: Restraints.* Pub. No. 41043.

Cooper, C., Selwood, A., & Livingston, G. (2008). The prevalence of elder abuse and neglect: A systematic review. *Age Ageing, 37,* 151–160.

Corrigan, J. M. (2005). Crossing the quality chasm. In P. P. Reid, W. D. Compton, & J. H. Grossman (Eds.), *Building a better delivery system: A new engineering/health care partnership.* National Academies Press.

Coward, H., & Sidhu, T. (2000). Bioethics for clinicians: 19. Hinduism and Sikhism. *Canadian Medical Association Journal, 163*(9), 1167–1170.

Curtis, E., Jones, R., Tipene-Leach, D., et al. (2019). Why cultural safety rather than cultural competency is required to achieve health equity: A literature review and recommended definition. *International Journal for Equity in Health, 18*(174), 1–17.

de Jonge, V., Sint Nicolaas, J., van Leerdam, M. E., et al. (2011). Overview of the quality assurance movement in health care. *Best Practice & Research Clinical Gastroenterology, 25*(3), 337–347.

Disclosure Working Group. (2008). *Canadian disclosure guidelines.* Canadian Patient Safety Institute. http://www.patientsafetyinstitute.ca/disclosure.html

Dupuis, S. L., & Luh, J. (2005). Understanding responsive behaviours: The importance of correctly perceiving triggers that precipitate residents' responsive behaviours. *Canadian Nursing Home, 16*(1), 29–34.

Echenberg, H., & Kirkby, C. (2012). *Legislative summary: Bill C-36: An Act to amend the Criminal Code (Elder Abuse).* Parliamentary Information and Research Service, Library of Parliament.

Encyclopedia, T. (2020). Berger Commission. In *The Canadian Encyclopedia.* https://www.thecanadianencyclopedia.ca/en/article/berger-commission

Emergency Health Services Branch, Ontario Ministry of Health and Long-Term Care. (2007). *Training bulletin: Do not resuscitate (DNR) standard.* https://www.health.gov.on.ca/en/pro/programs/emergency_health/docs/ehs_training_blltn108_en.pdf

Emergency Health Services Branch, Ontario Ministry of Health and Long-Term Care. (2017). *Basic life support patient care standards.* Version 3.0.1.

End of Life Planning Canada. (2016). *Advance care planning kit, Nova Scotia edition.* https://elplanning.ca/wp-content/uploads/2016/03/acp_nova-scotia-ap29.pdf

First Nations Health Authority. (2022). *Cultural safety and humility.* https://www.fnha.ca/wellness/wellness-and-the-first-nations-health-authority/cultural-safety-and-humility

Foerschner, A. M. (2010). The history of mental illness: From skull drills to happy pills. *Inquiries Journal/Student Pulse, 2*(9), 1–4. http://www.inquiriesjournal.com/articles/1673/the-history-of-mental-illness-from-skull-drills-to-happy-pills

Fryer, S., & Leblanc-Laurendeau, O. (2019). *Understanding federal jurisdiction and First Nations: Background paper.* Library of Parliament: Parliament of Canada. https://lop.parl.ca/sites/PublicWebsite/default/en_CA/ResearchPublications/201951E

Fulmer, T., Patel, P., Levy, N., et al. (2020). Moving toward a global age-friendly ecosystem. *Journal of the American Geriatrics Society, 68*(9), 1936–1940.

Galik, E. M., Resnick, B., & Pretzer-Aboff, I. (2009). "Knowing what makes them tick": Motivating cognitively impaired older adults to participate in restorative care. *International Journal of Nursing Practice, 15*(1), 48–55.

Gallant, N. L., Hardy, M., Beogo, I., et al. (2022). Improving family presence in long-term care during the COVID-19 pandemic [Special issue]. *Healthcare Quarterly, 25,* 34–40.

Geddes, G. (2017). *Medicine unbundled: A journey through the minefields of Indigenous health care.* Heritage House.

Glasdam, S., Sandberg, H., Stjernswärd, S., et al. (2022). Nurses' use of social media during the COVID-19 pandemic—A scoping review. *PLoS One, 17*(2), e0263502.

Government of Canada. (n.d.). *Indigenous peoples and communities: First Nations in Canada.* https://www.aadnc-aandc.gc.ca/eng/130 7460755710/1307460872523#chp4

Government of Canada. (2012). *Elder abuse: It's time to face the reality.* https://www.canada.ca/en/public-health/services/health-promotion/stop-family-violence/prevention-resource-centre/prevention-resources-older-adults/elder-abuses-time-face-reality.html#Wha

Government of Canada. (2021). *Indian Residential Schools Settlement Agreement.* https://www.rcaanc-cirnac.gc.ca/eng/1100100015576/1571581687074

Government of Canada. (2023). *Indigenous health care in Canada.* https://www.sac-isc.gc.ca/eng/1626810177053/1626810219482

Haddock, J. (1996). Towards further clarification of the concept "dignity". *Journal of Advanced Nursing, 24*(5), 924–931.

Hardcastle, L. (2017). Legal mechanisms to improve quality of care in Canadian hospitals. *Alberta Law Review, 54*(3), 681. https://albertalawreview.com/index.php/ALR/article/view/777/770

Hein, L. C., & Levitt, N. (2014). Caring for transgender patients. *Nursing Made Incredibly Easy! 12*(6), 28–36.

Hicks, T. (2017). *Social media's role in privacy breaches: Educate your medical employees on social media HIPAA.* https://www.verywellhealth.com/social-medias-role-in-privacy-breaches-2317518

Hicock, L., & Lewis, J. (2004). *Beware the grieving warrior: A child's preventable death, a father's fight for justice.* ECW Press.

Hofmann, H., Schorro, E., Haastert, B., et al. (2015). Use of physical restraints in nursing homes: A multicentre cross-sectional study. *BMC Geriatrics, 15*(1), 129.

Indigenous Corporate Training. (2017). *A brief look at Indian hospitals in Canada.* https://www.ictinc.ca/blog/a-brief-look-at-indian-hospitals-in-canada-0

Indigenous Services Canada. (2022). *Indigenous Services Canada flowing $125M in COVID-19 public health funding directly to First Nations communities.* https://www.canada.ca/en/indigenous-services-canada/news/2022/01/indigenous-services-canada-flowing-125m-in-covid-19-public-health-funding-directly-to-first-nations-communities.html

Institute of Medicine (US) Committee on Quality of Health Care in America. (2000). *To err is human: Building a safer health system.* National Academies Press. https://www.ncbi.nlm.nih.gov/books/NBK225182/. doi:10.17226/9728

International Nurse Regulator Collaborative. (2017). *Social media use: Common expectations for nurses.* https://inrc.com/Social+Media+Use+Common+Expectations+for+Nurses.page

Johnston, P., Keatings, M., & Monk, A. (2022). Experiences of essential care partners during the COVID-19 pandemic [Special issue]. *Healthcare Quarterly,* 25, 41–47.

Jones, A. (2022). Variations in long-term care home resident hospitalizations before and during the COVID-19 pandemic in Ontario. *PLoS One, 17*, e0264240.

Keatings, M., Martin, M., McCallum, A., et al. (2006). Medical errors: Understanding the parent's perspective. *Pediatric Clinics of North America, 53*(6), 1079–1089.

King, T. (2012). *The inconvenient Indian.* Anchor Canada.

Kon, A. A., Shepard, E. K., Sederstrom, N. O., et al. (2016). Defining futile and potentially inappropriate interventions: A policy statement from the Society of Critical Care Medicine Ethics Committee. *Critical Care Medicine, 44*(9), 1769–1774.

Konder, R. M., & Christie, T. (2019). Medical Assistance in Dying (MAiD) in Canada: A critical analysis of the exclusion of vulnerable populations. *Healthcare Policy, 15*(2), 28–38.

Lambda Legal. (2013). *Creating equal access to quality health care for transgender patients: Transgender-affirming hospital policies.* http://www.lambdalegal.org/publications/fs_transgender-affirming-hospital-policies

Lancaster, J. (2017, October 6). *Seeing red:* How did a mild-mannered nurse from small-town Ontario become one of Canada's worst serial killers? *CBC News.* https://www.cbc.ca/news2/interactives/sh/TBk79oWhpi/elizabeth-wettlaufer-nurse-senior-deaths/

LaSala, C. A. (2009). Moral accountability and integrity in nursing practice. *Nursing Clinics of North America, 44*(4), 423–434.

Lawrence, B. (2016). Enslavement of Indigenous people in Canada. In *Historica Canada.* https://www.thecanadianencyclopedia.ca/en/article/slavery-of-indigenous-people-in-canada/

Luce, J. M. (1995). Physicians do not have a responsibility to provide futile or unreasonable care if a patient or family insists [Special article]. *Critical Care Medicine, 23*(4), 760–766.

Lux, M. K. (2016). *Separate beds: A history of Indian hospitals in Canada, 1920s–1980s.* University of Toronto Press.

Maggio, M., Colizzi, E., Fisichella, A., et al. (2013). Stress hormones, sleep deprivation and cognition in older adults. *Maturitas, 76*(1), 22–44.

Marsh, J. (2023). James Bay Project. In *The Canadian Encyclopedia.* https://www.thecanadianencyclopedia.ca/en/article/james-bay-project

McGaffigan, P. (2019). *Why Florence Nightingale's improvement lessons still matter today.* Institute for Health Care Improvement. http://www.ihi.org/communities/blogs/why-florence-nightingales-improvement-lessons-still-matter-today

McGilton, K. S. (2004). Relating well to persons with dementia: A variable influencing staffing and quality of care outcomes. *Alzheimer's Care Today, 5*(1), 71–80.

McGilton, K. S., Vellani, S., Yeung, L., et al. (2018). Identifying and understanding the health and social care needs of older adults with multiple chronic conditions and their caregivers: A scoping review. *BMC Geriatrics, 18*(1), 231.

Missildine, K., Bergstrom, N., Meininger, J., et al. (2010). Sleep in hospitalized elders: A pilot study. *Geriatric Nursing, 31*(4), 263–271.

Möhler, R., & Meyer, G. (2014). Attitudes of nurses towards the use of physical restraints in geriatric care: A systematic review of qualitative and quantitative studies. *International Journal of Nursing Studies, 51*(2), 274–288.

Möhler, R., Richter, T., Köpke, S., et al. (2012). Interventions for preventing and reducing the use of physical restraints in long-term geriatric care—A Cochrane review. *Journal of Clinical Nursing, 21*(21–22), 3070–3081.

Morath, J. M. (2006). Patient safety: A view from the top. *Pediatric Clinics, 53*(6), 1053–1065.

National Steering Committee on Patient Safety. (2002). *Building a safer system: A national integrated strategy for improving patient safety in Canadian health care.* https://era.library.ualberta.ca/items/eda9644a-1f91-4ec9-880a-7b69c651bf0c/view/501053b2-43cf-4add-a1fd-9d032c52f6e3/building_a_safer_system_e%20(2).pdf

Ngai, E. W. T., Tao, S. S. C., & Moon, K. K. L. (2015). Social media research: Theories, constructs, and conceptual frameworks. *International Journal of Information Management, 35*(1), 33–44.

O'Leary, L., Erikainen, S., Peltonen, L. M., et al. (2022). Exploring nurses' online perspectives and social networks during a global pandemic COVID-19. *Public Health Nursing, 39,* 586–600.

Ontario Human Rights Commission. (n.d.-a). *Ageism and age discrimination (fact sheet).* http://www.ohrc.on.ca/en/ageism-and-age-discrimination-fact-sheet

Ontario Human Rights Commission. (n.d.-b). *Gender identity and gender expression.* https://www.ohrc.on.ca/en/policy-preventing-discrimination-because-gender-identity-and-gender-expression/3-gender-identity-and-gender-expression

Ontario Ministry of the Attorney General. (2018). *Child protection.* https://www.attorneygeneral.jus.gov.on.ca/english/family/divorce/child_protection/

The Canadian Museum for Human Rights. (2023). *The Doctrine of Discovery. (Story written by Travis Tomchuch)* https://humanrights.ca/story/doctrine-discovery

The Provincial Court of Manitoba. (2015). *In the matter of The Fatality Inquiries Act, C.C.S.M. c. F52 and in the matter of an inquest into the death of Heather Dawn Brenan.* https://www.manitobacourts.mb.ca/site/assets/files/1051/heather_brenan_inquest_report_-_december_22_2015_wiebe.pdf.

Rankin, D. (2004). *Disclosure of harm: Good medical practice.* Medical Council of New Zealand. http://www.menz.org.nz/portals/1/guidance/disclosure_of_harm

Re Heather Dawn Brenan (Inquest) Man. Prov. Ct., Dec 22, 2015.

Reason, J. (2000). Human error: Models and management. *BMJ, 320*(7237), 768–770.

Rousseau, S., Turner, S., Chochinov, H. M., et al. (2017). A national survey of Canadian psychiatrists' attitudes toward medical assistance in death. *Canadian Journal of Psychiatry, 62*(11), 787–794.

Standing Senate Committee on Human Rights. (2022). *The scars that we carry: Forced and coerced sterilization of persons in Canada—Part II.* https://sencanada.ca/content/sen/committee/441/RIDR/reports/2022-07-14_ForcedSterilization_E.pdf

Stanford Encyclopedia of Philosophy. (2014). *Feminist perspectives on trans issues.* https://plato.stanford.edu/entries/feminism-trans/#Con

Stratton, D., & Tadd, W. (2005). Dignity and older people: The voice of society. *Quality in Ageing & Older Adults, 6*(1), 37–48.

Tanner, R. (2018). An ethical-legal analysis of Medical Assistance in Dying for those with mental illness. *Alberta Law Review, 56,* 149.

Thompson, E., McMahon, M., Loates, K., et al. (2022). What we have heard: Next steps for long-term care pandemic preparedness in Canada [Special issue]. *Healthcare Quarterly, 25,* 53–58.

Trottier, J. P. (2015, May 1). The Ontario DNR Confirmation Form—What your patients need to know about their DNR order. Blog in *Physician's Update: In partnership with the Academy of Medicine Ottawa.* https://blogs.ottawa.ca/physicians/2015/05/01/the-ontario-dnr-confirmation-form-what-your-patients-need-to-know-about-their-dnr-order/

Truth and Reconciliation Commission of Canada. (2015). *Honouring the truth, reconciling for the future: Summary of the final report of the Truth and Reconciliation Commission of Canada.* https://ehprnh2mwo3.exactdn.com/wp-content/uploads/2021/01/Executive_Summary_English_Web.pdf

Tye, J. (2020). Florence Nightingale's lasting legacy for health care. *Nurse Leader, 18*(3), 220–226.

United Nations. (n.d.). *Global issues: Human rights.* https://www.un.org/en/global-issues/human-rights

United Nations. (1948). *Universal Declaration of Human Rights.* https://www.un.org/sites/un2.un.org/files/2021/03/udhr.pdf

United Nations. (2006). *Convention on the Rights of Persons with Disabilities.* https://www.ohchr.org/en/instruments-mechanisms/instruments/convention-rights-persons-disabilities

United Nations. (2015). *Transforming our world: The 2030 agenda for sustainable development.* https://www.bing.com/search?form=MOZLBR&pc=MOZD&q=+United+Nations%2C+Transforming+our+world%3A+the+2030+agenda+for+sustainable+development+

Uys, L. R., & Smit, J. H. (1994). Writing a philosophy of nursing? *Journal of Advanced Nursing, 20*(2), 239–244.

Vellani, S., Puts, M., Iaboni, A., et al. (2022a). Acceptability of the voice your values, an advance care planning intervention in persons living with mild dementia using videoconferencing technology. *PLoS One, 17*(4), e0266826.

Vellani, S., Puts, M., Iaboni, A., et al. (2022b). Voice your values, a tailored advance care planning intervention in persons living with mild dementia: A pilot study. *Palliative and Supportive Care,* 1–9. doi:10.1017/S1478951522000475.

Ventura, C. A., & Austin, W. (2017). Mental health professionals, Medical Assistance in Dying and mental illness: Challenges and possible alternatives. *Editor's Forum, 25*(1), 13.

Wang, X. M., Brisbin, S., Loo, T., et al. (2015). Elder abuse: An approach to identification, assessment and intervention. *Canadian Medical Association Journal, 187*(8), 575–581.

Weijer, C., Singer, P. A., Dickens, B. M., et al. (1998). Bioethics for clinicians: 16. Dealing with demands for inappropriate treatment. *Canadian Medical Association Journal, 159*(7), 817–821.

Wesp, M., Scheer, M., Ruiz, M., et al. (2018). An emancipatory approach to cultural competency: The application of critical race, postcolonial, and intersectionality theories. *Advances in Nursing Science, 41*(4), 316–326.

Wong, J. S., Breslau, H., McSorley, V. E., et al. (2020). The social relationship context of elder mistreatment. *Gerontologist, 60*(6), 1029–1039.

Wong, T. K. S., & Pang, S. M. C. (2000). Holism and caring: Nursing in the Chinese health care culture. *Holistic Nursing Practice, 15*(1), 12–21.

World Health Organization. (2018). *The global network for age-friendly cities and communities: Looking back over the last decade, looking forward to the next.* World Health Organization.

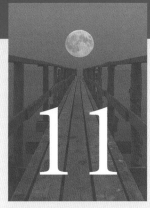

11

PERSPECTIVES ON THE RIGHTS OF NURSES

LEARNING OBJECTIVES

The purpose of this chapter is to enable you to understand:

- The rights of nurses as citizens, professionals, and employees
- Conscientious objections and when they can be invoked
- The accountabilities of nurses as employees
- The issues of concern to nurses regarding discrimination and sexual or physical abuse
- The importance of a healthy and supportive work environment and how this contributes to the retention and engagement of nurses
- The nature of workplace violence and how it should be prevented and addressed
- The role of labour relations and collective bargaining in nursing
- Occupational health and safety standards

INTRODUCTION

Along with all other residents of Canada, under the *Canadian Charter of Rights and Freedoms* (1982), nurses have the right to privacy, respect, and freedom of expression—to think, say, write, or otherwise act in accordance with their beliefs. However, these rights are not absolute. For nurses, professional rules and regulations, and ethical responsibilities to patients, may limit individual freedom. For example, when caring for a patient whose values and religious beliefs differ from their own, it is not professionally or ethically appropriate for nurses to attempt to influence patients toward their

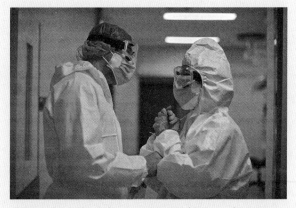

Nurses have the right to practise within a work environment where risks of harm are minimized. *Source: iStock.com/ xavierarnau.*

opinions, values, and beliefs, especially as it relates to a person's health care choices.

Nurses are entitled to respect from one another, from other health care professionals, from their employers, from government, and from patients. As individuals and as employees, they are entitled to freedom from any form of discrimination, harassment (sexual or otherwise), and physical or sexual abuse. They have the right to practise within a work environment in which risks of harm are minimized. This chapter explores some of these rights.

CONSCIENTIOUS OBJECTION

As employees, nurses are under a contractual obligation to provide competent care to patients. There are times, however, when the duty to provide care may

345

conflict with nurses' personal values—for example, having to participate in a procedure or provide care (e.g., elective abortion or Medical Assistance in Dying [MAiD]) that they find objectionable on moral or religious grounds.

Refusal to participate in a procedure does not always relate to conscientious factors. Non-conscientious-based factors such as previous experiences or discomfort in working with dying patients, fear of potential post-traumatic stress disorder (PTSD) and burnout, legal uncertainty, concerns that palliative care resources were not accessed, potential negative responses from colleagues and the community, and lack of experience, among other concerns, were all mentioned in research

on nurses refusing to participate in MAiD (Brown, 2022). What would be the response if the refusal is a based on a personal moral or religious conflict?

Such situations will usually not be emergencies. In an emergency, the nurse's foremost ethical obligation is to help patients and to protect them from harm. Refusing to act would go against the ethical principles of beneficence and nonmaleficence and of their professional duties and responsibilities. Therefore, in an emergency, a nurse with a conscientious objection nurse is bound to help the patient until alternative care is available. Note that the issue of conscientious objection is also discussed in Chapter 8 in the context of MAiD. Consider Case Scenario 11.1.

CASE SCENARIO 11.1

REFUSAL TO CARE . . . MY RIGHT?

M. F., a registered nurse of 5 years' standing, works in the obstetrics department of a public hospital in a large urban centre. Deeply religious and opposed to abortion, M. F. accepted her position with the understanding that no therapeutic abortions would be performed in the department. In this hospital, abortions are usually performed in the gynecology department; some such procedures involve saline injections. The understanding was that M. F. would never be asked or required to work on this unit.

Recent cutbacks in funding to the hospital have meant staff reductions and bed closures. Consequently, when beds are scarce, an abortion might occasionally be performed in the obstetrical department. One afternoon, M. F. is assigned to assist in a second-trimester saline abortion that is to take place in the department later that day. Angry and upset, M. F. approaches her manager: "There's no way I'm going to assist with this! Find another nurse!"

Issues

1. What are the hospital's ethical and legal obligations to M. F. and to the patient seeking the abortion?
2. How can the conflict between these interests be resolved?

Discussion

Whenever possible, employers are obliged to respect the conscientious objections of employees who decline to participate in certain actions on moral or religious grounds. The issue is not about indulging the employee's prejudices. The employee has the right not to be forced to engage in actions to which they object on ethical grounds. In this scenario, the treatment is not considered an emergency. If it were, M. F. would be ethically bound to render any and all assistance needed—it would take priority over her conscientious objections. For example, if the patient were suffering complications as a result of an abortion, such as internal bleeding after a saline injection, regardless of M. F.'s personal opinion of the patient's actions, M. F. would have the duty to render assistance. Although M. F. can refuse to participate in the abortion, they would be compelled to render emergency life-saving treatment after the fact.

In a different circumstance, a nurse working in a palliative care unit caring for a male patient with acquired immunodeficiency syndrome (AIDS) cannot ethically refuse to treat him on the grounds that he may be homosexual or a drug abuser. This would be a clear case of prejudice, and the employer is not obliged to accommodate requests that are unethical and unprofessional.

Problems relating to conscientious objection are best avoided by prospective nursing employees informing themselves of all expectations related to functions, roles, duties, and responsibilities. Once employment is accepted, nurses have no option but to provide the care required. Thus, an applicant for a position in the gynecology department of a secular hospital should be informed that their duties may include assisting during abortions. The informed nurse may then decline such employment.

However, if the nature of the nurse's role changes after employment, the agency or the hospital is obligated to reassign that nurse to areas where the objectionable activities are not performed. However, there are no guarantees, because in emergency situations nurses are ethically obliged to provide care. The nurse may withdraw from such situations only when doing so does not endanger the patient or when others are available to provide the required care. In smaller facilities, it may not be possible to reassign nurses or to guarantee exemptions based on a conscientious objection. In these cases, nurses may face the difficult choice of seeking employment elsewhere.

The ethical principles that apply in these circumstances are justice (the patient's right to be treated fairly and equitably), beneficence (the nurse's obligation to do good for the patient), and nonmaleficence (the nurse's duty to do the patient no harm). For example, if nurses were to withdraw their services arbitrarily because of an ethical objection, and thereby place the patient in danger, that nurse would be violating the principle of nonmaleficence and the duty to prevent harm.

It is clearly stated in the Canadian Nurses Association (CNA) *Code of Ethics for Registered Nurses* (2017) that nurses are not obliged to act on the wishes of a patient when those actions pose a serious moral conflict for the nurse. However, the nurse is obliged to ensure that other arrangements are available to a patient when the care required conflicts with the nurse's beliefs but is legally acceptable:

If nursing care is requested that is in conflict with the nurse's moral beliefs and values but in keeping with professional practice, the nurses should provide safe, compassionate, competent and ethical care until alternative care arrangements are in place to meet the person's needs or desires. If nurses can anticipate

a conflict with their conscience, they have an obligation to notify their employers or, if the nurse is self-employed, persons receiving care in advance so that alternative arrangements can be made. (CNA, 2017, p. 17)

In circumstances where the refusal of care is not related to conscientious objection but to other factors, such as those raised by nurses refusing to participate in MAiD based on concerns not related to conscientious objection, nurses should seek resolutions of these issues with their leaders. For example, if a nurse is concerned that a particular patient did not receive the benefit of palliative care prior to making a MAiD decision, then this should be addressed from a system perspective and also from the specific circumstances of the patient involved.

The Canadian Nurse Protective Society (CNPS), which provides insurance to nurses to protect them from liability, offers the following advice in an article about MAiD:

in the event a nurse refuses to participate in MAiD because it does not fall within their scope of practice, for moral or religious reasons, or because they are concerned about legal risk, it would be prudent for the nurse to consult with their regulatory body and/ or employer for guidance on what to do in these circumstances. (CNPS, 2021)

This advice is broadly applicable to all situations where a nurse is unwilling to participate in a procedure. If faced with a request to participate in a procedure that the nurse is unwilling to be part of, the nurse must "provide safe, compassionate, competent and ethical care until alternative care arrangements are in place to meet the person's needs" (CNA, 2017, p. 17). Ultimately, the nurse will have to consult their regulator and employer to determine whether they can be excused from the procedure or whether they will have to leave their employment in order to avoid being expected to participate.

DISCRIMINATION ISSUES IN EMPLOYMENT

Case Scenario 11.1 also raises an employment law issue and illustrates the competing interests of employees' and employers' rights. Legally, the matter involves the application of human rights legislation.

This legislation is virtually identical in all Canadian jurisdictions, and is essentially designed to prohibit discrimination against persons based on race, sexual and gender orientation, creed, religion, age, physical or mental disability, nationality, or ethnic origin. The thrust of the legislation is that employers are obliged, to the greatest extent possible, to structure work conditions and requirements to cause the least possible interference with the religious or cultural views, or the physical or mental characteristics, of their employees. For example, employers must accommodate work conditions such that no employee is unduly inconvenienced only by reason of gender, as in the case of providing adequate washroom facilities.

In Case Scenario 11.1, the religious views of the nurse conflicted with the employer's work requirements. If the circumstances were altered and the nurse was reassigned to the unit by a supervisor who thought the nurse's religious views were offensive, ignored these objections, and used threats to force the nurse to participate in the abortion, the nurse would have valid grounds for a complaint before the provincial Human Rights Commission. If it was found that the nurse's rights had been infringed upon, M. F. could be awarded compensation, depending on the laws of the particular province or territory. Nurses should not be forced to work in a setting they object to on moral or religious grounds, subject, of course, to the ethical rules and legal considerations discussed earlier.

Discrimination

While discrimination on the basis of race violates human rights codes, such discrimination and racism exist and have an impact on nurses, their profession, and the institutions within which they work. In recent years, the existence of racial discrimination in health care (as discussed in Chapter 10), as well as other parts of Canadian society, has been recognized, and this has been accompanied by an acknowledgement of the importance of including race information in data collection.

At the time of writing, the Canadian Nursing Association did not offer a race-based breakdown of nurses in Canada on its public website. Statistics Canada does have information about immigrants and their employment in health care that includes data on race. Their data indicate that visible minority immigrants are as likely to find work as white immigrants in professional nursing capacities (i.e., registered nurse, nurse practitioner, licensed practical nurse/registered practical nurse) (StatsCan, 2019).

However, visible minority immigrants are much more likely to be employed in the unregulated sector of health care, in lower-paying positions, than white immigrants.

Since 2020, major initiatives have been taken to address racism within the nursing profession. While nursing has been working toward more diverse, inclusive, and equitable workplaces and educational settings for many years, under-represented minority nurses have faced and still face discriminatory and inequitable treatment from employers, educators, co-workers, and patients (Hantkie et al., 2022). Minority nurses have reported institutional discrimination, racism, and microaggressions, leading to feelings of isolation, moral distress, and burnout (Çayır, 2021). Nurses find that their experiences of discrimination and racism use up their emotional capital and negatively affect their ability to engage in self-care and patient care (Cottingham et al., 2018).

The idea that racism is embedded in the profession of nursing has been accepted by the Registered Nurses' Association of Ontario (RNAO) and the Canadian Association of Schools of Nursing (CASN), among other groups. In 2022, the RNAO president noted: "Racism is a public health crisis that cannot be ignored. It threatens the health and well-being of racialized nurses. It limits their capacity to fully advance their careers and contributions to the health care system. And it can compromise their ability to provide safe and compassionate care for . . . Canadians" (RNAO, 2022b)

Black nurses and RNAO. https://rnao,ca/infocus/black-nurses-and-rnao issued a statement in response to the murder of George Floyd in the United States. A past president of the RNAO was appointed to a new Black Nurses Task Force (BNTF) with the mandate to interrupt complicity and lead transformational change resolving anti-Black racism and discrimination.

In 2022, the RNAO released the BNTF's report on anti-Black racism and discrimination in nursing (RNAO, 2022a). Black nurses are one of the largest visible minority groups in nursing in Ontario. Despite this, few Black nurses are in leadership or advanced practice roles. In a survey of Black nurses commissioned by the RNAO, cited in the report:

- 88.3% of respondents said that they had experienced racism or discrimination as a Black nurse in Ontario.
- 60.5% of respondents agreed that they were made to feel uncomfortable or very uncomfortable in

their academic or workplace settings because of their race, colour, or ethnicity as a Black nurse.
■ Racial microaggressions and systemic discrimination had affected the mental health of 63% of respondents (RNAO, 2022a).

RNAO is advocating for changes in nursing to eliminate racism and has proposed changes to its own internal structures to reduce racism.

The Canadian Association of Schools of Nursing (CASN) has developed a framework of strategies for nursing education to respond to the Truth and Reconciliation Commission's Calls to Action. The CASN proposal includes increasing the number of Indigenous professionals in nursing and requiring nursing educational programs to have courses on the legacy of Indigenous peoples in Canada included in their programs (CASN, 2020). Initiatives to attract Indigenous persons to the profession CASN/ACESI, 2020 have been in place for a number of years, and examples are highlighted in Chapter 5.

The British Columbia College of Nurses and Midwives has also taken steps to address systemic racism in health care in the province. A study of discrimination against Indigenous persons conducted for the government highlighted numerous problematic issues between Indigenous people and the provincial health care system. The report detailed a "B.C. health care system with widespread systemic racism against Indigenous peoples" (Turpel-Lafonte, 2020). The report included several recommendations, including changing educational programs to encourage Indigenous person enrollment, the establishment of senior civil service positions for Indigenous health, and the active promotion and recruitment of Indigenous staff within the health care system. The College has developed a new antiracism standard and is developing policies to address the engagement of Indigenous people in nursing.

THE RIGHT OF NURSES TO A RESPECTFUL, HEALTHY, AND SAFE PROFESSIONAL WORK SETTING

The Importance of a Healthy Work Environment

Nursing in Canada has moved beyond legislation to address the fundamental factors that influence nurses' work environment. A key study illustrating the components of a healthy work environment for nurses is *Commitment and Care: The Benefits of a Healthy Workplace for Nurses, Their Patients and the System* (Baumann et al., 2001). This Canada-wide study emphasized the importance of key attributes of the work environment necessary to ensure a satisfied and sustainable nursing workforce. This document continues to have relevance as a guiding framework for leaders and includes the following recommendations for a healthy nursing culture:

■ Ensure appropriate staffing is in place.
■ Reward effort and achievement.
■ Strengthen organizational structures.
■ Support nursing leadership and professional development.
■ Promote workplace health and safety.
■ Ensure a learning environment.
■ Promote effective recruitment and retention.

Chapter 12 addresses the importance of nursing leadership and having ethical organizational structures to support and engage nurses, and an ongoing health human resources plan for nurses that ensures:

■ Consistent and appropriate staffing levels to ensure a safe workload for nurses and optimal patient care
■ Strategies for attracting, retaining, and engaging nurses
■ The rights of nurses to an effective transition to practice or to a new work setting
■ The rights of professional nurses to ongoing education and learning
■ Strategies to ensure supportive leadership in ensuring a moral and safe climate and the avoidance of moral distress
■ Engagement of nurses in decision making and assurance that their efforts are recognized and rewarded

A healthy work environment is essential in all work settings—even more so in a health care environment, where the safety of patients is significantly affected by the overall health and well-being of the individuals and teams who provide care (CNA & CFNU, 2014; Laschinger & Leiter, 2006). A positive and healthy work culture results in reduced absenteeism, improved ability to attract and retain new employees, and high levels of staff satisfaction (CNA & CFNU, 2014; Laschinger et al., 2009). When staff morale is high and when engagement in and commitment to the organization are sustained, the setting becomes recognized as a workplace of choice. In a health care environment, employer savings associated with low absenteeism and turnover rates are then available to invest in additional strategies to improve the work environment and to advance patient care (Agency for Healthcare Research and Quality, 2003; Bargagliotti, 2012; Dugan et al., 1996; Estabrooks et al., 2005; Lundstrom et al., 2002; Purdy et al., 2010).

The National Quality Institute (NQI; http://www.nqi.ca), founded in 1992 and rebranded as Excellence Canada in 2011, and Health Canada, in collaboration with health care professionals, developed criteria to guide and evaluate the health of work environments. The model has evolved and now integrates four dimensions: (1) psychological well-being; (2) physical well-being and occupational health and safety; (3) health and lifestyle practices; and (4) corporate social responsibility. The model recognizes that the individual, the organization, and the system all share the responsibility for a healthy work environment (Excellence Canada, 2022).

Psychological Well-Being

The model endorses a healthy culture that values relationships and communication patterns that create a healthy culture. Essential to this is having leadership that nurtures the ability of people to fully use their talents and resources and the creation of a work environment that is open to receiving input and feedback and is transparent regarding its decisions and strategies (Excellence Canada, 2022).

Physical Well-Being and Occupational Health and Safety

The attributes of the physical environment and health and safety are not only aligned with legislation and directives that guide a safe workplace; they also challenge the workplace to exceed these expectations. Safety challenges for staff include excessive physical work demands, risks of exposure to infectious disease, radiation, chemotherapy, and other toxic substances—some known and some that may not yet be identified (Excellence Canada, 2022).

Health and Lifestyle Practices

The model recognizes the value of healthy lifestyle behaviours and the role of workplaces in encouraging good health practices among their employees. Examples include health promotion and illness prevention programs, healthy eating awareness, and fitness opportunities. The goal is to help staff balance work and life and to build this balance into the organizational culture (Excellence Canada, 2022).

Corporate Social Responsibility

Interrelationships between community, the workplace, and employees influence the health and performance of the employee and the organization. Activities are largely voluntary and involve workplace aspects like occupational health, human rights, community development, environment, and emergency response (Excellence Canada, 2022).

Registered Nurses' Association of Ontario's Healthy Work Environment Guidelines

An important outcome from *Ensuring the Care Will Be There: Report on Nursing Retention and Recruitment in Ontario* (Registered Nurses' Association of Ontario & Registered Practical Nurses Association of Ontario, 2000) was the establishment of the Healthy Work Environment initiative by the RNAO. The Ontario Ministry of Health and Long-Term Care provided funding to the RNAO (http://www.rnao.org) in 2003 to develop evidence-informed guidelines to facilitate the creation of healthy work environments and to thereby support the recruitment and retention of nurses. The Health Canada Office of Nursing Policy partnered with the RNAO to establish these Healthy Work Environment Guidelines in part to address priorities identified by the Canadian Nursing Advisory Committee (2002). These Best Practice Guidelines (BPGs) have been adopted not only by nursing organizations across Canada but internationally. They are also relevant to professions other than nursing. The guidelines are updated on a regular basis as the evidence evolves at the RNAO website.

Organizing Framework for the RNAO Healthy Work Environments Best Practice Guideline Project

A healthy work environment is described as "a practice setting that maximizes the health and well-being of nurses, quality patient outcomes and organizational and system performance" (RNAO, n.d.). The achievement of a healthy work environment for nurses (Fig. 11.1) benefits all interprofessional team members, positively

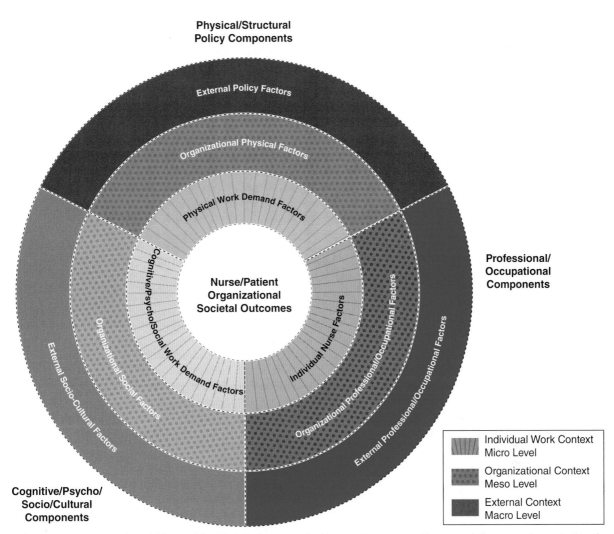

Fig. 11.1 ■ Conceptual Model for Healthy Work Environments for Nurses—Components, Factors and Outcomes. *Source: Registered Nurses' Association of Ontario (April 2007), Healthy Work Environments Best Practice Guidelines: Embracing Cultural Diversity in Health Care: Developing Cultural Competence. Retrieved from https://rnao.ca/sites/rnao-ca/files/Embracing_Cultural_Diversity_in_Health_Care_-_Developing_Cultural_Competence.pdf.*

influences recruitment and retention, and results in positive patient care outcomes. The guidelines are based on a conceptual model that describes the components and elements of a healthy work environment.

The framework conceptualizes a healthy work environment as a complex system with multiple dimensions and components that interact with one another. Also, it highlights the interdependence between the individual, the organization, and the external system (e.g., government, regulatory bodies). Because nurses function in a system mediated and influenced by these interactions, interventions to create and sustain a healthy work environment within this model focus on these dimensions and their interactions with one another. With the model as a foundation, evidence-informed guidelines have been developed that focus on leadership, professionalism, collaborative practice, cultural diversity, prevention of violence, and more.

As an example, the guideline *Professionalism in Nursing* (RNAO, 2007) demonstrates the interacting attributes of knowledge, a spirit of inquiry, accountability, autonomy, advocacy, innovation and vision, collegiality and collaboration, and ethics and values. The guideline acknowledges that nurses succeed when they work in an environment that supports and values ethical reflection and discourse. Within the guideline, recommendations are made to ensure that systems and processes are in place to meet this standard, which would not be possible were they isolated from all the components and attributes that make up a healthy work environment.

Safety in the Work Setting

Health care environments can pose multiple risks to nurses and other employees. These risks may be in the form of exposure to chemical and medical agents, such as disinfectants (e.g., glutaraldehyde [Cidex]), antineoplastic agents, anaesthetic gases, radiation, and electromagnetic fields) (Charney & Schirmer, 1990). Exposure to infectious diseases is also a growing concern, as was evident during the SARS crisis and the COVID-19 pandemic. Other risks are less tangible. Health care is a highly stressful environment, predisposing nurses not only to the effects of their own personal stress but also to the consequences of stress in others. Nurses may experience the effects of a disrespectful and nonsupportive work environment through the actions of their leaders, peers, other team members, and patients and families who may exhibit racist behaviour toward them. Nurses may also be at risk of physical harm from patients who may be cognitively impaired because of their illness or treatment. Nurses interact with patients' family members under extreme stress and who may cope and respond in varying ways. These multiple risks in the health care environment must be recognized, and interventions need to be put in place to minimize and manage these appropriately (RNAO, 2008).

A number of strategies, including legislation and workplace standards and guidelines, exist to ensure a healthy and safe environment for nurses.

Occupational Health and Safety

The understanding that occupational hazards may affect the health of workers has been understood for centuries. Legislation to protect workers generally began in the twentieth century. The field of occupational health and safety (OH&S) has grown significantly in the past 30 years.

In an effort to ensure that working conditions are safe and healthy, all provinces have enacted occupational health and safety (OH&S) legislation. (See the Evolve site for the laws for each province and territory.) These statutes mandate the establishment of health and safety committees comprising representatives of management and nonmanagerial employees. The object of these committees is to identify and recommend solutions to potentially hazardous conditions in the workplace. Furthermore, many provinces' statutes provide for the selection of OH&S representatives to make inquiries into and inspect hazardous working conditions, materials, substances, or unsafe equipment.

As with all employers, hospitals and other employers of health care professionals are legally obligated to provide safe working environments for their employees. In Ontario, for example, the *Health Care and Residential Facilities Regulation* (O. Reg. 67/93, s. 9), made under the *Occupational Health and Safety Act* (1990), requires employers of nurses and other health care professionals, among other things, to have written plans, policies, and procedures for such matters as infection control, proper hygiene, protection against biological and chemical hazards in the workplace, the use and wearing of personal protective equipment, and so forth. The same type of legislation exists in many other provinces, including Nova Scotia and New Brunswick.

In addition to this, the *Occupational Health and Safety Act* allows workers to refuse to work in circumstances in which "the physical condition of the workplace or the part thereof in which he or she works or is to work is likely to endanger himself or herself" (*Occupational Health and Safety Act*, 1990, s. 43(3)(b)). Despite this, a person employed in a hospital or health care facility does not have this right if the condition of the workplace "is inherent in the worker's work or is a normal condition of the worker's employment" or if "the worker's refusal to work would directly endanger the life, health or safety of another person" (*Occupational Health and Safety Act,* 1990, ss. 43(1), (2)). Thus, in a grave situation, such as the SARS outbreak or the COVID-19 pandemic discussed earlier, a nurse working in a hospital providing care for such patients would not likely have a right to refuse to work because of the conditions, because it is fairly certain that in a nurse's work, there is an inherent risk of infection when working with infected patients in a highly infectious environment. This does not mean, however, that a hospital is absolved of its legal responsibility to provide a safe work environment and to have proper procedures and protocols in place to minimize the risk of infection in the workplace. Employees have similar rights (with some minor differences) in all other provinces and territories.

It is the responsibility of the government and the organizations to put strategies in place to prevent harm to caregivers in high-risk situations. As a result of the SARS outbreak, and in preparation for future lethal outbreaks or pandemics, many strategies were implemented. The COVID-19 pandemic showed that many of these strategies were not followed, or if followed, they were insufficient to protect health care practitioners and patients from infection during the early stages of the pandemic (Liu et al., 2020; Marchand-Senécal et al., 2020).

Workplace Violence

The rights of nurses to be protected from harm in the workplace include having a violence-free work environment. One of the most serious contributors to moral distress and an unhealthy work environment is **workplace violence.** Nurses may experience many forms of violence in their work environments. Unfortunately, much of this violence may go unrecognized.

Nurses are at risk of violence from many perspectives. They work with seriously ill patients whose illnesses may predispose them to unintentional violence. They may encounter patients or family members who, because of their personalities or previous experiences, inflict physical or verbal abuse as a means of self-assertion. Nurses may also experience violence in the form of disrespectful behaviour, racism, bullying, or harassment by other nurses, their leaders, or other members of the team. Evidence-informed strategies are available to individual nurses,

leaders, and organizations (Braverman, 1999; RNAO, 2019) to prevent and manage these forms of violence.

Violence-related lost time injuries for front-line health workers is more than double the number of similar injuries experienced by police and correctional officers (RNAO, 2019).

Safeguards and protections that organizations can put in place to reduce the risk of harm include:

- Assessing the workplace to determine areas of risk
- Ensuring that prevention strategies are in place, including appropriate education to identify the potential for violence
- Ensuring employees have the knowledge and skills to defuse violent situations and to respond appropriately when assistance is needed

For example, nurses visiting patients in their homes may be vulnerable because of the isolated environment, and nurses in mental health settings and emergency departments, where patients may be cognitively impaired because of their illnesses and where families may be under immense stress, are at higher risk of violence. At the same time, employers have the responsibility to recognize and minimize the risk of harm to nurses regardless of where they work, but especially in high-risk environments.

The CNA and the Canadian Federation of Nurses Unions (CFNU) issued a joint position statement on workplace violence in 2019. It stated that it is the "right of all nurses to work in an environment that is free from violence" (CNA & CFNU, 2019, p. 1). The definition of *violence* set out in the statement is:

the exercise of physical force by a person against a worker, in a workplace, that causes or could cause physical injury to the worker. (CNA & CFNU, 2019, p. 1)

The statement also outlines the serious implications of workplace violence, including:

- Risks to patient safety
- Injury, and emotional and psychological trauma
- Impacts on staff retention, absenteeism, morale, productivity, among other factors

The RNAO BPG related to violence includes a list of the many factors "that may predict violent or aggressive behaviours" (RNAO, 2019, p. 125). The risk factors are broken down into four broad groups with references to the studies that have documented these risks:

1. Behavioural or psychological factors, such as whether patients are agitated, anxious, have violent histories, are restless, pacing, yelling, are cognitively impaired, or have experienced substance abuse
2. Biological factors, such as whether patients have a raised respiratory or heart rate, are younger than 35, have escalating illness, or low cholesterol levels
3. Environmental or situational factors, such as the physical layout of the environment (e.g., nurses working in isolation, lack of privacy, unfamiliarity, use of catheters or restraints)
4. Socioeconomic factors, such as poor social functioning, homelessness, social isolation (RNAO, 2019)

There are circumstances in which a nurse may be threatened or assaulted by a confused, disoriented, or delusional patient. Although nurses often understand that the behaviour of the patient may be a result of illness, response to treatment, medication, or sleep deprivation, workplaces should have strategies in place to prevent and neutralize violence and to call security personnel if this becomes necessary. When a high-risk patient is identified, a clear strategy for managing that patient needs to be determined. When faced with patients who are confused, agitated, or mentally ill, nurses must recognize that their behaviours may result from illness, fear, or stress. Thus, nurses need the knowledge and skills to identify patients who are medically or psychiatrically predisposed to violence; to recognize the triggers that precipitate violence; and to devise and initiate appropriate strategies for the prevention and effective management of violent behaviours if this becomes necessary. There are specific standards and guidelines related to the management of persons who are cognitively impaired and to better understand their responsive behaviours. It is also important to ensure that structures and processes are in place to prevent delirium in acute care settings, not only for patients' best interests, but also to avoid harm to nurses (Cohen-Mansfield, 2001; Dupuis & Luh, 2005; Galik et al., 2009; McGilton, 2004; Resnick et al., 2013).

Nurses who work in the community may be at further risk if they are sent alone to areas where there is known criminal activity. Backup should be provided and nurses should not be put in a position of danger without adequate support and security measures.

Unfortunately, violence in the workplace occurs frequently between peers and in supervisor–employee relationships. Significantly under-reported (Farrell, 1997, 1999; O'Connell et al., 2000), workplace violence may involve misuse of power and control (Deans, 2004; Farrell, 1999; MacIntosh, 2003) and may take the form of physical, psychological, or sexual abuse; harassment; bullying; or aggression. It may involve the interaction of people in different roles and power relationships (Deans, 2004) and is more likely to be verbal, be passive, and have a top-down element (Burnazi et al., 2005).

Most troubling is the extent of peer-to-peer violence, especially when it goes unrecognized and unreported, which is often the case. Causes for this include peer pressure not to report, lack of awareness that it constitutes violence, perception that it is part of the job, fear of being blamed for causing the violent act, and fear of job loss (McKoy & Smith, 2001).

Nurse-to-nurse violence is well documented in the literature; it begins early during nursing education and extends across all health care work environments. Bullying (e.g., passive–aggressive behaviour, personal diminishment) and incivility (e.g., rudeness, lack of respect, gossip) are the most common forms of violence in the workplace. Bullying includes behaviour toward others that is intimidating, lacking in respect, coercive, critical, and belittling. Incivility includes condescending and insulting behaviour and ignoring or humiliating the victim (Pejic, 2005).

Targets of bullying behaviour are often competent, committed employees who are trying to do their best. They do not always perceive the bullying event, but it tends to be recognized by other colleagues (M. Lewis, 2006; M. A. Lewis, 2006; Lewis et al., 2002). Bullies themselves are often insecure, fearful, or jealous. They bully to protect themselves and often lack insight into their own behaviour (MacIntosh, 2003). Bullying is most often found in organizations with a negative social climate and unsupportive leadership (Hansen et al., 2006).

Sustained exposure to workplace violence can have serious physical and psychological consequences

(MacIntosh, 2003, 2005; McKenna et al., 2003). Abused nurses report feeling unwanted or devalued, having thoughts about leaving their jobs, not wanting to go to work, having difficulty sleeping, experiencing anxiety and feelings of worthlessness, and being more critical of the organizational climate within which they work (Quine, 2003).

A review of 110 studies undertaken over 21 years comparing the consequences of **sexual harassment** and bullying at work concluded that although both can poison the work environment, the latter has worse consequences:

> *Victims of bullying, incivility or interpersonal conflicts are more likely to quit jobs, feel worse, and be less happy with their jobs and leaders than those who were sexually harassed. Society has deemed sexual harassment to be illegal and reaches out to victims in contrast to bullying and incivility leaving victims to fend for themselves. Bullying can be very subtle, making it difficult to deal with and punish.* (Stephens, 2008, p. L11)

RNAO Best Practice Guideline: Preventing Violence, Harassment and Bullying Against Health Workers

In 2019, the RNAO released the second edition of the healthy work environment BPG *Preventing Violence, Harassment and Bullying Against Health Workers*. The updated BPG makes recommendations for health service organizations, academic institutions, health workers, and students. These recommendations are aimed at recognizing, preventing, and managing violence, harassment, and bullying in the workplace.

Within the guideline, *violence* is defined as "the use, or attempted use, of physical force against a person that causes, or could cause, physical injury. Sexual aggression, verbal statements, nonverbal behaviours, or acts that are reasonably interpreted as a threat of physical force that can lead to physical harm are also considered violence" (RNAO, 2019, p. 8).

The intent of the guideline is to define and describe violence, identify strategies that help in the recognition and prevention of violence, and to monitor and evaluate outcomes associated with it. The guideline sets out a number of key recommendations to health service

organizations, academic institutions, health workers, and students for the prevention and management of workplace violence. These include:

- Ensuring policies and procedures are in place to prevent, and respond to workplace violence
- Undertaking risk assessments to identify the vulnerable areas and environments and individuals
- Ensuring staff awareness of what constitutes workplace violence
- Having reporting processes in place
- Following up on every incident
- Providing education to all health workers (regulated and nonregulated professionals, support staff, and students) (RNAO, 2019)

Because this culture seems to be pervasive in health care, nursing leaders in all settings need to address these problematic issues if nursing is to be sustained in the future and safe and ethical care is to be ensured for patients. If bullying behaviour exists among nurses, what then is the bully's approach to patients and families? How do we ensure a viable health care system in the future if we cannot ensure a safe and supportive environment for nurses?

Responsive Legislation

An extreme example of violence toward a nurse was the 2005 murder of Lori Dupont (Office of the Chief Coroner of Ontario, 2007). She was murdered, while at work, by her former partner, an anaesthesiologist who practised at the same hospital. This tragedy demonstrated the need for health care facilities and employers to follow up on disruptive and inappropriate behaviours and complaints brought forward by nurses and other employees. It was revealed during the inquest that numerous officials at the hospital were aware of the anaesthesiologist's disrespectful and aggressive conduct toward this nurse and others, yet they failed to take adequate steps to address his behaviour. The coroner's jury made numerous recommendations to ensure a safe and violence-free workplace and urged that labour legislation be amended to give the Ontario Ministry of Labour the authority to investigate workplace harassment and abuse claims. In response to this recommendation and the growing concern regarding workplace violence, the Ontario legislature introduced amendments to Ontario's *Occupational Health and*

Safety Act (OHSA) with the goal of protecting workers from violence and harassment. The *OHSA* now outlines penalties for all employers in Ontario who fail to meet their responsibilities and duties under the law.

Employers are required to assess risks of workplace violence and harassment, to develop corresponding policies and procedures for investigating and handling complaints and incidents, and to implement open communication and strategies to protect workers. The Act also requires that employers establish and deliver regular harassment and violence prevention training for their workers, including those who exercise managerial functions, and it requires workers to attend the training that is provided (*OHSA*, 1990, s. 32.0).

Nova Scotia has specifically enacted regulations pursuant to its *Occupational Health and Safety Act* (1996) that provide a positive duty on employers to protect employees from workplace violence (see *Violence in the Workplace Regulations*, N.S. Reg. 209/2007 made under the *Occupational Health and Safety Act* of Nova Scotia). This regulation specifically applies to a wide range of "healthcare workplaces."

Employers are required to conduct a violence risk assessment of the workplace and prepare a report on any such risk and the extent of the risk in that workplace. Where a risk of violence is found, the employer must prepare and implement policies and procedures designed to minimize the risks and to provide for the reporting, documentation, and investigation of incidences of workplace violence. New Brunswick has enacted a regulation under its *Occupational Health and Safety Act* (1983) that establishes a code of practice to protect workers who work alone from risks arising from or in connection with their work (*Code of Practice for Working Alone Regulation*, N.B. Reg. 92–133).

In the Lori Dupont case, the coroner's jury found that the hospital had allowed the existence of a culture in which the doctor could continue his outrageous and harassing conduct, which included throwing a computer across the room while a conscious patient was being prepared for surgery. The inquest raised concerns that there was no plan to address his inappropriate behaviour. It also identified a pervasive culture of "physician dominance" leading to double standards whereby inappropriate conduct by physicians was left unchallenged at the expense of a poisoned and potentially unsafe work environment for nurses and other health care workers. The jury recommended, among other things, that hospitals be given the requisite authority over physicians working in their facilities to enable management to better deal with such disruptive behaviour.

Federal Legislation

A growing awareness of the many issues related to harassment, including sexual harassment in the workplace, led the federal government to introduce Bill C-65, *An Act to amend the Canada Labour Code (harassment and violence), the Parliamentary Employment and Staff Relations Act and the Budget Implementation Act, 2017, No. 1.* This Act amends the *Canada Labour Code* to strengthen the existing framework for the prevention of harassment and violence, including sexual harassment and sexual violence, in the workplace. Bill C-65 followed a year-long public consultation commissioned by the Ministry of Employment, Workforce Development, and Labour. The consultation concluded that harassment and violence in workplaces is under-reported and not dealt with effectively. Bill C-65 also extended the protections of the *Canada Labour Code* to the nonpolitical employees of the Parliament of Canada (Government of Canada & Employment and Social Development Canada, 2017). This legislation was also motivated, in part, by sexual harassment complaints raised by a number of staff members working for elected politicians.

When proclaimed, Bill C-65 imposed several new duties on employers to investigate, record, and report all incidents of harassment or violence. It also addressed how employers should prevent and protect against harassment and violence, respond to complaints, and offer support to employees affected by harassment and violence.

WORKPLACE HEALTH: MINIMIZING MORAL DISTRESS

To illustrate the significance of healthy work environments in supporting ethical practice, let us once again consider the notion of moral distress (discussed in detail in Chapter 2).

Moral distress is defined as the emotional and psychological pain that occurs when "one knows the right thing to do, but institutional constraints make it nearly impossible to pursue the right course of action" (Jameton, 1984, p. 6). Moral distress often arises in situations in which nurses are faced with moral uncertainties or dilemmas, and power imbalances exist within the team in making the difficult ethical decisions. The CNA describes *moral distress* as:

> *situations in which nurses cannot fulfill their ethical obligations and commitments (i.e., their moral agency), or they fail to pursue what they believe to be the right course of action, or fail to live up to their own expectation of ethical practice, for one or more of the following reasons: error in judgment, insufficient personal resolve or other circumstances truly beyond their control. They may feel guilt, concern or distaste as a result.* (CNA, 2017, p. 6)

To minimize moral distress, the CNA encourages a climate of openness that encourages peer support, trust, respect, open communication, and facilitation of dialogue in which all team members are participants. Moral distress is minimized further in environments in which mentorship is provided, leaders are role models in demonstrating accountability for the disclosure of adverse events, nurses are provided with knowledge and tools to understand and address ethical challenges, and individual values and beliefs are respected (CNA, 2003). These are all descriptors of a healthy work environment.

Evidence suggests that certain situations in the workplace contribute to moral distress. These situations may include a lack of necessary resources, rule-oriented environments, conflicts of interest, and minimal support systems (Solomon et al., 1993). If issues of moral distress are not addressed in the workplace, the consequences may be serious: nurses may choose to leave the organization or, unfortunately, the profession. Distress may result in positive coping strategies (e.g., compassion and self-reflection) or negative coping strategies (e.g., negativity, despair, loss of integrity, or fractured relationships) (American Association of Critical-Care Nurses, 2006; Rushton, 2006). Those who remain in the workplace may lack trust, fail to collaborate with others, and experience or exhibit negative behaviour and disrespectful communication.

An ethical and healthy work environment can be achieved by leaders if attention is paid to important issues, such as:

- Acknowledging and responding to moral distress in a respectful and compassionate manner
- Addressing practice environment issues, such as systems of care, supports, and resources
- Ensuring collaborative, respectful relationships with shared authority and responsibility
- Influencing the culture of the work environment by setting standards for norms and behaviours, ensuring effective communication processes, and introducing processes and frameworks for resolving ethical conflicts (American Association of Critical-Care Nurses, 2006; Rushton, 2006)

CASE SCENARIO 11.2

WHY DO NURSES "EAT THEIR YOUNG"?

L. L. is a new graduate living in a small rural town and was thrilled to graduate at a time when the local hospital had a rare nursing vacancy.

Initially excited about this opportunity, L. L. was soon disappointed. Most of the nurses had worked there for many years and had developed strong friendships and affiliations. Not used to working with new graduates, they were surprised that L. L. was not as clinically competent as they believed they were when they graduated. As a result, they were highly critical of L. L. and the modern theoretical approach to education.

L. L. felt isolated from the team, was not included in breaks, and any requests for help were ignored. L. L. experienced constant monitoring and criticism from the team.

L. L. became extremely stressed and was having trouble sleeping at night. L. L. was reluctant to confide in others, as in this small town everyone knew each other, and the manager of the unit had a close friendship with most of the nurses.

Continued on following page

CASE SCENARIO 11.2 *(Continued)*

L.L.'s stress and sleeplessness increased, and one day, when unable to focus, made a serious medication error. Fearing the consequences, L.L. was worried about reporting the error. Before L. L. could disclose the error, one of the other nurses reported it to the manager.

Observing all of this in the background was a member of the cleaning staff, who was also part of the local community. As a subordinate to the nurses, this employee had experienced some alienation and was sensitive to what L. L. was experiencing, and they wanted to bring forward these concerns to the manager but were fearful of the consequences.

Questions

1. Does this scenario highlight a form of workplace violence?
2. What options are available to L. L. and the cleaner?
3. What are the ethical issues involved?
4. Do you think this is an isolated incident?
5. What strategies would you use to improve your work environment when you graduate as a nurse?
6. As a student, have you been exposed to workplace violence? What types? How have you dealt with these incidences?
7. What would you do if you experienced bullying in your existing environment?

CASE SCENARIO 11.3

A RISKY ENCOUNTER?

R. C. is a visiting nurse in a poor area of a major Canadian city, known for a great deal of criminal activity. R. C. is sent to the home of a young woman to ensure that her nutritional needs are being met. This young woman suffered major weight loss after undergoing serious abdominal surgery. The woman lives alone, but each time R. C. visits, a male neighbour is present. R. C. is concerned because this patient continues to lose weight, and, in spite of financial support, there is little evidence of food in the home. The neighbour is dominating and aggressive, and R. C. finds this intimidating. R C. is worried about the neighbour's influence and is concerned that the

woman's money is being used to support this neighbour's previously disclosed substance abuse issue. R. C. is uncertain about the next step and feels that by taking a stand on the issues they will be placed at personal risk. R. C. is also worried about the risks of harm to the woman, given the aggressive behaviours exhibited by the neighbour.

Questions

1. Do you think this is an unsafe work environment for R. C.?
2. What support should R. C. receive from her employer?
3. What strategies should be taken to address this issue while preventing both of them from harm?

LABOUR RELATIONS AND COLLECTIVE BARGAINING

Most nurses in Canada work in public hospitals and other health care facilities in which the employees are unionized. Therefore, nurses should have a basic understanding of labour relations concepts such as union formation, collective bargaining, grievance procedures, arbitration, and the right to strike. An exhaustive study of labour law and labour relations is beyond

the scope of this book. However, a brief review of the basics, and some of the related procedures, is provided to promote a general understanding of this subject.

Union Formation and Certification

It should be noted that not all health care settings are represented by unions. In settings without unions, structures and processes are often in place to ensure the appropriate input from and support for nurses. These may take the form of self-governance models or councils (Manuel & Bruinse, 2005; Rotstein & Peskun, 2008).

Unions: Mandate, Structures, and Processes

The recognition of labour unions in Canada and the concomitant rights of workers to organize and to bargain collectively with their employers came about as a result of a long struggle fraught with social unrest, strikes, and violence throughout the late nineteenth and early twentieth centuries. Gradually, unions and the principle of collective bargaining came to be accepted as valid means to equalize the bargaining power of employees with that of the often large, wealthy, and powerful corporations who employed them. Unions, recognized as protectors of workers' interests, could ensure that those workers received fair wages and achieved better and safer working conditions.

A **union** is a certified group of employees, in most cases having a common employer. Unions operate within the jurisdiction of their employer. As a result, employees of provincial organizations, such as hospitals or public health authorities, organize themselves under the labour relations legislation of that province or territory. Employees in federally regulated industries organize themselves under the *Canada Labour Code.* Despite the different jurisdictions, the basic rules are similar in most jurisdictions.

Unionized employees often work in common or related activities in the businesses or undertakings of these employers. The object of uniting is to provide bargaining influence, power, and leverage, by force of numbers, in negotiations pertaining to the terms of employment affecting each member (e.g., wages, hours of work, benefits, work scheduling, layoff and termination, disciplinary matters and procedures, seniority, and job security). Thus, with a common interest in the terms of their employment, the employees, through their union, negotiate the terms and conditions of the employment contract collectively for the benefit of all members.

All provinces have passed labour relations legislation dealing with union certification, procedures for collective bargaining, procedures for strike votes (in some cases), definition of unfair labour practices, and prohibition of strike breaking, as well as the establishment of labour relations boards, their duties and powers. (See the Evolve site for a list of laws for each province and territory.)

In workplaces where a group of employees wish to be represented by a union, they typically approach or are sought out by existing unions. Where there is no existing union willing to apply for certification on behalf of a group of employees, those employees may themselves form a new union.

Typically, the employees who join the union are in the nonmanagement category. Beyond management, those with highly confidential positions, in human resources, for example, are usually excluded from participation in a union with other employees.

When a union is formed, it seeks formal recognition as the workers' representative (certification) by the relevant labour relations board. The question as to whether a union is properly constituted usually arises during certification proceedings before the labour relations board. The board is charged, as part of its overall duties under the labour statute, with reviewing the union's application for certification and ensuring that all procedural formalities have been met. If the board is satisfied that the application is in order, it will organize and administer a vote of the potential members within the organization. If the majority vote in favour of unionization, the union is certified and becomes the exclusive representative for the employees in the bargaining unit.

After certification, the union will seek to negotiate a contract with the employer. In some cases, this is quite straightforward as the union and the employer are familiar with each other. For example, a newly established hospital and the Ontario Nurses' Association will know the contracts in existence in other workplaces in the province and can usually agree that many of their terms are acceptable. In other circumstances, particularly in industries where unionization of the workforce is rare, the road to certification and the first contract can be much more challenging.

Certification

All provinces and the federal government have some form of **certification** process that must be passed before a union can represent the employees of a particular employer. The size and membership of the group of employees will usually be examined by the particular provincial labour board to determine whether it is appropriate for collective bargaining—that is, whether its members are truly employees, and the group is of an appropriate size.

Once certified, the union becomes the exclusive **bargaining agent** for its employees. That union alone is then authorized to negotiate a collective agreement on behalf of the employees in the **bargaining unit** (the specific group of employees of a specific employer or group of employers whom it was certified to represent).

The labour relations statutes usually do not apply to managerial employees, who are seen to represent employers. To allow managers to participate in union formation, membership, and activities would create a conflict of interest because managers are usually charged with executing the employer's administrative, disciplinary, and evaluative policies. These activities are regarded as being inconsistent with the interests of workers in collective bargaining. Some employers with large groups of managerial employees may have separate unions representing management staff where this can be done without conflict of interest concerns. The provincial and federal governments have such bargaining units.

In some provinces, closed shops are permitted. A **closed shop** is a place of employment that requires all employees to be members of the union as a condition of employment. This stipulation will appear among the terms of the collective agreement. Alternatively, the contract may simply provide that although union membership is not mandatory (i.e., the place of employment is an **open shop**), preference in hiring will be given to union members over nonmembers.

In some provinces, such as Saskatchewan, certification may be automatic upon the union demonstrating that it has achieved a certain level of membership. Not all employees of an employer need be members of the union seeking certification. But if a large majority of them are, this may be sufficient, in some provinces, for automatic certification. In Alberta, for example, it is possible for an employer to voluntarily recognize a union as the bargaining agent for a group of employees without the union being certified (see Alberta's *Labour Relations Code,* 2000, s. 42).

Decertification

A union may also lose its right to act as bargaining agent for a group of workers, or it may be dissolved. This is usually referred to as **decertification**. For example, a union can lose its rights by failing to negotiate a collective agreement in good faith within a certain period. A group of the union's members can then apply for a declaration from the provincial labour relations board that the union no longer represents the bargaining unit and, thus, can no longer negotiate for the employees in a given bargaining unit.

In some provinces, a minimum number of employees may have to consent to such a declaration before the board may decertify the union. The union may also lose its certification if it fails to give the employer notice, within a certain period, of its desire to begin negotiations for a new collective agreement or to renew an existing agreement.

It is important for nurses who are members of labour unions to know that in all cases, their employers are not free to give them individual advice if nurses are dissatisfied with the manner in which their union is representing them. At all times, nurses in such a situation have the right to consult with a labour lawyer. A legal professional can best advise the nurse or nurses on all appropriate courses of action and their legal rights.

Collective Bargaining

Collective bargaining is a process whereby workers, through their union representatives, meet with their employers to negotiate the terms and conditions of employment applicable to the members of the bargaining unit. It is a right that was not recognized historically in common law and was even prohibited in past times as a "conspiracy in restraint of trade." Today, collective bargaining is fully recognized and promoted in the various labour relations statutes, both federal and provincial.

Under the laws of all provinces and the federal government, the parties to an expired collective agreement are obliged to negotiate a new contract when one of the parties serves the other with a notice to bargain for a new agreement (or, where there is no prior agreement and a union is newly certified, the first collective agreement). The notice begins the process of collective bargaining.

In collective bargaining, each side puts forth its desired terms and conditions for a new employment contract. Such terms may include wages; hours of work; work schedules; vacation pay; sick leave; pensions and other employee benefits; mechanisms for settling disputes that arise from the application, administration, interpretation, or alleged violation of the collective agreement (called *grievance procedures*); and employer and employee representation on the joint OH&S committee for the workplace.

Often, negotiations become mired in disagreement over one or more terms. These disputes, if not settled promptly, can lead to strike action by employees or a lockout of employees by an employer. Thus, the labour relations statutes contain several procedures that both sides must comply with before any strike or lockout can occur.

In all provinces, once a notice to bargain has been given, the employer cannot change the existing terms or conditions of employment, including wages, unless it has the permission of its board of directors and the union, or the provisions of the collective agreement permit it.

The Collective Agreement

The contract that emerges from the collective bargaining negotiations is called a **collective agreement**. The agreement must be effective for a minimum duration of 1 year and must be in writing, but it need not be embodied in a single document. For example, an exchange of letters, notes, and memoranda may constitute the collective agreement if the parties set out the agreed-upon terms.

If the collective agreement expires before a new one is in place, the terms and conditions of the old agreement usually continue to apply provided that there is no evidence that the parties intended otherwise. Some contracts specify that they will continue after the expiry date until and unless either party notifies the other of its desire to terminate the agreement. In all provinces, except Quebec and Nova Scotia, no employee is permitted to strike, nor may any employer lock out its employees, during the life of the contract. This is to preserve labour peace. This condition applies even after the agreement has expired and until a specified period has elapsed from the time a **conciliator** is appointed by the minister of labour (or other authorized person) to the time a conciliator's report is released to the parties. This is colloquially known as a **cooling-off period**.

Grievance Procedures and Arbitration

Because workers are not permitted to strike during the collective agreement and employers are not permitted to lock out workers, there must be a means of resolving disputes arising from the application, administration, interpretation, or alleged violation of the terms of the agreement. The violence of past labour disputes has shown the necessity and desirability of having effective and timely dispute resolution procedures in place before matters get out of hand. Indeed, all provincial labour statutes except Saskatchewan's require that collective agreements contain procedures for settling management–labour disputes. If they do not, the legislation deems certain provisions to be part of the agreement.

Such grievance procedures will be negotiated as part of the terms of the collective agreement. Many agreements provide relatively informal mechanisms for the presentation of a grievance. As well, many workplaces have grievance committees, which consist of employee representatives and employer representation.

Some hospitals have hospital association committees comprising members of the hospital's management and nonmanagerial nurse employees. They meet on a regular basis to review any grievances in an attempt to resolve them in an informal, cooperative setting before they become adversarial and part of a formal grievance process. However, if informal mechanisms fail, grievance procedures are implemented.

The following grievance procedures are not necessarily followed uniformly across Canada, but they are fairly common in many labour relations settings. They usually involve a progressive three-step process.

Step 1: Written Submission

In the event that the nurse's grievance is not settled satisfactorily after it is brought to the supervisor's attention, then, within a specified time, the grievance must be submitted in writing to the immediate supervisor for a response. Failing a settlement, it must then be filed within a specified time to the director of nursing for resolution. If it is still not settled, the procedure provides that it be submitted to the hospital administrator or other authorized hospital official within a set period for a meeting.

Step 2: Meeting With the Grievance Committee

The administrator, the person who filed the grievance, the grievance committee, and a representative of the union meet. Within a specified time, the hospital must then decide as to how it will deal with the grievance. Thus, the procedure provides for the grievance's being submitted to a progressively higher authority as long as it remains unsettled. (In many hospitals, this procedure is managed through the human resources department.) The collective agreement will also provide that any settlement reached through these procedures is binding on the parties.

Step 3: Binding Arbitration

If the decision rendered by the hospital administrator does not settle the issue, then the matter is submitted to binding arbitration.

Binding arbitration is a procedure mandated by the labour relations statutes of many provinces. Usually, the parties have a specified time from the rendering of the hospital administrator's decision to have the matter submitted to binding arbitration. At that time, the party requesting arbitration will nominate a person to be part of a three-member arbitration board.

The party to whom the notice is given then has a specified time within which to nominate a second person to that board. These two persons choose a third person to chair and complete the board. If they cannot agree, then the minister appoints a chair. In many contracts, the parties will agree in advance on a single arbitrator who will hear grievances to reduce costs and make the process less cumbersome.

Recent years have seen disputes over workloads and the right of nurses to refuse to provide services once the number of patients placed in their care exceeds their ability to provide adequate care. In the *Re Mount Sinai Hospital and Ontario Nurses' Association* (1978) case (which will be described in more detail later in this chapter), the nurses refused to care for an additional patient assigned to their unit. The nurses were disciplined, and the disciplinary measures were upheld upon arbitration under the collective agreement. The arbitration board felt that the nurses had not had just cause under the circumstances to refuse to care for the additional patient. Such a situation is now addressed in the professional responsibility clause of most collective agreements.

A matter may be submitted to arbitration only after all preliminary grievance procedures have been exhausted. All time limits for the giving of notice must be strictly observed; if notice that a party wishes the

matter submitted to binding arbitration is not given within a specified time, the grievance is deemed to have been abandoned. Alternatively, the parties may agree that the matter be settled by a single arbitrator.

Thus, through arbitration, every attempt is made to resolve disputes arising out of the collective agreement. This procedure has been referred to as *quid pro quo*— that is, something in return for the fact that the right to strike or to lock out is suspended during the life of the agreement.

There are numerous cases involving nurses disciplined for unprofessional conduct. In many of these, the nurse grieved the matter according to the union's collective agreement.

In *Re Ontario Cancer Institute and Ontario Nurses' Association (Priestley)* (1993), a nurse was discharged after striking a terminally ill patient. The nurse, through her union, brought a grievance against the hospital employer for unjust discharge. The union argued that the patient had provoked the nurse. Although there were no witnesses to the incident, the nurse had admitted the act to two colleagues and said that "it felt good" (*Re Ontario Cancer Institute and Ontario Nurses' Association (Priestley)*, 1993, p. 129).

The evidence presented at the hearing suggested that patient load had been very heavy in the unit for some months and that stress levels among staff were high. The patient struck by the nurse required the most attention in the unit and was very demanding of the nurses' time and attention. He had had a tracheotomy and was often confused, restless, and incontinent. The nurse admitted to striking the patient hard across the legs, being frustrated with his restless behaviour the night before. In finding that the nurse's discharge was justified, the arbitrator stated, in part:

> *I heard much evidence about what a difficult and heavy care patient [the patient] was. I accept that evidence.... However, the actions of a patient who is terminally ill and not in control of his mental or physical faculties cannot constitute provocation that would excuse a health care professional's physical retaliation. (Re Ontario Cancer Institute and Ontario Nurses' Association (Priestley), 1993, pp. 135–136)*

The arbitrator declined to interfere with the hospital's decision to dismiss the nurse.

Similarly, in *Re Vancouver General Hospital (Health and Labour Relations Assn.) and British Columbia Nurses Union* (1993), a nurse was discharged for continuing to feed a patient in an inappropriate manner despite having been shown the correct way by an occupational therapist. This nurse had previously been suspended for improperly responding to a patient's seizure because they were in a hurry to go home. In the second incident, which led to the dismissal, the nurse attempted to feed milk to a patient who was improperly positioned and already had food in her mouth, causing a great risk of aspiration. Moreover, the patient was drowsy after surgery and insufficiently alert to be fed orally. The arbitrator held that the hospital had just cause for disciplinary action given the nurse's record.

In *Newfoundland and Labrador Nurses' Union v. Eastern Regional Integrated Health Authority* (2014), Ms. King, a registered nurse, grieved her termination for breaching the privacy policy of the employer. Ms. King had accessed 29 confidential records on 64 occasions over a 4-month period. She had a variety of reasons for looking at the records. Some were personal or family records, some were of friends who asked her to check their records, some were of persons that she thought might be suitable candidates for her service, and some she could not explain. She was remorseful and had suffered personally as a result of her termination. The arbitrator decided that considering all of the circumstances, termination was too harsh, and he substituted it with a 2-year suspension without pay.

Right to Strike

Traditionally, common law did not recognize the right of employees to refuse to work. Gradually, collective action by workers came to be accepted as part of the give-and-take of industrial relations. Today, the right to strike has expanded beyond the industrial sector to many areas of society and has been recognized as one of the fundamental rights protected by the *Canadian Charter of Rights and Freedoms* (s. 2(d), freedom of association) (*Saskatchewan Federation of Labour v. Saskatchewan,* 2015.

Nurses have initiated strike action in the past. For example, in late 2000, nurses in Saskatchewan went on strike in support of a demand for a pay raise beyond

what the provincial government was willing to offer. The government ordered the nurses back to work via legislation, but the nurses continued their strike in defiance of the legislation (CBC News, 1999). In response, Saskatchewan eventually enacted the *Public Service Essential Services Act,* which provided that certain public services, such as nursing in hospitals, are deemed essential services. Public-sector employers, such as hospitals and health care authorities that provide such services, are required to enter into an essential services agreement with their unionized employees, including nurses, to set out which services are deemed essential and to provide for a certain number of unionized employees (including nurses) who must continue to provide services in the event of a strike. Many other provinces have enacted similar legislation. The effect of this legislation was that nurses' right to strike was very limited in most provinces.

In *Saskatchewan Federation of Labour v. Saskatchewan* (2015), the Saskatchewan Federation of Labour challenged the power of the province to ban nurses from going on strike. When the validity of such a law was heard in the Supreme Court of Canada, the Court held that the *Public Service Essential Services Act* amounted to a universal ban on striking by health care workers and was unconstitutional. The province had the power to ban strikes by essential employees—in other words, those employees necessary to maintain sufficient services for public safety and well-being. The province did not have the power to remove the right to strike from nurses and other health care workers, but it could identify "essential" employees who should not be allowed to strike in the public interest. The limit on striking had to meet the section 1 exception (reasonable limits prescribed by law as can be demonstrably justified in a free and democratic society) in the Charter. The province had to be able to justify the claim that the workers it designated as essential were actually essential to the operation of the health care system.

In many provinces, laws still broadly define nurses and other hospital employees as essential employees and try to restrict the right to strike. In return for the elimination of the right to strike, the legislation provides for arbitration of issues that cannot be settled between the parties. Where the provincial legislation has been challenged on constitutional grounds, as in

Alberta, Saskatchewan, and British Columbia, the definition of "essential employees" is less extensive.

Although the restrictions on striking may not affect nurses who are not employed at hospitals (which are defined in detail in the statutes), any nurse working at an institution that falls within the definition of a hospital would be prevented from going on strike. (See, for example, Ontario's *Hospital Labour Disputes Arbitration Act,* 1990, s. 11(1), as amended.)

As an example, in 2016, the Alberta government passed essential services legislation to replace an earlier ban on nurses' right to strike in an attempt to achieve a reasonable balance between the right to strike and the need to protect services where interruption could result in risks to life, personal safety, or public health. The Alberta legislation establishes a process through which employers and unions determine which workers provide essential services and how to deliver them during a strike (*Public Service Employee Relations Act,* 2000, as amended). The union treats the right to strike as a last resort when all other attempts to obtain a fair collective agreement have failed. Similar legislation exists in Saskatchewan and Nova Scotia.

Unionized nurses who are not providing essential services do have the right to strike. In practice, this means that nursing strikes are few and far between, and when they occur, they are between nursing unions and employers providing services outside a hospital environment, namely public health, clinic, and community care nurses. For example, 3,000 employees of the community care access centres in Ontario went on strike for 2 weeks in 2015.

Similarly, hospitals are not permitted to lock out their employees at any time. A **lockout** is a practice whereby an employer shuts out or refuses to continue to employ union employees as a means to pressure and influence them during negotiations for a collective agreement. A lockout, like the strike, is a coercive tactic. These provisions are designed to ensure that vital hospital services are not compromised and that services to the public are not diminished as a result of labour disputes.

For employees with the right to strike, strikes can be legal or illegal, depending on the circumstances around which the strike occurs. In most provinces, during the life of any collective agreement, employees may not strike, nor may an employer lock out employees. For

example, in 2014, nurses in several hospitals in Halifax, Nova Scotia, went on an illegal strike to protest proposed legislation restricting their right to strike. A legal strike deadline was only days away, but 140 nurses failed to show up for scheduled shifts, causing the cancellation of numerous surgeries. The Nova Scotia Labour Relations Board immediately ordered the illegally striking nurses to return to work.

Even after the expiration of the agreement, employees still cannot legally strike, and employers cannot lock them out. They must wait for the expiry of a cooling-off period after the expiry of the collective agreement before a lawful strike or lockout can occur.

Once the collective agreement has expired, its terms continue while the parties negotiate a new agreement. However, if no agreement is reached, in some provinces, the provincial minister of labour may be requested or may decide to appoint a conciliation board in an attempt to settle outstanding issues and to effect a new collective agreement. Such board or conciliator (if one person is appointed) must file a report on the results (or lack thereof) of any conciliation efforts to the minister of labour, who then releases the report to the parties.

Once a specified period has elapsed after the report's release or, if no conciliator has been appointed, and after the minister has notified the parties that they consider it inappropriate to appoint a conciliator, the union may then lawfully call a strike. Similarly, the employer may lawfully lock out employees.

Certain activities during the life of the collective agreement may or may not constitute a strike according to the applicable labour relations statute. Employees may vote to work to rule (i.e., to work only as much as is specified by the terms of their employment) as a form of protest; for example, they may refuse to work overtime or provide voluntary labour when requested to do so. If such conduct has the effect of stopping all work to pressure an employer to accede to union demands, it may be deemed a strike by the applicable labour relations board. However, refusal to work because of hazardous working conditions would likely not be deemed a strike because it is not intended to affect collective bargaining, but rather is intended to avoid potentially serious injury to workers.

Strike breaking—that is, the use of non-union labour to replace striking workers in an effort to pressure striking employees to abandon a lawful strike or to yield in contract negotiations—is prohibited in all provinces.

Depending on the province, a strike vote among employees may be required before a strike can begin. If a strike vote is held, all employees in the bargaining unit may vote. Voting is usually by secret ballot. A vote may also be held to ratify an agreement concluded between management and the union's negotiators.

A strike is an action of last resort for the union. The members on strike lose their salaries and may also lose their benefits. They have to picket, often in adverse weather conditions and in the face of hostility from the public and their co-workers who are not on strike. Striking workers receive some money from the union ("strike pay"), but this is far less than the striker's salary, is tied to the size of the striker's family, and can run out quite quickly.

The purpose of the strike is to bring pressure to bear on employers to negotiate and reach a collective agreement. If the employer is unable to replace the striking employees, pressure to settle will rise very quickly. The strike can be ended by the union at any time, but given the high cost to their members, unions prefer to have an agreement in place before ending the strike.

Unfair Labour Practices

All provinces have prohibited unfair management tactics, which, in previous times, were used by employers to pressure workers into returning to work or to induce employees to accept certain terms and conditions of employment. For example, it is illegal for an employer to discipline a worker for taking part in a lawful strike or in lawful union activities, such as encouraging new employees to join the union. Similarly, employers are prohibited from participating in or funding the creation of a union. Such prohibition is intended to avoid conflict of interest.

It is likewise illegal for an employer to discriminate in any way against employees because they either are or are not members of a union; to discipline them for exercising their rights under a labour relations statute; to use any form of intimidation against them for participating in union activity; or to induce them to join a particular union. Another illegal labour practice is the "yellow dog" contract, by which it is made a condition of a person's employment that they will not join a union or participate in any union activities.

If an employee alleges that an employer has engaged in an unfair labour practice, the employee can bring the matter to the attention of the union representative. The matter may be taken up as a grievance by the union, or if it is serious enough, it may be reported to a labour inspector appointed by the provincial labour relations board. The labour relations board of most provinces are given wide powers to order employers to cease and desist from engaging in such practices.

Professional Accountability and the Influence of Unionization

Nurses are accountable to their profession, their regulatory body, their patients, and their employers. These multiple accountabilities can, at times, pose conflicts for the nurse. Nurses in some settings have another dimension added to these complex relationships—that of a union or collective bargaining unit.

Mentioned earlier, the situation that occurred in Toronto in the mid-1970s illustrates the conflict that can arise between nurses' rights as employees and union members under a collective agreement and their duties and responsibilities as professionals. In *Re Mount Sinai Hospital and Ontario Nurses' Association* (1978), the staff of the Mount Sinai Intensive Care Unit was informed one evening of the urgent need to admit a patient with cardiac problems from the emergency department. This occurred during the night shift, when the intensive care unit (ICU) was already working at maximum capacity. The nurses informed the admitting resident that they could not handle another patient. They claimed, further, that they were not obliged to take an additional patient under the terms of the union's collective agreement with the hospital. The medical staff, despite the nurses' refusal to help, brought the patient to the unit. Although told by their supervisor to accept this patient, none of the nurses on the night shift assisted the admitting resident, who was required to care for this very ill patient by himself for the duration of the night. As a result of their refusal to care for the additional patient, the nurses were disciplined and suspended for three tours of duty. They grieved the matter, according to the grievance and arbitration procedures set out in their respective collective agreement, and the issue was passed on to an arbitrator. The arbitrator ruled in favour of the hospital and found that the nurses had been insubordinate because they had refused a direct order by their supervisor to provide care. They were not entitled, under the collective agreement, to refuse such an order.

Quite apart from the labour aspect, this case raises ethical concerns regarding standards of care. For example, the nurses had not reevaluated the allocation of their resources. They had not reassessed their workload and staffing, nor had they tried to determine whether some patients in their unit could be discharged to make room for the new admission. As they had not attempted to restructure their assignments to accommodate the patient, they violated the principles of beneficence and nonmaleficence. Further, they had not accorded the patient justice, fairness, or equity.

The rule that evolved from this case is now termed the "obey and grieve" rule. It provides that even if nurses have a legitimate grievance under the terms of a collective agreement or with respect to workload or working conditions, they must obey the orders of the supervisor and provide the needed care and *then* grieve the matter to the union if they feel there is a legitimate complaint. There is plenty of opportunity for such complaints to be heard and adjudicated upon at a more appropriate time, using the collective agreement's grievance procedures. In the present moment, however, the rights and needs of the patient must come first, and the fact that a nurse has a complaint must not be permitted to interfere with proper patient care. This approach is further supported in the Canadian Nurses Association code of ethics:

When resources are not available to provide appropriate or safe care, nurses collaborate with others to adjust priorities and minimize harm. Nurses keep persons receiving care informed about potential and actual plans regarding the delivery of care. They inform employers about potential threats to the safety and quality of health care. (CNA, 2017, p. 9)

The employee, during regular hours of work, has accountability to the employer. There are ample mechanisms to protect the employee's rights should these be violated by the employer, but the patient's care is paramount, especially given the fact that the health care facility is under a legal duty to provide competent and proper nursing care once a patient is admitted. This implies a corresponding right of the employer to discipline the employee and even to terminate the employment of a nurse who repeatedly fails to meet proper nursing standards. The employee in such a situation has the right to grieve or, if not unionized, to have recourse in the courts in an action for wrongful dismissal.

SUMMARY

This chapter has explored the rights of nurses as professionals, individuals, and employees. The varied contexts within which nurses engage in practice may pose varying ethical and legal challenges that have an impact on their values, beliefs, and well-being. Although nurses have the right to respect and should be able to practise in a safe work environment free from harm, discrimination, harassment, or physical and sexual abuse, the reality is that some will face such difficult situations. It is important that nurses have the knowledge and skills to address these challenging issues and to know where to seek support and guidance when necessary.

Employers have an obligation to represent the interests and rights of nurses. They must be aware of the risks to nurses and ensure that appropriate prevention strategies are in place. They must also be prepared to respond appropriately if nurses are harmed as a result of these risks. When this obligation is not fulfilled, then the collective agreement and collective bargaining rights of nurses who are unionized may provide protection and a mechanism for dealing with some situations. In other cases, the advice of a competent legal professional may be required.

Nurses should be aware of their rights and the responsibilities and obligations of their employers with respect to working conditions. The nurse has the right to a safe and violence-free working environment. If nurses' rights are not protected in an environment based on mutual respect, then they will be unable to deliver high-quality care to patients consistent with the standards of their profession.

CRITICAL THINKING

The following case scenarios are provided to facilitate reflection, discussion, and analysis.

Discussion Points

1. As a nurse, do you have rights that may supersede those of your patients ? What rights may, at times, be in conflict?
2. Do nurses give up certain rights when they assume their professional role?
3. Have you ever experienced violence in the workplace? Was anything done about it? If it happened now, what would you do?

4. What role should unions play in establishing rules that govern professional practice and conduct?

5. What mechanisms are in place in your facility to ensure the appropriate balance between caregiver and patient rights?

CASE SCENARIO 11.4

RIGHT OR PRIVILEGE?

C. D., a nurse in a busy critical care unit, is scheduled to work nights on a weekend and is subsequently invited to attend an informal university class reunion. C. D. knows that it is too late to ask for the weekend off and that other nurses are unlikely to willingly switch shifts on such short notice. C. D. has taken little sick leave, and because there are days remaining in the sick bank, decides to call in sick

That night, a number of emergency patients are admitted to the unit. Because of C. D.'s absence, the nurses on duty must take on double assignments of patients. One of the nurses, aware of C. D.'s reason for calling in sick, is upset and discloses this information to the nurse manager the following Monday.

Questions

1. Is C. D. entitled to take this time off? If not, what disciplinary action may ensue?
2. If the manager chooses to discipline C. D., can this action be grieved?
3. What ethical principles, if any, were breached?
4. How could this situation have been prevented?

CASE SCENARIO 11.5

SAFETY IN THE WORKPLACE?

A public health nurse is assigned to a young single mother and her 8-month-old son. This family receives welfare and lives in a subsidized housing unit.

During one of the nurse's regular visits, the mother's estranged boyfriend arrives. He has been drinking and becomes belligerent toward the mother. When the nurse—concerned about the patient's safety—intervenes, the boyfriend hits the nurse on the head, causing a fall that results in a serious head injury.

Although the head injury resolves, the mental state of this nurse is so badly affected that this nurse is unable to practise nursing again.

Questions

1. What obligations did the nurse's employer have to ensure a safe working environment?
2. What responsibilities does the employer have with respect to the nurse's permanent disability?
3. What charges can be laid against the boyfriend?
4. What obligations do employers have to educate nurses with respect to such potentially violent and dangerous situations?
5. How could this situation have been prevented?

CASE SCENARIO 11.6

RIGHT TO STRIKE?

R. B. is a registered nurse working in a long-term care facility. Recently, contract discussions between the union and the facility have broken down. Neither side is willing to compromise, and the staff have voted to strike. A plan is in place for a minimal number of nurses to be available in emergencies.

R. B. is concerned about the strike decision and is worried about the residents. Knowing how difficult and confusing the strike will be for them, R. B. decides to cross the picket line and go to work, and while entering the building, is heckled by colleagues.

Questions

1. What are R. B.'s rights and responsibilities in this situation?
2. Is the behaviour of the nurses on the picket line justifiable?
3. What would you do in this situation?
4. How could this situation have been prevented?

REFERENCES

Statutes

Canada Labour Code, R.S.C. 1985, c. L-2 (Canada).

Canadian Charter of Rights and Freedoms, Part I of the *Constitution Act*, 1982, being Schedule B to the *Canada Act 1982* (UK), 1982, c. 11.

Hospital Labour Disputes Arbitration Act, R.S.O. 1990, c. H.14 (Ontario).

Public Service Employee Relations Act, RSA 2000, c. P-43 (Alberta).

Labour Relations Code, R.S.A. 2000, c. L-1 (Alberta).

Occupational Health and Safety, An Act Respecting, R.S.Q. c. S-2.1 (Quebec).

Occupational Health and Safety Act, S.A. 2017, c. O-2.1 (Alberta).

Occupational Health and Safety Act, S.N.B. 1983, c. O-0.2 (New Brunswick).

Occupational Health and Safety Act, R.S.N.L. 1990, c. O-3 (Newfoundland and Labrador).

Occupational Health and Safety Act, S.N.S. 1996, c. 7 (Nova Scotia).

Occupational Health and Safety Act, R.S.O. 1990, c. O.1 (Ontario).

Public Service Employee Relations Act, RSA 2000, c. P-43 (Alberta).

Regulations

Code of Practice for Working Alone Regulation, NB Reg 92-133 (New Brunswick).

Health Care and Residential Facilities Regulation, O. Reg. 67/93 (Ontario).

Violence in the Workplace Regulations, NS Reg 209/2007 (Nova Scotia).

Case Law

Newfoundland And Labrador Nurses' Union v. Eastern Regional Integrated Health Authority [2014] CanLII 83846 (NL LA). http://canlii.ca/t/ggnl8

Re Mount Sinai Hospital and Ontario Nurses' Association [1978] 17 L.A.C. (2d) 242 (Ont. Arb.).

Re Ontario Cancer Institute and Ontario Nurses' Association (Priestley) [1993] 35 L.A.C. (4th) 129 (Ont. Arb.).

Re Vancouver General Hospital (Health and Labour Relations Assn.) and British Columbia Nurses Union [1993] 32 L.A.C. (4th) 231 (B.C.).

Saskatchewan Federation of Labour v. Saskatchewan [2015] SCC 4 (CanLII). http://canlii.ca/t/gg40r

Coroner's Inquests

Office of the Chief Coroner of Ontario. (2007). *Verdict of coroner's jury serving on the inquest into the deaths of Lori Dupont and Dr. Marc Daniel.* http://www.mcscs.jus.gov.on.ca/stellent/groups/public/@mcscs/@www/@com/documents/webasset/ec063542.pdf

Texts and Articles

Agency for Healthcare Research and Quality. (2003). *The effect of health care working conditions on patient safety (summary).* Evidence Report/Technology Assessment: Number 74. AHRQ Publication No. 03-E024.

American Association of Critical-Care Nurses. (2006). *The 4 A's to rise above moral distress toolkit.*

Bargagliotti, L. A. (2012). Work engagement in nursing: A concept analysis. *Journal of Advanced Nursing, 68*(6), 1414–1428.

Baumann, A., O'Brien-Pallas, L., Armstrong-Stassen, M., et al. (2001). *Commitment and care: The benefits of a healthy workplace for nurses, their patients and the system—A policy synthesis.* Canadian Health Services Research Foundation and The Change Foundation.

Black nurses and RNAO. https://rnao,ca/infocus/black-nurses-and-rnao

Braverman, M. (1999). *Preventing workplace violence: A guide for employers and practitioners.* Sage Publications, Inc.

Brown, J. (2022, July 17). Health-care providers and MAID: The reasons why some don't offer medically assisted death. *The Conversation.*

Burnazi, L., Keashly, L., & Neuman, J. H. (2005, August). *Aggression revisited: Prevalence, antecedents, and outcomes* [Conference session]. Academy of Management Annual Meeting, Honolulu, HI, United States.

Canadian Association of Schools of Nursing CASN/ACESI (2020). Framework of Strategies for Nursing Education to Respond to the Calls to Action of Canada's Truth and Reconciliation Commission. https://www.casn.ca/wp-content/uploads/2020/11EN-TRC-RESPONSE

Canadian Nurses Association. (2003, October). Ethical distress in health care environments. *Ethics in Practice for Registered Nurses.*

Canadian Nurses Association. (2017). *Code of ethics for registered nurses.*

Canadian Nurses Association, & Canadian Federation of Nurses Unions. (2014). *Practice environments: Maximizing outcomes for clients, nurses and organizations.*

Canadian Nurses Association, & Canadian Federation of Nurses Unions. (2019). *Workplace violence. Joint position statement.* https://nursesunions.ca/wp-content/uploads/2019/10/Workplace-Violence-and-Bullying_joint-position-statement.pdf

Canadian Nurses Protective Society. (2021). *Medical Assistance in Dying: What every nurse should know.* https://cnps.ca/article/medical-assistance-in-dying-what-every-nurse-should-know/

Canadian Nursing Advisory Committee. (2002). *Our health, our future: Creating quality workplaces for Canadian nurses.* Advisory Committee on Health Human Resources.

CASN (2020). Framework of strategies for nursing education to respond to the Calls to Action of Canada's Truth and Reconciliation Commission. E-book

Çayır, E. (2021). Self-care, communal care, and resilience among underrepresented minority nursing professionals and students. In D. K. Cunningham & N. M. Tim (Eds.), *Self-care for new and student nurses* (pp. 114–139). Sigma Theta Tau International.

CBC News. (1999). *Saskatchewan nurses to pay up for illegal strike.* https://www.cbc.ca/news/canada/sask-nurses-to-pay-up-for-illegal- strike-1.183379.

Charney, W., & Schirmer, J. (1990). *Essentials of modern hospital safety.* Lewis Publishers, Inc.

Cohen-Mansfield, J. (2001). Nonpharmacologic interventions for inappropriate behaviors in dementia: A review, summary, and critique. *The American Journal of Geriatric Psychiatry, 9*(4), 361–381.

Cottingham, M. D., Johnson, A. H., & Erickson, R. J. (2018). "I can never be too comfortable": Race, gender, and emotion at the hospital bedside. *Qualitative Health Research, 28*(1), 145–158.

Deans, C. (2004). Nurses and occupational violence: The role of organisational support in moderating professional competence. *Australian Journal of Advancing Nursing, 22*(2), 14–18.

Dugan, J., Lauer, E., Bouquot, Z., et al. (1996). Stressful nurses: The effect on patient outcomes. *Journal of Nursing Care Quality, 10*(3), 46–58.

Dupuis, S. L., & Luh, J. (2005). Understanding responsive behaviours: The importance of correctly perceiving triggers that precipitate residents' responsive behaviours. *Canadian Nursing Home, 16*(1), 29–34.

Estabrooks, C. A., Midodzi, W. K., Cummings, G. G., et al. (2005). The impact of hospital nursing characteristics on 30-day mortality. *Nursing Research, 54*(2), 74–84.

Excellence Canada. (2022). *Elements of a healthy workplace.* https://excellence.ca/healthy-workplace-standard/

Farrell, G. (1997). Aggression in clinical settings: Nurses' views. *Journal of Advanced Nursing, 25*(3), 501–508.

Farrell, G. (1999). Aggression in clinical settings: A follow-up study. *Journal of Advanced Nursing, 29*(3), 532–541.

Galik, E. M., Resnick, B., & Pretzer-Aboff, I. (2009). "Knowing what makes them tick": Motivating cognitively impaired older adults to participate in restorative care. *International Journal of Nursing Practice, 15*(1), 48–55.

Government of Canada, & Employment and Social Development Canada. (2017). *Harassment and sexual violence in the workplace.* https://www.canada.ca/en/employment-social-development/services/health-safety/reports/workplace-harassment-sexual-violence.html and https://openparliament.ca/bills/42-1/C-65/

Hansen, A. M., Hogh, A., Persson, R., et al. (2006). Bullying at work, health outcomes and physiological stress response. *Journal of Psychosomatic Research, 60*(1), 63–72.

Hantke, S., St. Denis, V., & Graham, H. (2022). Racism and antiracism in nursing education: Confronting the problem of whiteness. *BMC Nursing, 21*, 146.

Jameton, A. (1984). *Nursing practice: The ethical issues.* Prentice-Hall.

Laschinger, H. K. S., & Leiter, M. P. (2006). The impact of nursing work environments on patient safety outcomes: The mediating role of burnout engagement. *Journal of Nursing Administration, 36*(5), 259–267.

Laschinger, H. K. S., Leiter, M., Day, A., et al. (2009). Workplace empowerment, incivility, and burnout: Impact on staff nurse recruitment and retention outcomes. *Journal of Nursing Management, 17*, 302–311.

Lewis, J., Coursol, D., & Herting, K. (2002). Addressing issues of workplace harassment: Counseling the targets. *Journal of Employment Counseling, 39*(3), 109–116.

Lewis, M. (2006). Organisational accounts of bullying: An interactive approach. In J. Randle (Ed.), *Workplace Bullying in the NHS* (pp. 25–46). Radcliffe Publishing.

Lewis, M. A. (2006). Nurse bullying: Organizational considerations in the maintenance and perpetration of health care bullying cultures. *Journal of Nursing Management, 14*(1), 52–58.

Liu, M., Maxwell, C. J., Armstrong, P., et al. (2020). COVID-19 in long-term care homes in Ontario and British Columbia. *CMAJ, 192*(47), E1540–E1546.

Lundstrom, T., Pugliese, G., Bartley, J., et al. (2002). Organizational and environmental factors that affect worker health and safety and patient outcomes. *American Journal of Infection Control, 30*(2), 93–106.

MacIntosh, J. (2003). Reworking professional nursing identity. *Western Journal of Nursing Research, 25*(6), 725–741.

MacIntosh, J. (2005). Experiences of workplace bullying in a rural area. *Issues in Mental Health Nursing, 26*(9), 893–910.

Manuel, P., & Bruinse, B. (2005, November 17–18). *A registered nurses' council: Cultivating a healthy community for nurses* [Conference session]. 5th Annual International Healthy Workplaces in Action Conference, Toronto, ON, Canada.

Marchand-Senécal, X., Kozak, R., Mubareka, S., et al. (2020). Diagnosis and management of first case of COVID-19 in Canada: Lessons applied from SARS-CoV-1. *Clinical Infectious Diseases, 71*(16), 2207–2210.

McGilton, K. S. (2004). Relating well to persons with dementia: A variable influencing staffing and quality of care outcomes. *Alzheimer's Care Today, 5*(1), 71–80.

McKenna, B. G., Smith, N. A., Poole, S. J., et al. (2003). Horizontal violence: Experiences of registered nurses in their first year of practice. *Journal of Advanced Nursing, 42*(1), 90–96.

McKoy, Y., & Smith, M. H. (2001). Legal considerations of workplace violence in health-care environments. *Nursing Forum, 36*(1), 5–14.

O'Connell, B., Young, J., Brooks, J., et al. (2000). Nurses' perceptions on the nature and frequency of aggression in general ward settings and high dependency areas. *Journal of Clinical Nursing, 9*(4), 602–610.

Pejic, A. R. (2005). Verbal abuse: A problem for pediatric nurses. *Pediatric Nursing, 31*(4), 271–279.

Purdy, N., Laschinger, H. K., Finegan, J., et al. (2010). Effects of work environments on nurse and patient outcomes. *Journal of Nursing Management, 18*(8), 901–913.

Quine, L. (2003). Workplace bullying, psychological distress, and job satisfaction in junior doctors. *Cambridge Quarterly of Healthcare Ethics, 12*(1), 91–101.

Registered Nurses' Association of Ontario. (n.d.). *Healthy work environments BPGs.* https://rnao.ca/bpg/guidelines/hwe

Registered Nurses' Association of Ontario (2007). *Professionalism in Nursing.* Toronto, Canada: Registered Nurses' Association of Ontario

Registered Nurses' Association of Ontario (2008). *Workplace Health, Safety and Well-being of the Nurse.* Toronto, Canada: Registered Nurses' Association of Ontario

Registered Nurses' Association of Ontario. (2019). *Preventing violence, harassment and bullying against health workers.* https://rnao.ca/bpg/guidelines/preventing-violence-harassment-and-bullying-against-health-workers

Registered Nurses' Association of Ontario. (2022). *Black nurses and RNAO.* https://rnao,ca/infocus/black-nurses-and-rnao

Registered Nurses' Association of Ontario, & Registered Practical Nurses Association of Ontario. (2000). *Ensuring the care will be there: Report on nursing recruitment and retention in Ontario.*

Resnick, B., Galik, E., & Boltz, M. (2013). Function focused care approaches: Literature review of progress and future possibilities. *Journal of the American Medical Directors Association, 14*(5), 313–318.

RNAO (2022b) Nursing report calls to end anti-Black racism and discrimination within the profession, *Media Release.*

Rotstein, M., & Peskun, C. (2008, November 21). *RN council as a forum to promote healthy work environments* [Conference session]. 7th International Healthy Workplaces in Action Conference, Toronto, ON, Canada.

Rushton, C. H. (2006). Defining and addressing moral distress: Tools for critical care nursing leaders. *AACN Advanced Critical Care, 17*(2), 161–168.

Solomon, M. Z., O'Donnell, L., Jennings, B., et al. (1993). Decisions near the end of life: Professional views on life-sustaining treatments. *American Journal of Public Health, 83*(1), 14–23.

Statistics Canada. (2019). *Diversity of the Black population in Canada: An overview.* https://www150.statcan.gc.ca/n1/pub/89-657-x/89-657-x2019002-eng.htm.

Stephens, L. (2008, March 8). Workplace bullies most poisonous: Even sexual harassment takes second place to the harm done by on-the-job bullying. *Toronto Star*, L11.

Turpel-Lafonte, M. (2020). *In plain sight: Addressing indigenous-specific racism and discrimination in B.C. Health Care.* Queens Printer. https://engage.gov.bc.ca/app/uploads/sites/613/2020/11/In-Plain-Sight-Summary-Report.pdf

12 ETHICAL ISSUES IN LEADERSHIP, THE ORGANIZATION, AND APPROACHES TO THE DELIVERY OF CARE

LEARNING OBJECTIVES

The purpose of this chapter is to enable you to understand:

- The influence of ethical leadership behaviour and organizational structures and processes on nursing practice and patient outcomes
- The ethical challenges facing leaders and organizations in the health care system
- Why a value-based ethical framework for organizations and leaders is required
- How organizational structures, including interprofessional practice models, patient/person and family-centred care, and delivery models enhance nursing practice
- The responsibility of leaders in promoting and improving the quality and safety of care
- The complexities of the diverse Canadian community and how this should influence leaders and organizations
- The responsibilities of leaders in combating bias and prejudice and ensuring cultural safety

INTRODUCTION

This chapter explores some of the ethical considerations related to leaders and organizations and their significant influence on the outcomes of care. Ethics is involved in the behaviour of leaders, their values, and in the strategy, processes, and operations of an organization. A moral organizational climate is essential in supporting nurses as they navigate the complex and challenging ethical issues related to practice and achieving optimal patient care. Ethical leaders support and enable a healthy and open environment and culture that supports the ethical practice of nurses and ensures that the needs of patients are met. Ethical principles of justice, nonmaleficence, and beneficence, as well as ethical theory can influence and guide a leader's approach to the systems and processes within the care environment, such as how they ensure the appropriate resources are in place, structure care delivery, interact with each other, respect differences, and collaborate to achieve positive patient and family outcomes.

LEADERSHIP AND ORGANIZATIONAL ETHICS

Nursing leaders must be aware of the ethical challenges nurses face in day-to-day practice and commit to ethical leadership and organizational practices. Nurses in all sectors should expect that the same moral standards they apply to clinical practice are applied to the ethical actions of their leaders.

A principled nursing leader understands how to:

- Ensure their leadership practices are value-based and meet high ethical standards
- Design an organization's structure and culture to influence an ethical climate
- Identify the ethical dimensions of decisions and challenges within the organization
- Identify and address the ethical issues related to allocation of resources

371

- Address human resource and diversity issues from an ethical perspective
- Prevent and mitigate moral distress and compassion fatigue within the team

Organizational Ethics

In any organization, how business is conducted matters. This is especially true in health care. Table 12.1 summarizes the key ethical issues and practices that are relevant to organizations. Beyond these elements, in the health care sector, there is the added dimension of responsibility for a vulnerable patient population and the extremely complex ethical issues that arise. Organizational systems and processes must meet the same ethical standards as those for clinical practice because

---

TABLE 12.1

Ethical Organizational Practices

In any organization, sound ethical practices need to exist with respect to:

- Human resources policies that pay attention to:
  - Recruitment and retention
  - Equitable compensation
  - Labour relations
  - Performance improvement and, when necessary, progressive discipline
- Ensuring a healthy work environment:
  - That is safe and supportive
  - In which there is mutual respect and opportunities for advancement
- Leadership practices and organizational structures that ensure:
  - **Support and mentorship for staff**
  - **Succession planning**
- The prevention of negative outcomes, such as moral distress, which are managed through:
  - **Processes by which ethical issues are identified and addressed**
  - **Education and awareness**
  - **Counselling**
  - **Transparency**
  - **Appropriate management of conflict**
  - **Processes to ensure a respectful work environment**
- Issues regarding human rights, which are managed through:
  - **Establishing human rights as a priority**
  - **Ensuring equity and fairness**
  - **Ensuring just processes and procedures are in place**
  - **Providing accommodation for illness and disability**

Extracted from Piette, M., Ellis, J. L., St. Denis, P., et al. (2002). Integrating ethics and quality improvement: Practical implementation in the transitional/extended care setting. *Journal of Nursing Care Quality, 17*(1), 35–42.

these systems and processes have a strong impact on the practice environment and the care patients receive (Piette et al., 2002; Wong & Cummings, 2007).

In recent decades, there has been growing attention to organizational ethics. To achieve ethical standards in the clinical practice environment, Brodeur (1998) suggested that leaders must first assess the ethical organizational life and infrastructure of the total organization. Instead, health care organizations tend to base their ethics agendas on specific clinical ethical issues, such as those related to death and dying, organ transplantation, and informed consent, rather than the organizational structures and processes that enable an ethical climate and culture (Sashkin & Williams, 1990; Worthley, 1999). It is challenging to act ethically within cultures where the norms and values of the total organization are unclear. For example, if clinical staff members perceive that the organization's practices, such as its approach to recruitment or resource allocation, are not guided by ethical principles or frameworks, then that organization will find it difficult to enforce standards with respect to the ethical care of patients. It is critical that clinical staff have ethical role models and perceive an ethical organization.

An overall approach to ethics might include a framework that includes the organization's recruitment practices, the support that staff receive from leaders, how resources are allocated and used, how issues of diversity and systemic racism are addressed, and how staff are supported through times of extensive organizational stress and change (Baumann, Keatings, et al., 2006; Baumann, Yan, et al., 2006; Sashkin & Williams, 1990; Worthley, 1999).

An organization's culture intersects with its ethics at the point of its organizational values—those underlying assumptions and principles that guide organizational life (Seeger, 2001). How an organization identifies its values and its ethical standards can influence how the organization is perceived both internally and externally (Lozano, 2003); the ethical culture of an organization influences its image and reputation, establishes (or not) the legitimacy of its role in society, and clarifies what it stands for (Seeger, 2001). An ethical culture or climate is one in which all persons within the organization share common values and beliefs; where there is trust, respect, openness, transparency, and accountability; where all team members participate; and where leaders are considered important role models. In an ethical culture, the ethics and values of an organization inform all of its actions and decisions (Clegg et al., 2007; Storch et al., 2009). Values shape the structure of an organization and its practices, formal statements, and policies. In many organizations, the organization's mission defines its purpose, the goal of which is to achieve excellence—the "good." For a true ethical culture, all persons within the organization must share common values; the influence of leaders, although important, is not enough. Both leaders and followers shape an ethical culture. One or the other can negatively shape the culture; therefore, both must embrace common and sound ethical practices (Grosenick, 1994). Hence, ethical organizational practices are those that are collaborative and sustained by qualities that enable effective teamwork and collaboration (Parsons et al., 2007).

Trust and a sense of fairness are instrumental to an ethical organization. Williams (2006) suggested that "trust is the adhesive that binds its members" and that "fairness is an essential ingredient in trusting relationships regardless of roles" (p. 30). Evolving evidence demonstrates the importance of trust in ensuring that nurses are engaged and committed to the organization (Laschinger et al., 2000, 2001). Trust encompasses the "positive expectations individuals have about the intent and behaviours of multiple organizational members based on organization roles, relationships, experiences, and interdependencies" (Shockley-Zalabak et al., 2000, p. 37). Organizational trust-building behaviours are those that nurses would judge as fair—for example, how decisions are made (Williams, 2006). When leaders seek input through an open and transparent consultation, this will be deemed a fair process even if the decision does not agree with the wishes of all involved. For example, engaging staff by obtaining their input on efficiencies and savings within an organization may influence how they accept changes, even if their ideas are not implemented.

Shockley-Zalabak et al. (2000) developed a model of organizational trust that considers five key dimensions that influence employee satisfaction and the perception that the organization is effective. These dimensions are (1) leadership concern for employees, (2) an open and honest culture, (3) employee connection or engagement within the organization,

(4) meaningful relationships between leaders and employees, and (5) the reliability and competence of leaders (Shockley-Zalabak et al., 2000).

Principles of fairness and justice play a strong role in ensuring organizational trust. Williams (2006) suggested that organizational justice has two components: distributive and procedural justice. **Distributive justice** relates to such outcomes as the appropriate allocation of resources, salaries, benefits, and work conditions, whereas **procedural justice** refers to the perception that processes have been fair and inclusive regardless of the outcome. For example, as mentioned earlier, when key decisions are made, are the significant stakeholders included? In what manner are they involved? Is the process open and transparent (Williams, 2006)?

Renz and Eddy (1996) proposed a model that can guide organizations in creating a sound ethical culture and a strong ethics infrastructure. A summary of this model, which is based on four key building blocks, follows (Box 12.1).

It takes time to move a culture in a positive direction and effort to sustain this change. Change and sustainability are influenced by trust, respect, transparency, and open communication. As mentioned, in an ethical culture, all members, leaders, and followers participate. An ethical culture ensures the development of leaders who engage their teams in decision making and share with them accountability for outcomes (Keatings, 2005).

Ethical Leadership

Leaders are instrumental in the creation of an ethical climate that is transparent, supports a healthy work environment, and promotes successful interprofessional collaboration. Nursing leaders must:

- Not only meet the ethical standards of the profession but also be ethical leaders and role models
- Ensure a climate and culture that support high standards of ethical nursing practice
- Model and advance a humanistic culture that is sensitive to the needs of staff, patients, and families
- Ensure processes are in place to address the ethical challenges and concerns of their employees (Brown, 2003)

Leaders must model ethical behaviour if they expect the delivery of ethical care. Through their actions

BOX 12.1
CREATING AN ETHICAL CULTURE

LINK VALUES TO MISSION AND VISION

The strategy is to integrate the values, mission, and vision of the organization into its ethical framework. It is important to engage employees by encouraging their involvement in the development and design of the framework by using approaches such as retreats and focus groups. These approaches encourage team building and sharing of perspectives and contribute to a shared commitment to the values, mission, and vision of the organization.

FACILITATE COMMUNICATION AND LEARNING ABOUT ETHICS

This strategy includes communication of the framework (i.e., values, mission, and vision) through multiple processes, such as posting statements in highly visible areas, offering education sessions that encourage interaction, role playing, and value clarification. These types of sessions should occur on an ongoing basis and should not be restricted to the launch of such an initiative.

CREATE STRUCTURES THAT SUPPORT AN ETHICAL ENVIRONMENT

An ethical environment is enhanced through the establishment of multiple processes and venues in which ethical issues can be addressed (e.g., creating ethics committees, introducing such roles as executive champion and ethicist, and building ethics into quality and performance management processes).

MONITOR AND EVALUATE ETHICAL PERFORMANCE

Implementation alone does not create a successful ethical culture; processes must be in place to constantly evaluate the effectiveness of these strategies. Such processes may include evaluating outcomes, eliciting regular feedback from employees, and reviewing and updating the framework on a regular basis.

---

and approaches, leaders can demonstrate and influence desired attributes, such as compassion, flexibility, openness, and engagement. Nursing leaders can do this by ensuring that challenging ethical issues and ethics in general are discussed regularly, possibly during rounds or team meetings (Brown, 2003); reward and recognize good practice; and encourage ongoing advancements in care.

At the same time, nurses share accountability with leaders in ensuring sound ethical practice, a healthy work environment, and staff satisfaction to create an ethical culture and climate. Leaders are responsible for supporting their staff, and staff are responsible for supporting each other and their leader. Without this shared accountability and support, an ethical climate will not be achieved (Kupperschmidt, 2004).

Nursing leaders must also be sensitive to the emotional and psychological stresses that nurses experience when dealing with ongoing or unresolved ethical issues. In these circumstances, nurses are at risk of moral distress, which can lead to compassion fatigue. Compassion fatigue manifests as work-related physical and emotional symptoms. Indicators include headaches, anxiety, mood swings, increased sick time, avoidance of certain patient situations, and lack of empathy. It is important that nursing leaders not only implement strategies to prevent such situations but also

be equipped to recognize them when they arise. It is often the most caring and empathetic nurses who are at most risk. Nurses experiencing compassion fatigue need the support and guidance of their leader or mentor. When necessary, a consultant or professional counsellor may be required to undertake a comprehensive assessment and to develop an action plan specific to the needs of a particular nurse (Lombardo & Eyre, 2011).

During the height of the COVID-19 pandemic, a major source of distress for nurses working in acute and long-term care settings was the large number of people who died on a daily basis. Many patients of all ages decompensated quickly, frequently dying alone without the presence of a caring friend or family member. Nurses who were pulled in so many directions, impeded by infection control requirements, and coping with staff shortages, could not always be there with them. These experiences were contrary to the values of nurses and their commitment to give compassionate care, and were hence a source of moral distress. In one study, more than 80% of providers working in long-term care reported an increase in moral distress (Haslam-Larmer et al., 2023). Direct care staff described challenges with workload and the emotional burden of caring for residents facing significant isolation, illness, and death (Glowinski, 2022). Factors that influenced their stress included poor communication and demoralizing media coverage of long-term care versus hospitals (White et al., 2021).

Leaders also experienced profound distress and reported challenges with constantly changing public health orders and the chaos associated with redeployment to pandemic-related activities. Some leaders indicated that their experience signalled an unanticipated end to their careers (Savage et al., 2022). This reinforces the importance of self-care; nurses cannot care for their patients, and leaders cannot support their team, without first caring for themselves.

During these times, leadership support was essential. Leaders were required to promote and acknowledge the significance of the nursing role, to be present, and to provide open and transparent communication crucial to ensuring that nurses were adequately informed and supported.

In addition to these challenges, on a personal level, nurses were fearful of infecting others, including their families, during the early days of the pandemic when protective equipment was in limited supply. Some felt unprepared to provide care for COVID-19 patients as these settings struggled to build capacity for the high volume of patients. To mitigate moral distress, it is important in challenging circumstances to engage nurses in decision making, especially because they are the ones who ultimately must enforce and act on policy decision. Nurses must provided with ongoing education, emotional and mental health support, and most especially have leaders who listen and are present. (Godshall, 2021; Ness et al., 2021; Prestia, 2020).

Nursing leaders must understand the key principles of leadership, but they also need the structures and resources to support their leadership practices. The Canadian Nursing Advisory Committee (2002) made important recommendations related to nursing leadership. These recommendations make it explicit that:

- Leaders must have an appropriate span of control (Wong et al., 2015).
- Leaders must sustain ongoing contact with their staff.
- Leaders must have the resources in place to support them.
- Novice leaders must have an appropriate orientation, education, and mentorship in order to transition effectively to their roles (Baharum et al., 2022; Baumann et al., 2019; McGillis-Hall & Donner, 1997; Rush et al., 2015).
- Succession planning strategies must be in place to ensure the development of future leaders.

In summary, nursing leaders are instrumental in ensuring the engagement of staff through the development of trusting relationships, collaboration, transparency, the provision of opportunities for professional advancement, and consistency in the approach to addressing ethical challenges. Through these means, leaders contribute to positive outcomes for patients and their families. Nurses manage relationships with patients and ensure that these relationships are built on respect, transparency, and trust; these same principles apply to the relationships among the nurse leader, the team, and the individual professional (Kupperschmidt, 2004; Laschinger et al., 2001).

Consider Case Scenarios 12.1 to 12.3.

CASE SCENARIO 12.1

WHEN LIFE INTERSECTS WITH WORK

S. D., a nurse in a rehabilitation setting, is experiencing stress at home, and this is influencing their work. S. D. is in a common-law relationship, and their partner is threatening to leave. S. D. has a 4-year-old from a previous relationship and is worried about not being able to care for the child alone. Having been distracted for the past few weeks, S. D. has recently made three medication errors. The manager has spoken with S. D. about this and told them that their performance must improve or they may be subject to disciplinary action and even termination.

Questions

1. What responsibility do leaders have to understand the stresses their staff may be experiencing?
2. Do you think stress has an impact on patient safety?
3. How might the manager be supportive in managing this situation? Given that the manager is also a nurse, does the manager have additional responsibilities?

CASE SCENARIO 12.2

PLEASE KEEP ME SAFE!

H. L. is a manager for a home nursing agency in an urban area that has the highest crime rate in the city. Recently, nurses in the agency have been expressing concerns regarding their safety, especially when they work evenings. A staff member recommends that the agency supply the nurses with tracking devices so that they can be located if an emergency situation arises. H. L. takes this idea to their director, who says it is an expensive and foolish proposal. The director notes that not one nurse has experienced a problem in recent months.

Questions

1. What responsibility does the manager and director have to ensure the safety of the staff?
2. If you were this manager, what next steps would you take given the lack of support you are receiving from the director? What supports should be in place for the manager?

CASE SCENARIO 12.3

PEER RESPONSIBILITY?

A critical care nurse has just returned to work after recovering from a work-related back injury. This nurse is returning to modified duties and has been advised not to turn or lift patients. The unit manager has developed a plan that involves assigning two other nurses to assist this nurse given these restrictions. Some of the unit nurses have become irritated with this expectation and are ignoring their colleague. This nurse is experiencing a great deal of stress, which increases after hearing that some nurses have complained to the manager and are threatening to grieve these expectations.

Questions

1. How should the unit manager respond to this challenge?
2. What support should be provided to this nurse?
3. Do you think this is a form of bullying? How should bullying be managed?
4. If you were a nurse on this unit, what would you do?

LEADERSHIP AREAS OF INFLUENCE

The good leader is key to a culture that engages and supports staff to think and act ethically. Good leaders act ethically when they introduce best practices related to programs and approaches to care. Some of these have been discussed in previous chapters, including strategies such as the prevention of violence in the workplace and the use of best practice guidelines. Good leaders must also be aware of the ethical issues involved in approaches to the management of nursing resources, recruitment, cultural safety, the elimination of bias and prejudice in health care, and the establishment of care models that support interprofessional practice and person- and family-centred care.

Managing Nursing Resources

Nursing and nursing leaders of today face many challenges. Of paramount importance is the challenge of ensuring there are enough nurses to meet the current and future needs of health care. There are longstanding cyclical patterns of nursing shortages and excesses, not only in Canada but worldwide. Nursing human resource strategies should be at the forefront of the agenda of nursing leaders across the country and should not be abandoned when the situation is perceived to be stable. This recurring cycle was demonstrated once more in response to the COVID-19 pandemic, when the shortage of nurses intensified to serious levels, again reinforcing the need for a resilient system that is able to mitigate and respond to such challenges. Though the situation was unprecedented, it might have been mitigated had best practices associated with the engagement of nurses been consistently adopted by governments and health care organizations prior to this crisis.

The potential for nursing shortages increases when long-term human resource plans are not in place. Many studies have pointed to the factors that result in shortages and have offered strategies for their prevention and mitigation. Nursing leaders have a significant role in ensuring the implementation and success of these best practices (Baumann et al., 2004; Tomblin Murphy et al., 2005). It is imperative that nursing leaders and nurses institute and sustain strategies to improve the culture of health care so as to retain and engage nurses in the workplace and the profession.

Nursing shortages in the past were, in large measure, brought on by institutional efforts to cut costs during periods of fiscal constraints. These efforts resulted in massive layoffs, loss of full-time positions, casualization of the nursing workforce, increased use of unregulated health care workers, use of more expensive agency staff, fewer nursing student positions, closure of nursing education programs, and cutbacks in numbers of students accepted into nursing programs (Baumann et al., 2004; Tomblin Murphy et al., 2005). Looking ahead, demographic trends are emerging that promise new challenges to nursing and health care delivery. The consequences of the COVID-19 pandemic on the nursing profession demonstrates more acutely the urgency of forward planning and preparedness.

The aging of the general population in Canada is having two important consequences for nursing. First, an aging population creates an increased demand on health care services. Second, aging of the population means that there are fewer young people in the overall population and an ever-shrinking number of those entering the profession. Thus, there are two considerable and opposing pressures being exerted simultaneously on the nursing labour market (Baumann et al., 2004; Tomblin Murphy et al., 2005).

Beyond the impact of demographics, advances in technology have meant that lives that would have previously been lost are being saved. That same technology, however, has resulted in an ongoing need for specialized education for nurses. In many cases, the development of new technology has meant a considerable increase in the workload of nurses, particularly those in critical care and acute care settings. As care is moved to the community, there are increasing demands on nursing in that sector. With an aging population, challenges are emerging in long-term care, with a high nurse-to-resident ratio and the increasing complexity of the resident population.

An effective nursing human resource plan includes the following elements: forecasting need, attraction to the profession, access to educational programs, transition to practice, engagement and retention, and strong professional environments. Studies that have examined trends in the nursing labour market and predicted possible outcomes have also produced a number of strategies designed to address the concerns already outlined. Those strategies include the following:

- Ensure a stable supply of nurses through a pan-Canadian approach to nursing education in collaboration with the provincial, territorial, and federal governments to prepare the number of qualified graduates needed. Enhance data collection to help predict future trends and health care human resources needs.
- Use a health care human resources planning framework based on population health care needs to plan for nursing resources.
- Adopt evidence-informed practices to inform staffing decisions, including retention and recruitment decisions. Implement effective and efficient mechanisms to address workload issues.
- Create healthy work environments that influence positive patient, nurse, and system outcomes.
- Improve and maintain the health and safety of nurses.
- Introduce and sustain engagement strategies, including the support needed to prevent and mitigate moral distress and moral residue.
- Develop innovative approaches to expand clinical experiences in nursing education (Durrant et al., 2009). New graduate nurses need adequate clinical preparation to ensure quality of patient care, to avoid excessive strain on existing mentoring and teaching resources, and to help make the transition from student nurse to independent practitioner a positive experience (Baumann et al., 2018, Lalonde & McGillis-Hall, 2017).
- Maximize the ability of nurses to work to their full scope of practice and ensure career advancement programs are available.
- Create and enhance opportunities for nurses to have meaningful involvement in decision making at various levels in health care organizations, especially when those decisions influence nursing and patient care (Baumann et al., 2004; Tomblin Murphy et al., 2005).

A number of factors influence whether young people are attracted to nursing as a career. When there are cutbacks, young people become reluctant to enter a profession because they perceive limited employment opportunities. Also, possibly because of sociocultural changes or technological changes, women, in particular, now have a much greater pool of careers from which to choose than ever before (Baumann et al., 2004; Tomblin Murphy et al., 2005).

These recurring challenges in health care result in serious nursing shortages, bed closures, cancelled surgeries, deferral of critical cases, longer wait times, and challenges in transferring patients home and to long-term care settings. These outcomes have grave implications for patient safety and the quality of care. There are other negative consequences, such as lowered morale, moral distress, and frustration, to such an extent that nurses leave the profession. There is an added cost to the system from increased sick time, overtime, and turnover. In fact, considering the costs, both human and financial, associated with serious nursing shortages, there it is indeed greater return on investment to ensure more than adequate nursing resources. Leaders in nursing and the health care system have the moral imperative to introduce innovative and sustainable long-term human resource strategies that maintain a strong positive nursing workforce and thus end the recurring cycle (Baumann, Keatings, et al., 2006; Baumann, Yan, et al., 2006).

The evidence demonstrates that important considerations in an effective nursing human resource strategy include not only the engagement of nurses and the maintenance of strong professional practice environments, but also evidence-informed transition-to-practice programs, staffing models that focus on the creation of full-time positions, appropriate nurse-to-patient ratios, and the appropriate skill mix of staff to meet the needs of patients (Baumann et al., 2018). These approaches would ensure committed nurses, continuity of care, and patient safety.

To ensure a strong professional environment, nurses need continued mentorship and professional development from peers, managers, and leadership teams. Nurses are knowledge workers. They are taught to be lifelong learners and should be offered ongoing professional development, educational support, and involvement in decision making at the unit and organizational level. Performance evaluation and review is a useful

opportunity to review career advancement planning and to support future leadership. Additional aspects of a professional environment include things such as recognition programs, creative scheduling, professional development and advancement, collaborative work environments, and engagement in decision making.

Some provincial governments, including Ontario (Ministry of Health and Long-Term Care [MOHLTC], 2017) and British Columbia (British Columbia Ministry of Health & Ministry of Advanced Education, 2008; Island Health, 2005), have introduced policy initiatives and funding in an attempt to stabilize the nursing workforce. These governments agreed with provincial nursing leaders that the growing trend toward part-time and casual work for nurses was a serious concern. This trend in employment discourages people from entering the nursing profession, denies pensions and benefits and thus disrespects those affected, and subsequently has the potential to negatively influence the quality of patient care. Too much reliance on casual and part-time staff results in interruptions in the continuity of patient care, and this is known to influence quality and safety. Also, in the case of new graduates, they are not able to consolidate their knowledge and competencies in a stable environment through a supportive transition to practice (Baharum et al., 2022; Baumann et al., 2019; McGillis-Hall & Donner, 1997; Rush et al., 2015).

In Ontario, the Nursing Graduate Guarantee (NGG) program was launched in 2007 to provide the opportunity for health care organizations to recruit and transition new graduates into the workforce. The initiative provided funding to support new graduates during an extended orientation/mentorship program.

This comprehensive government initiative was designed to support new Ontario nursing graduates in obtaining full-time employment upon graduation. Funding enabled employers to hire new graduate nurses into temporary full-time, supernumerary (above staff complement) positions for up to 6 months (Baumann et al., 2016). Employers committed to providing new graduates with an extended orientation and ongoing mentorship to ease their transition to independent practice. The goal was to transition them to permanent full-time positions at the end of the 6 months (Baumann et al., 2016). If a full-time position was not available, then the employer was required to support the new graduate in a full-time position for an additional 6 weeks. The importance of such programs is not only that it encouraged the creation of full-time positions but it ensures an effective transition of the student to independent professional practice (Baumann et al., 2018). Utilization of this initiative was not consistent across the province, where in many settings new graduates continued to be recruited into casual or part-time positions.

Transition to Practice

The complexity of health care today, in relation to advancing science and technology, diversity, and the many ethical challenges nurses face, is such that educational programs in nursing cannot possibly prepare graduate nurses who are immediately ready to practise. Yet, in many circumstances, new graduates are introduced to complex environments without an appropriate transition to practice in a safe and respectful manner and that would enable them to develop into confident and competent nurses (Baumann et al., 2018). Innovative programs, such as the NGG, facilitate these transitions. Such programs are embraced by ethical nursing leaders because they not only benefit the nurses but also ensure safe quality care for patients. Even without special funding, transition-to-practice programs are important investments because safe quality care and an engaged and knowledgeable nursing profession are cost effective and better for the health care system across Canada.

An extended orientation or transition-to-practice program "that includes mentorship, a gradual increase in clinical responsibilities, and involvement in the professional role during the early stages of a nurse's career can enhance work readiness of new graduates" (Baumann et al., 2019, p. 823). The four characteristics of work readiness are personal characteristics, clinical characteristics, relational characteristics, and organizational acuity (Fig. 12.1). Ensuring an appropriate transition program improves the new graduate's readiness to practice and their effective integration into the system. This model outlines this approach and demonstrates the processes and characteristics of an effective transition of a new graduate to practise, or work, readiness.

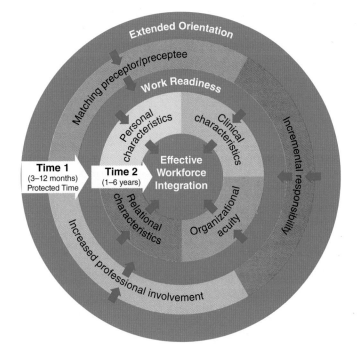

Fig. 12.1 ■ A strategy to address effective health workforces. *Source: Baumann, A., Crea-Arsenio, M., Hunsberger, M., Fleming-Carroll, B., & Keatings, M. (2019). Work readiness, transition, and integration: The challenge of specialty practice. Journal of Advanced Nursing, 75(4), 823–833.*

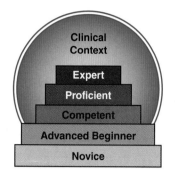

Fig. 12.2 ■ Five stages of proficiency. *Source: Kaminski, J. 2010. Theory applied to informatics — Novice to Expert. Canadian Journal of Nursing Informatics, 5(4).*

This approach to transition to practice recognizes the work of Dr. Patricia Benner, who introduced the concept that expert nurses develop skills and understanding of patient care over time through a sound educational base as well as a multitude of experiences. The model (Fig. 12.2) posits that in the acquisition and development of a skill, a learner passes through five stages of proficiency: novice, advanced beginner, competent, proficient, and expert (Fig. 12.2). These stages reflect three different aspects of skilled performance (Benner, 2000).

It has been demonstrated that a coherent strategy is important in ensuring a consistent and reliable nursing workforce. Over time, these strategies not only improve the quality of care but also ensure an organization's financial stability and the resilience of the system over time.

Aligning Staffing Resources to Patient Needs

Nursing leaders have many clients, including patients, their families, and the nurses within their teams. The needs of all groups are best met when scheduling, staff assignments, and nurse-to-patient ratios are designed to focus on the needs of patients/clients.

The principles of beneficence, nonmaleficence, and justice can be applied to these processes.

Leaders need to ensure that the qualifications of the team members are appropriate to the needs of the patients/clients and that valid evidence-informed tools are used to facilitate this process. Primarily, registered nurses, registered/licensed practical nurses, and personal support workers are used to provide direct care in hospitals, the community, and long-term care settings. The needs of the client population, not finances, should dictate the qualifications of the caregiver. In fact, having the most qualified caregiver is ultimately the most cost-effective approach. The same applies to nurse-to-patient ratios and assignments. When nurse-to-patient ratios are not appropriate, patient safety concerns arise, and fatigue caused by heavy and stressful assignments leads to increased sick time and overtime (Havaei et al., 2019). Other complexities arise with delivery models that use nonregulated providers who require supervision and where there is a risk of fragmented care. Ethical principles and frameworks can guide decisions to avoid these issues. Recognizing the significant impact that staff mix and nursing care delivery models have on outcomes and the work environment, the Canadian Nurses Association (CNA) promoted 10 principles to guide leaders in designing these processes and structures (CNA, 2012).

Fluctuations in acuity and patient care needs require that, at various times, more or less nurses are required. This fluctuation has led to the trend of increased use of casual and part-time staff. Innovative solutions, such as nursing resource teams, have been introduced as an alternative strategy, which also creates more full-time opportunities for nurses. Well-designed resource teams and strong orientation programs ensure that the competencies of the nurses match the various needs of the patients in the areas to which they are assigned (Baumann, 2005).

CASE SCENARIO 12.4

MANAGING WELL?

J. C. is the chief nurse at a community hospital in Ontario. A university close to the community offers a nursing program, and the hospital generally recruits its graduating students. The hospital has a strong focus on the management of its finances, and J. C. is always under pressure to be as efficient as possible with

the management of nursing resources. As a result, nurses are hired into casual positions in individual units because a consistent need for nurses does not exist and the hospital saves money by not paying for benefits. Because of the casual nature of the position, orientation is limited to 2 weeks of general orientation and a short time with a preceptor on the unit.

CASE SCENARIO 12.4 *(Continued)*

The hospital does not take advantage of the Nursing Graduate Guarantee (NGG) program because it does not believe it can offer full-time positions. One casual nurse who has been working in the hospital for 6 months is infrequently scheduled to shifts on the unit, and is usually called in at the last minute. This nurse averages about two to three 12-hour shifts weekly and is frequently reassigned elsewhere to unfamiliar units. This nurse, who's job satisfaction is low; does not feel engaged with the team, experiences anxiety when sent to other units; is terrified of

making mistakes and is thinking of leaving. Meanwhile, the chief nurse notices that sick time and overtime have increased, and many casual nurses are refusing shifts when called in at the last minute.

Questions

1. Are there ethical issues associated with this nursing resource management approach?
2. What would you do if you were a nurse working under these conditions?
3. Can you offer advice to the chief nurse?

Ethical Recruitment of Nurses

With the globalization of health care, there are greater risks of losing Canadian-educated nurses to other countries. One strategy for recruitment used by some countries is to recruit internationally educated nurses (IENs). Because this strategy is utilized in many countries, including Canada, the International Council of Nurses (ICN) believed it was important to establish a policy on ethical recruitment, a position that is endorsed by the CNA (ICN, 2001). As evident in the statement from the ICN, philosophically and ethically, nursing associations do not support the recruitment of nurses from developing countries—those countries that can little afford to lose what resources they have. However, IENs who chose to immigrate to Canada should be welcomed and supported in their transition to health care in this country. There are considerable challenges that prevent or delay IENs from integrating in a timely and seamless way into the nursing profession (Allan & Westwood, 2016; McGillis-Hall et al., 2015).

Internationally Educated Nurses: Migration Versus Recruitment

There are many complex ethical issues related to nursing migration (the movement of nurses from one

country to another). Some of these issues relate to the aggressive recruitment of nurses from developing countries and those with shortages, and the transition of nurses who make a choice to immigrate to Canada (Griffith, 2001; Keatings, 2006; McGuire & Murphy, 2005; Yi & Jezewski, 2000). Interest in attracting IENs grows at times of nursing shortages in Canada, as demonstrated in response to the human resources consequences of the COVID-19 pandemic. A joint report issued by the International Council of Nurses (ICN) and the World Health Organization (WHO) cautioned against affluent countries recruiting nurses from developing countries and hence creating more health disparities across the globe. Rather, they promoted the notion that each country ought to invest in the education of nurses, the creation of employment opportunities and leadership development for nurses (ICN & WHO, 2020). In 2022 ICN called for stronger ethical codes for the recruitment of nursing and investment in nursing education (ICN, 2022).

Consider Case Scenarios 12.5 and 12.6, adapted from *Nurses on the Move: Migration and the Global Health Care Economy* (Kingma, 2006). The first story illustrates some of the factors that would "push" a nurse to immigrate to another country.

CASE SCENARIO 12.5

FATIMA'S STORY

Fatima, a member of a minority ethnic community in her home country, was frequently the butt of intolerable discriminatory remarks and actions from her

colleagues and hospital leadership. After 11 years as a nurse, she was never able to secure full-time status. In spite of many efforts to advance her qualifications through continuing education courses, her applications

Continued on following page

CASE SCENARIO 12.5 *(Continued)*

were consistently ignored. Yet, the country was suffering from a desperate shortage of nurses. This made Fatima's position even more untenable. Ultimately, she moved to Europe, and her career aspirations were fulfilled. "The decision to move was mine, and I would do it again," says Fatima.

Source: From Nurses on the Move: Migration and the Global Health Care Economy, by Mireille Kingma, an ILR Press book published by Cornell University Press. Copyright (c) 2005 by Mireilla Kingma. Reprinted by permission of the publisher.

Other nurses tell of the "pull factors," when aggressive recruitment agencies offer major financial and transition incentives, which, in some instances, disappear upon their arrival to the new country. Stories include those of nurses being forced to work in less than attractive clinical areas, accept cuts in pay, and cope with relentless processes and expenses associated with securing registration or licensure. Paradoxically, when incentives do materialize, IENs often experience the abuse of local nurses who perceive reverse discrimination because the perks are given only to immigrant nurses (Kingma, 2006).

The following story illustrates some of the factors that would "pull" a nurse to immigrate to another country.

CASE SCENARIO 12.6

VICKI'S STORY

Vicki faced many economic and social challenges in her country. A recruitment agency convinced her that she would experience better personal and professional life in a developed country. She was offered the opportunity to work in a private nursing home in the heart of a cosmopolitan city for an annual salary equivalent to $40,000. She was also told her immigration expenses would be covered. When she arrived, she found not only that her expenses were not covered but also that she had to sign a contract for an annual salary of about $28,000 and give up her passport. Also, her place of employment was a 2-hour commute each way from the part of the city where she could find an apartment.

Source: From Nurses on the Move: Migration and the Global Health Care Economy, by Mireille Kingma, an ILR Press book published by Cornell University Press. Copyright (c) 2005 by Mireilla Kingma. Reprinted by permission of the publisher.

Nurses choose to leave their country when they are not respected as professionals and when they are not appropriately compensated and therefore unable to provide sufficiently for themselves and their families. These are not simple issues but serious ethical challenges that nursing leaders need to address.

At the root of these push/pull factors is whether the international community is ready to address the conditions that push or pull nurses away. Of global concern is the tendency to utilize short-term solutions, such as migration, when the core issue is attracting and retaining local nurses within a positive environment, one in which they feel satisfied with the care they are able to provide (Kingma, 2006).

These case scenarios illustrate that, on the one hand, it would seem unethical to engage in aggressive recruitment strategies to lure nurses from developing countries where shortages already exist and that, on the other, nurses should have a right to choose to leave an unsupportive environment in which their career aspirations are not fulfilled, and their personal freedom is limited.

Many IENs who choose to immigrate to Canada are faced with significant challenges in securing registration. Nursing regulatory bodies in Canada have reviewed the transition processes to ensure a streamlined process for the immigrant nurse. This starts with the review of qualifications, continues with the delivery of education programs that enable them to meet Canadian standards and competencies, and concludes with the process of registration. For many, the process has been a bureaucratic nightmare and time consuming, but the situation is improving. As a profession, nursing has the ethical responsibility to respect IENs and to enable them to integrate and function well in the Canadian health care sector (McGillis-Hall et al., 2015; McGuire & Murphy, 2005).

Further challenges exist when the IEN enters the clinical setting and faces challenges with regard to integration, orientation, communication, discrimination, and marginalization. Furthermore, they often miss their home country and their life there, and they may experience distress associated with scope and practice differences (Moyce et al., 2016; Pung et al., 2017). Supportive transition programs have been introduced to provide meaningful support for these nurses (CARE Centre for Internationally Educated Nurses, 2019).

Leaders must consider that these nurses need additional support and mentoring during this difficult transition. Beyond the normal orientation to a new clinical environment, they are transitioning to a new culture, adapting to a new language (Canadian health care technical terms), and may have to adapt to a new model or approach to the delivery of care. The scope of practice of Canadian nurses may be broader or narrower than that in their home country. IENs need to understand the Canadian health care environment and the challenges faced by nurses within this culture and

system. Nurses educated in Canada working with IENs have the opportunity to welcome a new perspective and to learn about different cultures and traditions. Nurses educated in other countries with diverse cultural and ethnic perspectives are therefore a positive addition to the multicultural model, which values diversity in a rich and vibrant Canadian community (Griffith, 2001; McGuire & Murphy, 2005; Yi & Jezewski, 2000).

Consider Case Scenario 12.7.

ETHICAL ISSUES ASSOCIATED WITH DIVERSITY

Considering the diversity of the Canadian community, it is imperative that organizations ensure that the systems, processes, and structures are in place to provide nurses and the team with the resources to provide culturally competent and respectful care. In all health care settings, nurses form professional relationships with patients from multiple backgrounds and cultures, and therefore engage with people and communities who may live in and interpret their worlds in many different ways (Arnold & Bruce, 2006).

Not only must nursing leaders be culturally competent and be strong role models, but also must ensure

---

CASE SCENARIO 12.7

AN ETHICAL CULTURAL TRANSITION?

M. V. emigrated from Estonia to Canada 5 years ago. They applied for registration in one of the provinces shortly after arrival. Even though M. V. had 10 years of experience in pediatric nursing in Estonia, including 2 years as a nurse manager, it took M. V. 5 years to become registered in Canada. M. V. applied for a pediatric nurse position in a local community hospital. Things did not go well. They were given the same orientation as for all new nurses but was confused by the "jargon" and how nurses interacted with the rest of the team. For example, M. V. was not used to challenging the physicians on the team or making suggestions to the team regarding the care of a patient. Because M. V. had not been working for some time, they had misgivings about their competence, especially because technology had advanced

since M. V. had last practised. M. V.'s preceptor was frustrated with M. V., and M. V. worried about what action the preceptor would take.

Questions

1. Should there be a restriction on recruitment of IENs? Should this restriction apply to all recruitment or only to developing countries? Under what circumstance should recruitment from developing countries be ethically justified?
2. What support policies and process should the health care institution have in place to help IENs?
3. Should there be a unique orientation for IENs? Can the system afford this?
4. What strategies might leaders introduce to facilitate the recruitment and transition of IENs?

that the systems, structures, and processes are in place to ensure cultural safety. For example, leaders should ensure access to interpreters who understand the culture and the health care issues facing patients, and they must facilitate access to traditional cultural approaches to care when this is requested.

Patients and families who come from diverse cultural backgrounds are at greater risk not only when language barriers are present, but also when there is not a shared understanding by the team of what is meaningful and important to them. Illness and associated stressors compound these challenges of language and comprehension (Andrews & Boyle, 2002). To ensure culturally safe care, there needs to be a balance of power between providers and patients, as well as an acknowledgement of the social, political, and economic factors that influence and shape individual responses and trusting relationships. For example, Canada has welcomed many refugees over the past years, and their experiences prior to entering Canada may influence their interactions with the health care system. As discussed in Chapter 10, culturally safe care is possible when nurses respect the story of their patients and attempt to understand the health beliefs and practices of different cultural groups. As role models, nursing leaders should engage in actions that respect and empower the cultural identity and well-being of individuals, families, and communities.

To address the gaps in health care delivery and health status among diverse groups, it is important for leaders to ensure that nurses and the team first understand and reflect on the assumptions of the dominant Western cultural values that underlie health policies, research, and interactions and how they may conflict with the values and beliefs of other cultures (Andrews & Boyle, 2002; Nicholas et al., 2017; Racine, 2003).

In a country as diverse as Canada, it is impossible for nurses to be knowledgeable about all cultures and, more specifically, the values of the particular patients they care for. However, to provide culturally safe nursing care, nurses should undertake assessments that include the exploration of a patient's or family's culture, their values, and what is meaningful to them regarding care and involvement of the family. Leaders should ensure that this cultural assessment is included in the questions posed to patients. Further, even if a person is known to come from a particular ethnic background,

nurses cannot assume that the individual embraces the values and beliefs of that culture. A comprehensive cultural assessment reveals the unique values and perspectives of others and helps design care that is most consistent with their values and beliefs (Andrews & Boyle, 2002). Understanding values and beliefs of patients and families ensures that these values and beliefs are considered in the development, implementation, and evaluation of a mutual plan of care. A comprehensive cultural assessment is the foundation for culturally safe nursing care.

Nursing leaders must ensure that nurses have these tools, and have the knowledge and skills to use them effectively. Cultural sensitivity education ought to be a key component of nursing education, transition to practice, and ongoing professional development (Karmali et al., 2011).

Health care organizations in Canada have a duty to encourage diversity in their workforces. There is value in having a team that mirrors the cultural diversity in the community. Patients and families feel more comfortable in health care settings that represent their community. Also, such diversity facilitates shared learning within the team and advances cultural competence and mutual respect. Such programs are encouraged by government policy and are constitutionally protected by section 15 of the *Canadian Charter of Rights and Freedoms,* which ensures reverse discrimination programs designed to provide advantages to traditionally disadvantaged ethnic or minority groups. The test for reverse discrimination or affirmative action is that (1) the program has an ameliorative or remedial purpose and (2) the program targets a disadvantaged group identified by the enumerated (race, national or ethnic origin, colour, religion, gender, age, or mental or physical disability) or analogous grounds (*R. v. Kapp,* 2008).

Organizations and leaders can also engage with members of various cultural communities to facilitate the development of educational programs that increase awareness and understanding of the cultural norms and values that are important to them.

In many Canadian cities, more than 10 languages may be spoken by the population. Census data from 2021 revealed that the number of people who speak a language other than French or English at home grew to 4.6 million, or about 13% of the population

CASE SCENARIO 12.8

WHOSE BEST INTERESTS? WHEN CULTURAL PERSPECTIVES CLASH

A 15-year-old Indigenous male has been transported from northern Manitoba to an acute care facility in Winnipeg. He sustained serious injuries in a hunting accident when he tripped over brush and severely injured his right arm. Uncertain whether they can save the arm and worried about sepsis and gangrene setting in, the team members think it is in the young man's best interests to have it amputated. The problem is that doing so will significantly affect his future livelihood because hunting is his chosen career. He and his family are reluctant to make this decision and ask for a meeting of the community elders. Five leaders arrive at the hospital and request that the team members try their best to save the arm.

Questions

1. What are the rights of this young man? What are his best interests?
2. Hospital policy states that the substitute decision maker is the patient's next of kin—in this case, his parents. How would you manage this different view of who should provide consent?
3. What organizational supports should be in place to support the team, the patient, and his community in this circumstance?
4. What is the role of the nursing leader in helping to achieve a positive resolution in this case?

(Statistics Canada, 2022b). Therefore, it is important that interpreters be available, especially because barriers to communication can pose serious safety challenges. Also, information related to patient and family education should be available in the primary languages spoken in that community, whether through interpreters or technology. Collaboration across organizations is essential to efficiency in ensuring this information is readily available. Ensuring patients have access to this information is an important component of patient safety and quality of care.

DISCRIMINATION AND SYSTEMIC RACISM IN HEALTH CARE

It is critical for leaders to acknowledge that systemic and individual racism exists across the Canadian health care system. *Racism* refers to the beliefs, practices, and systems that affirm the superiority of one race over others. Structural, or systemic, racism includes those processes established in law, policy, and the norms of a society that reinforce inequality and provide advantages to one group over another. It is influenced by organizational cultures, policies, and practices that create barriers or exclusions to access important benefits or opportunities for marginalized and racialized groups (Government of Ontario, 2022; Wellesley Institute/Ontario Health, 2021). Systemic

and structural change requires leadership and the creation of new policies, structures, and resources to address racism and discrimination against racialized and marginalized communities. Examples of systemic racism in nursing from the past include the exclusion of Black students from Canadian nursing schools until the 1940s, the use of textbooks in nursing education where light-skinned patients were the default, insufficient or biased attention being given to the differences in illness and injury presentation in darker-skinned patients, and class discussion of case studies that highlighted racialized stereotypes of intoxicated Indigenous people and Black people with poor personal hygiene (Registered Nurses' Association of Ontario [RNAO], 2022).

A study of discrimination against Indigenous persons undertaken for the government of British Columbia highlighted numerous concerns and problems with the interactions between Indigenous people and the provincial health care system. The report detailed a "B.C. health care system with widespread systemic racism against Indigenous peoples that resulted in a range of negative impacts, harm, and even death" (Turpel-Lafonte, 2020).

In Canada, a substantial power imbalance exists between non-Indigenous health care providers and Indigenous people, which grounds many of the unacceptable experiences they face in the system. In previous chapters, Indigenous people's experiences in

"Indian hospitals" provided an illustration of Canada-wide systemic racism, and the recent experiences of Joyce Echaquan and Brian Sinclair provide examples of individual racism and highlight a culture that allows discrimination to continue. Also consider the experiences of Indigenous women who have been coerced into sterilization, as described in Chapter 10 (Boyer, 2017).

In its advocacy role, the CNA addressed the issue of racism in health care in two important declarations: *Nursing Declaration Against Anti-Black Racism in Nursing and Health Care* (Box 12.2) and *Nursing Declaration Against Anti-Indigenous Racism in Nursing and Health Care* (Box 12.3) (https://www.cna-aiic.ca/en/policy-advocacy/advocacy-priorities/racism-in-health-care).

The CNA asserts that racism is an important determinant of health and contributes to unacceptable health and social inequities and that racism and discrimination

---

BOX 12.2
NURSING DECLARATION AGAINST ANTI-BLACK RACISM IN NURSING AND HEALTH CARE

As nurses,

1. We unconditionally condemn all acts of racism and discrimination.
2. We will look inwards to identify and address the biases, fears, assumptions and privilege within ourselves, our organizations, across the profession of nursing, and across health care broadly.
3. In conducting our work, we will seek, recognize, and respect the leadership of voices from Black communities and learn from lived experiences of anti-Black racism in Canada.
4. We will advocate for policies that are anti-racist at the local, provincial, and national levels that address health and social inequity.
5. We acknowledge that cultural safety can only be achieved through cultural and structural competence and humility.

Canadian Nurses Association. (2021a). *Nursing Declaration Against Anti-Black Racism in Nursing and Health Care.* https://hl-prod-ca-oc-download.s3-ca-central-1.amazonaws.com/CNA/2f975e7e-4a40-45ca-863c-5ebf0a138d5e/UploadedImages/documents/Nursing_Declaration_Anti-Black_Racism_November_8_2021_FINAL_ENG_Copy.pdf

---

BOX 12.3
NURSING DECLARATION AGAINST ANTI-INDIGENOUS RACISM IN NURSING AND HEALTH CARE

As nurses,

1. We declare racism directed at Indigenous Peoples a national health crisis.
2. We commit to protect and care for those whose dignity, safety, and well-being are threatened based on their Indigenous identity.
3. We vow to combat bias and prejudice in our own interactions with others, as well as in our organizations and communities.
4. We will develop strategic plans with measurable goals to identify and close the gaps in health outcomes between Indigenous and non-Indigenous communities.
5. We will recognize, respect, and address the distinct healthcare needs of the Métis, Inuit, and off-reserve Aboriginal Peoples (TRC Call to Action #20).
6. We acknowledge that cultural safety can only be achieved through cultural competence.
7. We will advocate for policies at the local, regional, federal, provincial, territorial, and pan-Canadian levels that address health and social inequities.

Canadian Nurses Association. (2021b). *Nursing Declaration Against Anti-Indigenous Racism in Nursing and Health Care.* https://hl-prod-ca-oc-download.s3-ca-central-1.amazonaws.com/CNA/2f975e7e-4a40-45ca-863c-5ebf0a138d5e/UploadedImages/documents/Nursing_Declaration_Anti-Indigenous_Racism_November_8_2021_ENG_Copy.pdf

---

are root causes of health disparities that must be addressed at all levels.

The CNA asserts that nurses are obliged to respect and value each person's individual culture and consider how culture influences an individual's experience of health care and the health care system (CNA, 2018).

Using Race-Based Data

In recognition that the "people of African descent represent a distinct group whose human rights must be promoted and protected," the United Nations (2022) proclaimed the years between 2015 and 2024 as the decade "for People of African Descent." In 2007, *the United Nations Declaration on the Rights of Indigenous Peoples* was adopted to recognize the human rights of Indigenous peoples across the world and to establish minimal standards for their protection in existing and future policy and law. This declaration became law in Canada in 2021, with the Act providing a roadmap for healing, reconciliation, and collaboration (*United Nations Declaration on the Rights of Indigenous Peoples Act,* 2021). According to the 2021 census, 4.3% of the population in Canada identified as Black (Statistics Canada, 2022a), and 5% of the population as Indigenous (Statistics Canada, 2022c). These data raise questions regarding the extent to which Black, Indigenous, and people of colour (BIPOC) are represented in the nursing profession. Unfortunately, the statistics regarding race and ethnicity needed to inform strategy and action to achieve appropriate representation is lacking (Oudshoorn, 2020).

Nurses who are Black, Indigenous, and people of colour have encountered overt and systemic racism. The intent of the United Nations proclamations would require that leaders in nursing understand these experiences and take action to protect nurses and patients from racist and discriminatory practices.

In the nursing profession, interventions and actions are usually based on evidence and good data, yet the full extent of systemic racism in Canada is not known because there is ongoing debate regarding the collection, interpretation, and use of race-based data.

Historical arguments against collecting race-based data are centred around crime and policing; the atrocities that previously occurred in the name of race; concerns that race-based data collection would normalize racism; and that data may be abused to further justify racist attitudes or beliefs. Some express fear that such statistics would be used to justify discriminatory policies, and that reporting of racial data may contribute to racial profiling and the stigmatization of racialized communities, presupposing an association between race and crime (Millar & Owusu-Bempah, 2011; Owusu-Bempah & Millar, 2010). In response to these concerns, the most current data related to Indigenous health are collected and assessed by Indigenous groups and organizations rather than the national and provincial health authorities (Canadian Institute for Health Information [CIHI], 2022).

Those who support the collection of race-based data consider it a means to evaluate the extent of racism and discriminatory practices, and believe it is necessary when advocating for changes in practice and policy. They argue that race-based data can increase transparency and accountability within institutions and systems to track discrimination and inequity (Hasnain-Wynia et al., 2012; Nerenz, 2005; Owusu-Bempah & Millar, 2010).

The call for the collection of race-based data was renewed by the Black Lives Matter social movement (Dordunoo, 2021). As well, BIPOC activists and organizations have started to demand the systematic collection of race-based data. They argue that without the collection of race-based data, racism and discrimination can persist and that the data are in fact necessary to combat racism. They propose that race-based data be collected and interpreted in a way that is meaningful to the interests of these communities (Owusu-Bempah & Millar, 2010). For example, rather than stereotyping the BIPOC community as associated with crime, good data should lead to a review of the root causes, such as poverty and other social determinants of health, that contribute to such outcomes. Race-based data are now being used to assess policing in Canada and to determine whether policing is influenced by race.

Race-Based Data and Health Equity

A heath equity approach recognizes that the risk of illness and the ability to recover are linked to social factors, and that changes to the social determinants of health to improve the well-being of vulnerable populations are considered important health equity interventions. The achievement of health equity is evidence informed. Therefore, data are needed to understand the systemic barriers to such evidence-informed interventions being deployed. Collecting race-based data is a good first step toward equity, but it should not be the only one (Dordunoo, 2021). Good sociodemographic data and race-based data are important tools but must be linked to action (McKenzie, 2020). There are valid concerns about governance, accountability, and protections against misuse of data that must be addressed as good data must inform effective equitable interventions for vulnerable communities and populations. For example, data revealed that Black women were not being appropriately screened for certain cancers, leading Cancer Care Ontario (CCO) to implement an evidence-informed strategy to remedy this disparity (McKenzie, 2020).

There have been calls for race and ethnicity data collection to identify health disparities and promote heath equity in Canada for decades. Because, historically, race-based data have been used for stereotyping and discrimination, governments have been reluctant to use such data (Mulligan et al., 2020). Though racial and ethnic data are collected in Canada through the census across settings such as provincial health care systems, immigration, and crime and justice, there is a lack of population-wide, disaggregated, high-quality race-based data (Mulligan et al., 2020).

The COVID-19 pandemic revealed and exacerbated existing inequalities. During the pandemic, information from American and British research indicated that Black and Latino populations had been disproportionately impacted by the COVID-19 pandemic (Mojtehedzadeh, 2020; Mulligan et al., 2020). Despite calls by racialized communities to collect these data in order to identify inequities and guide the pandemic response, initially few Canadian governments gathered race-based data (Wellesley Institute/Ontario Health, 2021). At first, the Ontario Ministry of Health and Long-Term Care took the position that it would not collect race-based data because such collection was not authorized by law. In fact, this was incorrect, and the government later acknowledged that the collection of such data for health purposes was not illegal. At the time, many advocacy groups were already collecting and using such data for other purposes. Ironically, the Chief Medical Officer of Ontario had authored a report for the ministry in 2018 arguing that the collection of race-based health data was essential to the health of the province (Mulligan, 2020). Ultimately, Manitoba, Ontario, some municipalities, regional health units, and advocacy groups initiated race-based data collection, but the other provincial governments and the federal government did not (McKenzie, 2020; Wellesley Institute/Ontario Health, 2021).Where race-based data were not collected, efforts were made to gather information about racial aspects of the pandemic through indirect methods such as the analysis of heavily racialized neighbourhoods. The race-based information from direct and indirect sources highlighted the greater impact that COVID-19 had within non-White populations, confirming British and American studies using race-based data (Wellesley Institute/Ontario Health, 2021), The Ontario data revealed disparities in the epidemiology and impact of COVID-19. Compared to White populations, age-standardized per capita racialized groups had

a 1.2- to 7.1-fold higher rate of infection, a 1.7- to 9.1-fold higher rate of hospitalization, a 2.1- to 10.4-fold higher rate of intensive care admissions, and a 1.7- to 7.6-fold higher rate of death (Wellesley, 2021). The data collection did not include Indigenous populations in Ontario. The province chose to work with Indigenous partners on "the issues and considerations surrounding Indigenous data collection for COVID-19 and beyond, including data sovereignty for Indigenous communities" (Wellesley Institute/Ontario Health, 2021, p. 5).

Nurses and their leaders must engage in strategies to combat systemic racism. Nursing must play a leading role, as this is consistent with the values and commitments of the nursing profession (Danda et al., 2022). Self-reflection and acknowledgement that such racism and discrimination exist are first steps.

ACHIEVING QUALITY CARE

It is an ethical imperative for leaders to introduce evidence-informed structures and care delivery systems to ensure the quality of patient care.

Interprofessional Practice (IPP)

Interprofessional practice (IPP) has emerged as a health care priority in Canada and internationally (Pape et al., 2013; Reeves et al., 2010). IPP is defined as the continuous interaction of two or more professions, organized with a common goal of solving or exploring mutual issues with the best possible collaboration with patients and their family (Nicholas et al., 2010). It involves moving beyond the narrow focus of disciplines working autonomously and in isolation to working together as an interdependent team (Lingard et al., 2012; Reeves et al., 2010). There has been longstanding recognition of the need for teamwork in clinical practice, and finding new ways to ensure delivery of interprofessional care has been raised as an imperative for best practice (Curran, 2004; Davis, 1988; Reeves et al., 2010; Sicotte et al., 2002). With the introduction of new health care disciplines, team approaches evolved. Previous team or multidisciplinary models had involved members functioning independently. An interprofessional approach, however, involves team members planning and coordinating care delivery together.

Changes in the health care sector over the past number of decades have been driven by an increasing emphasis on measurable outcomes, best practices, continuity of care, and cost containment. Patients presenting with multifactorial problems and chronic diseases feel the impact of social determinants of health (e.g., poor nutrition, limited education, poverty) and are better managed with an interprofessional approach to care. This approach helps ensure good communication, cooperation, coordination, collaboration, and integration through the exchange of ideas, expertise, theories, and perspectives (Hall, 2005; Reeves et al., 2010; Thompson et al., 2007). There is immense value in obtaining input from all members of the professional team, who may define or explain a situation in different but qualitatively important ways.

Historically, there have been many challenges to interprofessional collaboration. These have included the perceived uniqueness of each profession and its professional self-interest versus sharing knowledge and scope. There is a growing acceptance that scopes of practice do overlap but that each professional discipline has a distinct expertise to offer to achieve the best outcomes for patients.

It is recognized that critical to the evolution is the fact that an individual team members must be confident in their own professional identity and competent in their role (Barker et al., 2005; Barker & Oandasan, 2005). Reinforcing the importance of the new graduate's transition to practice and advancement as a strong professional, Hewison and Sim (1998) proposed that professionals evolve through these levels of team functioning:

- **Unidisciplinarity**—feeling confident and competent in one's own discipline
- **Intradisciplinarity**—believing that you and fellow professionals in your discipline can make an important contribution to care
- **Multidisciplinarity**—recognizing that other disciplines also have important contributions to make
- **Interdisciplinarity**—willing and able to work with others in the joint evaluation, planning, and care of the patient
- **Transdisciplinarity**—making the commitment to teach and practise with other disciplines across traditional boundaries for the benefit of the patient's immediate needs (Hewison & Sim, 1998, p. 311)

Within one profession, although each member may have a unique perspective, there are usually some shared views. At the same time, if team members within the same profession have various areas of expertise, they may offer different perspectives regarding care. Furthermore, when several professions are involved, each provides input influenced by the knowledge and expertise of that discipline.

Multidisciplinary teams focus on the same patients and may understand the contribution of each member of the team. However, the care can become fragmented if each member is contributing to a component of care in isolation from other team members. This may result in confusion for the patient and family.

In an interprofessional model, professionals from within each discipline share their views and perspectives in pursuit of a common set of objectives and a shared plan for the patient and the family.

Interprofessional teams consult with each other, coordinate care as a team, and negotiate the role that each member will play with respect to the care of the patient. *Coordination,* essential to IPP, is the integration of the team members' plans and action, and requires effective communication and common decision-making processes. *Collaboration,* also essential to IPP, is the process through which team members make decisions together and reach consensus on moving forward with a plan (Parsons et al., 2007). This also implies shared responsibility and accountability for outcomes (Lessard et al., 2008).

Although the nursing profession values interprofessional collaboration, this does not mean that it should surrender its own identity. The success of interprofessional collaboration is dependent on connecting each profession's shared value base while still maintaining each one's unique identity and skills.

Interprofessional collaboration requires different professions to learn from and about each other to provide efficient patient-focused delivery of health care. At the same time, the integrity of each profession must be maintained (Barker et al., 2005; Irvine et al., 2002; Irvine et al., 2004).

There is emerging evidence that IPP offers many benefits for patients, families, and health care professionals. Examples of these benefits that are evident in the literature include:

- Improved staff engagement and morale
- Improvement in patient care and outcomes

- Efficiency in health care delivery
- Improved communication within and beyond the team
- Greater patient consultation and engagement
- Timely and appropriate referrals
- More professional accountability and responsibility
- Unique opportunities for professional development
- Meaningful collaboration within the team

In summary, IPP is conceptualized as the health care team's "sharing" in the delivery of patient and family-centred care. Within the vision of IPP, the health care team is viewed as a means for integrating knowledge and finding solutions to complex health problems, rather than working in isolation. The values of the team complement each other. They share decision-making data, planning, interventions, and care philosophies (Cowan et al., 2006).

CASE SCENARIO 12.9

DO YOU EVER TALK TO EACH OTHER?

A 65-year-old patient, R. O., is being discharged after a total knee replacement. The admission nurse did a comprehensive assessment of R. O.'s home and social situation and documented that they have been living alone since their spouse died 6 months earlier. R. O. lives in a two-story house that has a bathroom on the main floor, so R. O. plans to sleep at this level of the house until they are comfortable with climbing stairs. R. O.'s neighbour has indicated that they will assist R. O. with ambulation and ensure that R. O. has meals during the convalescence period.

The surgery went well, and R. O. is now ready for discharge. On the day of discharge, R. O. is visited by the physiotherapist, dietitian, and, finally, the home care coordinator. Each of them asks if R. O. lives alone, has any supports, and has to cope with stairs. When the home care coordinator asks the same questions, R. O. becomes extremely abrupt and asks whether the team members ever talk to each other. The coordinator asks the nurses if R. O. is always this grumpy!

Questions

1. A number of professionals are involved in this patient's care. Are they functioning as a team?
2. How would interprofessional practice (IPP) change the approach of these team members?

Shared Ethical Challenges of Interprofessional Teams

Evidence suggests that patients experience positive outcomes when professional members of the health care team work and learn together (Barker & Oandasan, 2005; Walsh et al., 1999; Zwarenstein & Reeves, 2000). This is especially true when the team faces complex ethical issues and challenges. Collaboration and open discussion among team members are essential to ensuring that ethical issues are addressed (Kenny, 2002). The interprofessional team members must enter into negotiations with one another when facing ethical decisions, as these issues are not isolated to one discipline (Botes, 2000) but involve all team members who are caring for that patient and their family. As with all aspects of patient care, there is greater value when the team listens and learns from one another to understand the lens through which each profession

views the issue or problem. Morality and ethics within the health care setting cannot be isolated to individual team members or disciplines. Together, the team has a greater influence on ethical practice and will be more likely to achieve the best outcomes for patients and their families.

There are various methods of encouraging team learning and facilitating team approaches to ethical discourse. Understanding one another's individual and professional values can be done through the narrative, as discussed in Chapter 2. As a tool, the narrative—or sharing of stories—helps both the individual and each profession as a whole to engage in moral reflection. It also offers a framework to facilitate understanding of the individual and professional lenses through which the issue is viewed (Verkerk et al., 2004).

Verkerk et al. (2004) offered a process whereby teams learn and understand each other's ethical perspectives. The initial phase of the model encourages shared decision-making regarding ethical choice and action:

1. Team members support each other in attaining "a heightened moral sensitivity to the vulnerabilities, values, and responsibilities they encounter in their work—a sensitivity acquired by identifying and developing a point of view that can be used as a touchstone for the decisions about the best way of proceeding" (Verkerk et al., 2004, p. 32).
2. Team members support each other "to understand that they are a part of a practice that involves multiple perspectives and positions" (Verkerk et al., 2004, p. 32), thereby acknowledging that individuals may have different views and perspectives, all of which may have merit.
3. Team members support each other to "appreciate that they are participants in a socially shared practice" (Verkerk et al., 2004, p. 32) that requires collective action and decision making.

Through the process outlined previously, the team becomes committed to a collaborative and supportive approach to ethical decision making. Verkerk et al. then provided a guide through which the perspectives of the various professionals involved are shared so that collectively they can decide on a plan and clarify their respective responsibilities as negotiated by the team (Verkerk et al., 2004):

1. The team members offer their initial reaction to the story.
2. The team members are guided to critically examine the moral particulars of the story.
3. The team members map out their professional responsibilities with respect to the situation.

This model serves to create a clearer understanding of the various perspectives of one's fellow professionals. Through this process, learning occurs, and greater clarity about the roles of the team and its individual members is achieved. Best courses of action can be decided upon, as can the respective responsibilities of each team member and the team as a collective. As a methodology, this serves to ensure that different perspectives are heard and respected and that the many moral dimensions of the issues are discussed and understood.

Some other approaches use codes of ethics as a foundation to enhance interprofessional discussion and collaboration. Interprofessional teams may focus on their respective codes of ethics to understand their various roles and perspectives. In doing so, they have the potential to learn more about both their individual responsibility and the shared responsibility for patient care.

For IPP to be effective, leaders must be invested in and committed to its success. They must champion the promotion, implementation, and maintenance of IPP through creative strategies that foster motivation and engage the staff, the patients, and their families in the process (Barker et al., 2005). Although leaders help create the climate and culture that supports IPP, other structural elements, such as scheduling, regular meetings, time, and space, are essential to ensure the ongoing success of the model (Barker et al., 2005; Parsons et al., 2007).

Quality Improvement and Safety

Since the time of Florence Nightingale, quality has been a core value of the nursing profession. The values and ethical standards of nursing that drive quality are fundamental to the societal obligations and commitments of members of a profession. Leadership is one of the most important factors in ensuring a culture that focuses on quality improvement and patient safety.

If safety is important in an organization, its leaders should be discussing it on a regular basis and actively participating in strategies to promote it (Morath, 2006). To create such a culture, leaders must demonstrate a commitment through clearly articulated values and actions.

Over the past few decades, the focus on quality and patient safety has strengthened and advanced in health care. As a result, the body of knowledge regarding quality and safety has grown, and various methods to promote improvement have been designed. Nursing leaders are not only experts in this area but contribute to the advancement of this knowledge and to a deeper understanding of quality and safety in health care. Specifically nursing leaders must:

■ Understand the key principles, theories and methodologies, and evolving evidence fundamental to quality management and improvement

- Utilize the various models for quality improvement and safety, including the tools and processes that facilitate improvement, maintenance, and measurement of quality
- Develop, implement, and evaluate quality improvement plans
- Be familiar with the legislative requirements related to quality and safety and the specific accountabilities of organizations and health professionals

The obligation for nurses to focus on quality and bring forward concerns regarding safe practice was first raised by Nightingale (La Sala, 2009; McGaffigan, 2019; Tye, 2020). She asserted that the entire health care team should be held accountable for safe, high-quality care. These same values and responsibilities are still made clear in professional standards and supported by ethical principles. The principle of nonmaleficence requires that we do no harm. Therefore, leaders must ensure a safe culture, and the principle of beneficence requires that leaders constantly find ways to do better. As professionals, nurses are prepared to be evidence-informed in their practice and to focus on the best practices designed to ensure the best quality care. The principles and methods associated with quality are grounded in systems theory and statistics, but the need for quality and constant improvement is rooted in the philosophy and goals of nursing—indeed what motivates us to do what is the best for patients.

Dr. Donald Berwick, a pioneer in the area of quality improvement and patient safety, linked quality to ethics, asserting that quality care is ethical care. He described it as simply "the degree to which the results of the work you do match the needs you intend to meet" (Berwick, 2022). Dr. W. Edward Deming, an early architect of quality management and improvement, promoted the role of leaders in sustaining a constancy of purpose toward continuous improvement. Rather than focus on inspection, he advocated for *leadership for change,* encouraging leaders to give more attention to team collaboration and self-improvement based on education and just-in-time learning. Recognizing that health care is constantly improving, he promoted a culture where transformation is everyone's job, where improvement and innovation is rewarded and

acknowledged, and where people take pride in the work they do (de Jonge et al., 2011).

Beyond the ethical imperative, there are many reasons why leaders and organizations must focus on quality and patient safety and develop and maintain quality programs. This requirement is embedded in the professional standards of regulatory colleges across the country. Part I of the CNA *Code of Ethics for Registered Nurses* (2017), "Nursing Values and Ethical Responsibilities," makes it clear that quality and safety are grounded in the values, principles, and theories that guide nursing as a profession. Nurses are expected to be critical thinkers and identify evidence-informed solutions to ensure safe, compassionate, and competent care. In some provinces, this is required by legislation. For example, the *Excellent Care for All Act*, introduced in Ontario in 2010, mandates continuous quality improvement and requires specific health care organizations to submit an annual quality improvement plan (QIP).

Were there none who were discontented with what they have, the world would never reach anything better.

~ FLORENCE NIGHTINGALE

A Culture of Patient Safety

As discussed in Chapter 10, errors in health care are most often the result of system problems rather than individual acts. Yet, historically, the tendency has been to blame individuals for errors and adverse events. When error is not acknowledged, there is a missed opportunity to learn, to improve patient safety, and to prevent this from happening again. There is also the risk of moral distress and residue when staff are not supported through this process. There is a growing focus on changing the systems and processes that contribute to or influence the occurrence of error or adverse events.

As mentioned previously, leadership is one of the most important factors in ensuring a culture of safety and transparency. Examples of such strategies include *safety huddles.* These are brief daily meetings that focus on patient safety and provide an opportunity for the team to discuss existing or anticipated concerns and plan for their prevention or resolution. The evidence suggests that critical to their success is the role of leaders as models and mentors (Di Vincenzo, 2017;

Fencl & Willoughby, 2019; Melton et al., 2017; Pimentel et al., 2021).

To create a culture that ensures patient safety, leaders must demonstrate a commitment to creating a culture in which adverse events or mistakes are openly reported and communicated, people are made accountable, and people are recognized for providing an opportunity for learning and ensuring the mistake does not happen again. Often, a series of events or missteps precedes errors, so, today, there is a greater focus on system issues rather than on individual blame, and recognition that failed processes may contribute to errors.

The culture is evolving into one in which health care professionals are obliged to disclose any errors or near-misses that may have occurred, without fear of criticism or discipline. A system-oriented focus evaluates the structures or processes that might have led to mistakes, rather than instantly attributing blame to an individual. A well-known example relates to dangerous drugs, such as narcotics, of various strengths in similar packaging. Many improvements have been made over the years, but as an illustration, consider the true story, presented in Case Scenario 12.10, of a nurse working in a post anaesthesia care unit (PACU). This incident occurred before such system factors were recognized.

At that time, if the wrong medication had been given, L. K. would have been blamed for this error, resulting in potentially serious career consequences. The emotional distress if harm or death had resulted would be immeasurable. Today, there would be a review of the systems and processes that led to the wrong drug being placed in the container and prevention strategies would be put in place. The Institute for Safe Medication Practices Canada (ISMP Canada) would be informed, and it would send out an alert to other hospitals and pharmaceutical companies to implement prevention strategies. Drug companies have improved their labelling, pharmacy assistants double-check when they are replenishing stock, high-risk drugs are not kept in proximity to each other, and computerized dispensing systems are in place.

In most organizations, a "just culture" ensures that nurses are not afraid to report errors. The "just culture" encourages open reporting of errors and participation in instituting prevention and improvement strategies. It recognizes that errors are often system related and that it is important to understand the root of the problem so that changes to designs and processes can be made. It promotes a culture of accountability wherein individuals are held responsible for their actions within the context of the system in which they occurred. That accountability may include involvement in the improvement strategy, coaching, education, counselling, or corrective action. In Case Scenario 12.10, L. K. was likely at risk of moral distress given such a near miss, so leaders should recognize these risks and take supportive and preventative action.

Corrective action may be warranted in a situation where there used to be total disregard for standards and policies and where attempts were made to cover up an incident or there was dishonesty.

CASE SCENARIO 12.10

ATTENTION PAID

L. K. was working an evening shift in a busy recovery room. A patient had just arrived from the operating room after a fairly minor surgical procedure. While assessing the patient, L. K. noted a low blood pressure and an irregular heart rhythm. L. K. immediately connected the patient to the heart monitor and called the anaesthetist. The patient was having frequent premature beats, so the anaesthetist ordered a bolus of lidocaine, a drug frequently used to treat such arrhythmias. L. K. went to the medication cupboard and took an ampule from the box labelled "Lidocaine." Because the situation was urgent, L. K. started to draw up the medication while also checking the label and was shocked to read that the ampule did not contain lidocaine but pancuronium (Pavulon), a paralyzing agent used to facilitate the intubation of patients. Had L. K. not noticed this, there would have been serious complications for this patient, including a possible cardiac arrest. The lidocaine ampule and the Pavulon ampule looked the same. Both ampules held 5 cc of the medication, were made of clear glass, and had similar blue lettering. Clearly, someone had placed the wrong medication in the container.

PATIENT- AND FAMILY-CENTRED CARE

Organizations and leaders play a significant role in establishing appropriate models of practice to ensure the delivery of not only the best care but also the most ethical care. One such model and philosophy is that of patient/person- and family-centred care, which recognizes the voice of the patient and that the family is essential to the well-being of the patient. It has been demonstrated that patients have better outcomes and cope better when they are supported by their families, as defined by them, especially during the difficult experiences of illness or injury (Ecenrod & Zwelling, 2000; Shelton, 1999; Van Riper, 2001).

Patient- and family-centred care is an approach to the planning, delivery, and evaluation of health care that ensures collaboration among health care providers, patients, and families with the goal of achieving better health care outcomes and enhanced satisfaction. Patients and their families are recognized for their expertise and for the experiences they have shared within the health care system (Nicholas et al., 2014).

Patient- and family-centred care applies to patients of all ages and should be practised in all health care settings (Shelton et al., 1987). In pediatrics, it is "a way of caring for children and their families within health services which ensures that care is planned around the whole family, not just the individual child/person, and in which all the family members are recognized as care recipients" (Shields et al., 2007, p. 1318).

It has not been that long since families—even the parents of hospitalized children—were restricted or limited in visiting inpatients. There were concerns regarding infection control, as well as worry that visiting family members would cause the patient distress when they had to leave. This was the case even in children's hospitals; in some settings, parents were permitted to only visit for a 2-hour period on Sunday afternoons. When they left, they invariably left their children crying. This practice did not change until the 1950s. Consider the following quotes from a focus group of nurses who graduated from the Hospital for Sick Children between the late 1930s and the early 1970s. The discussion can be viewed in the film, *Beyond the Dream: A Legacy of Nursing at SickKids* (The Hospital for Sick Children, 2006).

"The thing that's most interesting to me, having nursed for as long as I have, was how little attention was given to the family, really, what this experience meant in having a very ill child. It seemed to me that the children became ours— the institutions. And that was very slow to evolve, I think, to recognize the importance of the family as being central to the child's experience."

"Parents were thought to be a nuisance. . . . They certainly weren't encouraged to participate in any way."

"There were stories and descriptions of parents standing outside having to look in on children. The parents weren't allowed in the public wards except for 2 hours on Sunday, 2–4. And they barricaded the ward. If the parents brought in candy or food, it was taken from them. And then after they left, you could hear those children all the way to Bloor Street. Sunday night was bedlam."

"The physicians wanted to minimize the death rate so the children were not to get any infections. And so there were no visitors."

"My superior at Sick Children's was the assistant director of surgical nursing, (she) was the one who decided that . . . based on some research coming from England—it came out in the '50s actually, but it had to do with separation anxiety. And they realized that, in fact, children did need their parents with them, and it was an important facet to their cure and well-being."

[Note: The person quoted above may have been referring to findings from the Platt report from the Tavistock Clinic in the U.K. (Shields et al., 2007).]

"And (our approach) was so much ingrained in my lifestyle that I didn't know whether we could do this or not. . . . However, we did it. I agreed to it . . . and, of course, then we had to get permission from other powers that be, and so it was opened up for visiting."

"One of the things we started doing was liberalizing the visiting hours and, in fact, going the extra mile to establish what we call family-centred care, which involved the parents in the actual care of the children." (The Hospital for Sick Children, 2006)

In contrast, in today's children's hospitals, parents are considered active participants in their children's care and are integral members of the health care team (Ward, 2005). The Platt report recommended changes based on the emotional needs of the children, including unrestricted visiting, parents staying with their child, and the education of medical and nursing staff about the emotional needs of the children (Shields et al., 2007). Today, parents and the team collaborate to make the most appropriate decisions regarding a child's care. With the parents' knowledge of their child, combined with the professional expertise of the health care team, it is hoped that the best interests of the child and the family are served. Partnership-in-care models evolved over time, and now parents are considered the primary caregivers, with nurses playing a supporting role (Jolley & Shields, 2009). Although there are many benefits to this approach, nurses have a role in supporting the family/parents to ensure they have personal space, the time to reenergize, and the resources and education necessary to be effective in this role.

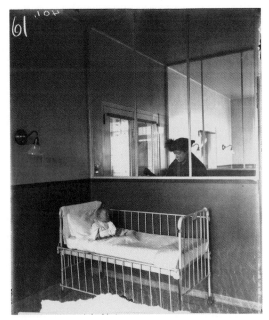

It hasn't been that long since families—even the parents of hospitalized children—were restricted from or limited in visiting. There were concerns regarding infection control, as well as worry that visiting family members would cause the patient distress when they had to leave. *Source: Hospital Archives, The Hospital for Sick Children, Toronto.*

Qualitative studies in neonatal intensive care unit (NICU) settings have reported findings that support the need for well-established family-centred structures and processes:

- Most parents want to be fully informed and involved in ethical decisions.
- Parents want even more involvement and participation in the care of their child.
- Some caregivers question whether parents are capable of making competent decisions in these stressful circumstances.
- Many parents did not believe they had received all the necessary information about their infant and had difficulty interpreting the information they did receive.
- Parents indicated that when they believe they are getting complete information about their infant, they are more likely to trust the caregivers.
- Patient units with less restrictive visiting reported greater parental involvement in decision making.
- The timing of discussions with parents and effective communication are significant factors in ensuring a better experience for the parents (Ward, 2005).

The Institute for Patient and Family-Centered Care has outlined the following elements that, together, ensure family-centred care (Shelton et al., 1987):

- Recognize the family as a constant in the child's life.
- Facilitate parent–professional collaboration at all levels of health care.
- Honour the racial, ethnic, cultural, and socio-economic diversities of families.
- Recognize family strengths and individuality, and respect different methods of coping.
- Share complete and unbiased information with families on a continuous basis.
- Encourage and facilitate family-to-family support and networking.
- Respond to child and family developmental needs as part of health care practices.
- Adopt policies and practices that provide families with emotional and financial support.
- Design health care that is flexible, culturally competent, and responsive to family needs.

Even though the previous discussion focuses on the roles of parents with respect to their children, these same principles apply to the relationships patients of all ages have with family members. Today, there are many views about who represents a person's "family." Families may be divorced, blended, adoptive, single-parent, or members of the 2SLGBTQI+ community. When the patient is a competent adult, the definition of their family should be made by that person. For example, although one is legally related to parents or siblings, some patients may identify their closest friends as their family and want their presence. Also, competent patients may designate a substitute decision maker, who might not be a relative.

Patients rarely live in isolation but are enmeshed in familial and other relationships and communities that influence their perspectives and provide them with comfort and reassurance. Family members share deep, personal connections and commitments and are mutually entitled to receive, and obligated to provide, support and care (Ward, 2005). They bring insights, share preferences regarding the best way to provide care, and, when listened to, contribute to assessing the needs and status of their family member. Consider the story in Case Scenario 12.11.

CASE SCENARIO 12.11

A DAUGHTER'S INTUITION

A daughter had been present with her mother throughout many hospital admissions over a 3-year period. After many investigations, it was discovered that her mother had a rare form of esophageal cancer, caused by exposure to metal fluids used in ammunition factories during the war. One afternoon, while her mother was sleeping, the daughter sensed that something was not quite right. It had something to do with her mother's breathing. Something seemed off. She went to the nursing station and asked one of the medical residents to come and assess her. The resident found her mother's heart rate, respiratory rate, and oxygen saturation to be normal. The daughter should have been reassured, but she was not. As her anxiety increased, she knew something was wrong. A short time later, her mother experienced acute pulmonary edema.

It is the right of patients to identify who, to them, is family, and the extent to which they want them involved in their care. Families may also be under stress and in crisis when dealing with the illness of a family member, and yet their needs may not always be identified by the health care team. The expertise of families with respect to their unique knowledge of the patient may not always be recognized. Indeed, each family is unique. Families cope in unique ways; for example, some may be information seekers, whereas others may not be. Some may express their emotions, whereas others may be stoic and reserved. Some families may challenge the authority of the team, and others may perceive that the team knows best and is "watching over them."

Sometimes, teams measure families against each other, and this may result in the labelling of some families as "difficult." Families become "difficult" when their needs are not being met, when there is a lack of trust, and when they are seriously worried about the care their family members are receiving. Nursing knowledge regarding family theory and an understanding and respect for family dynamics is important in these contexts (Shields et al., 2006). Being sensitive to a family's culture, beliefs, and values is also critical when partnering with patients and families from diverse backgrounds. A model of family-centred care that respects the family's knowledge and expertise, that recognizes them as both as recipients of care and as partners in care, enhances the therapeutic relationship and ultimately results in better care.

Roles That Family Members Can Play

Some family members play integral roles in care delivery. In many families, key individuals emerge as primary caregivers and, in this role, provide crucial and diverse care functions. They may participate in care delivery, simply be present, or be involved in planning and coordinating care. Yet, health care professionals may not fully appreciate the costs borne by these individuals or their families in providing this increased level of patient care. For instance, family caregivers might need to leave their jobs, which may cause precarious financial situations and increased stress. If families lack flexible workplace accommodations, substantial hardship may result. For nurses and other interprofessional team members, supporting the family caregiver and helping family members understand the role they can play in the context of the team may help them feel more comfortable as team members and, possibly, more able to articulate patient and family needs and challenges.

Most health care is delivered in the home by family members. A study of terminally ill patients found that family members, mainly women, provide the bulk of care for dying patients, with little help from paid caregivers or volunteers (Emanuel et al., 1999).

Clearly, families can play a variety of roles in supporting patients. They play an important role as advocates by ensuring that the best interests of the patient and the family members are identified and served. This is especially important when patients' capacity is compromised as a result of illness or hospitalization. Patient safety is enhanced when family members effectively assist in caregiving and ongoing monitoring of care (Burns, 2008; Canadian Patient Safety Institute, 2007; Fleming-Carroll et al., 2006; Stevens et al., 2005). In many settings, especially in the home, family caregivers may provide direct care. Whether this care is being provided by family caregivers or alternative care providers, such as trusted companions or substitute decision makers (Levine & Zuckerman, 1999), it is for nurses to not only know who is providing care but also consider ways to provide support and guidance.

Strategies for Involving Families

Tensions may be created with respect to the role of the family and their relationship with the team. Through an ethic of accommodation, health care professionals can better meet the needs of families by gaining greater knowledge and understanding of the family's needs and dynamics during times of crisis. Through negotiation and accommodation, the team can establish partnerships with families and keep avenues of communication and dialogue open. Learning what is important to families, recognizing the various roles that family members play, and sharing with family members are important means of supporting them through crisis and uncertainty (Levine & Zuckerman, 1999, 2000).

Negotiation and Roles

The delivery of patient and family-centred care requires a "process of negotiation between health professionals and the family, which results in shared decision-making" (Corlett & Twycross, 2006, p. 1308). An extensive review of the literature revealed three themes related to negotiation, familial expectations of participation in care, and power and control.

The literature emphasizes the importance of openness and communication regarding mutual understanding of expectations and roles. Although many family members want to participate in care, they differ in the level and extent of their participation. For example, parents who care for a child at home may want some respite; when a child's treatment is new, they may or may not want to participate in interventions usually provided by nurses. In the hospital setting, some parents feel they are losing their parental role and are reluctant to hand that role over to others. Some parents perceive nurses (whether the nurses are conscious of this or not) as the "gatekeepers" who determine the extent of parental involvement. They worry about who has control over their child.

The many nuances around family/caregiver inclusion and accommodation in health care provision are complex and multifaceted and call for careful and critical review of the practice of nurses.

Why Is Family-Centred Care Important?

Within the model of family-centred care, patients have a choice regarding the family's access. In keeping with this philosophy, the right thing to do as a nurse is to partner with patients and families. The health care environment is extremely complex and involves complicated technology; the family's ability to navigate this system is an essential component of keeping patients safe. Key points to consider when advocating for and inviting family involvement are as follows:

- They know the patient very well and can identify even the most subtle signs of discomfort, pain, or change in condition, and alert the team to that (as in the earlier story).
- They may have knowledge of the patient's history, which can be of assistance to the health care team. For example, in the hospital setting, a family member might be able to alert the team to a complication that may have arisen during a previous hospitalization, a reaction to a medication, or treatments that were effective or ineffective.

- When present with the patient most of the time, they can contribute to shift-to-shift reports and to team conferences regarding the patient's progress. Furthermore, parents and other family members can assist nurses and other health care professionals in monitoring patients and their response to treatment.
- When the patient is a child, or a vulnerable adult in long-term care who is unable to monitor their own care or respond to a treatment plan, a parent or essential family member can assume this role and alert the team when there is a risk of wrong medication or treatment being given.
- The health care team can collaborate with families and patients to ensure there is a clear understanding of discharge plans and other transitions (Johnson et al., 1992).

This approach to care ensures a shift in the power balance from the team to the patient and the family. Responsibilities are shared, resulting in positive benefits for all concerned. As the patient and the family become members of the team, there are many benefits related to patient safety, timely sharing of information, improved communication satisfaction, and quality of life (Bamm & Rosenbaum, 2008). The investment results in greater efficiency and cost-effectiveness (MacKean et al., 2005). Patient- and family-care should not be about shifting responsibility to save money, though the achievement of better outcomes and safe care is cost-effective. Frequently, more nursing resources are invested to provide support, educate, and address the complexities of diversity and family dynamics. Nurses collaborating with families are still accountable for safe practice.

Feelings of frustration and anger arose among patients and their families during the SARS epidemic and the COVID-19 pandemic as patients were isolated from their family members (Johnston et al., 2022). During SARS, psychological as well as physical effects emerged in patients when family visits and presence in the hospital are withdrawn (Maunder et al., 2003). A positive response to the challenges associated with family presence during COVID-19 was the design of innovative strategies for family-centred care, in long-term care settings that will hopefully make a difference in the future (Gallant et al., 2022; Hsu et al., 2022). The conseuences of the pandemic in these settings re-enforced the value of the presence of an essential family member.

Opportunities to Advance Family-Centred Care

Mounting evidence invites us to consider ways that leaders can ensure family presence and, conversely, challenge and change traditional practices.

Consider the practice of family members being kept out of the patient's room during emergency or resuscitation procedures, even though many studies have pointed to the benefits of their presence (Tsai, 2002). This is a challenging ethical area that is the focus of continued debate among health care professionals, and the notion is garnering variable support (Sacchetti et al., 2003). The ethical conflict is between the wishes of the family to be present and health care professionals' concern that the family might find the experience disturbing (Nibert, 2005). Although it may not always be possible and some families may choose not to be present, there are documented positive benefits of family presence. Surviving patients have reported feeling comfort and support from the presence of family members, and in cases of the patient's death, family members have reported that their presence at the death helped in the bereavement process.

Studies have suggested that up to 80% of family members would like to have been offered the opportunity to be present during resuscitation, but only 11% were given the opportunity. Families present during emergency and resuscitative procedures reported that they found it helpful to be present. Most families want to be present if there is a chance that their loved one may die. It makes sense that they would want the opportunity to say goodbye while the patient is still alive and that they would want to be present to ensure that all possible efforts are made to save their loved one (Back, 1991).

In advocating for family presence in these care situations, leaders may face a substantial challenge in responding to the attitudes of physicians and nurses (Osuagwu, 1991). These professionals express concern that the family might interfere, detracting from their focus on saving the person's life and causing stress for the team and the family. Although the experience of team stress is not uncommon during emergency situations, this can be balanced by the satisfaction that the patient and family have been helped by having their relational and support needs met.

Some institutions have introduced progressive programs to facilitate family presence in these circumstances. These programs offer an assessment process, education for the team and families, and support for the family during the emergency. This offers families greater opportunity for closure and a chance to say goodbye in the event of death (Nibert, 2005).

Barriers to overcome related to ensuring family presence include concerns about the potential negative impacts on patient care, negative psychological impacts on family members, the possibility of family interference in care, and an increase in staff stress that will influence performance (O'Connell et al., 2007). Studies have suggested that family presence does not interfere but can offer great comfort to both the patient and the family (Nibert, 2005). In a study of 197 family members present during emergencies, no incidents of family interference were identified. Accordingly, nurses have advocated for family presence (Nibert, 2005).

At this point, it might be worthwhile to reflect once more on "My Story" shared in Chapter 2.

As leaders seek to build patient- and family-centred care into the fabric and culture of their organization, they also have a role in establishing the structures and processes for enabling this philosophy and approach. Examples of structural strategies include creating space for families within patients' rooms and in nearby locations. These might include investment in lounging chairs in rooms so that family members might sleep over, laundry facilities, and lounges dedicated to family use. Ronald McDonald House Charities Canada has created "family rooms" in many settings across the country to support families from out of town (Ronald McDonald House Charities Canada, 2018). When staff members observe and benefit from these investments, they are more likely to embrace their own roles and responsibilities. It is also important that leaders engage patients and families to receive their input and encourage their contribution to the decision-making process. Engagement is facilitated through surveys, focus groups, organizational and program-specific councils, or advisory groups. In some settings, the family/patient representatives are included on committees and even on boards to ensure that their voices are heard.

Ethical Considerations

Ethical theories and principles support patient- and family-centred care. Utilitarians would consider the positive outcomes associated with this model, including patient safety, cost-effectiveness, the healing

power of family presence and support, and so on. Deontologists would consider this model as treating all persons involved as ends not means. They would consider this approach as one that values and respects persons and that acknowledges the duty of health care professions to do what is right and virtuous. Ethical principles, such as beneficence, nonmaleficence, autonomy, and justice, would endorse such a model. Feminist perspectives may vary. They would want the resources to be put in place to support the female family members but would not accept that women be the only participants in care. They would want systems to be put in place to protect the employment of both men and women caring for family members.

Conclusion

At the crux of patient- and family-centred care is the belief that the family (as defined by the patient) is essential to the management of illness or injury and is a cornerstone of a thoughtful, philosophical approach to care. Patients cope better when supported by the presence of those they love. The health care environment is extremely complex and involves high technology, and the role of families in navigating the system is an essential component of keeping patients safe. It calls for attention to and innovation in altering processes for partnerships in care; fosters decision making that ensures the best interests of patients and families; and emphasizes the moral responsibility of team members to facilitate family-centred care in an interprofessional health care environment.

SUMMARY

In any organization, how business is conducted matters, and this is especially true in health care. In the health care sector, there is the added dimension of having responsibility for a vulnerable population and aiming to provide the best care possible. The continuum of patient care is influenced by organizational and clinical systems and processes that must meet the same ethical standards as does practice.

In this chapter, organizational ethics and leadership ethics were explored as vital to ensuring the engagement of staff through the development of trusting relationships, collaboration, transparency, the provision of opportunities for professional advancement, ensuring appropriate resources, and the maintenance of a consistent approach to addressing ethical challenges. Leaders also contribute to positive patient and family outcomes by ensuring that important processes and structures are in place to address the many challenges in health care today.

Canada is culturally diverse; health care is changing; and technology is expanding and influencing the globalization of health care. These factors, in turn, influence the nature of health care and the need for and availability of nurses now and into the future. Nursing leaders must implement a nursing human resources plan that fosters a healthy and ethical work environment and sustains high-quality patient care.

In a country as diverse as Canada, it is impossible for nurses to be knowledgeable about all cultures. However, to provide culturally safe nursing care, assessments should include the exploration of a patient's or family's culture, values, and what is meaningful regarding care and the involvement of family.

There are positive outcomes for patients when health care professionals work and learn together, and this is especially true when interprofessional teams face complex ethical issues and challenges. Collaboration and open discussion among team members are essential to ensuring that ethical issues are addressed. Interprofessional practice is strongly aligned to family-centred care, in which the right thing to do is to partner with patients and families. The health care environment is extremely complex and involves high technology; the role of the family in navigating this system is an essential component of keeping patients safe. Ethical leaders and ethical organizations ensure all of these processes are in place and, in doing so, ensure a positive, healthy, and ethical culture.

CRITICAL THINKING

The following case scenarios are provided to facilitate reflection, discussion, and analysis.

Discussion Points

1. This chapter discussed leadership, diversity, interprofessional practice, and patient- and family-centred care. How are they related to one another? Are they integrated? Can excellence in any of these domains be achieved to the exclusion of another?
2. Consider the clinical environments within which you have had experience and evaluate them from the perspective of leadership, human resource planning, approaches to diversity, patient-centred care, and interprofessional practice.
3. What strategies should be implemented in the clinical environment to advance leadership, approaches to diversity, patient-centred care, and interprofessional practice?
4. Consider a leader whom you value and look up to, and reflect on why.
5. Do you see yourself as different from others? In what ways are you different? In what ways are you the same?

CASE SCENARIO 12.12

STAY WITH ME

A 80-year-old patient has just been transferred via ambulance to the emergency department. The patient is extremely short of breath and is experiencing some chest pain. The patient is accompanied by and adult child who proceeds to follow their parent but is stopped by the receptionist, who tells them to stay in the waiting room until called. The patient is upset about this, but they are told that the physician must complete the assessment first. The patient starts to cry. The adult child says they have information to share with the team and is told they will interview them later.

Questions

1. Do you have concerns about this scenario?
2. How can the emergency department become more family centred?
3. Are there patient safety issues here?
4. Do you think patient's emotional stress will influence the outcome?
5. If the patient is admitted, how might this experience influence the role the adult child with the health care team?

CASE SCENARIO 12.13

WHO IS MOST COMPETENT?

L. M. is a 16-year-old with cerebral palsy. All their life, they have been cared for at home by their parents with the support of community agencies. L. M. is not ambulatory, needs assistance with feeding, and has trouble being understood by anyone other than their parents.

L. M. has had some trouble recently with a chest infection and has been admitted to the local hospital for pneumonia. The hospital has relatively open visiting hours, but family members are not allowed to stay during the night unless the patient is in palliative care.

L. M.'s parents are very worried about leaving L. M. alone, especially because L. M. may not be able to communicate effectively with the nurses during the night. They are also concerned that they are not permitted to assist with L. M.'s care and are asked to leave the room when care is provided. When they ask whether they might hire one of the community nurses to remain with L. M. during the night, they are told that it is against hospital policy to have non-hospital-employed nurses providing care.

Questions

1. Is L. M. at risk in this situation? If so, what are those risks?
2. What might the leaders in this organization do to change practice?

REFERENCES

Statutes

Excellent Care for All Act, 2010, S.O. 2010, c. 14.
United Nations Declaration on the Rights of Indigenous Peoples Act, 2021, S.C. 2021, c. 14.

Case Law

R. v. Kapp [2008] SCC 41 (CanLII).

Texts and Articles

Allan, H. T., & Westwood, S. (2016). English language skills requirements for internationally educated nurses working in the care industry: Barriers to UK registration or institutionalised discrimination? *International Journal of Nursing Studies, 54*, 1–4.

Andrews, M. M., & Boyle, J. S. (2002). Transcultural concepts in nursing care. *Journal of Transcultural Nursing, 13*(3), 178–180.

Arnold, O. F., & Bruce, A. (2006). Nursing practice with Aboriginal communities: Expanding worldviews. *Nursing Science Quarterly, 18*(3), 259–263.

Back, K. J. (1991). Sudden, unexpected pediatric death: Caring for the parents. *Pediatric Nursing, 17*(6), 571–575.

Baharum, H., Ismail, A., McKenna, L., et al. (2022). *Success Factors of adaptation of newly graduated nurses: A scoping review*. Research Square. Submitted for publication.

Baharum H, Ismail A, McKenna L, Mohamed Z, Ibrahim R, Hassan NH. *Success factors in adaptation of newly graduated nurses: a scoping review*. BMC Nurs. 2023 Apr 18;22(1):125. doi: 10.1186/s12912-023-01300-1. PMID: 37069647; PMCID: PMC10111715.

Bamm, E. L., & Rosenbaum, P. (2008). Family-centered theory: Origins, development, barriers, and supports to implementation in rehabilitation medicine. *Archives of Physical Medicine and Rehabilitation, 89*, 1618–1624.

Barker, K. K., Bosco, C., & Oandasan, I. F. (2005). Factors in implementing interprofessional education and collaborative practice initiatives: Findings from key informant interviews. *Journal of Interprofessional Care, 19*(Suppl. I), 166–176.

Barker, K. K., & Oandasan, I. (2005). Interprofessional care review with medical residents: Lessons learned, tensions aired—A pilot study. *Journal of Interprofessional Care, 19*(3), 207–214.

Baumann, A. (2005). *Nursing resource teams can recruit and retain nurses: New strategy could create full-time jobs in nursing*. https://fhs.mcmaster.ca/main/news/news_archives/nursingteams.htm

Baumann, A., Blythe, J., Kolotylo, C., et al. (2005). The international nursing labour market report. In Fuse Communications and Public Affairs Inc., (Ed.), *Building the future: An integrated strategy for nursing human resources in Canada*. The Nursing Sector Study Corporation.

Baumann, A., Crea-Arsenio, M., Akhtar-Danesh, N., et al. (2016). Strategic workforce planning for health human resources: A nursing case analysis. *Canadian Journal of Nursing Research, 48*(3-3), 93–99.

Baumann, A., Crea-Arsenio, M., Hunsberger, M., et al. (2019). Work readiness, transition, and integration: The challenge of specialty practice. *Journal of Advanced Nursing, 75*(4), 823–833. https://doi.org/10.1111/jan.13918

Baumann, A., Hunsberger, M., Crea-Arsenio, M., et al. (2018). Policy to practice: Investment in transitioning new graduate nurses to the workplace. *Journal of Nursing Management, 26*(4), 373–381.

Baumann, A., Keatings, M., Holmes, G., et al. (2006). *Better data, better decisions: A profile of the nursing workforce at Hamilton health sciences, 2002-2003*. Nursing Health Services Research Unit: Human Resources Series Number, 4. https://fhs.mcmaster.ca/nhsru/documents/SeriesReport4BetterDataBetterDecisions-AProfileoftheNursingWorkforce.pdf

Baumann, A., Yan, J., Degelder, J., et al. (2006). *Retention strategies for nursing: A profile of four countries*. Nursing Health Services

Research Unit: Human Resources Series Number, 5. https://www.fhs.mcmaster.ca/nhsru/documents/SeriesReport5RetentionStrategiesforNursingAProfileofFour Countries.pdf

Benner, P. (2000). *From novice to expert*. Pearson.

Berwick, D. (2022). *Quality mercy, and the moral determinants of health*. [Video]. YouTube. https://www.youtube.com/watch?v=GX7vjL6dIuM

Botes, A. (2000). An integrated approach to ethical decision-making in the health team. *Journal of Advanced Nursing, 32*(5), 1076–1082.

Boyer, Y. (2017). Healing racism in Canadian health care. *Canadian Medical Association Journal, 189*(46), E1408–E1409.

British Columbia Ministry of Health, & Ministry of Advanced Education. (2008). *B.C.'s nursing strategy*. https://archive.news.gov.bc.ca/releases/news_releases_2005-2009/2008HEALTH0058-000754-Attachment1.htm

Brodeur, D. (1998). Health care institutional ethics: Broader than clinical ethics. In J. F. Monagle & D. C. Thomasma (Eds.), *Health care ethics: Critical issues for the 21st century* (pp. 497–504). Aspen Publishers.

Brown, J. (2003). Women leaders: A catalyst for change. In R. Adlam & P. Villiers (Eds.), *Leadership in the twenty-first century: Philosophy, doctrine and developments* (pp. 174–187). Waterside Press.

Burns, K. K. (2008). Canadian patient safety champions: Collaborating on improving patient safety. *Healthcare Quarterly, 11*(Special Issue), 95–100.

Canadian Institute for Health Information. (2022). *Guidance on the use of standards for race-based and indigenous identity data collection and health reporting in Canada*.

Canadian Nurses Association. (2012). *Staff mix decision making framework for quality care*.

Canadian Nurses Association. (2017). *Code of ethics for registered nurses*.

Canadian Nurses Association. (2018). *Code of ethics for registered nurses and licensed practical nurses*.

Canadian Nurses Association. (2021a). *Nursing Declaration Against Anti-Black Racism in Nursing and Health Care*. https://hl-prod-ca-oc-download.s3-ca-central-1.amazonaws.com/CNA/2f975e7e-4a40-45ca-863c-5ebf0a138d5e/UploadedImages/documents/Nursing_Declaration_Anti-Black_Racism_November_8_2021_FINAL_ENG_Copy.pdf

Canadian Nurses Association. (2021b). *Nursing Declaration Against Anti-Indigenous Racism in Nursing and Health Care*. https://hl-prod-ca-oc-download.s3-ca-central-1.amazonaws.com/CNA/2f975e7e-4a40-45ca-863c-5ebf0a138d5e/UploadedImages/documents/Nursing_Declaration_Anti-Indigenous_Racism_November_8_2021_ENG_Copy.pdf

Canadian Nursing Advisory Committee. (2002). *Our health, our future: Creating quality workplaces for Canadian nurses*. Advisory Committee on Health Human Resources.

Canadian Patient Safety Institute. (2007). *Canadian Patient Safety Institute: Ask, talk, listen, be involved in your health care and safety*. http://www.patientsafetyinstitute.ca/uploadedFiles/Ask%20Talk%20Listen%20For%20Patients%20and%20Families.pdf

CARE Centre for Internationally Educated Nurses. (2019). *History of CARE Centre for IENs*. https://www.care4nurses.org/who-we-are/history-care/

Clegg, S., Kornberger, M., & Rhodes, C. (2007). Organizational ethics, decision making, undecidability. *Sociological Review, 55*(2), 393–409.

Corlett, J., & Twycross, A. (2006). Negotiation of parental roles within family-centred care: A review of the research. *Journal of Clinical Nursing, 15*(10), 1308–1316.

Cowan, M. J., Shapiro, M., Hays, R. D., et al. (2006). The effect of a multidisciplinary hospitalist/physician and advanced practice nurse collaboration on hospital costs. *Journal of Nursing Administration, 36*(2), 79–85.

Curran, V. (2004). Interprofessional education for collaborative patient-centred practice research synthesis paper. *Health Canada*. http://www.hc-sc.gc.ca/hcs-sss/hhr-rhs/strateg/interprof/synth-eng.php

Danda, M., Pitcher, C., & Key, J. (2022, May 24). Hearing our voices (part 2): Empowering nurses to take anti-racist action in health care: The time has come to stand together and change the system. *Canadian Nurse*. https://www.canadian-nurse.com/blogs/cn-content/2022/05/16/hearing-our-voices-part-1-facilitating-nurses-refl

Davis, C. (1988). Philosophical foundations of interdisciplinarity in caring for the elderly, or the willingness to change your mind. *Physiotherapy Practice, 4*, 23–25.

de Jonge, V., Sint Nicolaas, J., van Leerdamm, M. E., & et al. (2011). Overview of the quality assurance movement in health care. *Best Practice & Research Clinical Gastroenterology, 25*(3), 337–347.

Di Vincenzo, P. (2017). Team huddles: A winning strategy for safety. *Nursing, 47*(7), 59–60.

Dordunoo, D. (2021, April 12). Collecting race-based data is a good first step toward equity, but should not be the only one. *Canadian Nurse*. https://www.canadian-nurse.com/blogs/cn-content/2021/04/12/collecting-race-based-data-is-a-good-first-step-to

Durrant, M., Crooks, D., & Pietrolungo, L. (2009). A clinical extern program evaluation: Implications for nurse educators. *Journal for Nurses in Professional Development, 25*(6), E1–E8. https://doi.org/10.1097/NND.0b013e31819ad50d

Ecenrod, D., & Zwelling, E. (2000). A journey to family-centered maternity care. *American Journal of Maternal Child Nursing, 25*(4), 178–185.

Emanuel, E. J., Fairclough, D. L., Slutsman, J., et al. (1999). Assistance from family members, friends, paid care givers, and volunteers in the care of terminally ill patients. *New England Journal of Medicine, 341*(13), 956–963.

Fencl, J. L., & Willoughby, C. (2019). Daily organizational safety huddles: An important pause for situational awareness. *AORN Journal, 109*(1) 111–118.

Fleming-Carroll, B., Matlow, A., Dooley, S., et al. (2006). Patient safety in a pediatric centre: Partnering with families. *Healthcare Quarterly, 9*(Special Issue), 96–101.

Gallant, N. L., Hardy, M. S., Beogo, I., et al. (2022). Improving family presence in long-term care during the COVID-19 Pandemic. *Health Care Quarterly, 25*(Special Issue), 34–40.

Glowinski, B. J. (2022).The Canadian long-term care sector collapse from COVID-19: Innovations to support people in the workforce. *Healthcare Quarterly, 25*(Special Issue), 20–26.

Godshall, M. (2021). Coping with moral distress during COVID-19. *Nursing, 51*(2) 55–58.

Government of Ontario. (2022). *Data standards for the identification and monitoring of systemic racism.* https://www.ontario.ca/document/data-standards-identification-and-monitoring-systemic-racism/context

Griffith, H. (2001). So long home: Hello Canada. *Nursing BC, 33*(2), 16–19.

Grosenick, L. E. (1994). Governmental ethics and organizational culture. In T. L. Cooper (Ed.), *Handbook of administrative ethics* (pp. 183–197). Marcel Dekker.

Hall, L. M., Lalonge, M., Strudwick, G., et al. (2015). Not very welcoming: A survey of internationally educated nurses employed in Canada. *Journal of Nursing and Health Care, 2*(2). doi:10.5176/2010-4804_2.2.78

Hall, P. (2005). Interprofessional teamwork: Professional cultures as barriers. *Journal of Interprofessional Care, 19*(Suppl. 1), 188–196.

Haslam-Larmer, L., Grigorovich, A., Quirt, H., et al. (2023). Prevalence, causes, and consequences of moral distress in healthcare providers caring for people living with dementia in long-term care during a pandemic. *Dementia, 22*(1), 5–27.

Hasnain-Wynia, R., Weber, D. M., Yonek, J. C., et al. (2012). Community-level interventions to collect race/ethnicity and language data to reduce disparities. *American Journal of Managed Care, 18*(Suppl. 6), S141–S147.

Havaei, F., Dahinten, S., & MacPhee, M. (2019). Effect of nursing care delivery models on registered nurse outcomes. *SAGE: Open Nursing, 5*, 1–10.

Hewison, A., & Sim, J. (1998). Managing interprofessional working: Using codes of ethics as a foundation. *Journal of Interprofessional Care, 12*(3), 309–321.

The Hospital for Sick Children (Producer). (2006). *Beyond the dream: A legacy of nursing at SickKids* [Documentary DVD].

Hsu, A. T., Mukerji, G., Levy, A. M., et al. (2022). Pandemic preparedness and beyond: Person-centred care for older adults living in long-term care during the COVID-19 pandemic. *Health Care Quarterly, 25*(Special Issue), 13–19.

International Council of Nurses. (2001). *Position statement: Ethical nurse recruitment.* http://www.icn.ch/ psrecruit01.htm

International Council of Nurses. (2022). *ICN calls for stronger codes for ethical recruitment of nurses and investment in nursing education.* https://www.icn.ch/news/icn-calls-stronger-codes-ethical-recruitment-nurses-and-investment-nursing-education

International Council of Nurses, & World Health Organization. (2020). *State of the world's nursing.* https://apps.who.int/iris/bitstream/handle/10665/331673/9789240003293-eng.pdf

Irvine, R., Kerridge, I., & McPhee, J. (2004). Towards a dialogical ethics of interprofessionalism. *Journal of Postgraduate Medicine, 50*(4), 278–280.

Irvine, R., Kerridge, I., McPhee, J., et al. (2002). Interprofessionalism and ethics: Consensus or clash of cultures? *Journal of Interprofessional Care, 16*(3), 199–210.

Island Health. (2005). *New graduate transition.* http://www.viha.ca/professional_practice/new_grad.htm

Johnson, B. H., Seale Jeppson, E., & Redburn, L. (1992). *Caring for children and families: Guidelines for hospitals* (1st ed.). Association for the Care of Children's Health.

Jolley, J., & Shields, L. (2009). The evolution of family-centered care. *Journal of Paediatric Nursing, 24*(2), 164–170.

Karmali, K., Grobovsky, L., & Levy, J. (2011). Enhancing cultural competence for improved access to quality care. *Healthcare Quarterly, 14*(Special Issue 3), 52–57. https://doi.org/10.12927/hcq.2011.22578

Keatings, M. (2005, February 23). Values: Shaping organizational culture. In *Bioethics Seminar presented at the Joint Centre for Bioethics.* University of Toronto.

Keatings, M. (2006). Reframing policies for global nursing migration in North America—A Canadian perspective. *Policy Politics and Nursing Practice, 7*(Suppl. 3), 62S–65S. https://doi.org/10.12927/hcq.2011.22578

Kenny, G. (2002). The importance of nursing values in interprofessional collaboration. *British Journal of Nursing, 11*(1), 65–68.

Kingma, M. (2006). *Nurses on the move: Migration and the global health care economy.* Cornell University Press.

Kupperschmidt, B. R. (2004). Making a case for shared accountability. *Journal of Nursing Administration, 34*(3), 114–116.

Lalonde, M., & McGillis-Hall, L. (2017). The socialisation of new graduate nurses during a preceptorship programme: Strategies for recruitment and support. *Journal of Clinical Nursing, 26*(3), 774–783.

La Sala, C. A. (2009). Moral accountability and integrity in nursing practice. *Nursing Clinics of North America, 44*(4), 423–434.

Laschinger, H. K. S., Finegan, J., Shamian, J., et al. (2000). Organizational trust and empowerment in restructured health care settings: Effects on staff nurse commitment. *Journal of Nursing Administration, 30*(9), 413–425.

Laschinger, H. K. S., Shamian, J., & Thomson, D. (2001). Impact of magnet hospital characteristics on nurses' perceptions of trust, burnout, quality of care and work satisfaction. *Nursing Economics, 19*, 209–219.

Lessard, L., Morin, D., & Sylvain, H. (2008). Understanding teams and teamwork. *Canadian Nurse, 104*(3), 12–13.

Levine, C., & Zuckerman, C. (1999). The trouble with families: Toward an ethic of accommodation. *Annals of Internal Medicine, 130*(2), 148–152.

Levine, C., & Zuckerman, C. (2000). Hands on/hands off: Why health care professionals depend on families but keep them at arm's length. *Journal of Law Medicine & Ethics, 28*(1), 5–18.

Lingard, L., Vanstone, M., Durrant, M., et al. (2012). Conflicting messages: Examining the dynamics of leadership on interprofessional teams. *Academic Medicine, 87*(12), 1762–1767.

Lombardo, B., & Eyre, B. (2011). Compassion fatigue: A nurse's primer. *Online Journal of Issues in Nursing, 16*(1), 3.

Lozano, J. M. (2003). An approach to organizational ethics. *Ethical Perspectives, 10*(1), 46–65.

MacKean, G. L., Thurston, W. E., & Scott, C. M. (2005). Bridging the divide between families and health professionals' perspectives on family-centred care. *Health Expectations, 8*, 74–85.

Maunder, R., Hunter, J., Vincent, L., et al. (2003). The immediate psychological and occupational impact of the 2003 SARS outbreak in a teaching hospital. *Canadian Medical Association Journal, 168*(10), 1245–1251.

McGaffigan, P. (2019). *Why Florence Nightingale's improvement lessons still matter today.* Institute for Health Care Improvement. http://www.ihi.org/communities/blogs/why-florence-nightingales-improvement-lessons-still-matter-today

McGillis-Hall, L. M., & Donner, G. J. (1997). The changing role of hospital nurse managers: A literature review. *Canadian Journal of Nursing Administration, 10*(2), 114–139.

McGuire, M., & Murphy, S. (2005). The internationally educated nurse. *Canadian Nurse, 101*(1), 25–29.

McKenzie, K. (2020). *Race and ethnicity data collection during COVID-19 in Canada: If you are not counted you cannot count on the pandemic response.* Wellesley Institute. https://rsc-src.ca/en/race-and-ethnicity-data-collection-during-covid-19-in-canada-if-you-are-not-counted-you-cannot-count

Melton, L., Lengerich, A., Collins. M., et al. (2017). Evaluation of huddles: A multisite study. *Health Care Manager, 36*(3), 282–287.

Millar, P., & Owusu-Bempah, A. (2011). Whitewashing criminal justice in Canada: Preventing research through data suppression. *Canadian Journal of Law and Society, 26*(3), 653–661. doi:10.3138/cjls.26.3.653

Ministry of Health and Long-Term Care. (2017). *Ontario guidelines for participation in the nursing graduate guarantee.* MOHLTC: Nursing Policy and Innovation Branch.

Mojtehedzadeh, S. (April 21, 2020). Toronto public health to start collecting COVID-19 data on race in a bid to track health inequities: Some public health units will also start tracking cases by occupation, as critics blast "flabbergasting" provincial response to COVID-19 data collection. *Toronto Star.* https://www.thestar.com/news/gta/2020/04/21/toronto-public-health-to-start-collecting-covid-19-data-on-race-in-a-bid-to-track-health-inequities.html

Morath, J. M. (2006). Patient safety: A view from the top. *Pediatric Clinics, 53*(6), 1053–1065.

Moyce, S., Lash, R., & de Leon Siantz, M. (2016). Migration experiences of foreign educated nurses: A systematic review of the literature. *Journal of Transcultural Nursing, 27*(2), 181–188.

Mulligan, K., Rayner, J., & Nnorom, O. (April 20, 2020). Race-based health data urgently needed during the coronavirus pandemic. *The Conversation.* https://theconversation.com/race-based-health-data-urgently-needed-during-the-coronavirus-pandemic-136822

Nerenz, D. R. (2005). Health care organizations' use of race/ethnicity data to address quality disparities. *Health Affairs (Millwood), 24*(2), 409–416.

Ness, M. M., Saylor, J., DiFusco, L. A., et al. (2021). Leadership, professional quality of life and moral distress during COVID-19: A mixed-methods approach. *Journal of Nursing Management, 29*(8), 2412–2422.

Nibert, A. T. (2005). Teaching clinical ethics using a case study: Family presence during cardiopulmonary resuscitation. *Critical Care Nurse, 25*(1), 38–44.

Nicholas, D., Keilty, K., & Karmali, K. (2014). Paediatric patient-centred care: Evidence and evolution. In R. Zlotnik Shaul (Ed.), *Paediatric patient and family-centred care: Ethical and legal issues. International Library of Ethics, Law, and the New Medicine, vol 57.* Springer.

Nicholas, D., Fleming-Carroll, B., Durrant, M., et al. (2017). Examining pediatric care for newly immigrated families: Perspectives of health care providers. *Social Work in Health Care, 56*(5), 335–351.

Nicholas, D., Fleming-Carroll, B., & Keatings, M. (2010). Examining organizational context and a developmental framework in advancing interprofessional collaboration: A case study. *Journal of Interprofessional Care, 24*(3), 319–322.

O'Connell, K. J., Farah, M. M., Spandorfer, P., et al. (2007). Family presence during pediatric trauma team activation: An assessment of a structured program. *Pediatrics, 120*(3), 565–574.

Osuagwu, C. C. (1991). ED codes: Keep the family out. *Journal of Emergency Nursing, 17*(6), 363–364.

Oudshoorn, A. (2020, August 20). The unbearable whiteness of nursing. *Canadian Nurse.* https://www.canadian-nurse.com/blogs/cn-content/2020/08/20/the-unbearable-whiteness-of-nursing

Owusu-Bempah, A., & Millar, P. (2010). Research note: Revisiting the collection of "Justice Statistics by Race" in Canada. *Canadian Journal of Law and Society, 25*(1), 97–104.

Pape, B., Thiessen, P. S., Jakobsen, F., et al. (2013). Interprofessional collaboration may pay: Introducing a collaborative approach in an orthopaedic ward. *Journal of Interprofessional Care, 27*(6), 496–500.

Parsons, M. L., Clark, P., Marshal, M., et al. (2007). Team behavioral norms: A shared vision for a healthy patient care workplace. *Critical Care Nursing Quarterly, 30*(3), 213–218.

Piette, M., Ellis, J. L., St. Denis, P., et al. (2002). Integrating ethics and quality improvement: Practical implementation in the transitional/extended care setting. *Journal of Nursing Care Quality, 17*(1), 35–42.

Pimentel, C. B., Snow, A. L., Carnes. S. L., et al. (2021). Huddles and their effectiveness at the frontlines of clinical care: A scoping review. *Journal of General Internal Medicine, 36*(9), 2272–2283.

Prestia, A. S. (2020). The moral obligation of nurse leaders: COVID-19. *Nurse Leaders, 18*(4), 326–328.

Pung, L. X., Lee, A., & Lin, Y. L. (2017). Challenges faced by international nurses when migrating: An integrative literature review. *International Nursing Review, 64*, 146–165.

Racine, L. (2003, June). Implementing a postcolonial feminist perspective in nursing research related to non-Western populations. *Nursing Inquiry, 10*(2), 91–102.

Reeves, S., Lewin, S., Espin, S., et al. (2010). *Interprofessional teamwork for health and social care.* Wiley-Blackwell.

Registered Nurses' Association of Ontario. (2022). *Black Nurses Task Force report.* https://rnao.ca/in-focus/black-nurses-and-rnao#BNTF-report

Renz, D. O., & Eddy, W. B. (1996). Organizations, ethics, and health care: Building an ethics infrastructure for a new era. *Bioethics Forum, 12*(2), 29–39.

Ronald McDonald House Charities Canada. (2018). *Ronald McDonald family rooms.* https://www.rmhccanada.ca/what-we-do/family-rooms

Rush, K. L., Adamack, M., Gordon, J., et al. (2015). Orientation and transition programme component predictors of new graduate workplace integration. *Journal of Nursing Management, 23*(2), 143–155.

Sacchetti, A. D., Guzzetta, C. E., & Harris, R. H. (2003). Family presence during resuscitation attempts and invasive procedures:

Is there science behind the emotion? *Clinical Pediatric Emergency Medicine, 4*(4), 292–296.

Sashkin, M., & Williams, R. L. (1990, Spring). Does fairness make a difference? *Organizational Dynamics, 19*(2), 56–71.

Savage, A., Young, S., Titley, H., et al. (2022). This was my Crimean War: COVID-19 experiences of nursing home leaders. *Journal of the American Medical Directors Association, 23*(11), 1827–1832.

Seeger, M. W. (2001). Ethics and communication in organizational contexts: Moving from the fringe to the center. *American Communication Journal, 5*(1), 1827–1832.

Shelton, T. L. (1999). Family-centered care in pediatric practice: When and how? *Journal of Developmental and Behavioral Pediatrics, 20*(2), 117–119.

Shelton, T. L., Jeppson, E. S., & Johnson, B. H. (1987). *Family-centered care for children with special health care needs.* Association for the Care of Children's Health.

Shields, L., Pratt, J., Davis, L. M., et al. (2007). Family-centred care for children in hospital. *Cochrane Database of Systematic Reviews, 1,* CD004811.

Shields, L., Pratt, J., & Hunter, J. (2006). Family-centred care: A review of qualitative studies. *Journal of Clinical Nursing, 15*(10), 1317–1323.

Shockley-Zalabak, P., Ellis, K., & Winograd, G. (2000). Organizational trust: What it means, why it matters. *Organizations Development Journal, 18*(4), 35–48.

Sicotte, C., D'Amour, D., & Moreault, M. P. (2002). Interdisciplinary collaboration within Quebec community health care centres. [Evaluation Studies. Journal Article]. *Social Science & Medicine, 55*(6), 991–1003.

Statistics Canada. (2022a). *The Canadian census: A rich portrait of the country's religious and ethnocultural diversity.* https://www150.statcan.gc.ca/n1/daily-quotidien/221026/dq221026b-eng.htm

Statistics Canada. (2022b). *Language statistics.* https://www.statcan.gc.ca/en/subjects-start/languages

Statistics Canada. (2022c). *Statistics on Indigenous peoples.* https://www.statcan.gc.ca/en/subjects-start/indigenous_peoples

Stevens, P., Matlow, A., & Laxer, R. (2005). Building from the blueprint for patient safety at the Hospital for Sick Children. *Healthcare Quarterly, 8*(Special Issue), 132–139.

Storch, J., Rodney, P., Varcoe, C., et al. (2009). Leadership for Ethical Policy and Practice (LEPP): Participatory action project. *Nursing Leadership, 22*(3), 68–80.

Thompson, B. M., Schneider, V. F., Haidet, P., et al. (2007). Team-based learning at ten medical schools: Two years later. *Medical Education, 41*(3), 250–257.

Tomblin Murphy, G., Maaten, S., Smith, R., et al. (2005). Review of concurrent research on nursing labour market topics. In Fuse Communications and Public Affairs Inc., (Ed.), *Building the future: An integrated strategy for nursing human resources in Canada.* The Nursing Sector Study Corporation.

Tsai, E. (2002). Should family members be present during cardiopulmonary resuscitation? *New England Journal of Medicine, 346*(13), 1019–1021.

Turpel-Lafonte, M. (2020). *In plain sight: Addressing Indigenous-specific racism and discrimination in B.C. health care.* Queens Printer.

Tye, J. (2020). Florence Nightingale's lasting legacy for health care. *Nurse Leader, 18*(3), 220–226.

United Nations. (2007). *United Nations Declaration on the Rights of Indigenous Peoples.* https://www.un.org/development/desa/indigenouspeoples/wp-content/uploads/sites/19/2018/11/UNDRIP_E_web.pdf

United Nations. (2022). *International decade for people of African Descent: 2015–2024.* https://www.un.org/en/observances/decade-people-african-descent

Van Riper, M. (2001). Family-provider relationships and well-being in families with preterm infants in the NICU. *Heart & Lung, 30*(1), 74–84.

Verkerk, M. A., Lindemann, H., Maeckelberghe, E., et al. (2004). Enhancing reflection: An interpersonal exercise in ethics education. *Hasting Center Report, 34,* 31–38.

Walsh, M., Brabeck, M., & Howard, K. (1999). Interprofessional collaboration in children's services: Toward a theoretical framework. *Children's Services: Social Policy Research and Practice, 2*(4), 183–208.

Ward, F. R. (2005). Parents and professionals in the NICU: Communication within the context of ethical decision making—An integrative review. *Neonatal Network, 24*(3), 25–33.

Wellesley Institute/Ontario Health. (2021). *Tracking COVID-19 through race-based data.*

White, E. M., Wetle, T. E., Reddy, A., et al. (2021). Front-line nursing home staff experiences during the COVID-19 pandemic. *Journal of the American Medical Directors Association, 22*(1), 199–203.

Williams, L. L. (2006). The fair factor in matters of trust. *Nursing Administration Quarterly, 30*(1), 30–37.

Wong, C. A., & Cummings, P. G. (2007). The relationship between nursing leadership and patient outcomes: A systematic review. *Journal of Nursing Management, 15*(5), 508–521.

Wong, C., Elliott-Miller, P., Laschinger, H., et al. (2015). Examining the relationship between span of control and manager job and unit performance outcomes. *Journal of Nursing Management, 23*(2), 156–168. https://doi.org/10.1111/jonm.12107

Worthley, J. A. (1999). Compliance in the organizational ethics context. *Frontiers of Health Services Management, 16*(2), 41–44.

Yi, M., & Jezewski, M. A. (2000). Korean nurses' adjustment to hospitals in the United States of America. *Journal of Advanced Nursing, 32*(3), 721–729.

Zwarenstein, M., & Reeves, S. (2000). What's so great about collaboration? *British Medical Journal, 320,* 1022–1023.

GLOSSARY

Abortion: The interruption of a pregnancy either spontaneously or intentionally by means of medical intervention. (Ch. 4)

Action: A *lawsuit* or court proceeding in which an injured party asserts a claim for damages or some other relief against a another. (Ch. 4)

Actus reus: The physical element of a criminal offence that results in physical or other harm (e.g., in assault touching another person deliberately without consent or a lawful excuse). (Ch. 4)

Adjudicate: In law, the functions of a court or *administrative tribunal* in hearing evidence in a legal controversy between two or more parties, assessing the evidence, making findings of fact and credibility, and rendering a decision (e.g., a verdict of guilty or not guilty in a criminal trial, or a finding of liability and assessment of damages against a defendant in a civil trial). (Ch. 4)

Administrative tribunals: boards, agencies, councils, and commissions established under legal authority from the government and charged with administration of a particular area of law (e.g., professional misconduct property taxes, human rights complaints, energy rates, transport licences). These often operate like courts in that they decide claims, grant licences, and so on. (Ch. 4)

Advance directive: A document made and signed by a mentally competent adult, detailing specific medical treatments that are to be administered or withheld in the event that the maker later becomes incapable of expressing such wishes as a result of mental or physical illness (e.g., Alzheimer's disease, coma). (Ch. 6)

Appeal: A legal proceeding in which a superior *appellate court* is asked by one or more parties to the original proceedings to review those proceedings to determine whether the inferior court or administrative tribunal committed any errors of law, misconstrued the evidence before it, exceeded its powers, or otherwise acted contrary to law in adjudicating upon the matter. This is not a retrial but a review of the proceedings at trial or at the hearing. (Ch. 5)

Appellate court: A court that hears appeals or reviews decisions of lower or inferior courts. (Ch. 4)

Applied ethics: The application of particular *ethical theories* to actual problems or issues. (Ch. 2)

Assisted insemination: A form of *donor insemination*, typically used when the male partner's sperm count is low, in which sperm are extracted and concentrated before being artificially introduced into the recipient's uterus. (Ch. 9)

Assisted suicide: Any aid directed at terminating the life of persons who, because of severe physical limitations or illness, cannot carry out the act by themselves. (Chs. 4, 8)

Autonomy: An *ethical principle* founded on respect for persons that assumes that a capable and competent person is free to determine a self-chosen plan unless that plan interferes with the rights of others. (Ch. 2)

Bargaining agent: In labour relations, a *union* certified by statute and authorized to negotiate collectively on behalf of a group of employees. (Ch. 11)

Bargaining unit: In labour relations, a single group of employees who are members of a *union* and who are bound by the terms of a *collective agreement* (employment contract) negotiated by the union on their behalf with their employer. The members of a bargaining unit must have similar interests so that the union can properly represent them. A single employer might have several different bargaining units representing different types of employees. (Ch. 11)

Battery: Harmful or offensive and nonconsensual contact with the person or clothing of another. (Ch. 7)

Beneficence: A principle that obliges us to act in such a way as to produce some good or benefit for another. (Ch. 2)

Best Practice Guidelines (BPGs): These guidelines are a product of the Registered Nurses' Association of Ontario's *Nursing Best Practice Program,* which was launched in 1999. These documents, informed by a systemic review of the evidence, are developed by clinical experts with input from key stakeholders. They provide guidance (recommendations and tools) for nurses to ensure they meet the highest standards of evidence-informed clinical practice. (Ch. 3)

Bill: A draft or proposed law that is not yet passed and must be voted upon by Parliament or a legislature; usually introduced by the governing party, but any member of a legislative assembly may introduce a bill. (Ch. 4)

Biomedical ethics: A field of ethics that focuses on issues associated with science, medicine, and health care. (Ch. 2)

Burden of proof: The obligation on a party to litigation (i.e., a criminal or civil lawsuit) to prove a certain fact or facts to a judge or jury. (Ch. 4)

Canadian Charter of Rights and Freedoms: A portion of Canada's *Constitution Act* that sets out the fundamental rights and freedoms of all persons in Canada and limits the rights of the state to infringe upon these rights. Laws or governmental actions that violate these rights without proper justification are null and void. (Ch. 4)

Case law: The law as set forth in decided cases. This is called *jurisprudence* in civil law systems. (See also *Precedent.*) (Ch. 4)

Categorical imperative: In Kantian ethics, a supreme principle that must be followed by a law of morality. (Ch. 2)

Causation: In negligence law, a series of related successive events, each of which is dependent upon the previous one, that ultimately result in damage or injury to persons or property. (Ch. 7)

Certification: In labour relations law, the process whereby a particular *union* is legally recognized as the official representative for collective bargaining and labour relations purposes of a certain group of employees in a certain industry or workplace. (Ch. 11)

Civil code: A central written and formal source of *civil law* principles and rules used in the province of Quebec and in other countries with a Roman Law tradition. (Ch. 4)

Closed shop: In labour relations, a place of employment in which, as a condition of employment, a worker is required to belong to the *union* representing the employees. (Ch. 11)

Codify: To formally arrange legal rules and principles into a central written source of law known as a code. (Ch. 4)

Collective agreement: A written contract of employment between an employer and a unionized group of employees. It binds all employees, lasts for at least 1 year, and sets out conditions of employment (e.g., wages, hours of work, benefits, sick leave, pension, layoffs, termination, disciplinary action, arbitration of grievances). (Ch. 11)

Collective bargaining: In labour relations, the process by which a *union* (the *bargaining agent*) negotiates the conditions of employment of a group of non-managerial employees (the *bargaining unit*) with an employer or group of employers. (Ch. 11)

Common law: English system of law dating back to the eleventh century, based on unwritten principles derived from judicial *precedents*. (Ch. 4)

Compensatory justice: requires compensation or payment for harm that has been done to an individual or a group. Compensation is provided because of a breach of a duty (such as contract, negligence, malpractice) that has damaged the claimants.

Complainant: In professional disciplinary matters, a person who complains, through a formal disciplinary procedure, about the conduct of by a member of a self-governing profession (e.g., a physician, nurse, dentist, lawyer). (Ch. 5)

Conciliator: In labour relations, a person usually appointed by the minister of labour to intervene in a strike or other labour dispute in an attempt to work out a settlement agreeable to both sides, to narrow the issues under dispute, and to canvass possible solutions. (Ch. 11)

Consent: The permission given by a person to allow someone else to perform an act upon the person giving such permission. Consent can be explicit (expressed verbally or in writing) or implicit (implied by the circumstances or the conduct of the person giving it). (Chs. 6, 7)

Constitution: A written law that sets forth the fundamental rules and principles defining how a country is organized, how its laws are passed, and the extent of the power of its government and its courts. (Ch. 4)

Constitutional convention: In British, Canadian, and Commonwealth constitutional law, a practice that is not a part of the legal written *Constitution* yet is followed by tradition. For example, it is a convention that the King (or the Governor General, the King's representative in Canada) always follows and accepts the advice of his ministers and give royal assent to all legislation submitted to him (or the Governor General). Although the King can legally decline to give such assent, to do so would create a constitutional crisis and political impasse. (Ch. 4)

Contract: An oral or written agreement between two or more parties that creates legally binding, mutual obligations and rights. (Ch. 4)

Contributory negligence: A situation in which a *plaintiff* is held partly responsible for the damage or injury sustained because they are partly at fault. (Ch. 7)

Controlled act: In Ontario (under the *Regulated Health Professions Act, 1991*, S.O. 1991, c. 18, s. 27), a specific medical act or procedure that may be performed only by a person who is a member of a health care profession (e.g., a nurse, doctor, dentist) and who is authorized by a health care profession act (e.g., the *Nursing Act, 1991*, S.O. 1991, c. 32) to perform such an act. (See Chapter 5.) Also called *restricted act* in Manitoba. (Ch. 10)

Cooling-off period: In labour relations, the period between the breakdown in negotiations and the time in which unionized employees may legally commence a strike against the employer or after which the employer may legally lock out the employees. Its purpose is to attempt to settle tensions between labour and management and assist in the resumption of negotiations. (Ch. 11)

Coroner's inquest: An inquiry convened under the authority of a coroner to investigate the circumstances of a death under suspicious circumstances, as a result of wrongdoing, possible negligence, or accident (i.e., not through natural causes). The inquest is presided over by a deputy coroner, and determinations of fact and recommendations are made by a jury. (Ch. 7)

Court of first instance: See *Original jurisdiction*. (Ch. 4)

Criminal Code: An act of Parliament that lists and defines all criminal offences and sets out procedural rules for trying such offences and punishing convicted persons. (Chs. 1, 4)

Criminal law: The body of law that prohibits certain specified conduct or acts set out in a criminal code or other statute and includes sanctions (punishment), such as imprisonment or fines, for breach. It includes all rules of criminal procedure used in trying accused persons charged with offences; regulates relationships between the state (society) and the individual; and aims to keep and maintain order. (Ch. 4)

Criminal negligence: Conduct in which the actor (the accused) has acted intentionally in a reckless or wanton manner, showing disregard for the rights or safety of others who might reasonably be expected to suffer harm or damage as a result of such conduct, and in which damage or harm ensues. (Ch. 4)

Crown: Crown refers to His Majesty, King Charles III, in right of Canada, or one of his provinces or territories and the rights, duties, and prerogatives belonging to him. The government exercises the powers of the sovereign, and the term "Crown" usually is a reference to the government. The term "Crown" is used to represent the state in relation to its citizens. The Crown Attorney is the lawyer who represents the state in the prosecution of offences. (Ch. 4)

Cryopreservation: The freezing of tissue for later use. For example, sperm or embryos may be preserved for use in *assisted insemination*. (Ch. 9)

Cultural relativism: The view that individual and group responses to morality are relative to the norms and values of that particular culture or society, or to the specific situation. Also called *normative relativism*. (Ch. 2)

Custom: In law, practice or rules of a particular trade or industry given force of law by the courts in the absence of specific statute law, case law, or doctrine governing the particular area. (Ch. 4)

Damages: A sum of money awarded by a court to a plaintiff at the end of a civil trial as compensation for an injury to person or property caused by the defendant. (Ch. 4)

Decertification: In labour law, the process by which a union loses its right to represent a group of employees and to bargain collectively on employees' behalf, either through its failure to take steps to negotiate a collective agreement or through a vote of the members themselves. (Ch. 11)

Defendant: A person or party against whom a lawsuit is brought; the party sought to be made responsible for the plaintiff's damages. (Ch. 4)

Delegation: In health care, the assignment by a health care professional to another person of a certain act or procedure that the professional is authorized by law and by his or her professional regulatory body to perform. Delegation is lawful if the person to whom the task is delegated is adequately trained to perform the act and properly supervised. (Ch. 5)

Delict: In the *civil law* system of Quebec, a civil wrong, such as an assault. *Delict* corresponds to the word *tort* in common law. (Ch. 7)

Democratic rights: Rights enshrined in the *Canadian Charter of Rights and Freedoms,* which provide for democratic participation of citizens in government. These include the right to vote; a maximum 5-year term limit on the life of Parliament or a provincial legislature (i.e., an election at least every 5 years); and the requirement that Parliament or a legislative assembly sit at least once per year (i.e., no rule by decree or dispensing with legislative approval of laws). (Ch. 4)

Descriptive ethics: A systematic explanation of moral behaviour or beliefs. (Ch. 2)

Detain: To hold in police custody or control without freedom to leave. (Ch. 4)

Directive: See *Advance directive.* (Ch. 6)

Disclosure: The obligation of each party to a lawsuit under the rules of civil procedure to reveal to the other party or parties all evidence, documents, reports, records, and so on that will be relied upon at trial. (Ch. 10)

Distributive justice: A process for deciding how resources are allocated. (Ch. 12)

Doctrine: Texts, journal articles, treatises, restatements of the law, and other learned writings of legal scholars on any legal subject; used by lawyers and judges as an aid in interpreting or developing the law. (Ch. 4)

Donor insemination: A therapeutic procedure in which sperm from a healthy donor (who may or may not be the woman's partner) are artificially introduced into a fertile woman's uterus. (Ch. 9)

Double effect: A morally correct action intended for good purposes resulting in a negative, unintended outcome (e.g., the provision of appropriate pain relief with the good intention to eliminate pain, and a subsequent effect of that good intention is the hastening of the person's death). (Ch. 8)

Dual procedure offence: In criminal law, an offence that may be tried either as a *summary conviction offence* or an *indictable offence* at the option of the Crown attorney. The choice usually depends on the seriousness of the facts surrounding the laying of charges. (Ch. 4)

Due process: The right of every citizen, regardless of race, gender, colour, creed, or religion, to receive fair treatment according to established procedures and rules of natural justice. (Ch. 4)

Duty of care: A legal obligation imposed on an individual to act or refrain from acting in a way such as to avoid causing harm to the person or property of another who might reasonably be affected and whose rights and well-being ought to be considered by the actor. (Ch. 7)

Ectogenesis: The maintenance of an embryo in an artificial womb. (Ch. 9)

Embryo donation: The making available of surplus cryopreserved embryos that are no longer needed or wanted by the couple who originated them (i.e., by in vitro fertilization). The alternatives are to destroy the embryos or to use them for research purposes. (Ch. 9)

Equality rights: The right to be treated equally by and before the law regardless of one's race, gender, sexual orientation, religion, ethnic origin, physical or mental disability, age, or skin colour. These rights are specifically enshrined in the *Canadian Charter of Rights and Freedoms.* (Ch. 4)

Ethical dilemma: A situation in which the most ethical course of action is unclear, in which there is a strong moral reason to support each of several positions, or in which a decision must be made based on the most right or the least wrong choice of action. (Ch. 2)

Ethical principles: A set of values based on ethical theory and intended to guide right action. Derived from moral theory, ethical principles or rules, guide moral conduct and provide a framework for ethical decision making. They are expressed in many professional codes of ethics. (Ch. 2)

Ethical theory: A framework of assumptions and principles intended to guide decisions about morality. (Chs. 1, 2)

Ethics: The philosophical study of questions regarding what is morally right and wrong. (Ch. 2)

Euthanasia: Based on the Greek language, *eu* for "good," and *thanatos* for "death", in its strictest sense *euthanasia* is defined as a painless death. The term is used in a number of situations including active voluntary or involuntary euthanasia, in which steps are taken with consent to actively end the life of a dying patient, and situations of passive euthanasia, in which the person is allowed to die; that is, no active steps are taken to preserve the life of a dying person. (Ch. 8)

Evidence: The material with which a party builds its case against another and proves a fact or set of facts. It may take the form of oral testimony given under oath by witnesses, documentary or real physical evidence, such as DNA, blood samples, hair and clothing fibres, photographs, and so on. (Ch. 4)

Examination for discovery: A preliminary oral examination at which the lawyer for each party in a trial has the opportunity to ask relevant questions of the other party or parties, under oath, to obtain full disclosure of all evidence and facts that will be relied upon at trial. (Ch. 4)

Feminist ethics: Attempts to re-frame traditional ethics that de-value the experience and contribution of women. It is committed to eliminating the subordination of women and raising the moral question about what this means for women. (Ch.2)

Fidelity: A guiding principle of relationships based on loyalty, promise keeping, and truth telling. (Ch. 2)

Findings of fact: In law, conclusions drawn by a trier of fact (i.e., a judge or jury) as to what actually occurred, and in what sequence, in a given case. These are based upon an examination and assessment of the evidence adduced at trial by the parties to the litigation (whether criminal or civil). For example, in a civil action in a motor vehicle accident case, one witness may testify that the person drove his vehicle through the intersection against a red light, whereas another witness may say that the light was green. The trier of fact will assess the evidence given by these two witnesses, determine which is more credible, and make a finding of fact as to which colour the light was when the accident occurred. (Ch. 4)

Fundamental rights: Specific rights enshrined in the *Canadian Charter of Rights and Freedoms* that are considered to be basic and necessary in every democratic society (e.g., the freedoms of religion, conscience, thought and expression, press, peaceful assembly, association). (Ch. 4)

Grantor: A person of sound mind and usually (in most provinces) over the age of majority who signs a document giving another power to make medical treatment decisions on their behalf or decisions respecting their property or finances. (See also *Power of attorney for personal care.*) (Ch. 6)

Harm: Negative consequences to persons, usually as a result of action or nonaction, related to their physical, emotional, and psychological well-being. (Ch. 10)

Health disciplines board: A provincial regulatory body that governs a health care profession with respect to licensing members and that ensures appropriate educational and professional qualifications, standards of practice, and ethical conduct by members. This body's name varies among provinces. (Ch. 4)

Homicide: The death of a human being caused by the actions or omissions of another. (Ch. 7)

Hybrid offence: In criminal law, an offence that can be tried either by indictment or summarily at the option of the Crown. (See also *Dual procedure offence.*) (Ch. 4)

Indictable offence: The most serious of criminal offences; usually triable by a jury but only after a preliminary hearing at which the accused is ordered to stand trial. Punishment ranges from heavy fines and/or several years' to life imprisonment. (Ch. 4)

Inferior court: A level of court that is judicially subordinate to a superior one; usually a trial court, which is bound by previous decisions of an appeal court. (Ch. 4)

Informed consent: In health care, a legally capable person's consent to a specific medical treatment, the nature and purpose of which, material risks and benefits of which, and material risks of not proceeding with which the person is informed by the health care practitioner. A material risk is one that a person would reasonably wish to know prior to making the decision of whether to undergo or forgo the proposed treatment. (Chs. 2, 6)

Injunction: A court order obtained by one party against one or more other parties that directs those others to refrain from a specific conduct or to perform a specific act. (Ch. 4)

Interdisciplinarity: When more than one discipline is involved in the care of the client, but planning and implementation are undertaken collaboratively. (Ch. 12)

Interprofessional practice: The continuous interaction of two or more health care professionals, organized with a common goal of solving or exploring mutual issues and achieving the best outcomes, with the best possible inclusion of the patient and family. (Ch. 12)

Intradisciplinarity: Individuals or teams within a specific discipline collaborating toward the achievement of positive client outcomes (e.g., a team of nurses planning the patient's care together). (Ch. 12)

In vitro fertilization: A process whereby fertilization occurs outside the body and without sexual intercourse. (Ch. 9)

Jurisdiction: The authority of a court to hear and decide a legal dispute (e.g., civil or criminal) in a particular territory, as well as the types of orders and judgements it may make. Also the territory and subject matter within the authority of a government. For example, regulation of health care is within the jurisdiction of the provinces. (Ch. 4)

Jurisprudence: Judges' written decisions in past court cases, which serve as *precedents* for future decisions in civil law systems; not binding, but seen as evidence of how past courts have interpreted a civil code provision or legal principle. (See also *Case law.*) (Ch. 4)

Juror: Member of a jury. (Ch. 4)

Jury: A group of 12 (in criminal juries) or fewer depending on the province (in civil juries) citizens over the age of majority who are convened to hear evidence, make findings of fact, and ultimately deliver a verdict in a criminal or civil trial. (Ch. 4)

Justice: A principle that focuses on the fair treatment of individuals and groups within society. (Ch. 2)

Lawsuit: See *Action.* (Ch. 4)

Legal rights: Rights of all persons residing in Canada that are invoked upon arrest or detention or when such persons are charged with a criminal offence. These are enshrined in the *Canadian Charter of Rights and Freedoms* and include the right to life, liberty, and security of the person (e.g., the right not to be compelled to give evidence against oneself in a police investigation and the right to remain silent); the right to be secure against unreasonable search and seizure (e.g., having one's home searched by the police without permission, without good reason, and without a warrant issued by a justice of the peace); the right not to be arbitrarily detained or imprisoned; the right to be informed of the reason for one's arrest and to be informed of the charge; the right to speak to a lawyer in private and to be informed of this right; the right to have the legality of one's detention determined by an impartial court and to be immediately released if that detention is judged to be unlawful; and the right to be tried within a reasonable time by an impartial court, to be presumed innocent until proven guilty, to reasonable bail, and to a jury trial if the punishment for the offence with which one is charged is 5 or more years' imprisonment. If acquitted or convicted of a criminal offence, a resident of Canada has the right not to be tried again for the same offence (the "double jeopardy" rule). Residents have the right, when punished for an offence of which they have been convicted, not to be subjected to cruel or unusual punishment (e.g., torture or degrading punishment and treatment, inhumane treatment or living conditions while in prison, and, arguably, capital punishment). (Ch. 4)

Legislative assembly: A provincial parliament consisting of only one house. Also called *the legislature.* (Ch. 4)

Liability: The legal responsibility owed by a party at fault to another for *damages* incurred or injury suffered by that other. (Ch. 4)

Licensing: The granting by a nursing regulatory body, such as a college of nurses or provincial nursing association, to an otherwise qualified nurse, of the right to practise within the province in accordance with recognized standards of care and ethics and subject to any restrictions specified in the licence. (Ch. 5)

Living will: A written document signed by a mentally competent person setting forth specific instructions regarding medical treatments to be applied or withheld in the event that the maker later becomes incapable of expressing those wishes. For example, the document might indicate whether resuscitation should be attempted in the event of a cardiac arrest. (Ch. 6)

Lockout: In labour relations, the employer's equivalent of the strike, in which the employer locks out its unionized employees from the workplace or refuses to continue to employ them, in an effort to pressure them to concede during contract negotiations or in labour disputes. In most provinces, a lockout, like a strike, may occur only after the expiry of a *collective agreement* and only after a *cooling-off period* under the applicable provincial labour statute. (Ch. 11)

Malfeasance: In law, doing an act that is one's duty but doing it poorly, incorrectly, or negligently. (Ch. 4)

Mens rea: The mental element of a criminal offence (i.e., the accused's state of mind when he or she is alleged to have committed a crime); the requirement that the accused was aware and willfully intended to commit the act, knew that the act was wrong, or was reckless as to the consequences of the act. (Ch. 4)

Metaethics: A philosophical focus on the meaning and nature of morality and ethics. (Ch. 2)

Misfeasance: Misfeasance, strictly, is not doing a lawful act in a proper manner, omitting to do it as it should be done. (Ch. 2)

Mobility rights: The rights of all persons legally resident in Canada to move in and out of Canada and between various provinces and cities, to take up residence anywhere in the country to pursue employment or educational and other opportunities. These rights are enshrined in the *Canadian Charter of Rights and Freedoms.* (Ch. 4)

Moral distress: Stress caused by situations in which one is convinced of what is morally right but is unable to act; results when moral issues are unresolved and when supportive processes are not in place. (Chs. 2, 11)

Morality: That which defines what is good, or moral. It is the distinction between what is right and what is wrong conduct or behaviour based on the tradition of beliefs and norms within a culture or society. (Ch. 2)

Multidisciplinarity: The involvement of professionals from more than one discipline (e.g., a nurse, physician, and physiotherapist) in the care of a patient. (Ch. 12)

Narrative: The examination of stories for the purpose of revealing notions of morality and helping to clarify one's moral perspectives. (Ch. 2)

Negligence: The nonintentional category of *tort* law wherein one person has, through carelessness, failed in a *duty of care* toward another such that that other has sustained injury to person or property as a result of the person's act or failure to act. (Ch. 4)

New reproductive technologies: Techniques to promote pregnancy by overcoming or bypassing infertility, including *donor insemination, assisted insemination, in vitro fertilization, cryopreservation,* ovum and *embryo donation,* and *surrogacy.* Advanced genetic technologies have also been developed that include sex selection, embryo research, prenatal diagnosis, and human embryo cloning. (Ch. 9)

Nightingale Pledge: Composed by a committee chaired by Lystra Gretter, a nursing instructor at the old Harper Hospital in Detroit, Michigan. Adapted from the Hippocratic Oath, it was first used by its graduating class in the spring of 1893.

I solemnly pledge myself before God and in the presence of this assembly, to pass my life in purity and to practice my profession faithfully. I will abstain from whatever is deleterious and mischievous, and will not take or knowingly administer any harmful drug. I will do all in my power to maintain and elevate the standard of my profession, and will hold in confidence all personal matters committed to my keeping and all family affairs coming to my knowledge in the practice of my calling. With loyalty will I endeavor to aid the physician, in his work, and devote myself to the welfare of those committed to my care. (Ch. 3)

Nonfeasance: Failing to do that which is one's legal duty or obligation to do. (Chs. 2, 4)

Nonmaleficence: A principle that obliges us to act in such a way as to prevent causing harm to others. (Ch. 2)

Normative relativism: See *Cultural relativism.* (Ch. 2)

Nursing ethics: The study of moral questions that fall within the sphere of nursing practice and nursing science. (Ch. 2)

Objective standard: The standard of the reasonable or "average" person against which someone's particular conduct in a given situation is judged. For example, a nurse performing a given task in a particular manner will have his or her methods of doing such task measured against the manner in which one would expect a reasonably competent and skilled nurse to perform it. (Ch. 7)

Obligation: In civil law (as opposed to common law), some act or course of conduct that the law requires an individual or individuals to perform, either for the benefit of another party or parties or for that of society in general. (See also *Duty.*) (Ch. 10)

Open shop: A place of employment in which *union* membership is not mandatory. (See also *Closed shop.*) (Ch. 11)

Original jurisdiction: The first court to hear a criminal or civil case (i.e., the court in which the litigation process begins). (Ch. 4)

Originating process: A document issued out of a court that begins a legal proceeding and must be formally served upon (delivered to) a *defendant* or responding party or parties. (See also *Statement of claim*) (Ch. 4)

Palliative care: Care intended to ensure that, through emotional and psychological support and effective symptom management, the patient experiences a quality dying process and a dignified death. (Ch. 8)

Personalized medicine: An emerging field of science and medicine whereby a person's genetic profile, lifestyle, and environment guides decisions regarding treatment and disease prevention. A deeper understanding of the genome provides greater insight into how a person's genetic and molecular structure influences and reacts to external factors that contribute to disease. This knowledge also guides treatment options by predicting a person's response to various treatments or interventions. (Ch. 9)

Plaintiff: The party who brings a lawsuit and seeks *damages* against another for breach of contract or other wrong done. (Ch. 4)

Pleadings: The court documents filed by each party to the lawsuit outlining the nature of the claim, the defence to the claim, and the issues to be tried in the action. (Ch. 4)

Political plurality: Where various views and ideological perspectives are considered and valued. This is demonstrated in Canada where various political perspectives are recognized in the parliamentary system. (Ch. 2)

Power of attorney for personal care: In Ontario, a legal document in which the maker appoints someone to make decisions on his or her behalf regarding medical treatment, care, feeding, clothing, shelter, hygiene, and so on, in the event that he or she becomes incapable because of physical or mental illness. This document takes legal effect only on the maker of the document becoming incapable of making treatment decisions and giving consent for themselves. (See also *Grantor.*) (Ch. 6)

Precedent: A judge's previous decision that serves as a guide or basis for deciding future cases having similar facts or legal issues. A higher-court precedent is usually binding on an inferior court. (See also *Case law.*)

Presumption of innocence: The principal of law that holds that a person charged with a criminal offence is not guilty until and unless proven guilty of the offence at trial. The Crown (i.e., the prosecution) is obliged to prove beyond a reasonable doubt that the accused committed the offence; the accused need not prove that they did not commit the offence. (Ch. 4)

Pretrial conference: A conference of all parties and their lawyers held before trial in the presence of a judge other than the one who will hear the trial. The judge reviews the facts of the case and the positions of each party, as well as the strengths and weaknesses of each party's case. Then, the judge advises the litigants how the case might be decided. This is a last attempt to reach a settlement without a lengthy and expensive trial. (Ch. 4)

Prima facie duties: Those duties that one must always act upon unless they conflict with those of equal or stronger obligation. (Ch. 2)

Principles: See *Ethical principles.* (Ch. 2)

Procedural law: Law that regulates how individual rights are asserted and enforced in the judicial system, such as which court hears the matter, what documents must be filed and when, and so on. (Ch. 4)

Procedural justice: The perception that processes (e.g., how decisions are made, who is involved, and what process is undertaken) have been fair and inclusive regardless of the outcome. (Ch. 12)

Professions Tribunal: In Quebec, an administrative tribunal that hears appeals (with leave) of disciplinary decisions involving members of the Ordre des infirmières et infirmiers du Québec and other professional regulatory bodies in the province. (Ch. 5)

Proxy: In health care, a person appointed or otherwise authorized by law to give consent to a specified medical treatment or procedure on behalf of another if the patient is unable to give such consent because of physical or mental incapacity. (Ch. 6)

Proxy consent: In health care, the consent given by a patient via another person authorized by the patient to give consent to medical treatment. (Ch. 6)

Rationality: The notion of thinking and reasoning, associated with comprehension, intelligence, or inference. Rationality requires explanations, or justifications, particularly for the purpose of supporting an opinion or conclusion. For example, a rational person would have reasons or arguments to support an ethical opinion. (Ch. 2)

Reasonable doubt: The standard of proof in a criminal case. This means that the Crown (the prosecution) must satisfy the trier of fact (either a judge or a jury) that the accused committed the offence with which he or she is charged, giving sufficient *evidence* such that no real or logically compelling reason exists in the trier's mind that the accused did not commit such act. (Ch. 4)

Recertification: Further training and further examination undertaken by a health care professional to demonstrate proficiency in certain professional skills or to maintain such proficiency as a condition of being licensed or certified to practise. (Ch. 7)

Registration: In the regulation of nursing practice, the recording of a nurse's name and other particulars and enrolment of that person as a member of a provincial nursing *regulatory body.* (Ch. 5)

Regulations: Detailed secondary laws passed by a federal or provincial cabinet pursuant to a specific statute. The statute usually gives the cabinet the power to make detailed rules to carry out the intent and purpose of the act which are too detailed and time-consuming for the legislature to enact. (Chs. 4, 7)

Sex Selection: When an embryos created through in vitro fertilization is chosen for implantation based on the desired sex of the offspring. This can also be accomplished through sex-selective abortion. Section 5(1) (e) of the *Assisted Human Reproduction Act* prohibits any action that would "ensure or increase the probability that an embryo will be of a p[articular sex".

Sexual harassment: Any unwanted conduct, language, or behaviour of a sexist or sexual nature directed by one person toward another. (Ch. 11)

Slippery slope: An argument that suggests that when an exception to the rule is made, exceptions will continue to be made until the rule no longer exists. For example, consider the notion of sanctity of life. If we were to allow physician-assisted suicide, soon euthanasia in all circumstances may become the norm. (Ch. 8)

Standard of care: Legal yardstick against which a person's conduct is measured to determine whether that person has been *negligent* and whether the person's conduct or actions in a given situation have met those expected of a competent health care professional. (Ch. 7)

Stare decisis: Rule of English common law whereby courts are legally bound to follow previous court decisions, which have the force of law. Usually, courts will follow *precedents* whose facts and legal issues are similar or identical to the case they are deciding unless there is good reason to depart from following the precedent (e.g., clear evidence that the court

that issued the precedent decision failed to consider relevant facts or another clearly applicable previous precedent). (See also *Precedent* and *Case law.*) (Ch. 4)

Statement of claim: A document prepared and filed by a *plaintiff* in a lawsuit initiating the court *action.* It sets out the *damages* and other relief sought from the court and the bare facts (but not the evidence) upon which the plaintiff relies to support a claim against a *defendant.* (Ch. 4)

Statement of defence: A document prepared and filed by the *defendant* in a lawsuit. It sets forth the defendant's version of the facts (but not the evidence) giving rise to the *action* and the legal grounds or reasons that the defendant is not liable for the *plaintiff's* damages. (Ch. 4)

Statute law: A formal written law passed by *Parliament* or a provincial legislature that takes precedence over and supersedes common law case law. Also found in *civil law* systems. (Ch. 4)

Stem cells: Cells that are able to renew themselves through cell division. Stem cells exist in the human embryo, where they differentiate to become a fetus and then a human being. Current research induces stem cells to differentiate to replace, for example, brain cells that have been damaged and can be stimulated to become cells with special functions, such as heart muscle and insulin-producing cells. (Ch. 9)

Substantive law: Law that sets out detailed rights and obligations of citizens in private dealings with one another and with society in general. (Ch. 4)

Summary conviction offences: In criminal law, offences of a less serious nature that are tried without a jury in a fairly rapid, straightforward way and for which the maximum punishment is 6 months' imprisonment or a fine of up to $2,000, or both. (Ch. 4)

Superior court: A higher trial court of a province or territory. (Ch. 4)

Surrogacy: An arrangement whereby a woman bears a child for another couple or individual. The gestational mother may be the biological mother (through sperm donation of either the male partner or a donor) or may carry the embryo of the couple, an embryo donated by another couple, or one created from a donor egg and donor sperm. (Ch. 9)

Tonic-clonic seizure: Generalized in that they involve all parts of the brain. They are also referred to as *grand mal seizures.* The tonic component involves the stiffening and contraction of muscles whereas the clonic component is the rhythmic twitching or jerking of muscles. (Ch. 7)

Tort: An intentional or nonintentional (i.e., negligent) wrongful act that causes damage or injury to another's person, reputation, or property. (Chs. 4, 7)

Transdisciplinarity: Disciplines crossing traditional boundaries to share roles with other professionals in the areas of education and practice (e.g., recognizing that more than one discipline may function in a particular role). (Ch. 12)

Trial court: See *Original jurisdiction.* (Ch. 4)

Unidisciplinarity: Confidence in one's own discipline and the contribution it makes, that then enables collaboration with others. For example, nurses must be secure in their role in order to work effectively with others. (Ch. 12)

Union: In labour law, a group of nonmanagerial employees in a common trade or industry organized in association with a constitution and membership for the purpose of advancing the common interests of its members respecting employment relations with a common employer or group of employers. (Ch. 11)

Utilitarianism: An ethical theory that considers an action to be right when it leads to the greatest possible number of good consequences or to the least possible number of bad consequences. (Ch. 2)

Utility: A term that considers the value of an outcome or consequence from many perspectives. (Ch. 2)

Value: An ideal that has significant meaning or importance to an individual, a group, or a society. (Ch. 2)

Veracity: A moral principle that emphasizes truth telling. (Ch. 2)

Virtue: A characteristic of the person that promotes good or high ethical standards. (Ch. 2)

Workplace violence: Violence that occurs in the course of work (e.g., bullying, disrespectful and threatening behaviour, verbal or physical abuse). It may occur between peers, be inflicted by a manager on staff, or be inflicted by clients, patients, or families on health care professionals. Workplace violence may result in psychological or physical harm. (Ch. 11)

Worldview: The way different cultures and societies view the world and the reality within which they exist. For example, one culture may view society as being made up of individuals who have individual choice and autonomy; others may view society as an interdependent community. (Ch. 12)

INDEX

Note: Page numbers followed by *f* indicate figures, *t* indicate tables, and *b* indicate boxes.